Handbook of
Experimental Pharmacology

Volume 177

Analgesia

Contributors

F. Benedetti, K. Brune, A. H. Dickenson, M. Diers, H. Flor,
J. Ghandehari, P. J. Goadsby, R. G. Hill, B. Hinz, R.-R. Ji,
Y. Kawasaki, I. J. Lever, M. Maze, V. Neugebauer, K. R. Oliver,
A. S. C. Rice, R. D. Sanders, J. Sawynok, H. G. Schaible, C. Stein,
G. R. Strichartz, Y.-R. Wen, J. N. Wood, F. Yanagidate, Y. Zhang,
Z.-Y. Zhuang, C. Zöllner

Editor
Christoph Stein

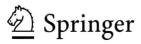
Springer

Prof. Dr. Christoph Stein
Department of Anesthesiology
and Critical Care Medicine
Charité – Campus Benjamin Franklin
Free University Berlin
Hindenburgdamm 30
12200 Berlin
Germany

Email: christoph.stein@charite.de

With 24 Figures and 8 Tables

ISSN 0171-2004

ISBN-10 3-540-33822-5 Springer Berlin Heidelberg New York

ISBN-13 978-3-540-33822-2 Springer Berlin Heidelberg New York

Springer is a part of Springer Science+Business Media
springer.com

© Springer-Verlag Berlin Heidelberg 2007

Editor: Simon Rallison, London
Desk Editor: Susanne Dathe, Heidelberg
Cover design: *design & production* GmbH, Heidelberg, Germany
Typesetting and production: LE-TEX Jelonek, Schmidt & Vöckler GbR, Leipzig, Germany
Printed on acid-free paper   27/3100-YL - 5 4 3 2 1 0

Preface

Analgesics are among the oldest drugs described, albeit not necessarily for medicinal use. For example, the Sumerians isolated opioids (probably for their euphoric effects) in the third millennium b.c. and the use of willow bark (salicin) for fever was first reported in the eighteenth century. Both types of drugs are still in use, but today they are supplemented by a wide array of substances ranging from antidepressants to ion channel blockers. Not all of these are prescribed by physicians. Many compounds are sold over the counter and thus available to the public for self-medication. As a result, analgesics are also the most misused class of drugs and are the culprit for a multitude of health problems due to untoward side effects.

This volume attempts to summarize the current state of knowledge on mechanisms underlying the various effects of these drugs, their side effect profiles, and their indications and contraindications in clinical use. It also gives insights into current efforts to discover novel mechanisms underlying different types of pain generation and the resulting development of new modulating compounds. These efforts have emerged mostly as a consequence of the more profound insights provided by molecular methods and of the now common use of animal models of pathological, rather than physiological, pain. These important issues are elaborated in the introductory chapter. In parallel, contemporary interdisciplinary treatment approaches have taught us that somatic mechanisms alone cannot explain pain; it is an experience shaped as well by social context, memory, and other psychological phenomena. Thus, the book closes with two chapters putting pharmacological strategies into a broader perspective. All of these advancements culminate in the contemporary common goal of developing mechanism-based rather than empiric approaches to the treatment of pain.

I would like to express my sincere gratitude to Susanne Dathe at Springer and to all authors for their hard work, patience, continuous support, and enthusiasm for this project.

Berlin,   C. Stein
June 2006

List of Contents

Part I. Introduction

Peripheral and Central Mechanisms of Pain Generation   3
   H.-G. Schaible

Part II. Drugs in Clinical Use

Opioids   31
   C. Zöllner, C. Stein

Antipyretic Analgesics: Nonsteroidal Antiinflammatory Drugs,
Selective COX-2 Inhibitors, Paracetamol and Pyrazolinones   65
   B. Hinz, K. Brune

Local Anesthetics   95
   F. Yanagidate, G. R. Strichartz

Serotonin Receptor Ligands: Treatments of Acute Migraine
and Cluster Headache 129
   P. J. Goadsby

Anti-convulsants and Anti-depressants 145
   A. H. Dickenson, J. Ghandehari

Part III. Compounds in Preclinical Development

Neuropeptide and Kinin Antagonists 181
   R. G. Hill, K. R. Oliver

Glutamate Receptor Ligands 217
   V. Neugebauer

Adrenergic and Cholinergic Compounds 251
   R. D. Sanders, M. Maze

Cannabinoids and Pain 265
   I. J. Lever, A. S. C. Rice

Part IV. Future Targets in Analgesia Research

Adenosine and ATP Receptors 309
    J. Sawynok

Ion Channels in Analgesia Research 329
    J. N. Wood

Protein Kinases as Potential Targets for the Treatment
of Pathological Pain   359
    R.-R. Ji, Y. Kawasaki, Z.-Y. Zhuang, Y.-R. Wen, Y.-Q. Zhang

Part V. Pain Management Beyond Pharmacotherapy

Placebo and Endogenous Mechanisms of Analgesia 393
    F. Benedetti

Limitations of Pharmacotherapy:
Behavioral Approaches to Chronic Pain 415
    H. Flor, M. Diers

Subject Index 429

List of Contributors

Addresses given at the beginning of respective chapters

Benedetti, F. , 393
Brune, K. , 65

Dickenson, A.H. , 145
Diers, M. , 415

Flor, H. , 415

Ghandehari, J. , 145
Goadsby, P.J. , 129

Hill, R.G. , 181
Hinz, B. , 65

Ji, R.-R. , 359

Kawasaki, Y. , 359

Lever, I.J. , 265

Maze, M. , 251

Neugebauer, V. , 217

Oliver, K.R. , 181

Rice, A.S.C. , 265

Sanders, R.D. , 251
Sawynok, J. , 309
Schaible, H.-G. , 3
Stein, C. , 31
Strichartz, G.R. , 95

Wen, Y.-R. , 359
Wood, J.N. , 329

Yanagidate, F. , 95

Zhang, Y.-Q. , 359
Zhuang, Z.-Y. , 359
Zöllner, C. , 31

Part I
Introduction

HEP (2006) 177:3–28
© Springer-Verlag Berlin Heidelberg 2006

Peripheral and Central Mechanisms of Pain Generation

H.-G. Schaible

Institut für Physiologie/Neurophysiologie, Teichgraben 8, 07740 Jena, Germany
Hans-Georg.Schaible@mti.uni-jena.de

1	**Introduction on Pain**	4
1.1	Types of Pain	4
1.2	The Nociceptive System: An Overview	5
2	**The Peripheral Pain System: Primary Afferent Nociceptors**	6
2.1	Responses to Noxious Stimulation of Normal Tissue	6
2.2	Changes of Neuronal Responses During Inflammation (Peripheral Sensitization)	7
2.3	Peripheral Neuronal Mechanisms of Neuropathic Pain	7
2.4	Molecular Mechanisms of Activation and Sensitization of Nociceptors	8
2.4.1	TRP Channels	9
2.4.2	Voltage-Gated Sodium Channels and ASICs	9
2.4.3	Receptors of Inflammatory Mediators (Chemosensitivity of Nociceptors)	10
2.4.4	Neuropeptide Receptors and Adrenergic Receptors	11
2.5	Mechanisms Involved in the Generation of Ectopic Discharges After Nerve Injury	12
3	**Spinal Nociceptive Processing**	12
3.1	Types of Nociceptive Spinal Neurons and Responses to Noxious Stimulation of Normal Tissue	12
3.2	Projections of Nociceptive Spinal Cord Neurons to Supraspinal Sites	15
3.3	Plasticity of Nociceptive Processing in the Spinal Cord	15
3.3.1	Wind-Up, Long-Term Potentiation and Long-Term Depression	16
3.3.2	Central Sensitization (Spinal Hyperexcitability)	16
3.4	Synaptic Transmission of Nociceptive Input in the Dorsal Horn	17
3.5	Molecular Events Involved in Spinal Hyperexcitability (Central Sensitization)	20
4	**Descending Inhibition and Facilitation**	21
4.1	Periaqueductal Grey and Related Brain Stem Nuclei	21
4.2	Changes of Descending Inhibition and Facilitation During Inflammation	21
4.3	Changes of Descending Inhibition and Facilitation During Neuropathic Pain	22
5	**Generation of the Conscious Pain Response in the Thalamocortical System**	22
	References	23

Abstract Pain research has uncovered important neuronal mechanisms that underlie clinically relevant pain states such as inflammatory and neuropathic pain. Importantly, both the peripheral and the central nociceptive system contribute significantly to the generation of pain upon inflammation and nerve injury. Peripheral nociceptors are sensitized during inflammation, and peripheral nerve fibres develop ectopic discharges upon nerve injury or disease. As a consequence a complex neuronal response is evoked in the spinal cord where neurons become hyperexcitable, and a new balance is set between excitation and inhibition. The spinal processes are significantly influenced by brain stem circuits that inhibit or facilitate spinal nociceptive processing. Numerous mechanisms are involved in peripheral and central nociceptive processes including rapid functional changes of signalling and long-term regulatory changes such as up-regulation of mediator/receptor systems. Conscious pain is generated by thalamocortical networks that produce both sensory discriminative and affective components of the pain response.

Keywords Nociceptive system · Nociceptors · Inflammatory pain · Neuropathic pain · Peripheral sensitization · Central sensitization · Ectopic discharges · Descending inhibition · Descending facilitation

1
Introduction on Pain

1.1
Types of Pain

In daily life the sensation pain is specifically evoked by potential or actual noxious (i.e. tissue damaging) stimuli applied to the body such as heat, squeezing a skin fold or over-rotating a joint. The predictable correlation between the noxious stimulus and the pain sensation causes us to avoid behaviour and situations that evoke pain. Pain during disease is different from "normal" pain. It occurs in the absence of external noxious stimuli, during mild stimulation or in an unpredictable way. Types of pain have been classified according to their pathogenesis, and pain research intends to define their neuronal mechanisms.

Cervero and Laird (1991) distinguish between three types of pain. Application of an acute noxious stimulus to normal tissue elicits *acute physiological nociceptive pain*. It protects tissue from being (further) damaged because withdrawal reflexes are usually elicited. *Pathophysiological nociceptive pain* occurs when the tissue is inflamed or injured. It may appear as spontaneous pain (pain in the absence of any intentional stimulation) or as hyperalgesia and/or allodynia. Hyperalgesia is extreme pain intensity felt upon noxious stimulation, and allodynia is the sensation of pain elicited by stimuli that are normally below pain threshold. In non-neuropathic pain, some authors include the lowering of the pain threshold in the term hyperalgesia. While nociceptive pain is elicited by stimulation of the sensory endings in the tissue, *pain!neuropathic* results from injury or disease of neurons in the peripheral or central nervous system. It does not primarily signal noxious tissue stimulation and often feels abnormal. Its character is often burning or electrical, and it can be persistent or occur in short episodes (e.g. trigeminal neuralgia). It may be combined with hyperalgesia and allodynia. During allodynia even touching the skin can cause intense pain. Causes of neuropathic pain are numerous, including axotomy, nerve or plexus damage, metabolic diseases such as diabetes mellitus, or herpes zoster. Damage to central neurons (e.g. in the thalamus) can cause central neuropathic pain.

This relatively simple classification of pain will certainly be modified for several reasons. First, in many cases pain is not strictly inflammatory or neuropathic because neuropathy may involve inflammatory components and neuropathic components may contribute to inflammatory pain states. Second, pain research now addresses other types of pain such as pain during surgery (incisional pain), cancer pain, pain during degenerative diseases (e.g. osteoarthritis), or pain in the course of psychiatric diseases. This research will probably lead to a more diversified classification that takes into account general and disease-specific neuronal mechanisms.

An important aspect is the distinction between acute and chronic pain. Usually pain in patients is called "chronic" when it lasts longer than 6 months (Russo and Brose 1998). Chronic pain may result from a chronic disease and may then actually result form persistent nociceptive processes. More recently the emphasis with chronic pain is being put on its character. In many chronic pain states the causal relationship between nociception and pain is not tight and pain does not reflect tissue damage. Rather psychological and social factors seem to influence the pain, e.g. in many cases of low back pain (Kendall 1999). Chronic pain may be accompanied by neuroendocrine dysregulation, fatigue, dysphoria, and impaired physical and even mental performance (Chapman and Gavrin 1999).

1.2
The Nociceptive System: An Overview

Nociception is the encoding and processing of noxious stimuli in the nervous system that can be measured with electrophysiological techniques. Neurons involved in nociception form the nociceptive system. Noxious stimuli activate primary nociceptive neurons with "free nerve endings" (Aδ and C fibres, nociceptors) in the peripheral nerve. Most of the nociceptors respond to noxious mechanical (e.g. squeezing the tissue), thermal (heat or cold), and chemical stimuli and are thus polymodal (cf. in Belmonte and Cervero 1996). Nociceptors can also exert efferent functions in the tissue by releasing neuropeptides [substance P (SP), calcitonin gene-related peptide (CGRP)] from their sensory endings. Thereby they induce vasodilatation, plasma extravasation, attraction of macrophages or degranulation of mast cells, etc. This inflammation is called neurogenic inflammation (Lynn 1996; Schaible et al. 2005).

Nociceptors project to the spinal cord and form synapses with second order neurons in the grey matter of the dorsal horn. A proportion of second-order neurons have ascending axons and project to the brain stem or to the thalamocortical system that produces the conscious pain response upon noxious stimulation. Other spinal cord neurons are involved in nociceptive motor reflexes, more complex motor behaviour such as avoidance of movements, and the generation of autonomic reflexes that are elicited by noxious stimuli.

Descending tracts reduce or facilitate the spinal nociceptive processing. The descending tracts are formed by pathways that originate from brainstem nuclei (in particular the periaqueductal grey, the rostral ventromedial medulla) and descend in the dorsolateral funiculus of the spinal cord. Descending inhibition is part of an intrinsic antinociceptive system (Fields and Basbaum 1999).

2
The Peripheral Pain System: Primary Afferent Nociceptors

2.1
Responses to Noxious Stimulation of Normal Tissue

Nociceptors of different tissues are assumed to share most of their general properties. However, qualitative and quantitative differences of neurons supplying different tissues cannot be ruled out, e.g. the mechanical threshold of nociceptors may be quite different in different tissues because the potentially damaging stimuli may be of low (as in the cornea) or higher intensity (in the skin, muscle or joint). Furthermore, evidence was provided that dorsal root ganglion (DRG) neurons supplying fibres to different tissues differ in their passive and active electrophysiological properties (Gold and Traub 2004). Thus, subtle differences in nociceptor properties may be important for pain mechanisms in different tissues.

In skin, muscle and joint, many Aδ and C fibres have elevated thresholds for mechanical stimuli, thus acting as specific nociceptors that detect potentially or actually damaging mechanical stimuli. At least in the skin many nociceptors respond to noxious heat. The heat threshold may be below the frankly noxious range but the neurons encode different heat intensities by their response frequency. In some visceral organs such as the bladder, most slow-conducting fibres have thresholds in the innocuous range and stronger responses in the noxious range, raising the possibility that visceral noxious stimuli are also encoded by "wide dynamic range neurons" and not only by specific nociceptors. In addition, many nociceptors are sensitive to chemical stimuli (chemosensitivity). Most of the nociceptors are thus polymodal (cf. Belmonte and Cervero).

Nociceptors are different from afferents subserving other modalities. Most fast-conducting Aβ afferents with corpuscular endings are mechano-receptors that respond vigorously to innocuous mechanical stimuli. Although they may show their strongest response to a noxious stimulus, their discharge pattern does not discriminate innocuous from noxious stimuli. A proportion of Aδ and C fibres are warmth or cold receptors encoding innocuous warm and cold stimuli but not noxious heat and cold.

In addition to polymodal nociceptors, joint, skin and visceral nerves contain Aδ and C fibres that were named silent or initially mechano-insensitive nociceptors. These neurons are not activated by noxious mechanical and thermal stimuli in normal tissue. However, they are sensitized during inflammation and then start to respond to mechanical and thermal stimuli (Schaible and Schmidt 1988; Weidner et al. 1999). In humans this class of nociceptors exhibits a particular long-lasting response to algogenic chemicals, and such nociceptors are crucial in mediating neurogenic inflammation (Ringkamp et al. 2001). Moreover, they play a major role in initiating central sensitization (Kleede et al. 2003). These neurons have distinct axonal biophysical characteristics separating them from polymodal nociceptors (Orstavik et al. 2003; Weidner et al. 1999).

2.2
Changes of Neuronal Responses During Inflammation (Peripheral Sensitization)

During inflammation the excitation threshold of polymodal nociceptors drops such that even normally innocuous, light stimuli activate them. Noxious stimuli evoke stronger responses than in the non-sensitized state. After sensitization of "pain fibres", normally non-painful stimuli can cause pain. Cutaneous nociceptors are in particular sensitized to thermal stimuli; nociceptors in deep somatic tissue such as joint and muscle show pronounced sensitization to mechanical stimuli (Campbell and Meyer 2005; Mense 1993; Schaible and Grubb 1993). In addition, during inflammation initially mechano-insensitive nerve fibres become mechano-sensitive. This recruitment of silent nociceptors adds significantly to the inflammatory nociceptive input to the spinal cord. Resting discharges may be induced or increased in nociceptors because of inflammation, providing a continuous afferent barrage into the spinal cord.

2.3
Peripheral Neuronal Mechanisms of Neuropathic Pain

In healthy sensory nerve fibres action potentials are generated in the sensory endings upon stimulation of the receptive field. Impaired nerve fibres often show pathological ectopic discharges. These action potentials are generated at the site of nerve injury or in the cell body in DRG. The discharge patterns vary from rhythmic firing to intermittent bursts (Han et al. 2000; Liu et al. 2000). Ectopic discharges occur in Aδ and C fibres and in thick myelinated Aβ fibres. Thus, after nerve injury both low threshold Aβ as well as high threshold Aδ and C fibres may be involved in the generation of pain. Aβ fibres may evoke exaggerated responses in spinal cord neurons that have undergone the process of central sensitization (see Sect. 3.3.2). Recently, however, it was proposed that pain is not generated by the injured nerve fibres themselves but rather by intact nerve fibres in the vicinity of injured nerve fibres. After an experimental lesion in the L5 dorsal root, spontaneous action potential discharges were observed in C fibres in the uninjured L4 dorsal root. These fibres may be affected by the process of a Wallerian degeneration (Wu et al. 2001).

2.4
Molecular Mechanisms of Activation and Sensitization of Nociceptors

Recent years have witnessed considerable progress in the understanding of molecular events that lead to activation and sensitization of nociceptors. Nociceptors express ion channels for stimulus transduction and action potential generation, and a large number of receptors for inflammatory and other mediators (Fig. 1). These receptors are either coupled to ion channels or, more often, activate second messenger systems that influence ion channels. Sensitization of nociceptors by inflammatory mediators is induced within a few minutes. If noxious stimuli or inflammatory conditions persist, the expression of ion channels, receptors and mediator substances may change. An up-regulation of excitatory receptors may contribute to the maintenance of pain. Furthermore, some receptors exert trophic influences on the neurons regulating synthesis of mediators and expression of ion channels and receptors in these cells.

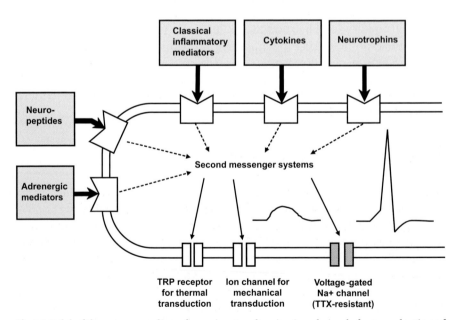

Fig. 1 Model of the sensory ending of a nociceptor showing ion channels for transduction of thermal and mechanical stimuli and action potential generation and metabotropic receptors subserving chemosensitivity

2.4.1
TRP Channels

The first cloned nociceptive ion channel was the TRPV1 receptor, which is expressed in about 40% of DRG cells. This ion channel is opened by binding of capsaicin, the compound in hot pepper that causes burning pain. In particular, Ca^{2+} flows through this channel and depolarizes the cell. The TRPV1 receptor is considered one of the transducers of noxious heat because it is opened by heat (>43°C). In TRPV1 knock-out mice, the heat response is not abolished but the mice do not exhibit thermal hyperalgesia during inflammation, showing the importance of TRPV1 for inflammatory hyperalgesia (Caterina et al. 2000; Davis et al. 2000). Up-regulation of TRPV1 transcription during inflammation explains longer-lasting heat hypersensitivity (Ji et al. 2002; Wilson-Gering et al. 2005). Following experimental nerve injury and in animal models of diabetic neuropathy, TRPV1 receptor is present on neurons that do not normally express TRPV1 (Rashid et al. 2003; Hong and Wiley 2005).

The TRPV1 receptor is a member of the TRP (transient receptor protein) family. Other TRP members may be transducers of temperature stimuli in other ranges (Papapoutian et al. 2003). The TRPV2 receptor in nociceptors is thought to be a transducer for extreme heat (threshold >50°C). TRPA1 could be the transducer molecule in nociceptors responding to cold (Peier et al. 2002). It is activated by pungent compounds, e.g. those present in cinnamon oil, mustard oil and ginger (Bandell et al. 2004). By contrast, TRPV3 and/or TRPV4 may be transduction molecules for innocuous warmth in warm receptors, and TRPM8 may transduce cold stimuli in innocuous cold receptors. Although the putative warmth transducer TRPV4 shows some mechano-sensitivity, it is still unclear whether TRPV4 is involved in the transduction of mechanical stimuli (Marchand et al. 2005).

2.4.2
Voltage-Gated Sodium Channels and ASICs

While most voltage-gated Na^+ channels are blocked by tetrodotoxin (TTX), many small DRG cells express TTX-resistant (R) Na^+ channels ($Na_V 1.8$ and $Na_V 1.9$) in addition to TTX-sensitive (S) Na^+ channels. Both TTX-S and TTX-R Na^+ channels contribute to the Na^+ influx during the action potential. Interestingly, TTX-R Na^+ currents are influenced by inflammatory mediators. They are enhanced e.g. by prostaglandin E_2 (PGE_2) that sensitizes nociceptors (McCleskey and Gold 1999). This raises the possibility that TTX-R Na^+ channels also play a role in the transduction process of noxious stimuli (Brock et al. 1998). $SNS^{-/-}$ knock-out mice (SNS is a TTX-R Na^+ channel) exhibit pronounced mechanical hypoalgesia but only small deficits in the response to thermal stimuli (Akopian et al. 1999).

Acid sensing ion channels (ASICs) are Na^+ channels that are opened by low pH. This is of interest because many inflammatory exudates exhibit a low pH. Protons directly activate ASICs with subsequent generation of action potentials (Sutherland et al. 2001).

2.4.3
Receptors of Inflammatory Mediators (Chemosensitivity of Nociceptors)

The chemosensitivity of nociceptors allows inflammatory and trophic mediators to act on these neurons. Sources of inflammatory mediators are inflammatory cells and non-neuronal tissue cells. The field of chemosensitivity is extremely complicated due to the large numbers of receptors that have been identified in primary afferent neurons (Gold 2005; Marchand et al. 2005). Receptors that are involved in the activation and sensitization of neurons are either ionotropic (the mediator opens an ion channel) or metabotropic (the mediator activates a second messenger cascade that influences ion channels and other cell functions). Many receptors are coupled to G proteins, which signal via the production of the second messengers cyclic AMP (cAMP), cyclic guanosine monophosphate (cGMP), diacylglycerol and phospholipase C. Other receptor subgroups include receptors bearing intrinsic protein tyrosine kinase domains, receptors that associate with cytosolic tyrosine kinases and protein serine/threonine kinases (Gold 2005). Table 1 shows the mediators to which receptors are expressed in sensory neurons (Gold 2005; Marchand et al. 2005). It is beyond the scope of this chapter to describe all the important mediators. Many of the mediators and their receptors will be addressed in the following chapters.

Functions of mediators are several-fold. Some of them activate neurons directly (e.g. the application of bradykinin evokes action potentials by itself) and/or they sensitize neurons for mechanical, thermal and chemical stimuli (e.g. bradykinin and prostaglandins increase the excitability of neurons so that mechanical stimuli evoke action potentials at a lower threshold than under control conditions). PGE_2, for example, activates G protein-coupled EP receptors that cause an increase of cellular cAMP. This second messenger activates protein kinase A, and this pathway influences ion channels in the membrane, leading to an enhanced excitability of the neuron with lowered threshold and increased action potential frequency elicited during suprathreshold stimulation. Bradykinin receptors are of great interest because bradykinin activates numerous Aδ and C fibres and sensitizes them for mechanical and thermal stimuli (Liang et al. 2001). Bradykinin receptor antagonists reverse thermal hyperalgesia, and Freund's complete adjuvant induced mechanical hyperalgesia of the rat knee joints. Some reports suggest that in particular bradykinin B1 receptors are up-regulated in sensory neurons following tissue or nerve injury, and that B1 antagonists reduce hyperalgesia. Other authors also found an up-regulation of B2 receptors during inflammation (Banik et al. 2001; Segond von Banchet et al. 2000).

Table 1 Receptors in subgroups of sensory neurons

Ionotropic receptors for
 ATP, H^+ (acid-sensitive ion channels, ASICs), glutamate (AMPA, kainate, NMDA
 receptors), acetylcholine (nicotinic receptors), serotonin (5-HT3)

Metabotropic receptors for
 Acetylcholine, adrenaline, serotonin, dopamine, glutamate, GABA, ATP
 Prostanoids (prostaglandin E_2 and I_2), bradykinin, histamine, adenosine, endothelin
 Neuropeptides (e.g. substance P, calcitonin gene-related peptide, somatostatin, opioids)
 Proteases (protease-activated receptors, PAR1 and PAR2)
 Neurotrophins [tyrosine kinase (Trk) receptors]
 Glial cell line-derived neurotrophic factor (GDNF)
 Inflammatory cytokines (non-tyrosine kinase receptors)

While prostaglandins and bradykinin are "classical" inflammatory mediators, the list of important mediators will be extended by cytokines. Some cytokines such as interleukin (IL)-1β are pro-nociceptive upon application to the tissue (Obreja et al. 2003). It is likely that cytokines play an important role in both inflammatory and neuropathic pain (Marchand et al. 2005; Sommer and Schröder 1995).

Neurotrophins are survival factors during the development of the nervous system, but during inflammation of the tissue, the level of nerve growth factor (NGF) is substantially enhanced. By acting on the tyrosine kinase A (trk A) receptors, NGF increases the synthesis of SP and CGRP in the primary afferents. NGF may also act on mast cells and thereby activate and sensitize sensory endings by mast cell degranulation (cf. Schaible and Richter 2004).

2.4.4
Neuropeptide Receptors and Adrenergic Receptors

Receptors for several neuropeptides have been identified in primary afferent neurons, including receptors for the excitatory neuropeptides SP (neurokinin 1 receptors) and CGRP, and receptors for inhibitory peptides, namely for opioids, somatostatin and neuropeptide Y (NPY) (for review see Bär et al. 2004; Brack and Stein 2004). These receptors could be autoreceptors because some of the neurons with these receptors also synthesize the corresponding neuropeptide. It has been proposed that the activity or threshold of a neuron results from the balance between excitatory and inhibitory compounds. Many nociceptive neurons, for example, seem to be under the tonic inhibitory influence of somatostatin because the application of a somatostatin receptor antagonist enhances activation of the neurons by stimuli (Carlton et al. 2001; Heppelmann and Pawlak 1999). The expression of excitatory neuropeptide receptors in the neurons can be increased under inflammatory conditions (Carlton et al. 2002; Segond von Banchet et al. 2000).

The normal afferent fibre does not seem to be influenced by stimulation of the sympathetic nervous system. However, primary afferents from inflamed tissue may be activated by sympathetic nerve stimulation. The expression of adrenergic receptors may be particularly important in neuropathic pain states (see the following section).

2.5
Mechanisms Involved in the Generation of Ectopic Discharges After Nerve Injury

Different mechanisms may produce ectopic discharges. After nerve injury the expression of TTX-S Na^+ channels is increased, and the expression of TTX-R Na^+ channels is decreased. These changes are thought to alter the membrane properties of neurons such that rapid firing rates (bursting ectopic discharges) are favoured (Cummins et al. 2000). Changes in the expression of potassium channels of the neurons have also been shown (Everill et al. 1999). Injured axons may be excited by inflammatory mediators, e.g. by bradykinin, NO (Michaelis et al. 1998) and cytokines (Cunha and Ferreira 2003; Marchand et al. 2005). Sources of these mediators are white bloods cells and Schwann cells around the damaged nerve fibres. Finally, the sympathetic nervous system does not activate primary afferents in normal tissue, but injured nerve fibres may become sensitive to adrenergic mediators (Kingery et al. 2000; Lee et al. 1999; Moon et al. 1999). This cross-talk may occur at different sites. Adrenergic receptors may be expressed at the sensory nerve fibre ending. Direct connections between afferent and efferent fibres (so-called "ephapses") is considered. Sympathetic endings are expressed in increased numbers in the spinal ganglion after nerve injury, and cell bodies of injured nerve fibres are surrounded by "baskets" consisting of sympathetic fibres (Jänig et al. 1996).

3
Spinal Nociceptive Processing

The spinal cord is the lowest level of the central nociceptive system. The neuronal organization of the spinal cord determines characteristic features of pain, e.g. the projection of pain into particular tissues. The spinal cord actively amplifies the spinal nociceptive processing because nociceptive spinal cord neurons change their excitability to inputs from the periphery under painful conditions. On the other hand the spinal cord is under the influence of descending influences. Figure 2 shows functionally important aspects of the nociceptive processing in the central nervous system.

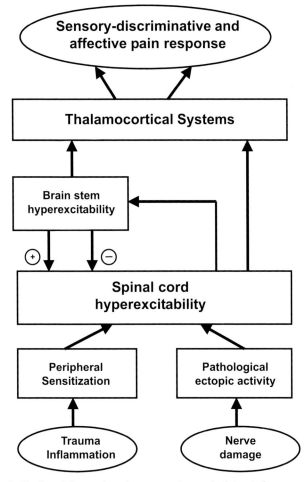

Fig. 2 Schematic display of the nociceptive processing underlying inflammatory and neuro-pathic pain

3.1
Types of Nociceptive Spinal Neurons and Responses to Noxious Stimulation of Normal Tissue

Nociceptive Aδ fibres project mainly to lamina I (and II). Some Aδ fibres have further projections into lamina V. Cutaneous C fibres project mainly to lamina II, but visceral and muscular unmyelinated afferents project to lamina II and also to deeper laminae. Visceral afferents distribute to a wider area of the cord, but the number of terminals for each fibre is much lower for visceral than for cutaneous fibres (Sugiura et al. 1989). By contrast, non-nociceptive primary afferents with Aβ fibres project to lamina III and IV. However, not only neurons in the superficial dorsal horn receive direct inputs from primary afferent neurons; dendrites of deep dorsal horn may extend dorsally into the superficial laminae and receive nociceptive inputs in superficial layers (Willis and Coggeshall 2004).

Neurons with nociceptive response properties are located in the superficial and deep dorsal and in the ventral horn. Both wide dynamic range neurons and nociceptive-specific neurons encode the intensity of a noxious stimulus applied to a specific site. Wide dynamic range neurons receive inputs from $A\beta$, $A\delta$ and C fibres and respond in a graded fashion to innocuous and noxious stimulus intensities. Nociceptive-specific neurons respond only to $A\delta$ and C fibre stimulation and noxious stimulus intensities.

A proportion of neurons receive only inputs from the skin or from deep tissue such as muscle and joint. However, many neurons exhibit convergent inputs from skin and deep tissue, and all neurons that receive inputs from the viscera also receive inputs from skin (and deep tissue). This uncertainty in the message of a neuron could in fact be the reason why, during disease in viscera, pain is felt as occurring in a cutaneous or subcutaneous area; the pain is projected into a so-called Head zone. Another encoding problem is that, in particular, wide dynamic range neurons often have large receptive fields, and a stimulus of a defined intensity may elicit different intensities of responses when applied to different sites of the receptive field. Quite clearly, the precise location of a noxious stimulus, its intensity and character cannot be encoded by a single nociceptive neuron. Presumably, encoding of a noxious stimulus is only achieved by a population of nociceptive neurons (see Price et al. 2003). By contrast, other authors propose that only lamina I neurons with smaller receptive fields are able to encode noxious stimuli, thus forming labelled lines from spinal cord to the cortex (for review see Craig 2003).

The response of a spinal cord neuron is dependent on its primary afferent input, its spinal connections and on descending influences. Evidence has been provided that loops of neurons involving the brain stem influence the responses of nociceptive neurons. These loops may mainly originate in neurons in projection neurons in lamina I (see the following section) and facilitate, via descending fibres from the brain stem, neurons in superficial and deep dorsal horn (Suzuki et al. 2002). In addition, descending inhibition influences responses of neurons (see Sect. 4.1).

Samples of activated neurons can be mapped by visualizing FOS protein in neurons (Willis and Coggeshall 2004). Noxious heat stimulation, for example, evokes expression of C-FOS within a few minutes in the superficial dorsal horn, and causes staining shifts to deeper laminae of the dorsal horn thereafter (Menetréy et al. 1989; Williams et al. 1990). Noxious visceral stimulation evokes C-FOS expression in laminae I, V and X, thus resembling the projection area of visceral afferent fibres, and injection of mustard oil into the muscle elicited C-FOS expression in laminae I and IV to VI (Hunt et al. 1987; Menetréy et al. 1989).

3.2
Projections of Nociceptive Spinal Cord Neurons to Supraspinal Sites

The axons of most dorsal horn neurons terminate in the same or adjacent laminae, i.e. they are local interneurons. However, a proportion of neurons projects to supraspinal sites. Ascending pathways in the white matter of the ventral quadrant of the spinal cord include the spinothalamic tract (STT), the spinoreticular tract (SRT), and the spinomesencephalic tract (SMT). Axons of the STT originate from neurons in lamina I (some lamina I STT cells may ascend in the dorsolateral funiculus), lamina V and deeper. Many STT cells project to the thalamic ventral posterior lateral (VPL) nucleus, which is part of the lateral thalamocortical system and is involved in encoding of sensory stimuli (see Sect. 5). Some STT cells project to thalamic nuclei that are not involved in stimulus encoding, and they have collaterals to the brain stem. Axons of the SRT project to the medial rhombencephalic reticular formation, the lateral and dorsal reticular nucleus, the nucleus reticularis gigantocellularis and others. SRT cells are located in laminae V, VII, VIII and X, and they have prominent responses to deep input. SMT neurons are located in laminae I, IV, V, VII and VIII and project to the parabrachial nuclei and the periaqueductal grey and others. The parabrachial projection reaches in part to neurons that project to the central nucleus of amygdala. STT, SRT and SMT cells are either low-threshold, wide dynamic range or nociceptive-specific.

In addition, several spinal projection paths have direct access to the limbic system, namely the spinohypothalamic tract, the spino-parabrachio-amygdalar pathway, the spino-amygdalar pathway and others. In some species there is a strong spino-cervical tract (SCT) ascending in the dorsolateral funiculus. SCT neurons process mainly mechano-sensory input, but some additionally receive nociceptive inputs (Willis and Coggeshall 2004). Finally, there is substantial evidence that nociceptive input from the viscera is processed in neurons that ascend in the dorsal columns (Willis 2005).

3.3
Plasticity of Nociceptive Processing in the Spinal Cord

Importantly, spinal cord neurons show changes of their response properties including the size of their receptive fields when the peripheral tissue is sufficiently activated by noxious stimuli, when thin fibres in a nerve are electrically stimulated, or when nerve fibres are damaged. In addition descending influences contribute to spinal nociceptive processing (see Sect. 4 and Fig. 2). In general it is thought that plasticity in the spinal cord contributes significantly to clinically relevant pain states.

3.3.1
Wind-Up, Long-Term Potentiation and Long-Term Depression

Wind-up is a short-term increase of responses of a spinal cord neuron when electrical stimulation of afferent C fibres is repeated at intervals of about 1 s (Mendell and Wall 1965). The basis of wind-up is a prolonged excitatory post-synaptic potential (EPSP) in the dorsal horn neuron that builds up because of a repetitive C fibre volley (Sivilotti et al. 1993). Wind-up disappears quickly when repetitive stimulation is stopped. It produces a short-lasting increase of responses to repetitive painful stimulation. Neurons may also show wind-down.

Long-term potentiation (LTP) and long-term depression (LTD) are long-lasting changes of synaptic activity after peripheral nerve stimulation (Randic et al. 1993; Rygh et al. 1999; Sandkühler and Liu 1998). LTP can be elicited at a short latency after application of a high-frequency train of electrical stimuli that are suprathreshold for C fibres, in particular when descending inhibitory influences are interrupted. However, LTP can also be elicited with natural noxious stimulation, although the time course is much slower (Rygh et al. 1999). By contrast, LTD in the superficial dorsal horn is elicited by electrical stimulation of Aδ fibres. It may be a basis of inhibitory mechanisms that counteract responses to noxious stimulation (Sandkühler et al. 1997).

3.3.2
Central Sensitization (Spinal Hyperexcitability)

In the course of inflammation and nerve damage neurons in the superficial, the deep and the ventral cord show pronounced changes of their response properties, a so-called central sensitization. This form of neuroplasticity has been observed during cutaneous inflammation, after cutaneous capsaicin application and during inflammation in joint, muscle and viscera. Typical changes of responses of individual neurons are:

- Increased responses to noxious stimulation of inflamed tissue.

- Lowering of threshold of nociceptive specific spinal cord neurons (they change into wide dynamic range neurons).

- Increased responses to stimuli applied to non-inflamed tissue surrounding the inflamed site.

- Expansion of the receptive field.

In particular, the enhanced responses to stimuli applied to non-inflamed tissue around the inflamed zone indicate that the sensitivity of the spinal cord neurons is enhanced so that a previously subthreshold input is sufficient to activate the neuron. After sensitization, an increased percentage of neurons in a segment respond to stimulation of an inflamed tissue. Central sensitization can persist for weeks, judging from the recording of neurons at different stages of acute and chronic inflammation (for review see Dubner and Ruda 1992; Mense 1993; Schaible and Grubb 1993).

Evidence for central sensitization has been observed in neuropathic pain states in which conduction in the nerve remains present and thus a receptive field of neurons can be identified. In these models more neurons show ongoing discharges and, on average, higher responses can be elicited by innocuous stimulation of receptive fields (Laird and Bennett 1993; Palacek et al. 1992a, b). In some models of neuropathy neurons with abnormal discharge properties can be observed.

During inflammation and neuropathy a large number of spinal cord neurons express C-FOS, supporting the finding that a large population of neurons is activated. At least at some time points metabolism in the spinal cord is enhanced during inflammation and neuropathy (Price et al. 1991; Schadrack et al. 1999).

The mechanisms of central sensitization are complex, and it is likely that different pain states are characterized at least in part by specific mechanisms, although some of the mechanisms are involved in all types of central sensitization. It may be crucial whether central sensitization is induced by increased inputs in sensitized but otherwise normal fibres (such as in inflammation), or whether structural changes such as neuronal loss contribute (discussed for neuropathic pain, see Campbell and Meyer 2005). Mechanisms of central sensitization are discussed in Sect. 3.5.

3.4
Synaptic Transmission of Nociceptive Input in the Dorsal Horn

Numerous transmitters and receptors mediate the processing of noxious information arising from noxious stimulation of normal tissue, and they are involved in plastic changes of spinal cord neuronal responses during peripheral inflammation and nerve damage (see Sect. 3.5). Transmitter actions have either fast kinetics (e.g. action of glutamate and ATP at ionotropic receptors) or slower kinetics (in particular neuropeptides that act through G protein-coupled metabotropic receptors). Actions at fast kinetics evoke immediate and short effects on neurons, thus encoding the input to the neuron, whereas actions at slow kinetics modulate synaptic processing (Millan 1999; Willis and Coggeshall 2004).

Glutamate is a principal transmitter of primary afferent and dorsal horn neurons. It activates ionotropic S-alpha-amino-3-hydroxy-5-methyl-4-isoxazolepropionic acid (AMPA)/kainate [non-N-methyl-D-aspartate (NMDA)] and NMDA receptors. In particular in the substantia gelatinosa, evoked synaptic activity is mainly blocked by antagonists at non-NMDA receptors whereas

NMDA receptor antagonists usually cause a small reduction of mainly later EPSP components. Both non-NMDA and NMDA receptors are involved in the synaptic activation of neurons by noxious stimuli (cf. Fundytus 2001; Millan 1999; Willis and Coggeshall 2004). ATP has been implicated in synaptic transmission of innocuous mechano-receptive and nociceptive input in the superficial dorsal horn. Purinergic ATP receptors are expressed in dorsal horn neurons and in DRG cells, mediating enhanced release of glutamate (cf. Willis and Coggeshall 2004).

Excitatory neuropeptides are co-localized with glutamate. Neuropeptide-mediated EPSPs usually occur after a latency of seconds and are long-lasting. They may not be sufficient to evoke action potential generation but act synergistically with glutamate (Urban et al. 1994). SP is released mainly in the superficial dorsal horn by electrical stimulation of unmyelinated fibres and during noxious mechanical, thermal or chemical stimulation of the skin and deep tissue. Neurokinin-1 (NK-1) receptors for SP are mainly located on dendrites and cell bodies of dorsal horn neurons in laminae I, IV–VI and X. Upon strong activation by SP, NK-1 receptors are internalized. Mice with a deletion of the preprotachykinin A have intact responses to mildly noxious stimuli but reduced responses to moderate and intense noxious stimuli. Mice with a deleted gene for the production of NK-1 receptors respond to acutely painful stimuli but lack intensity coding for pain and wind-up. In addition, neurokinin A (NKA) is found in small DRG cells and in the dorsal horn and spinally released upon noxious stimulation. CGRP is often colocalized with substance P in DRG neurons. It is spinally released by electrical stimulation of thin fibres and noxious mechanical and thermal stimulation. CGRP binding sites are located in lamina I and in the deep dorsal horn. CGRP enhances actions of SP by inhibiting its enzymatic degradation and potentiating its release. CGRP activates nociceptive dorsal horn neurons; blockade of CGRP effects reduces nociceptive responses. Other excitatory neuropeptides in the dorsal horn are vasoactive intestinal polypeptide (VIP), neurotensin, cholecystokinin (CCK, antinociceptive effects of CCK have also been described), thyrotropin-releasing hormone (TRH), corticotropin-releasing hormone (CRH) and pituitary adenylate cyclase-activating polypeptide (PACAP) (for review see Willis and Coggeshall 2004).

γ-Aminobutyric acid (GABA)ergic inhibitory neurons are located throughout the spinal cord. They can be synaptically activated by primary afferent fibres. Both the ionotropic $GABA_A$ and the metabotropic $GABA_B$ receptor are located pre-synaptically on primary afferent neurons or post-synaptically on dorsal horn neurons. Responses to both innocuous mechanical and noxious stimuli can be reduced by GABA receptor agonists. Some of the inhibitory effects are due to glycine, and the ventral and the dorsal horn contain numerous glycinergic neurons. Glycine may be co-localized with GABA in synaptic terminals. Many DRG neurons and neurons in the dorsal horn express nicotinergic and muscarinergic receptors for acetylcholine. Application of acetylcholine to the spinal cord produces pro- or anti-nociception (cf. Willis and Coggeshall 2004).

The dorsal horn contains leu-enkephalin, met-enkephalin, dynorphin and endomorphins 1 and 2. Enkephalin-containing neurons are particularly located in laminae I and II, with dynorphin-containing neurons in laminae I, II and V. Endomorphin 2 has been visualized in terminals of primary afferent neurons in the superficial dorsal horn and in DRG, but also in post-synaptic neurons. Opiate receptors

(μ, δ, κ) are concentrated in the superficial dorsal horn, and in particular μ and δ receptors are located in interneurons and on primary afferent fibres. Opioids reduce release of mediators from primary afferents (pre-synaptic effect), responses of neurons to (innocuous and) noxious stimulation and responses to ionophoretic application of excitatory amino acids showing post-synaptic effects of opioids (many dorsal horn neurons are hyperpolarized by opiates). In addition to these "classical" opiate receptors, nociceptin [orphanin fluoroquinolone (FQ)] receptors have been discovered. Nociceptin has similar cellular actions as classical opioid peptides. However, pro-nociceptive effects have also been described. A related peptide is nocistatin. At present it is unknown at which receptor nocistatin acts. Somatostatin is expressed in primary afferent neurons, dorsal horn interneurons and axons that descend from the medulla. It is released mainly in the substantia gelatinosa, by heat stimulation. It is an intriguing question whether inhibitory somatostatin is released in the spinal cord from primary afferent fibres or from interneurons. Galanin is expressed in a subpopulation of small DRG neurons, and galanin binding sites are also expressed on DRG neurons. Both facilitatory and inhibitory effects of galanin have been described in inflammatory and neuropathic pain states. NPY is normally only expressed at very low levels in DRG neurons, but DRG neurons express Y1 and Y2 receptors. It was proposed that Y1 and Y2 receptors contribute to pre-synaptic inhibition (for review see Willis and Coggeshall 2004).

Spinal processing is influenced by numerous other mediators including spinal prostaglandins, cytokines and neurotrophins. These mediators are produced in neurons and/or glia cells (Marchand et al. 2005; Vanegas and Schaible 2001). They are particularly important under pathophysiological conditions (see the following section). In addition, synaptic transmission is influenced by transmitters of descending systems (see Sect. 4.1).

Transmitter release is dependent on Ca^{2+}-influx into the pre-synaptic ending through voltage-dependent calcium channels. In addition, Ca^{2+} regulates neuronal excitability. Important for the nociceptive processing are high-voltage activated N-type channels, which are mainly located pre-synaptically but also on the post-synaptic side, and P/Q-type channels that are located on the pre-synaptic site. Blockers of N-type channels reduce responses of spinal cord neurons and behavioural responses to noxious stimulation of normal and inflamed tissue, and they reduce neuropathic pain. P/Q-type channels are mainly involved in the generation of pathophysiological pain states. A role for high-voltage activated L-type channels and low-voltage activated T-type channels has also been discussed (Vanegas and Schaible 2000).

3.5
Molecular Events Involved in Spinal Hyperexcitability (Central Sensitization)

A complex pattern of events takes place in the spinal cord that changes sensitivity of spinal nociceptive processing involving pre- and post-synaptic mechanisms. (1) During peripheral inflammation the spinal release of mediators such as glutamate, SP, neurokinin A and CGRP from nociceptors is increased (Schaible 2005). (2) Spinal cord neurons are sensitized by activation of NMDA receptors, and this process is supported by activation of metabotropic glutamate, NK-1 and CGRP receptors, and brain-derived neurotrophic factor plays a role as well (Woolf and Salter 2000). Antagonists to the NMDA receptor can prevent central sensitization and reduce established hyperexcitability (Fundytus 2001). Antagonists at NK-1 and CGRP receptors attenuate central sensitization. Ablation of neurons with NK-1 receptors was shown to abolish central sensitization (Khasabov et al. 2002). Important molecular steps of sensitization are initiated by Ca^{2+} influx into cells through NMDA receptors and voltage-gated calcium channels (Woolf and Salter 2000). Ca^{2+} activates Ca^{2+}–dependent kinases that e.g. phosphorylate NMDA receptors. (3) The subunits NR1 and GluR1 of glutamate receptors show an up-regulation of the protein and an increase of phosphorylation (also of the NR2B NMDA receptor subunit) thus enhancing synaptic glutamatergic transmission. First changes appear within 10 min after induction of inflammation and correlate well with behavioural hyperalgesia (Dubner 2005). (4) Expression of genes that code for neuropeptides is enhanced. In particular, increased gene expression of opioid peptides (dynorphin and enkephalin) have become known, suggesting that inhibitory mechanisms are up-regulated for compensation. However, dynorphin has both an inhibitory action via κ receptors and excitatory actions involving NMDA receptors. (5) Other mediators such as spinal prostaglandins and cytokines modify central hyperexcitability. As mentioned above, sources of these mediators are neurons, glia cells, or both (Marchand et al. 2005; Watkins and Maier 2005). Spinal actions of prostaglandins include increase of transmitter release (cf. Vanegas and Schaible 2001), inhibition of glycinergic inhibition (Ahmadi et al. 2002) and direct depolarization of dorsal horn neurons (Baba et al. 2001).

In the case of neuropathic pain, loss of inhibition is being discussed as a major mechanism of spinal hyperexcitability. Reduced inhibition may be produced by loss of inhibitory interneurons through excitotoxic actions and apoptosis (Dubner 2005, see, however, Polgár et al. 2004).

4
Descending Inhibition and Facilitation

4.1
Periaqueductal Grey and Related Brain Stem Nuclei

From brain stem nuclei, impulses "descend" onto the spinal cord and influence the transmission of pain signals at the dorsal horn (cf. Fields and Basbaum 1999; Ossipov and Porreca 2005). Concerning descending inhibition, the periaqueductal grey matter (PAG) is a key region. It projects to the rostral ventromedial medulla (RVM), which includes the serotonin-rich nucleus raphe magnus (NRM) as well as the nucleus reticularis gigantocellularis pars alpha and the nucleus paragigantocellularis lateralis (Fields et al. 1991), and it receives inputs from the hypothalamus, cortical regions and the limbic system (Ossipov and Porreca 2005). Neurons in RVM then project along the dorsolateral funiculus (DLF) to the dorsal horn. Exogenous opiates imitate endogenous opioids and induce analgesia by acting upon PAG and RVM in addition to the spinal dorsal horn (Ossipov and Porreca 2005). RVM contains so-called on- and off-cells. Off-cells are thought to exert descending inhibition of nociception, because whenever their activity is high there is an inhibition of nociceptive transmission, and because decreases in off-cell firing correlate with increased nociceptive transmission. On-cells instead seem to facilitate nociceptive mechanisms at the spinal dorsal horn. Thus, RVM seems to generate antinociception and facilitation of pain transmission (Gebhart 2004; Ossipov and Porreca 2005). Ultimately, spinal bulbospinal loops are significant in setting the gain of spinal processing (Porreca et al. 2002; Suzuki et al. 2002).

A particular form of descending inhibition of wide dynamic range (WDR) neurons is the "diffuse noxious inhibitory control" (DNIC). When a strong noxious stimulus is applied to a given body region, nociceptive neurons with input from that body region send impulses to structures located in the caudal medulla (caudal to RVM), and this triggers a centrifugal inhibition (DNIC) of nociceptive WDR neurons located throughout the neuraxis (Le Bars et al. 1979a, b).

4.2
Changes of Descending Inhibition and Facilitation During Inflammation

In models of inflammation, descending inhibition predominates over facilitation in pain circuits with input from the inflamed tissue, and thus it attenuates primary hyperalgesia. This inhibition descends from RVM, LC and possibly other supraspinal structures, and spinal serotonergic (from RVM) and noradrenergic (from LC) mechanisms are involved. By contrast, descending facilitation predominates over inhibition in pain circuits with input from neighbouring tissues, thus facilitating secondary hyperalgesia. Reticular nuclei located dorsally to RVM also participate in facilitation of secondary hyperalgesia. Lesion of these nuclei completely prevents secondary hyperalgesia (Vanegas and Schaible 2004).

In the RVM, excitatory amino acids mediate descending modulation in response to transient noxious stimulation and early inflammation, and they are involved in the development of RVM hyperexcitability associated with persistent pain (Heinricher et al. 1999; Urban and Gebhart 1999). As in the spinal cord, increased gene and protein expression and increased phosphorylation of NMDA and AMPA receptors take place in RVM (Dubner 2005; Guan et al. 2002).

A hypothesis is that messages from the inflamed tissue are amplified and relayed until they reach the appropriate brain stem structures. These in turn send descending impulses to the spinal cord, dampen primary hyperalgesia and cause secondary hyperalgesia. It is also possible that the "secondary neuronal pool" becomes hyperexcitable as a result of intraspinal mechanisms and that descending influences mainly play a contributing, yet significant, role in secondary hyperalgesia. Thus, during inflammation descending influences are both inhibitory and facilitatory, but the mix may be different for primary and secondary hyperalgesia and may change with time (Vanegas and Schaible 2004).

4.3
Changes of Descending Inhibition and Facilitation During Neuropathic Pain

Peripheral nerve damage causes primary hyperalgesia and allodynia that seem to develop autonomously at the beginning but need facilitation from RVM for their maintenance. CCK_B receptor activation, as well as excitation of neurons that express μ-opioid receptors in RVM, is essential for maintaining hyperexcitability in the primary neuronal pool (Porreca et al. 2002; Ossipov and Porreca 2005; Vanegas and Schaible 2004). "Secondary neuronal pools" are subject to a descending inhibition that is induced by the nerve damage and stems from the PAG. In contrast with inflammation, facilitation prevails in the primary while inhibition prevails in the secondary pool (Vanegas and Schaible 2004).

5
Generation of the Conscious Pain Response in the Thalamocortical System

The conscious pain response is produced by the thalamocortical system (Fig. 2). Electrophysiological data and brain imaging in humans have provided insights into which parts of the brain are activated upon noxious stimulation. As pointed out earlier, pain is an unpleasant sensory and emotional experience, and these different components of the pain response are produced by different networks. The analysis of the noxious stimulus for its location, duration and intensity is the sensory-discriminative aspect of pain. This is produced in the lateral thalamocortical system consisting of relay nuclei in the lateral thalamus and the areas SI and SII in the post-central gyrus. In these regions innocuous and noxious stimuli are discriminated (Treede et al. 1999).

The second component of the pain sensation is the affective aspect, i.e. the noxious stimulus is unpleasant and causes aversive reactions. This component is produced in the medial thalamocortical system, which consists of relay nuclei in the central and medial thalamus, the anterior cingulate cortex (ACC), the insula and the prefrontal cortex (Treede et al. 1999; Vogt 2005). These brain structures are part of the limbic system, and the insula may be an interface of the somatosensory and the limbic system. Even when destruction of the somatosensory cortex impairs stimulus localization, pain affect is not altered. It should be noted that limbic regions are not only involved in pain processing. In particular the ACC is activated during different emotions including sadness and happiness, and parts of the ACC are also involved in the generation of autonomic responses (they have projections to regions that command autonomic output systems). Other cingulate regions are involved in response selection (they have projections to the spinal cord and the motor cortices) and the orientation of the body towards innocuous and noxious somatosensory stimuli. A role of the ACC in the process of memory formation/access has also been put forward (Vogt 2005).

References

Ahmadi S, Lippross S, Neuhuber WL, Zeilhofer HU (2002) PGE2 selectively blocks inhibitory glycinergic neurotransmission onto rat superficial dorsal horn neurons. Nat Neurosci 5:34–40

Akopian AN, Souslova V, England S, Okuse K, Ogata N, Ure J, Smith A, Kerr BJ, McMahon SB, Boyce S, Hill R, Stanfa LC, Dickenson AH, Wood JN (1999) The tetrodotoxin-resistant sodium channel SNS has a specialized function in pain pathways. Nat Neurosci 2:541–548

Baba H, Kohno T, Moore KA, Woolf CJ (2001) Direct activation of rat spinal dorsal horn neurons by prostaglandin E2. J Neurosci 21:1750–1756

Bär KJ, Schurigt U, Scholze A, Segond von Banchet G, Stopfel N, Bräuer R, Halbhuber KJ, Schaible HG (2004) The expression and localisation of somatostatin receptors in dorsal root ganglion neurons of normal and monoarthritic rats. Neuroscience 127:197–206

Bandell M, Story GM, Hwang SW, Viswanath V, Eid SR, Petrus MJ, Earley TJ, Patapoutian A (2004) Noxious cold ion channel TRPA1 is activated by pungent compounds and bradykinin. Neuron 41:849–857

Banik RK, Kozaki Y, Sato J, Gera L, Mizumura K (2001) B2 receptor-mediated enhanced bradykinin sensitivity of rat cutaneous C-fiber nociceptors during persistent inflammation. J Neurophysiol 86:2727–2735

Belmonte C, Cervero E (1996) Neurobiology of nociceptors. Oxford University Press, Oxford

Brack A, Stein C (2004) Potential links between leukocytes and antinociception. Pain 111:1–2

Brock JA, McLachlan EM, Belmonte C (1998) Tetrodotoxin-resistant impulses in single nociceptor nerve terminals in guinea-pig cornea. J Physiol 512:211–217

Campbell JN, Meyer RA (2005) Neuropathic pain: from the nociceptor to the patient. In: Merskey H, Loeser JD, Dubner R (eds) The paths of pain 1975–2005. IASP Press, Seattle, pp 229–242

Carlton SM, Coggeshall RE (2002) Inflammation-induced up-regulation of neurokinin 1 receptors in rat glabrous skin. Neurosci Lett 326:29–36

Carlton SM, Du J, Zhou S, Coggeshall RE (2001) Tonic control of peripheral cutaneous nociceptors by somatostatin receptors. J Neurosci 21:4042–4049

Caterina MJ, Leffler A, Malmberg AB, Martin WJ, Trafton J, Petersen-Zeitz KR, Koltzenburg M, Basbaum AI, Julius D (2000) Impaired nociception and pain sensation in mice lacking the capsaicin receptor. Science 288:306–313

Cervero F, Laird JMA (1991) One pain or many pains? A new look at pain mechanisms. News Physiol Sci 6:268–273

Chapman CR, Gavrin J (1999) Suffering: the contributions of persistent pain. Lancet 353:2233–2237

Craig AD (2003) Pain mechanisms: labeled lines versus convergence in central processing. Annu Rev Neurosci 26:1–30

Cummins TR, Black JA, Dib-Hajj SD, Waxman SG (2000) Glial-derived neurotrophic factor upregulates expression of functional SNS and NaN sodium channels and their currents in axotomized dorsal root ganglion neurons. J Neurosci 20:8754–8761

Cunha FQ, Ferreira SH (2003) Peripheral hyperalgesic cytokines. Adv Exp Med Biol 521:22–39

Davis JB, Gray J, Gunthorpe MJ, Hatcher JP, Davey PT, Overend P, Harries MH, Latcham J, Clapham C, Atkinson K, Hughes SA, Rance K, Grau E, Harper AJ, Pugh PL, Rogers DC, Bingham S, Randall A, Sheardown SA (2000) Vanilloid receptor-1 is essential for inflammatory thermal hyperalgesia. Nature 405:183–187

Dubner R (2005) Plasticity in central nociceptive pathways. In: Merskey H, Loeser JD, Dubner R (eds) The paths of pain 1975–2005. IASP Press, Seattle, pp 101–115

Dubner R, Ruda MA (1992) Activity-dependent neuronal plasticity following tissue injury and inflammation. Trends Neurosci 15:96–103

Everill B, Kocsis JD (1999) Reduction in potassium currents in identified cutaneous afferent dorsal root ganglion neurons after axotomy. J Neurophysiol 82:700–708

Fields HL, Basbaum AI (1999) Central nervous system mechanisms of pain modulation. In: Wall PD, Melzack R (eds) Textbook of pain. Churchill Livingstone, London, pp 309–329

Fields HL, Heinricher MM, Mason P (1991) Neurotransmitters in nociceptive modulatory circuits. Annu Rev Neurosci 14:219–245

Fundytus ME (2001) Glutamate receptors and nociception. CNS Drugs 15:29–58

Gebhart GF (2004) Descending modulation of pain. Neurosci Biobehav Rev 27:729–737

Gold MS (2005) Molecular basis of receptors. In: Merskey H, Loeser JD, Dubner R (eds) The paths of pain 1975–2005. IASP Press, Seattle, pp 49–67

Gold MS, Traub JT (2004) Cutaneous and colonic rat DRG neurons differ with respect to both baseline and PGE2-induced changes in passive and active electrophysiological properties. J Neurophysiol 91:2524–2531

Guan Y, Terayama R, Dubner R, Ren K (2002) Plasticity in excitatory amino acid receptor-mediated descending pain modulation after inflammation. J Pharmacol Exp Ther 300:513–520

Han HC, Lee DH, Chung JM (2000) Characteristics of ectopic discharges in a rat neuropathic pain model. Pain 84:253–261

Heinricher MM, McGaraughty S, Farr DA (1999) The role of excitatory amino acid transmission within the rostral ventromedial medulla in the antinociceptive actions of systemically administered morphine. Pain 81:57–65

Heppelmann B, Pawlak M (1999) Peripheral application of cyclo-somatostatin, a somatostatin antagonist, increases the mechanosensitivity of the knee joint afferents. Neurosci Lett 259:62–64

Hong S, Wiley JW (2005) Early painful diabetic neuropathy is associated with differential changes in the expression and function of vanilloid receptor 1. J Biol Chem 280:618–627

Hunt SP, Pini A, Evan G (1987) Induction of c-fos-like protein in spinal cord neurons following sensory stimulation. Nature 328:632–634

Jänig W, Levine JD, Michaelis M (1996) Interactions of sympathetic and primary afferent neurons following nerve injury and tissue trauma. In: Kumazawa T, Kruger L, Mizumura K (eds) The polymodal receptor: a gateway to pathological pain. Progress in brain research, vol 113. Elsevier Science, Amsterdam, pp 161–184

Ji RR, Samad TA, Jin SX, Schmoll R, Woolf CJ (2002) p38 MAPK activation by NGF in primary sensory neurons after inflammation increases TRPV1 levels and maintains heat hyperalgesia. Neuron 36:57–68

Kendall NA (1999) Psychological approaches to the prevention of chronic pain: the low back paradigm. Baillieres Best Pract Res Clin Rheumatol 13:545–554

Khasabov SG, Rogers SD, Ghilardi JR, Pertes CM, Mantyh PW, Simone DA (2002) Spinal neurons that possess the substance P receptor are required for the development of central sensitization. J Neurosci 22:9086–9098

Kingery WS, Guo TZ, Davies ME, Limbird L, Maze M (2000) The alpha(2A) adrenoceptor and the sympathetic postganglionic neuron contribute to the development of neuropathic heat hyperalgesia in mice. Pain 85:345–358

Klede M, Handwerker HO, Schmelz M (2003) Central origin of secondary mechanical hyperalgesia. J Neurophysiol 90:353–359

Laird JMA, Bennett GJ (1993) An electrophysiological study of dorsal horn neurons in the spinal cord of rats with an experimental peripheral neuropathy. J Neurophysiol 69:2072–2085

Le Bars D, Dickenson AH, Besson JM (1979a) Diffuse noxious inhibitory controls (DNIC). I. Effects on dorsal horn convergent neurons in the rat. Pain 6:283–304

Le Bars D, Dickenson AH, Besson JM (1979b) Diffuse noxious inhibitory controls (DNIC). II. Lack of effect on non-convergent neurones, supraspinal involvement and theoretical implications. Pain 6:305–327

Lee DH, Liu X, Kim HT, Chung K, Chung JM (1999) Receptor subtype mediating the adrenergic sensitivity of pain behavior and ectopic discharges in neuropathic Lewis rats. J Neurophysiol 81:2226–2233

Liang YF, Haake B, Reeh PW (2001) Sustained sensitization and recruitment of cutaneous nociceptors by bradykinin and a novel theory of its excitatory action. J Physiol 532:229–239

Liu CN, Michaelis M, Amir R, Devor M (2000) Spinal nerve injury enhances subthreshold membrane potential oscillations in DRG neurons: relation to neuropathic pain. J Neurophysiol 84:205–215

Lynn B (1996) Neurogenic inflammation caused by cutaneous polymodal receptors. Prog Brain Res 113:361–368

Marchand F, Perretti M, McMahon SB (2005) Role of the immune system in chronic pain. Nat Rev Neurosci 6:521–532

McCleskey EW, Gold MS (1999) Ion channels of nociception. Annu Rev Physiol 61:835–856

Mendell LM, Wall PD (1965) Responses of single dorsal cord cells to peripheral cutaneous unmyelinated fibers. Nature 206:97–99

Menetréy D, Gannon JD, Levine JD, Basbaum AI (1989) Expression of c-fos protein in interneurons and projection neurons of the rat spinal cord in response to noxious somatic, articular, and visceral stimulation. J Comp Neurol 285:177–195

Mense S (1993) Nociception from skeletal muscle in relation to clinical muscle pain. Pain 54:241–289

Michaelis M, Vogel C, Blenk KH, Arnarson A, Jänig W (1998) Inflammatory mediators sensitize acutely axotomized nerve fibers to mechanical stimulation in the rat. J Neurosci 18:7581–7587

Millan MJ (1999) The induction of pain: an integrative review. Prog Neurobiol 57:1–164

Moon DE, Lee DH, Han HC, Xie J, Coggeshall RE, Chung JM (1999) Adrenergic sensitivity of the sensory receptors modulating mechanical allodynia in a rat neuropathic pain model. Pain 80:589–595

Obreja O, Rathee PK, Lips KS, Distler C, Kress M (2002) IL-1β potentiates heat-activated currents in rat sensory neurons: involvement of IL-1 RI, tyrosine kinase, and protein kinase C. FASEB J 16:1497–1503

Orstavik K, Weidner C, Schmidt R, Schmelz M, Hilliges M, Jørum E, Handwerker H, Torebjörk HE (2003) Pathological C-fibres in patients with a chronic painful condition. Brain 126:567–578

Ossipov MH, Porreca F (2005) Descending modulation of pain. In: Merskey H, Loeser JD, Dubner R (eds) The paths of pain 1975–2005. IASP Press, Seattle, pp 117–130

Palacek J, Dougherty PM, Kim SH, Paleckova V, Lekan V, Chung JM, Carlton SM, Willis WD (1992a) Responses of spinothalamic tract neurons to mechanical and thermal stimuli in an experimental model of peripheral neuropathy in primates. J Neurophysiol 68:1951–1966

Palacek J, Paleckova V, Dougherty PM, Carlton SM, Willis WS (1992b) Responses of spinothalamic tract cells to mechanical and thermal stimulation of skin in rats with experimental peripheral neuropathy. J Neurophysiol 67:1562–1573

Papapoutian A, Peier AM, Story GM, Viswanath V (2003) ThermoTRP channels and beyond: mechanisms of temperature sensation. Nat Rev Neurosci 4:529–539

Peier AM, Moqrich A, Hergarden AC, Reeve AJ, Andersson DA, Story GM, Earley TJ, Dragoni I, McIntyre P, Bevan S, Patapoutian A (2002) A TRP channel that senses cold stimuli and menthol. Cell 108:705–715

Polgár E, Gray S, Riddell JS, Todd AJ (2004) Lack of evidence for significant neuronal loss in laminae I-III of the spinal dorsal horn of the rat in the chronic constriction injury model. Pain 111:144–150

Porreca F, Ossipov MH, Gebhart GF (2002) Chronic pain and medullary descending facilitation. Trends Neurosci 25:319–325

Price DD, Mao J, Coghill RC, d'Avella D, Cicciarello R, Fiori MG, Mayer DJ, Hayes RL (1991) Regional changes in spinal cord glucose metabolism in a rat model of painful neuropathy. Brain Res 564:314–318

Price DD, Greenspan JD, Dubner R (2003) Neurons involved in the exteroceptive function of pain. Pain 106:215–219

Randic M, Jiang MC, Cerne R (1993) Long-term potentiation and long-term depression of primary afferent neurotransmission in the rat spinal cord. J Neurosci 13:5228–5241

Rashid MH, Inoue M, Bakoshi S, Ueda H (2003) Increased expression of vanilloid receptor 1 on myelinated primary afferent neurons contributes to the antihyperalgesic effect of capsaicin cream in diabetic neuropathic pain in mice. J Pharmacol Exp Ther 306:709–717

Ringkamp M, Peng B, Wu G, Hartke TV, Campbell JN, Meyer RA (2001) Capsaicin responses in heat-sensitive and heat-insensitive A-fiber nociceptors. J Neurosci 21:4460–4468

Russo CM, Brose WG (1998) Chronic pain. Annu Rev Med 49:123–133

Rygh LJ, Svendson F, Hole K, Tjolsen A (1999) Natural noxious stimulation can induce long-term increase of spinal nociceptive responses. Pain 82:305–310

Sandkühler J, Liu X (1998) Induction of long-term potentiation at spinal synapses by noxious stimulation or nerve injury. Eur J Neurosci 10:2476–2480

Schadrack J, Neto FL, Ableitner A, Castro-Lopes JM, Willoch F, Bartenstein B, Zieglgänsberger W, Tölle TR (1999) Metabolic activity changes in the rat spinal cord during adjuvant monoarthritis. Neuroscience 94:595–605

Schaible HG (2005) Basic mechanisms of deep somatic tissue. In: McMahon SB, Koltzenburg M (eds) Textbook of pain. Elsevier, London, pp 621–633

Schaible HG, Grubb BD (1993) Afferent and spinal mechanisms of joint pain. Pain 55:5–54

Schaible HG, Richter F (2004) Pathophysiology of pain. Langenbecks Arch Surg 389:237–243

Schaible HG, Schmidt RF (1988) Time course of mechanosensitivity changes in articular afferents during a developing experimental arthritis. J Neurophysiol 60:2180–2195

Schaible HG, Del Rosso A, Matucci-Cerinic M (2005) Neurogenic aspects of inflammation. Rheum Dis Clin North Am 31:77–101

Segond von Banchet G, Petrow PK, Bräuer R, Schaible HG (2000) Monoarticular antigeninduced arthritis leads to pronounced bilateral upregulation of the expression of neurokinin 1 and bradykinin 2 receptors in dorsal root ganglion neurons of rats. Arthritis Res 2:424–427

Sivilotti LG, Thompson SWN, Woolf CJ (1993) The rate of rise of the cumulative depolarization evoked by repetitive stimulation of small-calibre afferents is a predictor of action potential windup in rat spinal neurons in vitro. J Neurophysiol 69:1621–1631

Sommer C, Schröder JM (1995) HLA-DR expression in peripheral neuropathies: the role of Schwann cells, resident and hematogenous macrophages, and endoneurial fibroblasts. Acta Neuropathol (Berl) 89:63–71

Sugiura Y, Terui N, Hosoya Y (1989) Difference in the distribution of central terminals between visceral and somatic unmyelinated (C) primary afferent fibres. J Neurophysiol 62:834–840

Sutherland SP, Benson CJ, Adelman JP, McCleskey EW (2001) Acid-sensing ion channel 3 matches the acid-gated current in cardiac ischemia-sensing neurons. Proc Natl Acad Sci USA 98:711–716

Suzuki R, Morcuende S, Webber M, Hunt SP, Dickenson AH (2002) Superficial NK1-expressing neurons control spinal excitability through activation of descending pathways. Nat Neurosci 5:1319–1326

Treede RD, Kenshalo DR, Gracely RH, Jones AKP (1999) The cortical representation of pain. Pain 79:105–111

Urban L, Thompson SWN, Dray A (1994) Modulation of spinal excitability: cooperation between neurokinin and excitatory amino acid transmitters. Trends Neurosci 17:432–438

Urban MO, Gebhart GF (1999) Supraspinal contributions to hyperalgesia. Proc Natl Acad Sci USA 96:7687–7692

Vanegas H, Schaible HG (2000) Effects of antagonists to high-threshold calcium channels upon spinal mechanisms of pain, hyperalgesia and allodynia. Pain 85:9–18

Vanegas H, Schaible HG (2001) Prostaglandins and cyclooxygenases in the spinal cord. Prog Neurobiol 64:327–363

Vanegas H, Schaible HG (2004) Descending control of persistent pain: inhibitory or facilitatory? Brain Res Rev 46:295–309

Vogt BA (2005) Pain and emotion. Interactions in subregions of the cingulate gyrus. Nat Rev Neurosci 6:533–544

Watkins LR, Maier SF (2005) Glia and pain: past, present, and future. In: Merskey H, Loeser JD, Dubner R (eds) The paths of pain 1975–2005. IASP Press, Seattle, pp 165–175

Weidner C, Schmelz M, Schmidt R, Hansson B, Handwerker HO, Torebjörk HE (1999) Functional attributes discriminating mechano-insensitive and mechano-responsive C nociceptors in human skin. J Neurosci 19:10184–10190

Williams S, Ean GL, Hunt SP (1990) Changing pattern of c-fos induction following thermal cutaneous stimulation in the rat. Neuroscience 36:73–81

Willis WD (2005) Physiology and anatomy of the spinal cord pain system. In: Merskey H, Loeser JD, Dubner R (eds) The paths of pain 1975–2005. IASP Press, Seattle, pp 85–100

Willis WD, Coggeshall RE (2004) Sensory mechanisms of the spinal cord, 3rd edn. Kluwer Academic/Plenum Publishers, New York

Wilson-Gerwing TD, Dmyterko MV, Zochodne DW, Johnston JM, Verge VM (2005) Neurotrophin-3 suppresses thermal hyperalgesia associated with neuropathic pain and attenuates transient receptor potential vanilloid receptor-1 expression in adult sensory neurons. J Neurosci 25:758–767

Woolf CJ, Salter MW (2000) Neuronal plasticity: increasing the gain in pain. Science 288:1765–1768

Wu G, Ringkamp M, Hartke TV, Murinson BB, Campbell JN, Griffin JW, Meyer RA (2001) Early onset of spontaneous activity in uninjured C-fiber nociceptors after injury to neighbouring nerve fibers. J Neurosci 21 RC140:1–5

Part II
Drugs in Clinical Use

HEP (2006) 177:31–63

Opioids

C. Zöllner · C. Stein (✉)

Klinik für Anaesthesiologie und operative Intensivmedizin, Charité–Universitätsmedizin Berlin, Campus Benjamin Franklin, Hindenburgdamm 30, 12200 Berlin, Germany
christoph.stein@charite.de

1	History	32
2	Opioid Receptors	32
2.1	Molecular Biology	32
2.2	Structural Features of Opioid Receptors	35
2.2.1	Extracellular Loops	35
2.2.2	Transmembrane Domains	35
2.2.3	C-Terminal Tail	36
2.3	Signal Transduction	36
2.4	Opioid Tolerance	39
2.4.1	In Vitro	39
2.4.2	In Vivo	40
3	Opioid Receptor Ligands and Sites of Action	41
3.1	Endogenous Ligands	41
3.2	Exogenous Ligands	42
3.3	Sites of Action	43
3.3.1	Supraspinal and Spinal Sites	43
3.3.2	Peripheral Sites	44
3.3.3	Peripheral Opioid Receptors and Inflammation	45
4	Clinical Applications	45
4.1	Acute Pain	45
4.2	Chronic Pain	46
4.3	Pharmacokinetics	47
4.3.1	Absorption	47
4.3.2	Distribution	47
4.3.3	Metabolism and Excretion	48
5	Side Effects	49
5.1	Acute Opioid Application	49
5.1.1	Cardiovascular System	49
5.1.2	Respiratory System	49
5.1.3	Sedation	50
5.1.4	Nausea and Vomiting	50
5.1.5	Cough Suppression	51
5.1.6	Pupil Constriction	51
5.1.7	Skeletal Muscle Rigidity	51
5.1.8	Gastrointestinal System	52
5.1.9	Histamine Release	52

5.2   Chronic Opioid Application   53
5.2.1 Tolerance   53
5.2.2 Physical Dependence   54

References   54

Abstract Opioids are the most effective and widely used drugs in the treatment of severe pain. They act through G protein-coupled receptors. Four families of endogenous ligands (opioid peptides) are known. The standard exogenous opioid analgesic is morphine. Opioid agonists can activate central and peripheral opioid receptors. Three classes of opioid receptors (μ, δ, κ) have been identified. Multiple pathways of opioid receptor signaling (e.g., $G_{i/o}$ coupling, cAMP inhibition, Ca^{++} channel inhibition) have been described. The differential regulation of effectors, preclinical pharmacology, clinical applications, and side effects will be reviewed in this chapter.

Keywords Central and peripheral opioid receptors · Signal transduction · Clinical applications · Pharmacokinetics and side effects · Routes of administration

1
History

Opium is an extract of the exudate derived from seedpods of the opium poppy, *Papaver somniferum*. The poppy plant was cultivated in the ancient civilizations of Persia, Egypt, and Mesopotamia, and the first known written reference to the poppy appears in a Sumerian text dated around 4000 BC. Opium was inhaled or given through punctures in the skin, which subsequently led to analgesia, but also to respiratory depression and death due to variable rates of absorption. Opium is a complex chemical cocktail containing sugars, proteins, fats, water, plant wax, latex, gums, and numerous alkaloids, most notably morphine (10%–15%), codeine (1%–3%), noscapine (4%–8%), papaverine (1%–3%), and thebaine (1%–2%). Many alkaloids are used medicinally to treat pain (morphine, codeine), cough (noscapine, codeine), and visceral spasms (papaverine). The chemist Sertürner was the first to publish the isolation of morphine, which he named after the god of dreams (Schmitz 1985). Morphine is a potent analgesic and it was more predictable than opium, which subsequently led to its widespread use in the treatment of acute and chronic pain.

2
Opioid Receptors

2.1
Molecular Biology

Early binding studies and bioassays defined three types of opioid receptors (Lord et al. 1977; Martin et al. 1976; Pert and Snyder 1973), the μ-, δ- and κ-receptors. A number of other receptor types have been proposed (e.g., sigma, epsilon, orphanin) but are currently not considered "classical" opioid receptors (Kieffer and Gavériaux-Ruff 2002). The identification of opioid receptor complementary DNA (cDNA) allowed for the independent study of individual opioid receptor types with regard to pharmacological profile, cellular effector coupling, anatomical distribution, and regulation of expression. The first cDNA encoding an opioid receptor was isolated simultaneously by two laboratories in 1992 (Evans et al. 1992; Kieffer et al. 1992). When expressed in transfected cells, the protein showed the expected pharmacological profile of the δ-receptor. Expression in mammalian cells indicated that the δ-receptor has structural characteristics similar to the family of seven transmembrane G protein-coupled receptors (GPCRs) (Fig. 1). Subsequently, the μ- and the κ-receptor were cloned (Meng et al. 1993; Wang et al. 1993). The μ-receptor gene shows approximately 50%–70% homology to the genes encoding for the δ-receptor and κ-receptor.

The concept of receptor subtypes has emerged from classical pharmacological data to explain biphasic binding characteristics of opioid receptor ligands

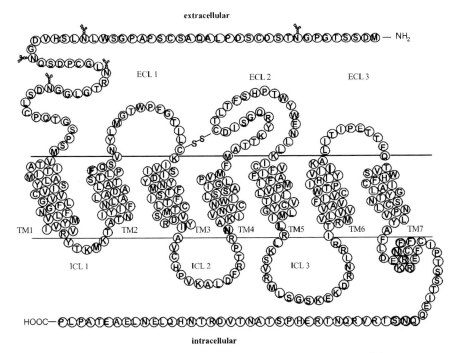

Fig. 1 The seven α-helical transmembrane (*TM*) domains characteristic of the μ-receptor. N-terminal tail and extracellular loops (*ECL*) are *above* the TM domains. A disulfide bond connects ECL1 and ECL2. The intracellular loops (*ICL*) 1–3 and the C terminal tail contain multiple serines and threonines that are potential phosphorylation sites for protein kinases

(Pasternak 2004). Using radiolabeled agonists and antagonists different high-affinity binding sites were detected and termed as μ_1- and μ_2-receptor (Pasternak 2004). In vivo pharmacological studies proposed δ_1- and δ_2-receptor subtypes (Mattia et al. 1991) and κ_1-, κ_2, and κ_3-receptor subtypes (Attali et al. 1982). However, only three opioid receptor genes have been characterized so far. Subtypes may result from alternative processing, splice variants, or a combination of the two. Splicing of μ-receptor messenger RNA (mRNA) has been observed in a variety of species. The cytoplasmic tail of the rat μ-receptor undergoes alternative splicing leading to two isoforms, μ-receptor1 and μ-receptor1B. These receptor variants share 100% amino acid sequence identity up to amino acid 386, but differ from residue 387 to the carboxyl terminus. When expressed in human embryonic kidney (HEK293) cells, both isoforms exhibit similar pharmacological profiles; however, μ-receptor1B appears to be more resistant to agonist-induced desensitization than μ-receptor1 (Koch et al. 1998). In addition to alternative splicing, posttranslational modifications of the gene product (glycosylation, palmitoylation, phosphorylation) or receptor dimerization to form homomeric and heteromeric complexes might explain pharmacologically defined differences in opioid receptor binding (Gavériaux-Ruff and Kieffer 1999b).

In addition to classic pharmacological methodology, the contribution of each receptor to opioid actions in vivo can be assessed by genetic approaches. For example, synthetic antisense oligodeoxynucleotides hybridize to complementary sequences in the target gene or its mRNA, thereby leading to reduced transcription, translation, and protein levels. Antisense studies have confirmed the contribution of μ-, δ-, and κ-receptors in opioid-induced analgesia (Kieffer 1999). The availability of techniques to knock out genes now permits unprecedented selectivity in the removal of responses mediated by the respective encoded protein. While this approach circumvents some shortcomings of conventional pharmacology (e.g., limited duration of action and variable selectivity of agonists, antagonists, or antibodies) it is itself limited by compensatory developmental changes during embryogenesis and adolescence and by variable genetic backgrounds (Kieffer and Gavériaux-Ruff 2002). Knockout studies have shown that the removal of any single opioid receptor does not result in major changes of basal pain thresholds or other behaviors, but they have confirmed that all three classes of opioid receptors mediate analgesia induced by their respective agonists, and that there is only one gene encoding for each receptor (Kieffer 1999). Those data have also demonstrated a critical role of the μ-receptor in cannabinoid and alcohol reinforcement, an important role for the δ-receptor in emotional behaviors, and an involvement of κ-receptors in dysphoric responses (Gavériaux-Ruff and Kieffer 2002). Mice lacking all three opioid receptors are viable and healthy (Simonin et al. 2001). Triple mutants allow for exploration of the molecular basis of unusual opioid receptor subtypes or nonclassical opioid responses. For example, it was shown that κ-2 receptor binding is most likely related to binding to the three known opioid receptors and that no additional receptor is required to explain κ-2 receptor pharmacology (Simonin et al. 2001). In addition, it was shown that the immunosuppressive action of naltrindole is not mediated by opioid receptors (Gavériaux-Ruff et al. 2001). Triple knockout mutants may also help us to explore the molecular basis for nonopioid activity of different opioid peptides (Narita and Tseng 1998).

2.2
Structural Features of Opioid Receptors

2.2.1
Extracellular Loops

Among GPCRs, bovine rhodopsin is the only receptor whose structure has been solved at high resolution (Palczewski et al. 2000). Comprehensive biochemical and mutational analyses of the transmembrane segments of all three opioid receptors and the ability to align receptor sequences by highly conserved residues in each helix support the use of the rhodopsin structure as a template to model other GPCRs, including the opioid receptors. Opioid receptors have a high similarity in transmembrane (TM) domain 2, 3, 5, 6, and 7, the three intracellular loops, and a short region of the C-terminal tail (Fig. 1). Almost no homology is found in the extracellular loops (ECL) or in the N-terminal tails. One of the few features preserved throughout the GPCR family is a disulfide bond connecting the second extracellular loop and TM 3. This disulfide bridge is found in more than 90% of all GPCRs and may be important in receptor function (Karnik et al. 2003). We demonstrated that an intact disulfide bond between a highly conserved cysteine residue in the second ECL and an equally well-conserved cysteine residue in the third ECL is an important regulator of μ-receptor activity (Zhang et al. 1999). For the chemoattractant C5a receptor, another GPCR, it was suggested that the ECL act as a filter and regulate the ability of the ligand to interact with the binding pocket (Massotte and Kieffer 2005). Evidence supports the notion that, in addition to guiding ligands on their way to the binding pocket, the ECL may regulate the "on-off" transition in the absence of ligands (Klco et al. 2005).

2.2.2
Transmembrane Domains

TM residues within the lipophilic environment of the cell membrane are key in ligand recognition and/or signal transduction and are expected to be oriented toward a relatively hydrophilic central cavity (Surratt et al. 1994). Structural motives important for ligand binding and subtype specificity have been identified for the opioid receptors from experimental mutagenesis studies and computer modeling. A current view of how GPCRs achieve the transition between resting and active conformations to convey external signals across the cell membrane is that ligands bind with hydrophilic and aromatic residues within the helical core. This triggers outward movements of TM helices 3, 6, and 7 to promote the formation of the active receptor state that results in G protein coupling and signal transduction, as it was shown for the structurally related muscarinic receptor (Hulme et al. 1999). Charged and polar amino acid residues are useful starting points in identifying important residues for agonist and antagonist binding within the binding pocket. For opioid receptors, histidine, asparagine, and tyrosine residues within TM 3, 6, and 7 are critical for receptor activation (Mansour et al. 1997). Random mutagenesis is another tool to identify important structure–function relationships. Such a strategy with the entire δ-receptor revealed 30 point mutations leading to a constitutive activity of the receptor (Decaillot et al. 2003). Mutagenesis studies are useful tools to identify potential domains important for ligand binding. However, they do not allow the definitive identification of binding sites, because the mutation of single amino acids could affect the amino acid side-chain interaction and subsequently the secondary and/or tertiary structure of the entire receptor.

2.2.3
C-Terminal Tail

The C-terminal portion of the opioid receptor determines coupling to second messenger molecules and is important for receptor trafficking. μ-receptor point mutations of any of the Ser/Thr within the C-terminal tail result in significant reductions in the rate of receptor internalization in HEK cell lines (Koch et al. 1998, 2001). This was confirmed using CHO-K1 cells expressing μ-receptors and a mutant form, in which all Ser and Thr residues from the third cytoplasmic loop and C-terminal were changed to alanine (Capeyrou et al. 1997; Wang 2000).

2.3
Signal Transduction

Opioid receptors are prototypical G_i/G_o-coupled receptors. Opioid signals are efficiently blocked by pertussis toxin that adenosine diphosphate (ADP)-

$\longrightarrow$

Fig. 2a Opioid ligands induce a conformational change at the receptor which allows coupling of G proteins to the receptor. The heterotrimeric G protein dissociates into active G_α and $G_{\beta\gamma}$ subunits (*a*) which can subsequently inhibit adenylyl cyclase (*b*), decrease the conductance of voltage-gated Ca^{2+} channels, open rectifying K^+ channels (*c*), or activate the PLC/PKC pathway (*d*) that modulates Ca^{2+} channel activity in the plasma membrane (*e*). **b** Opioid receptor desensitization and trafficking is activated by G protein-coupled receptor kinases (*GRK*). After arrestin binding, the receptor is in a desensitized state at the plasma membrane (*a*). Arrestin-bound receptors can then be internalized via a clathrin-dependent pathway, and either be recycled to the cell surface (*b*) or degraded in lysosomes (*c*)

ribosylates and inactivates the α-subunits of G_i/G_o proteins. After opioid agonists bind to the receptor, dissociation of the trimeric G protein complex into
G_α- and $G_{\beta\gamma}$-subunits can subsequently lead to the inhibition of cyclic $3'5'$
adenylyl cyclase (cAMP) and/or to direct interaction with K^+, Ca^{2+}, and other
ion channels in the membrane (Fig. 2a). Ion-channel regulation by opioids

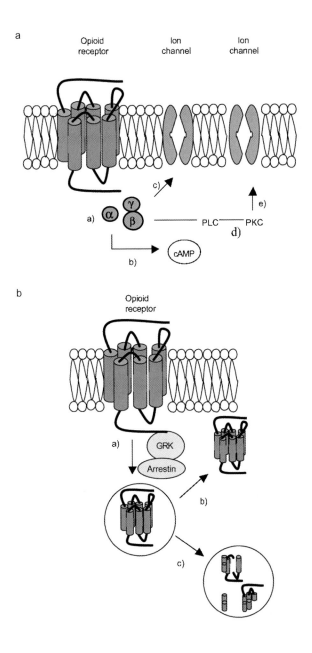

is mainly mediated via direct G protein $\beta\gamma$-subunits (Herlitze et al. 1996). All three opioid receptors couple to various N, T-type and P/Q-type Ca^{2+} channels, suppress Ca^{2+} influx and subsequently the excitation and/or neurotransmitter release in many neuronal systems. A prominent example is the inhibition of (pronociceptive) substance P release from primary afferent sensory neurons in the spinal cord and from their peripheral terminals (Kondo et al. 2005). At the postsynaptic membrane, opioid receptors mediate hyperpolarization by activating K^+ channels, thereby preventing excitation or propagation of action potentials. Four families of potassium channels play important roles in antinociception, including voltage-gated K^+ channels (K_v), inward recti-fier K^+ channels (K_{ir}), calcium-activated K^+ channels (K_{Ca}), and two-pore K^+ channels (K_{2P}) (Ocana et al. 2004). In the central nervous system (CNS), opioid-induced antinociception is associated with activation of voltage-gated K^+ channels of the K_{ir} channel family (Ocana et al. 1995). Some opioids also induce opening of calcium-activated K^+ channels (Stretton et al. 1992).

Apart from Ca^{2+} and K^+ channels, opioid receptors may regulate the functions of other ion channels. For example, opioids suppress tetrodotoxin-resistant sodium-selective and nonselective cation currents, which are mainly expressed in nociceptors (Gold and Levine 1996; Ingram and Williams 1994). In addition, a number of studies indicate that opioids can directly modulate N-methyl-D-aspartate (NMDA) receptors at presynaptic and postsynaptic sites within the CNS (Mao 1999). NMDA receptors can be blocked at the same site where Mg^{2+} and ketamine interfere with the ion channel. In addition, we recently showed that activation of opioid receptors modulates the transient receptor potential vanilloid type 1 (TRPV1), a member of the ligand gated ion channels (J. Endres-Becker, P.A. Heppenstall, S.A. Mousa, A. Oksche, M. Schäfer, C. Stein, C. Zöllner, submitted for publication). TRPV1 is involved in thermosensation and nociception and is mainly expressed in peripheral sensory neurons. It was also suggested that opioid receptors regulate the phos-pholipase Cβ (PLCβ) pathway via $G_{\beta\gamma}$-subunits (Chan et al. 1995) or G_q proteins (Rubovitch et al. 2003). PLC activation mobilizes phosphokinase C (PKC) that opens calcium channels in the plasma membrane. The entry of Ca^{2+} into the cell stimulates calcium-activated adenylyl cyclases to produce cAMP. However, the physiological relevance of such a potential bidirectional regulation of in-tracellular cAMP by opioid receptors is not completely solved at the moment and most data indicate that opioids mainly inhibit cAMP production.

Mitogen-activated protein kinase (MAPK), also known as extracellular signal-regulated kinase (ERK), is regarded as a major pathway for growth factor signaling from the cell surface to the nucleus (Seger and Krebs 1995). MAPK activation has been noted in response to agonist stimulation of many GPCRs, including all opioid receptor types (Belcheva et al. 1998; Ignatova et al. 1999; Schulz et al. 2004a). A suggested mechanism includes the activation of PLC, generating diacylglycerol that binds to PKCϵ, leading to its phosphory-lation. PKCϵ can then signal to matrix metalloproteinases, which can cleave membrane-anchored epidermal growth factor receptor (EGF)-type ligands, thereby initiating EGF receptor transactivation and ultimately activation of the MAPK phosphorylation cascade (Belcheva et al. 2005; Pierce et al. 2001). So far, little is known about the functional significance of this phenomenon. Besides an impact of opioids on neural development, the MAPK pathway might be involved in homologous desensitization of the μ-receptor (Polakiewicz et al. 1998; Schmidt et al. 2000). Future studies might investigate the role of the MAPK cascade in opioid tolerance and dependence.

2.4
Opioid Tolerance

2.4.1
In Vitro

On the cellular level long-term opioid treatment can result in the eventual loss of opioid receptor-activated function (i.e., desensitization). Three general mechanisms are associated with desensitization of GPCRs: (1) receptor phosphorylation, (2) receptor internalization and/or sequestration, and (3) receptor downregulation (i.e., a reduced total number of receptors). Opioid receptors are substrates for second messenger kinases (i.e., PKC) and for members of the GPCR kinases (GRK). Opioid receptor phosphorylation by these kinases increases the affinity to arrestin molecules. Arrestin-receptor complexes sterically prevent coupling between receptor and G proteins and promote internalization via clathrin-dependent pathways (Fig. 2b; Law et al. 2000). Agonist-induced internalization of the receptor via the endocytic pathway has been thought to contribute directly to tolerance by decreasing the number of opioid receptors on the cell surface. However, more recent studies have shown that morphine fails to promote endocytosis of opioid receptors in cultured cells (Eisinger et al. 2002) and native neurons (Sternini et al. 1996), although it is highly efficient in inducing tolerance in vivo (Sim et al. 1996). Moreover, endocytosis and recycling of the opioid receptor was shown to dramatically decrease opioid tolerance and withdrawal (Koch et al. 2005). These findings suggest that desensitization and receptor internalization might be a protective mechanism and prevent the development of tolerance. Drugs that do not cause receptor internalization, such as morphine, may have higher propensities to induce tolerance. In contrast to full agonists such as [D-Ala(2)-MePhe(4)-Gly-ol]enkephalin (DAMGO), morphine stimulated a selective phosphorylation of the carboxy-terminal residue 375, indicating that morphine-desensitized receptors remained at the plasma membrane in a Serin-375-phosphorylated state for prolonged periods (Schulz et al. 2004b). Recycling of opioid receptors to the plasma membrane promotes rapid resensitization of signal transduction, whereas targeting to lysosomes leads to proteolytic downregulation. A protein that binds preferentially to the cytoplasmic tail of opioid receptors was identified and named as GPCR-associated sorting protein (GASP) (Whistler et al. 2002). It was suggested that GASPs modulate lysosomal sorting and functional downregulation of GPCRs.

2.4.2
In Vivo

Tolerance in vivo describes the phenomenon that the magnitude of a given opioid effect decreases with repeated administration of the same opioid dose, or that increasing doses of an opioid are needed to produce the same effect. All opioid effects (e.g., analgesia, respiratory depression, sedation, constipation) can be subject to tolerance development. It is evident that opiate-induced adaptations occur at multiple levels in the nervous and other organ systems, beginning with regulation of opioid receptors themselves and extending to complex networks including learned behavior and genetic factors (von Zastrow 2004). The importance of opioid receptor endocytosis for chronic adaptation of the intact nervous system is not yet understood. Indirect evidence that arrestin-dependent μ-receptor desensitization contributes to morphine tolerance in vivo comes from studies in arrestin-3 and GRK3 knockout mice. Functional deletion of the arrestin-3 gene resulted in remarkable potentiation and prolongation of the analgesic effect of morphine (Bohn et al. 2000; Bohn et al. 2002) but had no effect on the acute antinociceptive potency of etorphine, fentanyl, or methadone (Bohn et al. 2004). However, to date the majority of studies on opioid tolerance have been performed in the absence of painful tissue injury. This may explain some of the discrepancies between experimental (Smith et al. 2003) and clinical studies (Stein et al. 1996). Tolerance is not ubiquitously observed in clinical routine and is in many cases explained by increasing nociceptive stimulation with progressing disease (e.g., cancer pain; Zech et al. 1995). Animal models of pathological situations have also produced evidence for a reversal of tolerance to morphine, e.g., during intestinal inflammation (Pol and Puig 1997). These findings indicate differences in the development of opioid tolerance (and possibly in receptor desensitization and recycling) under pathological situations. Future studies are necessary on the development of opioid receptor tolerance in the presence of postoperative pain, arthritis, or other types of inflammatory and chronic pain.

Several investigators have focused on the concept that tolerance can be counteracted by NMDA receptor antagonists (Mao 1999; Price et al. 2000). NMDA receptors are a subclass of excitatory amino acid receptors that, once activated, facilitate calcium influx into neurons. Although it has been shown NMDA receptor antagonists, e.g., MK801, inhibit tolerance to the analgesic effects of repeated morphine administration (Elliott et al. 1995; Price et al. 2000), the underlying mechanisms have not been fully elucidated.

3
Opioid Receptor Ligands and Sites of Action

3.1
Endogenous Ligands

Pentapeptides that mimic opioid activity and activate opioid receptors were initially isolated from brain extracts. Two isoforms were identified: Met-enkephalin (Tyr-Gly-Gly-Phe-Met) and Leu-enkephalin (Tyr-Gly-Gly-Phe-Leu) (Hughes et al. 1975). The same and other opioid peptides (endorphins, END; dynorphins, DYN) were later isolated from brain, spinal cord, pituitary gland, adrenals, immune cells, and other tissues. The amino-terminal of these opioid peptides contains the Tyr-Gly-Gly-Phe-[Met/Leu] sequence. Three distinct opioid precursors have been identified so far: prodynorphin (PDYN), proopiomelanocortin (POMC), and proenkephalin (PENK) (Comb et al. 1982; Kakidani et al. 1982; Nakanishi et al. 1979). Each of these precursors undergoes processing by proteolytic enzymes into DYN, END, and ENK, respectively. The POMC gene is transcribed and translated into a prohormone of 267 amino acids. Posttranslational processing of this large precursor peptide produces several smaller peptides, including β-endorphin, α-melanocyte-stimulating hormone (α-MSH), and ACTH. Posttranslational processing of PENK results in Met-enkephalin, Leu-enkephalin, and a number of other enkephalins, including bovine adrenal medulla peptide 22. The PDYN gene produces a prohormone of 254 amino acids, which encodes the opioid peptides dynorphin A and B (Höllt 1993). END, ENK, and DYN can bind to any of the known opioid receptors with varying affinities. In addition, a novel family of endogenous opioid peptides have been discovered and termed endomorphins (Zadina et al. 1997). Endomorphin-1 (Tyr-Pro-Trp-Phe) and endomorphin-2 (Tyr-Pro-Phe-Phe) bind to the μ-receptor with high affinity (Horvath 2000).

Endogenous opioid peptides can be released from neurons and axon terminals by depolarization and can exert pre- and postsynaptic effects. In addition, endogenous opioids are produced in many nonneuronal tissues, notably also in lymphocytes, monocytes, and granulocytes in inflamed tissue (Rittner et al. 2001). In models of inflammatory pain, opioid peptide-containing immune cells migrate from the circulation to the injured tissue. Selectins and integrins have been identified as important adhesion molecules which regulate the migration of opioid-containing immune cells (Machelska et al. 1998, 2002). Upon exogenous stressful stimuli or releasing agents (e.g., cold water swim stress, postoperative pain, corticotropin releasing factor, catecholamines), these peptides can be locally released and subsequently bind to opioid receptors on sensory neurons. By inhibiting the excitability of these neurons, they can increase nociceptive thresholds (i.e., produce analgesia; Stein et al. 1993). Preclinical research using protease ("enkephalinase") inhibitors to increase concentrations of endogenous opioid peptides in various central and peripheral tissues is ongoing but has not resulted in clinical applications for pain treatment so far (Roques 2000).

3.2
Exogenous Ligands

Exogenous opioid ligands can be classified into three groups: full agonists, partial agonists/antagonists, and full antagonists. The standard to which all other opioid analgesics are compared is morphine. Although the alkaloid morphine was isolated in the early 1800s the structure of morphine was identified only in 1925 by Gullard and Robinson (Fig. 3a). It was hypothesized that the piperidine ring is essential for its pharmacological activity. The nitrogen atom of this ring is normally positively charged and can interact with

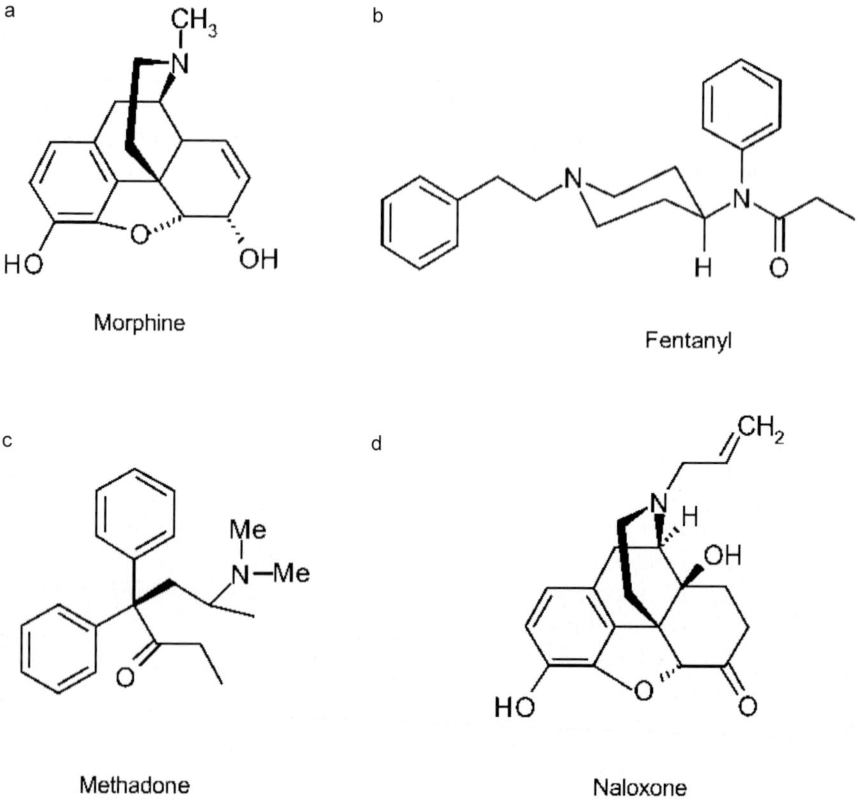

Fig. 3a–d Structures of classical opioid receptor agonists: **a** morphine, **b** the 4-phenylpiperidine fentanyl, and **c** the diphenylpropylamine methadone. **d** Structure of the classical opioid receptor antagonist naloxone

a negatively charged counterpart. Many pharmacologists and chemists tried to produce more potent synthetic opioids with less physical and psychological dependence. The 4-phenylpiperidines (e.g., fentanyl; Fig. 3b), the diphenyl-propylamines (e.g., methadone; Fig. 3c), and many derivatives (e.g., alfentanil, sufentanil, remifentanil) have different structures from morphine. Ligands at μ-receptors produce potent analgesia; however, they also produce side effects like respiratory depression, constipation, physical dependence, and tolerance. In 1942 the substitution of an allyl group for the methyl group on the nitrogen atom of morphine produced the first opioid receptor antagonist, nalorphine. Nalorphine not only countered the effects of morphine but also produced limited analgesia mediated through κ-opioid receptors. An additional member of this mixed agonist/antagonist group is buprenorphine, a semi-synthetic opiate derivative of thebaine. Buprenorphine is a partial agonist at the μ-receptor. At low doses it produces typical morphine-like effects, and at higher doses it has a reduced intrinsic activity compared to pure agonists (Cowan et al. 1977). Buprenorphine also has the properties of a κ-receptor antagonist (Negus et al. 1989). Naloxone was developed as a pure opioid receptor antagonist, which has a structure similar to that of morphine (Fig. 3d). Several newer compounds with restricted access to the CNS have been synthesized. These were designed with the aim to activate peripheral opioid receptors exclusively, without the occurrence of central side effects (Binder et al. 2001; Furst et al. 2005; Kumar et al. 2005; Whiteside et al. 2004).

3.3
Sites of Action

3.3.1
Supraspinal and Spinal Sites

Various major brain regions containing opioid peptides and opioid receptors have been identified including the periaqueductal gray, the locus coeruleus, and the rostral ventral medulla (Heinricher and Morgan 1999; Fig. 4a). All three opioid receptors are also present in the dorsal horn of the spinal cord, which is in another area important for opioid-induced analgesia (Fig. 4b). The μ-, δ-, and κ-opioid receptors are mainly located in the upper laminae, particularly the substantia gelatinosa (laminae I and II). In addition, δ-opioid receptors are found in the deeper laminae of the dorsal horn and in the ventral horn (Gouarderes et al. 1993). Opioid receptor activation mostly results in depression of neuronal firing. Presynaptically, opioids inhibit Ca^{2+} influx and the subsequent release of glutamate and neuropeptides (e.g., substance P, calcitonin gene-related peptide) from primary afferent terminals. Postsynaptically, opioids hyperpolarize ascending projection neurons by increasing K^+ conductance.

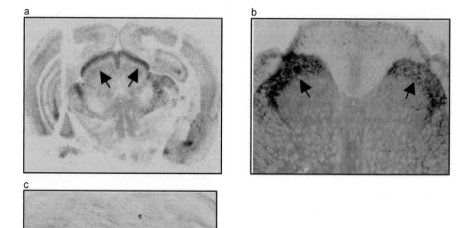

Fig. 4a An autoradiographic receptor binding technique showing the distribution of µ-receptors within rat brain slices. An increase in µ-receptor density (indicated with *arrows*) shows their distribution in various regions, including the cortex, thalamus, hypothalamus, and brainstem. **b** Immunocytochemical studies showing µ-receptors within laminae I–II of spinal cord dorsal horns from rats (kindly provided by Dr. S. Mousa). **c** Immunocyto-chemical studies from rat hindpaw preparations indicating µ-receptors on primary afferent neurons (also kindly provided by Dr. S. Mousa)

3.3.2
Peripheral Sites

It became clear in the late 1980s that opioid receptors and opioid peptides are also located in the peripheral nervous system, including primary afferent neurons and dorsal root ganglia (DRG) (Stein et al. 1989; Stein et al. 2003). Opioid receptors have been shown mainly on small- to medium-diameter neuronal cell bodies of sensory neurons (Mousa et al. 2000). After synthesis in the DRG, opioid receptors are transported to the peripheral nerve terminals of primary afferent neurons (Hassan et al. 1993; Fig. 4c). Opioid receptors are also expressed by neuroendocrine (pituitary, adrenals), immune, and ecto-dermal tissues (Slominski et al. 2000). Although opioids increase potassium currents in the CNS it is still controversial whether this occurs in DRG neurons. Rather, it was shown that the modulation of Ca^{2+} currents is the principal mechanism for the inhibitory effect of opioids on sensory neurons (Akins and

McCleskey 1993). Recently, G protein-coupled inwardly rectifying potassium channels (GIRK2) and μ-opioid receptors were colocalized on sensory nerve endings in epidermis, and it was proposed that endothelin-B receptors trigger the release of endorphin from keratinocytes, suppressing pain via opioid receptors coupled to GIRK channels (Khodorova et al. 2003). In addition, it was shown that opioids activate inhibitory $G_{i/o}$ proteins, which leads to a decrease of cAMP in peripheral sensory neurons (Chen et al. 1997).

3.3.3
Peripheral Opioid Receptors and Inflammation

In animal experiments, local application of opioid receptor agonists elicits a more pronounced antinociceptive effect under painful inflammatory conditions than in noninflamed tissue. It was shown that subcutaneous inflammation can induce an upregulation of μ-opioid receptor mRNA within the lumbar spinal cord (Maekawa et al. 1996) and DRG (Puehler et al. 2004). In addition, the expression of opioid receptors in sensory neurons increases time-dependently during inflammation (Zöllner et al. 2003). Subsequently, the axonal transport of opioid receptors to the peripheral nerve terminals is augmented (Hassan et al. 1993; Laduron and Castel 1990). This increase might be related to cytokines (e.g., interleukin 4) through the binding of STAT-6 transcription factors to the μ-opioid receptor gene promoter (Kraus et al. 2001). Other potential mechanisms contributing to enhanced antinociceptive efficacy include an increase in the number of opioid receptor bearing peripheral sensory nerve terminals (Stein et al. 2003), an increase in G protein coupling (Shaqura et al. 2004; Zöllner et al. 2003), a disruption of the perineural barrier (Antonijevic et al. 1995), and an enhanced opioid receptor trafficking to the neuronal membrane (Patwardhan et al. 2005).

4
Clinical Applications

4.1
Acute Pain

Opioids are the most broadly effective analgesics and are used in both acute and chronic pain. Typical acute pain situations include intraoperative, postoperative, and posttraumatic pain. In those situations opioids are used preemptively (i.e., before occurrence of an anticipated noxious stimulus, e.g., during induction of anesthesia) or therapeutically (i.e., after occurrence of noxious stimulation). Whereas acute pain is generally amenable to drug therapy, chronic pain is a complex disease in its own right and needs to be differentiated into malignant (cancer-related) and nonmalignant (e.g., neuropathic, inflammatory) pain. Acute and cancer-related pain are commonly responsive to opioids. Chronic nonmalignant pain requires a multidisciplinary approach encompassing various pharmacological and nonpharmacological (e.g., psychological, physiotherapeutic) treatment strategies. Various routes of opioid administration (e.g., oral, intravenous, subcutaneous, intrathecal, epidural, topical, intraarticular, transnasal) are used, depending on the clinical circumstances. The opioid effect is a selective one on nociception. Touch, pressure, and other sensory modalities are generally unaffected. After systemic administration, forebrain mechanisms play a prominent role in the clinical effects, and a common clinical manifestation of opioid analgesia is a change in the affective response to pain. Spinal mechanisms become proportionally more important when opioids are given by neuraxial injection. Patients given systemic opioids will typically say that pain is still present, but the intensity is reduced and it no longer bothers them as much. Mental clouding and dissociation from pain is often accompanied by mood elevation.

4.2
Chronic Pain

The use of opioids for chronic noncancer pain (e.g., neuropathic pain, musculoskeletal pain) is controversial. Despite the fact that many patients have received opioids chronically (Portenoy et al. 1991), we do not really know how well they work. Opioid efficacy in musculoskeletal pain and neuropathic pain has been claimed in a number of case reports and uncontrolled open studies. Few controlled studies investigating the efficacy and side effects of opioids in these clinical settings are available (Caldwell et al. 1999; Moulin et al. 1996; Peloso et al. 2000; Watson and Babul 1998). At the moment, the maximum duration of opioid treatment investigated in a double-blind placebo-controlled study is 9 weeks (Moulin et al. 1996). Most trials found a reduction in subjective pain scores, but only one study examined in detail much more important parameters such as psychosocial features, quality of life, drug dependence, and functional status (Moulin et al. 1996). No significant improvements in any of the latter parameters were detected, and there was a lack of overall patient preference for the opioid. Most authors concluded that morphine may confer analgesic benefit with a low risk of addiction, but that it is unlikely to yield psychological or functional improvement (Watson and Babul 1998). Adverse opioid side effects were reported in all of these investigations and led to the drop-out of large numbers (up to 60%) of patients. Thus, there is a lack of prospective controlled studies examining the long-term (at least several months) administration of opioids. Future studies need to demonstrate positive outcomes, not only in subjective pain reports, but, more importantly, also in terms of reduced depression, functional improvement, reemployment and decreased use of the healthcare system.

Many recent studies have focused on the activation of opioid receptors outside the CNS. One of the most extensively studied and most successful applications is the intraarticular injection of morphine (Kalso 2002). In dental surgery, peripheral antinociception was detected after local morphine application (Likar et al. 1998). In patients with chronic arthritis local morphine has also been shown to reduce pain and possibly inflammation (Likar et al. 1997; Stein et al. 1999). The topical application of opioids produces antihyperalgesic effects when applied to painful ulcers and skin lesions, after burn injuries, and in cutaneous pain (Kolesnikov et al. 2000; Krajnik et al. 1999; Long et al. 2001; Twillman et al. 1999). The local application of morphine in patients with corneal abrasion also showed analgesic effects (Peyman et al. 1994). Novel peripherally restricted κ-agonists have been investigated in humans with chronic painful pancreatitis (Eisenach et al. 2003). In addition, some studies have suggested a relatively reduced development of opioid tolerance in inflamed tissue (Stein et al. 1996).

4.3
Pharmacokinetics

4.3.1
Absorption

Almost all opioids are rapidly absorbed after oral administration and many undergo substantial first-pass metabolism in the liver. Much effort has been directed at delaying absorption with sustained-release opioid preparations because adequate duration of analgesia is a bigger clinical problem than slow onset. Sometimes almost no absorption is desirable: For example, loperamide and diphenoxylate are potent opioids used in the treatment of diarrhea (and recently for topical application) because they are poorly absorbed and produce minimal effects in the CNS. Opioid drugs vary tremendously in their lipid solubility, and this largely determines the efficiency of absorption from peripheral sites. For example, after sublingual administration, the bioavailability of morphine is only 12%, while highly lipid soluble drugs like fentanyl and buprenorphine are 60%–70% absorbed into the bloodstream (Gong and Middleton 1992; Weinberg et al. 1988). Lipophilic opioids are now commercially available in buccal, intranasal, and transdermal preparations. Using a special nebulizer apparatus, it is possible to administer morphine by inhalation and achieve 63% bioavailability (Dershwitz et al. 2000).

4.3.2
Distribution

All opioids are rapidly and extensively distributed throughout the body. After a bolus intravenous injection, the rapid increase and decrease in plasma concentration looks quite similar for morphine and fentanyl. The difference in onset and duration of effect for these two drugs is a function of the rate at which plasma concentrations equilibrate with those in brain, at least in situations where activation of central opioid receptors is the predominant mechanism of action (i.e., without major peripheral tissue injury). CNS concentration of a lipophilic opioid like fentanyl closely follows the concentration in plasma, rising then falling rapidly as the drug is redistributed from highly perfused tissues into muscle and fat (Hug and Murphy 1979; Lotsch 2005b). Its short duration is due to the rapidity of physical translocation out of the CNS. In comparison, the slow onset and offset of morphine are because it enters and exits the CNS slowly. Brain concentrations of morphine lag far behind those in plasma. When an opioid is administered intrathecally or epidurally, the onset of effect is determined by the rate at which the drug penetrates to reach opioid receptors in the dorsal horn. Since little metabolism occurs in the CNS, the effects are terminated by redistribution into blood vessels. Recent animal studies into the relative contribution of peripheral versus central opioid receptors indicate that, depending on the presence and extent of tissue injury and on the types of opioid receptors involved, up to 80% of an analgesic effect following systemic opioid administration may be mediated by peripheral opioid receptors (D. Labuz, S.A. Mousa, M. Schäfer, C. Stein, H. Machelska, submitted). Similar observations were made in human studies using the peripherally restricted agonist morphine-6-glucuronide (Tegeder et al. 2003; Hanna et al. 2005).

4.3.3
Metabolism and Excretion

All clinically available opioids undergo extensive hepatic metabolism to polar metabolites that are excreted by the kidney (Lotsch 2005a). The notable exception is remifentanil, which is rapidly hydrolyzed by nonspecific esterases in peripheral tissues and plasma (Servin 2003). In general, morphine and its close congeners mainly undergo synthetic biotransformation to glucuronides, while meperidine and the fentanyl derivatives undergo oxidative metabolism by cytochrome P450 enzymes. Both morphine and fentanyl have high hepatic extraction ratios (0.7 and 0.6, respectively). This means that the clearance of these drugs is sensitive to factors that alter liver blood flow. On the other hand, clearance is relatively unaffected by inducers or inhibitors of liver enzymes. The major metabolite of morphine is the 3-glucuronide, but about 15% forms morphine 6-glucuronide (M6G), a compound that has substantial opioid agonist activity (Kilpatrick and Smith 2005). It is likely that this highly polar metabolite does not easily enter the CNS (Portenoy et al. 1991) but may produce analgesia via peripheral opioid receptors (Hanna et al. 2005; Tegeder et al. 2003).

5
Side Effects

5.1
Acute Opioid Application

5.1.1
Cardiovascular System

High doses of morphine, fentanyl, sufentanil, remifentanil, and alfentanil are associated with a vagus-mediated bradycardia. Severe bradycardia or even asystole is possible, especially in conjunction with the vagal stimulating effects of intubation (Bowdle 1998). With the exception of meperidine, opioids do not depress cardiac contractility. Arterial blood pressure often falls as a result of bradycardia and decreased sympathetic reflexes. However, opioids have depressant effects in patients with congestive heart failure (Liang et al. 1987) and in myocardial ischemia/reperfusion-induced arrhythmias (Lee 1992). Recent evidence has also implicated opioids as having cardioprotective effects ("ischemic preconditioning"), in that tissue damage after brief periods of coronary artery occlusion was prevented by opioids (Schultz et al. 1997). Suggested mechanisms include the activation of mitochondrial ATP-sensitive K channels (K_{ATP} channels) in cardiomyocytes. Opening of mitochondrial K_{ATP} channels is thought to be protective by preservation of mitochondrial integrity, by dissipation of mitochondrial membrane potential, and consequent reduction of calcium overload and apoptotic cell death (Cao et al. 2005; Cao et al. 2003). In isolated cardiomyocytes as well as sympathectomized intact rat hearts, it was suggested that opioid receptors functionally and physically crosstalk with β-adrenergic receptors, including heterodimerization of these receptors, counterbalance of functionally opposing G protein signaling, and interference with downstream signaling events. As a result, the β-adrenergic receptor-mediated positive inotropic effect and an increase in cAMP are markedly attenuated after opioid receptor activation (Pepe et al. 2004).

5.1.2
Respiratory System

Respiratory depression is the adverse effect most feared by clinicians. These effects are mediated by μ- and δ-receptors through the direct inhibition of rhythm-generating respiratory neurons in the pre-Boetzinger complex (PBC) of the brainstem (Manzke et al. 2003). Opioids produce a dose-dependent depression of the ventilatory response to hypercarbia and hypoxia (Ladd et al. 2005; Weil et al. 1975). Respiratory depressant effects may be detectable well before clinically apparent changes in respiratory rate and depth. With increasing opioid doses, respiratory rate slows and tidal volume initially increases and then eventually decreases. High doses can produce apnea, and a small number of patients still die each year from opioid-induced respiratory depression. The potential is greatest in heavily co-medicated (e.g., with sedatives) patients who are unstimulated and unmonitored. In a classic study, Forrest and Belleville showed that natural sleep greatly increases the respiratory depressant effects of morphine (Forrest and Bellville 1964). Fentanyl, alfentanil, and sufentanil have all been reported to produce "recurrent" respiratory depression in postoperative patients who initially seemed to be breathing well (Becker et al. 1976). It seems likely that these episodes were actually due to variations in the level of postoperative (e.g., nociceptive) stimulation. Recently it was shown that serotonin 4(a) [5-HT4(a)] receptors are expressed in respiratory PBC neurons, their selective activation protects spontaneous respiratory activity, and 5-HT(4a) receptors and μ-receptors affect the intracellular concentration of cyclic AMP in opposite ways (Manzke et al. 2003). Treatment of rats with a 5-HT4 receptor-specific agonist prevented fentanyl-induced respiratory depression without loss of fentanyl's analgesic activity (Manzke et al. 2003). These findings might stimulate novel therapeutic developments in the future (Eilers and Schumacher 2004).

5.1.3
Sedation

Sedation is a frequent and serious side effect of opioid analgesics, sometimes reported as fatigue or tiredness by patients (Shaiova 2005). Importantly, small subanalgesic doses of opioids can multiply the sedative potency of midazolam (Kissin et al. 1990). Similar interactions have been demonstrated with propofol (Short et al. 1992) and barbiturates. Thus, for the clinician it is important to remember that patients receiving multiple sedative medications simultaneously are at increased risk and need to be monitored adequately.

5.1.4
Nausea and Vomiting

Opioids stimulate nausea and vomiting by a direct effect on the chemoreceptor trigger zone in the area postrema in the brainstem (Apfel et al. 2004; Wang and Glaviano 1954). This effect is increased by labyrinthine input, so patients who are moving are much more likely to be nauseated than those lying quietly. Prophylactic antiemetic interventions include the avoidance of other emetogenic drugs (e.g., inhalational anesthetics) by total intravenous anesthesia (e.g., with propofol). Serotonin antagonists, dexamethasone, and droperidol can be used to treat opioid-induced nausea and vomiting (Apfel et al. 2004).

5.1.5
Cough Suppression

Opioids depress cough by direct effects on medullary cough centers (e.g., raphe nuclei; Chou and Wang 1975; Schug et al. 1992). The structure-activity requirements for the antitussive effects are not the same as those for typical µ-receptor-mediated analgesic effects. The greatest activity is seen with drugs like codeine and heroin—morphine congeners with bulky substitutions at the 3 position. The stereospecificity of the response is different as well: cough suppression is produced by dextroisomers of opioids (e.g., dextromethorphan) that do not have analgesic activity (Chung and Chang 2002; Lal et al. 1986).

5.1.6
Pupil Constriction

The miotic effect of opioids occurs through a direct action on the autonomic (Edinger–Westphal) nucleus of the oculomotor nerve to increase parasympathetic tone. This effect can be detected after extremely small (subanalgesic) doses. Relatively little tolerance occurs to this effect, so even patients taking very high doses of opioids for extended periods of time (e.g., for chronic cancer pain) will continue to have constricted pupils. Pupil responses have proved useful for simultaneous pharmacokinetic–pharmacodynamic modeling of opioids (Zacny 2005).

5.1.7
Skeletal Muscle Rigidity

This phenomenon, often incorrectly termed "truncal" or "chest wall" rigidity, is actually a generalized hypertonus of striated muscle throughout the body (Benthuysen et al. 1986). It is usually seen when potent opioids are administered rapidly (e.g., during induction of anesthesia) and is most commonly produced by fentanyl and its congeners (Bowdle 1998). The mechanism appears to be an inhibition of striatal γ-aminobutyric acid (GABA) release and an increase in dopamine production (Costall et al. 1978). Selective antagonism at the nucleus raphe magnus in the rat can completely prevent the increase in muscle tone (Weinger et al. 1991). During induction of anesthesia, opioid-induced muscle rigidity can render a patient difficult to ventilate. Some authors have claimed that the problem does not seem to be loss of chest wall compliance but rather hypertonus of the pharyngeal and laryngeal musculature leading to narrowing of the laryngeal inlet (Arandia and Patil 1987; Bowdle and Rooke 1994). When rigidity is recognized, it must be treated with a muscle relaxant or reversed with naloxone.

5.1.8
Gastrointestinal System

Opioids can seriously disturb gastrointestinal function. Opioid receptors are found throughout the enteric nervous system in the nervous plexus of the bowel, in the sacral plexus, along the biliary tree, and in ureters and bladder. Opioids stimulate tonic contraction of smooth muscle at all of these sites, while reducing normal propulsive activity. This can be a source of significant morbidity: Inhibition of normal intestinal secretions and peristalsis can lead to increased water absorption and constipation. Very little tolerance develops to this effect, so patients taking opioids chronically can develop severe ongoing constipation. This is a very common problem in cancer patients. The inhibitory effect of opioids on peristalsis is mediated by the enteric nerve pathway and by the blockade of presynaptic release of acetylcholine (De Luca and Coupar 1996). Besides inhibiting peristalsis, opioids contract intestinal muscles and induce tonic spasms in the intestine. These effects may involve depression of nitric oxide release from inhibitory enteric neurons or direct activation of smooth muscle cells that express opioid receptors (Townsend et al. 2004). Opioid-induced bowel dysfunction can be prevented by selectively targeting intestinal opioid receptors with orally administered opioid receptor antagonists (Holzner 2004). A new µ-receptor selective antagonist with a peripherally restricted site of action was developed recently (Schmidt 2001). This compound (alvimopan) is characterized by low systemic absorption and it prevents morphine-induced delays in oral-cecal transit time without antagonizing centrally mediated opioid effects. Alvimopan was found to improve the management of postoperative ileus in patients who underwent abdominal surgery and received opioids for acute postoperative pain (Taguchi et al. 2001). Opioid stimulation of smooth muscles along the gall bladder and cystic duct and opioid-induced contraction of the sphincter of Oddi may increase intrabiliary pressure and lead to episodes of biliary colic and false positive cholangiograms. These effects can be completely reversed by naloxone. In addition, opioids can cause urinary retention by decreasing bladder detrusor tone and increasing tone in the urinary sphincter. They also decrease awareness of bladder distension and inhibit the reflex urge to void. This complication is more common in males and more likely to occur when opioids are given by epidural or intrathecal injection.

5.1.9
Histamine Release

Like many other low molecular weight basic drugs, morphine, codeine, and meperidine can cause displacement of histamine from tissue mast cells, resulting in several undesirable effects, such as hypotension, urticaria, pruritus, and tachycardia (Barke and Hough 1993). This is a nonimmunological response that is most often seen as local itching, redness, or hives near the site of i.v. injection. Although functional opiate receptors may exist on mast cells and may be capable of modulating IgE-mediated histamine release, there is no evidence that these receptors account for opiate-induced histamine release. Fentanyl and its congeners do not typically release histamine. Patients who have experienced hives and itching will frequently report that they are allergic to the drug, although true allergy to opioids is extremely rare. Itching may be produced by other mechanisms as well. Opioid receptor-dependent processes activate inhibitory circuits in the CNS and regulate the extent of intensity and quality of perceived itch (Greaves and Wall 1996). Opioids frequently cause itching and warmth over the neck and face, especially over the malar area. Epidural opioids can produce troublesome generalized itching (Chaney 1995; Ballantyne et al. 1989). These dysesthesias appear to be opioid-specific effects since they can be reversed by naloxone and are produced by opioids like fentanyl, which do not release histamine (Kjellberg and Tramer 2001).

5.2
Chronic Opioid Application

5.2.1
Tolerance

As discussed in Sect. 2.4.2, repeated or prolonged exposure to opioids can result in apparent tolerance, a phenomenon that can be due to opioid receptor alterations or to progressively increasing nociceptive stimulation. Cross-tolerance to other agonists can occur, but this cross-tolerance is often incomplete. Tolerance usually develops most rapidly to opioid depressant effects like analgesia and respiratory depression and very slowly to stimulant effects like constipation or miosis. There is a striking difference between the profound degree of tolerance to the analgesic effect of opioids observed in animal models and the relative stability of opioid dose-response relationships in patients with ongoing pain. Dose escalation is common in long-term opioid treatment for the management of cancer pain, but tumor growth could be the reason for this increase. Many clinical studies indicate that opioid tolerance is of minor relevance and develops less frequently in patients experiencing pain (Adriaensen et al. 2003). A survey of over 2,000 cancer patients showed that less than 50% had increased their daily morphine dose over 1 year of treatment (Zech et al. 1995). These differences between clinical and laboratory investigations caution against generalization from the laboratory to the clinic.

5.2.2
Physical Dependence

As with many other drugs, the continuous application of opioids over of longer periods of time produces physical (and psychological) dependence. Stopping the drug abruptly causes a stereotypical withdrawal syndrome that includes restlessness, mydriasis, gooseflesh, runny nose, diarrhea, shaking chills, and drug seeking (Heit 2003). The rate of onset of these symptoms depends upon the rate at which the opioid is eliminated. Administration of an opioid antagonist can cause an immediate "precipitated" withdrawal. The symptoms of withdrawal are terminated rapidly by administering opioid agonists. Physical dependence must be distinguished from psychological dependence or addiction, which includes the dimension of compulsive drug-seeking behavior (Enck 1991). However, some investigations suggest that addiction resulting from appropriate medical treatment is a very unusual event (Porter and Jick 1980).

Acknowledgements   We thank Dr. Stefan Schulz for critical reading of the manuscript.

References

Adriaensen H, Vissers K, Noorduin H, Meert T (2003) Opioid tolerance and dependence: an inevitable consequence of chronic treatment? Acta Anaesthesiol Belg 54:37–47

Akins PT, McCleskey EW (1993) Characterization of potassium currents in adult rat sensory neurons and modulation by opioids and cyclic AMP. Neuroscience 56:759–769

Antonijevic I, Mousa SA, Schäfer M, Stein C (1995) Perineurial defect and peripheral opioid analgesia in inflammation. J Neurosci 15:165–172

Apfel CC, Korttila K, Abdalla M, Kerger H, Turan A, Vedder I, Zernak C, Danner K, Jokela R, Posock SJ, Trenkler S, Kredel M, Biedler A, Sessler DI, Roewer N (2004) A factorial trial of six interventions for the prevention of postoperative neusea and vomiting. N Engl J Med 350:2441–2451

Arandia HY, Patil VU (1987) Glottic closure following large doses of fentanyl. Anesthesiology 66:574–575

Attali B, Gouarderes C, Mazarguil H, Audigier Y, Cros J (1982) Evidence for multiple "Kappa" binding sites by use of opioid peptides in the guinea-pig lumbo-sacral spinal cord. Neuropeptides 3:53–64

Ballantyne JC, Loach AB, Carr DB (1989) The incidence of pruritus after epidural morphine. Anaesthesia 44:863

Barke KE, Hough LB (1993) Opiates, mast cells and histamine release. Life Sci 53:1391–1399

Becker LD, Paulson BA, Miller RD, Severinghaus JW, Eger EI 2nd (1976) Biphasic respiratory depression after fentanyldroperidol or fentanyl alone used to supplement nitrous oxide anesthesia. Anesthesiology 44:291–296

Belcheva MM, Bohn LM, Ho MT, Johnson FE, Yanai J, Barron S, Coscia CJ (1998) Brain opioid receptor adaptation and expression after prenatal exposure to buprenorphine. Brain Res Dev Brain Res 111:35–42

Belcheva MM, Clark AL, Haas PD, Serna JS, Hahn JW, Kiss A, Coscia CJ (2005) Mu and kappa opioid receptors activate ERK/MAPK via different protein kinase C isoforms and secondary messengers in astrocytes. J Biol Chem 280:27662–27669

Benthuysen JL, Smith NT, Sanford TJ, Head N, Dec-Silver H (1986) Physiology of alfentanil-induced rigidity. Anesthesiology 64:440–446

Binder W, Machelska H, Mousa S, Schmitt T, Riviere PJ, Junien JL, Stein C, Schäfer M (2001) Analgesic and antiinflammatory effects of two novel kappa-opioid peptides. Anesthesiology 94:1034–1044

Bohn LM, Gainetdinov RR, Lin FT, Lefkowitz RJ, Caron MG (2000) Mu-opioid receptor desensitization by beta-arrestin-2 determines morphine tolerance but not dependence. Nature 408:720–723

Bohn LM, Lefkowitz RJ, Caron MG (2002) Differential mechanisms of morphine antinociceptive tolerance revealed in (beta)arrestin-2 knock-out mice. J Neurosci 22:10494–10500

Bohn LM, Dykstra LA, Lefkowitz RJ, Caron MG, Barak LS (2004) Relative opioid efficacy is determined by the complements of the G protein-coupled receptor desensitization machinery. Mol Pharmacol 66:106–112

Bowdle TA (1998) Adverse effects of opioid agonists and agonist-antagonists in anaesthesia. Drug Saf 19:173–189

Bowdle TA, Rooke GA (1994) Postoperative myoclonus and rigidity after anesthesia with opioids. Anesth Analg 78:783–786

Caldwell JR, Hale ME, Boyd RE, Hague JM, Iwan T, Shi M, Lacouture PG (1999) Treatment of osteoarthritis pain with controlled release oxycodone or fixed combination oxycodone plus acetaminophen added to nonsteroidal antiinflammatory drugs: a double blind, randomized, multicenter, placebo controlled trial. J Rheumatol 26:862–869

Cao Z, Liu L, VanWinkle DM (2003) Activation of delta- and kappa-opioid receptors by opioid peptides protects cardiomyocytes via KATP channels. Am J Physiol Heart Circ Physiol 285:1032–1039

Cao Z, Liu L, Van Winkle DM (2005) Met5-enkephalin-induced cardioprotection occurs via transactivation of EGFR and activation of PI3 K. Am J Physiol Heart Circ Physiol 288:1955–1964

Capeyrou R, Riond J, Corbani M, Lepage JF, Bertin B, Emorine LJ (1997) Agonist-induced signaling and trafficking of the mu-opioid receptor: role of serine and threonine residues in the third cytoplasmic loop and C-terminal domain. FEBS Lett 415:200–205

Chan JS, Chiu TT, Wong YH (1995) Activation of type II adenylyl cyclase by the cloned mu-opioid receptor: coupling to multiple G proteins. J Neurochem 65:2682–2689

Chaney MA (1995) Side effects of intrathecal and epidural opioids. Can J Anaesth 42:891–903

Chen JJ, Dymshitz J, Vasko MR (1997) Regulation of opioid receptors in rat sensory neurons in culture. Mol Pharmacol 51:666–673

Chou DT, Wang SC (1975) Studies on the localization of central cough mechanism; site of action of antitussive drugs. J Pharmacol Exp Ther 194:499–505

Chung KF, Chang AB (2002) Therapy for cough: active agents. Pulm Pharmacol Ther 15:335–338

Comb M, Seeburg PH, Adelman J, Eiden L, Herbert E (1982) Primary structure of the human Met- and Leu-enkephalin precursor and its mRNA. Nature 295:663–666

Costall B, Fortune DH, Naylor RJ (1978) Involvement of mesolimbic and extrapyramidal nuclei in the motor depressant action of narcotic drugs. J Pharm Pharmacol 30:566–572

Cowan A, Lewis JW, Macfarlane IR (1977) Agonist and antagonist properties of buprenorphine, a new antinociceptive agent. Br J Pharmacol 60:537–545

De Luca A, Coupar IM (1996) Insights into action in the intestinal tract. Pharmacol Ther 69:103–115

Decaillot FM, Befort K, Filliol D, Yue S, Walker P, Kieffer BL (2003) Opioid receptor random mutagenesis reveals a mechanism for G protein-coupled receptor activation. Nat Struct Biol 10:629–636

Dershwitz M, Walsh JL, Morishige RJ, Connors PM, Rubsamen RM, Shafer SL, Rosow CE (2000) Pharmacokinetics and pharmacodynamics of inhaled versus intravenous morphine in healthy volunteers. Anesthesiology 93:619–628

Eilers H, Schumacher MA (2004) Opioid-induced respiratory depression: are 5-HT4a receptor agonists the cure? Mol Interv 4:197–199

Eisenach JC, Carpenter R, Curry R (2003) Analgesia from a peripherally active kappa-opioid receptor agonist in patients with chronic pancreatitis. Pain 101:89–95

Eisinger DA, Ammer H, Schulz R (2002) Chronic morphine treatment inhibits opioid receptor desensitization and internalization. J Neurosci 22:10192–10200

Elliott K, Kest B, Man A, Kao B, Inturrisi CE (1995) N-methyl-D-aspartate (NMDA) receptors, mu and kappa opioid tolerance, and perspectives on new analgesic drug development. Neuropsychopharmacology 13:347–356

Enck RE (1991) Understanding tolerance, physical dependence and addiction in the use of opioid analgesics. Am J Hosp Palliat Care 8:9–11

Evans CJ, Keith DE Jr, Morrison H, Magendzo K, Edwards RH (1992) Cloning of a delta opioid receptor by functional expression. Science 258:1952–1955

Forrest WH Jr, Bellville JW (1964) The effect of sleep plus morphine on the respiratory response to carbon dioxide. Anesthesiology 25:137–141

Furst S, Riba P, Friedmann T, Timar J, Al-Khrasani M, Obara I, Makuch W, Spetea M, Schutz J, Przewlocki R, Przewlocka B, Schmidhammer H (2005) Peripheral versus central antinociceptive actions of 6-amino acid-substituted derivatives of 14-O-methyloxymorphone in acute and inflammatory pain in the rat. J Pharmacol Exp Ther 312:609–618

Gavériaux-Ruff C, Kieffer BL (2002) Opioid receptor genes inactivated in mice: the highlights. Neuropeptides 36:62–71

Gavériaux-Ruff C, Filliol D, Simonin F, Matthes HW, Kieffer BL (2001) Immunosuppression by delta-opioid antagonist naltrindole: delta- and triple mu/delta/kappa-opioid receptor knockout mice reveal a nonopioid activity. J Pharmacol Exp Ther 298:1193–1198

Gavériaux-Ruff C, Kieffer BL (1999b) Opioid receptors: gene structure and function. In: Stein C (ed) Opioids in pain control. Cambridge University Press, Cambridge, pp 1–20

Gold MS, Levine JD (1996) DAMGO inhibits prostaglandin E2-induced potentiation of a TTX-resistant Na+ current in rat sensory neurons in vitro. Neurosci Lett 212:83–86

Gong L, Middleton RK (1992) Sublingual administration of opioids. Ann Pharmacother 26:1525–1527

Gouarderes C, Tellez S, Tafani JA, Zajac JM (1993) Quantitative autoradiographic mapping of delta-opioid receptors in the rat central nervous system using [125I][D.Ala2]deltorphin-I. Synapse 13:231–240

Greaves MW, Wall PD (1996) Pathophysiology of itching. Lancet 348:938–940

Hanna MH, Elliott KM, Fung M (2005) Randomized, double-blind study of the analgesic efficacy of morphine-6-glucuronide versus morphine sulfate for postoperative pain in maijor surgery. Anesthesiology 102:815–821

Hassan AH, Ableitner A, Stein C, Herz A (1993) Inflammation of the rat paw enhances axonal transport of opioid receptors in the sciatic nerve and increases their density in the inflamed tissue. Neuroscience 55:185–195

Heinricher M, Morgan M (1999) Supraspinal mechanisms of opioid analgesia. In: Stein C (ed) Opioids in pain control: basic and clinical aspects. Cambridge University Press, Cambridge, pp 46–69

Heit HA (2003) Addiction, physical dependence, and tolerance: precise definitions to help clinicians evaluate and treat chronic pain patients. J Pain Palliat Care Pharmacother 17:15–29

Herlitze S, Garcia DE, Mackie K, Hille B, Scheuer T, Catterall WA (1996) Modulation of Ca^{2+} channels by G-protein beta gamma subunits. Nature 380:258–262

Höllt V (1993) Regulation of opioid peptide gene expression. In: Herz A (ed) Opioids I. (Handbook of experimental pharmacology) Springer Verlag, New York, pp 307–346

Holzner P (2004) Opioids and opioid receptors in the enteric nervous system: from a problem in opioid analgesia to a possible new prokinetic therapy in humans. Neurosci Lett 361:192–195

Horvath G (2000) Endomorphin-1 and endomorphin-2: pharmacology of the selective endogenous mu-opioid receptor agonists. Pharmacol Ther 88:437–463

Hug CC Jr, Murphy MR (1979) Fentanyl disposition in cerebrospinal fluid and plasma and its relationship to ventilatory depression in the dog. Anesthesiology 50:342–349

Hughes J, Smith TW, Kosterlitz HW, Fothergill LA, Morgan BA, Morris HR (1975) Identification of two related pentapeptides from the brain with potent opiate agonist activity. Nature 258:577–580

Hulme EC, Lu ZL, Ward SD, Allman K, Curtis CA (1999) The conformational switch in 7-transmembrane receptors: the muscarinic receptor paradigm. Eur J Pharmacol 375:247–260

Ignatova EG, Belcheva MM, Bohn LM, Neumann MC, Coscia CJ (1999) Requirement of receptor internalization for opioid stimulation of mitogen-activated protein kinase: biochemical and immunofluorescence confocal microscopic evidence. J Neurosci 19:56–63

Ingram SL, Williams JT (1994) Opioid inhibition of Ih via adenylyl cyclase. Neuron 13:179–186

Kakidani H, Furutani Y, Takahashi H, Noda M, Morimoto Y, Hirose T, Asai M, Inayama S, Nakanishi S, Numa S (1982) Cloning and sequence analysis of cDNA for porcine beta-neo-endorphin/dynorphin precursor. Nature 298:245–249

Kalso E, Smith L, McQuay HJ, Andrew Moore R (2002) No pain, no gain: clinical excellence and scientific rigour-lessons learned from IA morphine. Pain 98:269–275

Karnik SS, Gogonea C, Patil S, Saad Y, Takezako T (2003) Activation of G-protein-coupled receptors: a common molecular mechanism. Trends Endocrinol Metab 14:431–437

Khodorova A, Navarro B, Jouaville LS, Murphy JE, Rice FL, Mazurkiewicz JE, Long-Woodward D, Stoffel M, Strichartz GR, Yukhananov R, Davar G (2003) Endothelin-B receptor activation triggers an endogenous analgesic cascade at sites of peripheral injury. Nat Med 9:1055–1061

Kieffer B, Befort K, Gaveriaux-Ruff C, Hirth C (1992) The δ-opioid receptor: isolation of a cDNA by expression cloning and pharmacological characterization. Proc Natl Acad Sci U S A 90:12048–12052

Kieffer BL (1999a) Opioids: first lessons from knockout mice. Trends Pharmacol Sci 20:19–26

Kieffer BL, Gaveriaux-Ruff C (2002) Exploring the opioid system by gene knockout. Prog Neurobiol 66:285–306

Kilpatrick GJ, Smith TW (2005) Morphine-6-glucuronide: actions and mechanisms. Med Res Rev 25:521–544

Kissin I, Vinik HR, Castillo R, Bradley EL Jr (1990) Alfentanil potentiates midazolam-induced unconsciousness in subanalgesic doses. Anesth Analg 71:65–69

Kjellberg F, Tramer MR (2001) Pharmacological control of opioid-induced pruritus: a quantitative systematic review of randomized trials. Eur J Anaesthesiol 18:346–357

Klco JM, Wiegand CB, Narzinski K, Baranski TJ (2005) Essential role for the second extracellular loop in C5a receptor activation. Nat Struct Mol Biol 12:320–326

Koch T, Schulz S, Schroder H, Wolf R, Raulf E, Hollt V (1998) Carboxyl-terminal splicing of the rat mu opioid receptor modulates agonist-mediated internalization and receptor resensitization. J Biol Chem 273:13652–13657

Koch T, Schulz S, Pfeiffer M, Klutzny M, Schroder H, Kahl E, Hollt V (2001) C-terminal splice variants of the mouse mu-opioid receptor differ in morphine-induced internalization and receptor resensitization. J Biol Chem 276:31408–31414

Koch T, Widera A, Bartzsch K, Schulz S, Brandenburg LO, Wundrack N, Beyer A, Grecksch G, Hollt V (2005) Receptor endocytosis counteracts the development of opioid tolerance. Mol Pharmacol 67:280–287

Kolesnikov YA, Chereshnev I, Pasternak GW (2000) Analgesic synergy between topical lidocaine and topical opioids. J Pharmacol Exp Ther 295:546–551

Kondo I, Marvizon JC, Song B, Salgado F, Codeluppi S, Hua XY, Yaksh TL (2005) Inhibition by spinal mu- and delta-opioid agonists of afferent-evoked substance P release. J Neurosci 25:3651–3660

Krajnik M, Zylicz Z, Finlay I, Luczak J, van Sorge AA (1999) Potential uses of topical opioids in palliative care—report of 6 cases. Pain 80:121–125

Kraus J, Borner C, Giannini E, Hickfang K, Braun H, Mayer P, Hoehe MR, Ambrosch A, Konig W, Höllt V (2001) Regulation of mu-opioid receptor gene transcription by interleukin-4 and influence of an allelic variation within a STAT6 transcription factor binding site. J Biol Chem 276:43901–43908

Kumar V, Guo D, Cassel JA, Daubert JD, Dehaven RN, Dehaven-Hudkins DL, Gauntner EK, Gottshall SL, Greiner SL, Koblish M, Little PJ, Mansson E, Maycock AL (2005) Synthesis and evaluation of novel peripherally restricted kappa-opioid receptor agonists. Bioorg Med Chem Lett 15:1091–1095

Ladd LA, Kam PC, Williams DB, Wright AW, Smith MT, Mather LE (2005) Ventilatory responses of healthy subjects to intravenous combinations of morphine and oxycodone under imposed hypercapnic and hypoxaemic conditions. Br J Clin Pharmacol 59:524–535

Laduron PM, Castel MN (1990) Axonal transport of receptors. A major criterion for presynaptic localization. Ann N Y Acad Sci 604:462–469

Lal J, Krutak-Krol H, Domino EF (1986) Comparative antitussive effects of dextrorphan, dextromethorphan and phencyclidine. Arzneimittelforschung 36:1075–1078

Law PY, Wong YH, Loh HH (2000) Molecular mechanisms and regulation of opioid receptor signaling. Annu Rev Pharmacol Toxicol 40:389–430

Lee AY (1992) Stereospecific antiarrhythmic effects of naloxone against myocardial ischaemia and reperfusion in the dog. Br J Pharmacol 107:1057–1060

Liang CS, Imai N, Stone CK, Woolf PD, Kawashima S, Tuttle RR (1987) The role of endogenous opioids in congestive heart failure: effects of nalmefene on systemic and regional hemodynamics in dogs. Circulation 75:443–451

Likar R, Schäfer M, Paulak F, Sittl R, Pipam W, Schalk H, Geissler D, Bernatzky G (1997) Intraarticular morphine analgesia in chronic pain patients with osteoarthritis. Anesth Analg 84:1313–1317

Likar R, Sittl R, Gragger K, Pipam W, Blatnig H, Breschan C, Schalk HV, Stein C, Schäfer M (1998) Peripheral morphine analgesia in dental surgery. Pain 76:145–150

Long TD, Cathers TA, Twillman R, O'Donnell T, Garrigues N, Jones T (2001) Morphine-Infused silver sulfadiazine (MISS) cream for burn analgesia: a pilot study. J Burn Care Rehabil 22:118–123

Lord JA, Waterfield AA, Hughes J, Kosterlitz HW (1977) Endogenous opioid peptides: multiple agonists and receptors. Nature 267:495–499

Lotsch J (2005a) Opioid metabolites. J Pain Symptom Manage 29:S10–24

Lotsch J (2005b) Pharmacokinetic-pharmacodynamic modeling of opioids. J Pain Symptom Manage 29:S90–103

Machelska H, Cabot PJ, Mousa SA, Zhang Q, Stein C (1998) Pain control in inflammation governed by selectins. Nat Med 4:1425–1428

Machelska H, Mousa SA, Brack A, Schopohl JK, Rittner HL, Schäfer M, Stein C (2002) Opioid control of inflammatory pain regulated by intercellular adhesion molecule-1. J Neurosci 22:5588–5596

Maekawa K, Minami M, Masuda T, Satoh M (1996) Expression of mu- and kappa-, but not delta-, opioid receptor mRNAs is enhanced in the spinal dorsal horn of the arthritic rats. Pain 64:365–371

Mansour A, Taylor LP, Fine JL, Thompson RC, Hoversten MT, Mosberg HI, Watson SJ, Akil H (1997) Key residues defining the mu-opioid receptor binding pocket: a site-directed mutagenesis study. J Neurochem 68:344–353

Manzke T, Guenther U, Ponimaskin EG, Haller M, Dutschmann M, Schwarzacher S, Richter DW (2003) 5-HT4(a) receptors avert opioid-induced breathing depression without loss of analgesia. Science 301:226–229

Mao J (1999) NMDA and opioid receptors: their interactions in antinociception, tolerance and neuroplasticity. Brain Res Brain Res Rev 30:289–304

Martin WR, Eades CG, Thompson JA, Huppler RE, Gilbert PE (1976) The effects of morphine- and nalorphine-like drugs in the nondependent and morphine-dependent chronic spinal dog. J Pharmacol Exp Ther 197:517–532

Massotte D, Kieffer BL (2005) The second extracellular loop: a damper for G protein-coupled receptors? Nat Struct Mol Biol 12:287–288

Mattia A, Vanderah T, Mosbert HI, Porreca F (1991) Lack of antinociceptive cross-tolerance between [D-Pen2, D-Pen5]enkephalin and [D-Ala2]deltorphin II in mice: evidence for delta receptor subtypes. J Pharmacol Exp Ther 258:583–587

Meng F, Xie GX, Thompson RC, Mansour A, Goldstein A, Watson SJ, Akil H (1993) Cloning and pharmacological characterization of a rat kappa opioid receptor. Proc Natl Acad Sci U S A 90:9954–9958

Moulin DE, Iezzi A, Amireh R, Sharpe WK, Boyd D, Merskey H (1996) Randomised trial of oral morphine for chronic non-cancer pain. Lancet 347:143–147

Mousa SA, Machelska H, Schäfer M, Stein C (2000) Co-expression of beta-endorphin with adhesion molecules in a model of inflammatory pain. J Neuroimmunol 108:160–170

Nakanishi S, Inoue A, Kita T, Nakamura M, Chang AC, Cohen SN, Numa S (1979) Nucleotide sequence of cloned cDNA for bovine corticotropin-beta-lipotropin precursor. Nature 278:423–427

Narita M, Tseng LF (1998) Evidence for the existence of the beta-endorphin-sensitive "epsilon-opioid receptor" in the brain: the mechanisms of epsilon-mediated antinociception. Jpn J Pharmacol 76:233–253

Negus SS, Picker MJ, Dykstra LA (1989) Kappa antagonist properties of buprenorphine in non-tolerant and morphine-tolerant rats. Psychopharmacology (Berl) 98:141–143

Ocana M, Del Pozo E, Barrios M, Baeyens JM (1995) Subgroups among mu-opioid receptor agonists distinguished by ATP-sensitive K$^+$ channel-acting drugs. Br J Pharmacol 114:1296–1302

Ocana M, Cendan CM, Cobos EJ, Entrena JM, Baeyens JM (2004) Potassium channels and pain: present realities and future opportunities. Eur J Pharmacol 500:203–219

Palczewski K, Kumasaka T, Hori T, Behnke CA, Motoshima H, Fox BA, Le Trong I, Teller DC, Okada T, Stenkamp RE, Yamamoto M, Miyano M (2000) Crystal structure of rhodopsin: a G protein-coupled receptor. Science 289:739–745

Pasternak GW (2004) Multiple opiate receptors: deja vu all over again. Neuropharmacology 47:312–323

Patwardhan AM, Berg KA, Akopain AN, Jeske NA, Gamper N, Clarke WP, Hargreaves KM (2005) Bradykinin-induced functional competence and trafficking of the delta-opioid receptor in trigeminal nociceptors. J Neurosci 25:8825–8832

Peloso PM, Bellamy N, Bensen W, Thomson GT, Harsanyi Z, Babul N, Darke AC (2000) Double blind randomized placebo control trial of controlled release codeine in the treatment of osteoarthritis of the hip or knee. J Rheumatol 27:764–771

Pepe S, van den Brink OW, Lakatta EG, Xiao RP (2004) Cross-talk of opioid peptide receptor and beta-adrenergic receptor signalling in the heart. Cardiovasc Res 63:414–422

Pert CB, Snyder SH (1973) Opiate receptor: demonstration in nervous tissue. Science 179:1011–1014

Peyman GA, Rahimy MH, Fernandes ML (1994) Effects of morphine on corneal sensitivity and epithelial wound healing: implications for topical ophthalmic analgesia. Br J Ophthalmol 78:138–141

Pierce KL, Tohgo A, Ahn S, Field ME, Luttrell LM, Lefkowitz RJ (2001) Epidermal growth factor (EGF) receptor-dependent ERK activation by G protein-coupled receptors: a co-culture system for identifying intermediates upstream and downstream of heparin-binding EGF shedding. J Biol Chem 276:23155–23160

Pol O, Puig MM (1997) Reversal of tolerance to the antitransit effects of morphine during acute intestinal inflammation in mice. Br J Pharmacol 122:1216–1222

Polakiewicz RD, Schieferl SM, Dorner LF, Kansra V, Comb MJ (1998) A mitogen-activated protein kinase pathway is required for mu-opioid receptor desensitization. J Biol Chem 273:12402–12406

Portenoy RK, Khan E, Layman M, Lapin J, Malkin MG, Foley KM, Thaler HT, Cerbone DJ, Inturrisi CE (1991) Chronic morphine therapy for cancer pain: plasma and cerebrospinal fluid morphine and morphine-6-glucuronide concentrations. Neurology 41:1457–1461

Porter J, Jick H (1980) Addiction rare in patients treated with narcotics. N Engl J Med 302:123

Price DD, Mayer DJ, Mao J, Caruso FS (2000) NMDA-receptor antagonists and opioid receptor interactions as related to analgesia and tolerance. J Pain Symptom Manage 19:S7–11

Puehler W, Zöllner C, Brack A, Shaqura M, Krause H, Schäfer M, Stein C (2004) Rapid upregulation of μ opioid receptor mRNA in dorsal root ganglia in response to peripheral inflammation depends on neuronal conduction. Neuroscience 129:473–479

Rittner HL, Brack A, Machelska H, Mousa SA, Bauer M, Schäfer M, Stein C (2001) Opioid peptide-expressing leukocytes: identification, recruitment, and simultaneously increasing inhibition of inflammatory pain. Anesthesiology 95:500–508

Roques BP (2000) Novel approaches to targeting neuropeptide systems. Trends Pharmacol Sci 21:475–483

Rubovitch V, Gafni M, Sarne Y (2003) The mu opioid agonist DAMGO stimulates cAMP production in SK-N-SH cells through a PLC-PKC-Ca^{++} pathway. Brain Res Mol Brain Res 110:261–266

Schmidt H, Schulz S, Klutzny M, Koch T, Handel M, Höllt V (2000) Involvement of mitogen-activated protein kinase in agonist-induced phosphorylation of the mu-opioid receptor in HEK 293 cells. J Neurochem 74:414–422

Schmidt WK (2001) Alvimopan (ADL 8-2698) is a novel peripheral opioid antagonist. Am J Surg 182:27–38

Schmitz R (1985) Friedrich Wilhelm Serturner and the discovery of morphine. Pharm Hist 27:61–74

Schug SA, Zech D, Grond S (1992) Adverse effects of systemic opioid analgesics. Drug Saf 7:200–213

Schultz JJ, Hsu AK, Gross GJ (1997) Ischemic preconditioning and morphine-induced cardioprotection involve the delta (delta)-opioid receptor in the intact rat heart. J Mol Cell Cardiol 29:2187–2195

Schulz R, Eisinger DA, Wehmeyer A (2004a) Opioid control of MAP kinase cascade. Eur J Pharmacol 500:487–497

Schulz S, Mayer D, Pfeiffer M, Stumm R, Koch T, Hollt V (2004b) Morphine induces terminal micro-opioid receptor desensitization by sustained phosphorylation of serine-375. EMBO J 23:3282–3289

Seger R, Krebs EG (1995) The MAPK signaling cascade. FASEB J 9:726–735

Servin F (2003) Remifentanil; from pharmacological properties to clinical practice. Adv Exp Med Biol 523:245–260

Shaiova L (2005) The management of opioid-related sedation. Curr Pain Headache Rep 9:239–242

Shaqura MA, Zöllner C, Mousa SA, Stein C, Schäfer M (2004) Characterization of mu opioid receptor binding and G protein coupling in rat hypothalamus, spinal cord, and primary afferent neurons during inflammatory pain. J Pharmacol Exp Ther 308:712–718

Short TG, Plummer JL, Chui PT (1992) Hypnotic and anaesthetic interactions between midazolam, propofol and alfentanil. Br J Anaesth 69:162–167

Sim LJ, Selley DE, Dworkin SI, Childers SR (1996) Effects of chronic morphine administration on mu opioid receptor-stimulated [^{35}S]GTPgammaS autoradiography in rat brain. J Neurosci 16:2684–2692

Simonin F, Slowe S, Becker JA, Matthes HW, Filliol D, Chluba J, Kitchen I, Kieffer BL (2001) Analysis of [^{3}H]bremazocine binding in single and combinatorial opioid receptor knockout mice. Eur J Pharmacol 414:189–195

Slominski A, Wortsman J, Luger T, Paus R, Solomon S (2000) Corticotropin releasing hormone and proopiomelanocortin involvement in the cutaneous response to stress. Physiol Rev 80:979–1020

Smith FL, Javed RR, Elzey MJ, Dewey WL (2003) The expression of a high level of morphine antinociceptive tolerance in mice involves both PKC and PKA. Brain Res 985:78–88

Stein A, Yassouridis A, Szopko C, Helmke K, Stein C (1999) Intraarticular morphine versus dexamethasone in chronic arthritis. Pain 83:525–532

Stein C, Millan MJ, Shippenberg TS, Peter K, Herz A (1989) Peripheral opioid receptors mediating antinociception in inflammation. Evidence for involvement of mu, delta and kappa receptors. J Pharmacol Exp Ther 248:1269–1275

Stein C, Hassan AH, Lehrberger K, Giefing J, Yassouridis A (1993) Local analgesic effect of endogenous opioid peptides. Lancet 342:321–324

Stein C, Pfluger M, Yassouridis A, Hoelzl J, Lehrberger K, Welte C, Hassan AH (1996) No tolerance to peripheral morphine analgesia in presence of opioid expression in inflamed synovia. J Clin Invest 98:793–799

Stein C, Schäfer M, Machelska H (2003) Attacking pain at its source: new perspectives on opioids. Nat Med 9:1003–1008

Sternini C, Spann M, Anton B, Keith DE Jr, Bunnett NW, von Zastrow M, Evans C, Brecha NC (1996) Agonist-selective endocytosis of mu opioid receptor by neurons in vivo. Proc Natl Acad Sci U S A 93:9241–9246

Stretton D, Miura M, Belvisi MG, Barnes PJ (1992) Calcium-activated potassium channels mediate prejunctional inhibition of peripheral sensory nerves. Proc Natl Acad Sci U S A 89:1325–1329

Surratt CK, Johnson PS, Moriwaki A, Seidleck BK, Blaschak CJ, Wang JB, Uhl GR (1994) -mu opiate receptor. Charged transmembrane domain amino acids are critical for agonist recognition and intrinsic activity. J Biol Chem 269:20548–20553

Taguchi A, Sharma N, Saleem RM, Sessler DI, Carpenter RL, Seyedsadr M, Kurz A (2001) Selective postoperative inhibition of gastrointestinal opioid receptors. N Engl J Med 345:935–940

Tegeder I, Meier S, Burian M, Schmidt H, Geisslinger G, Lotsch J (2003) Peripheral opioid analgesia in experimental human pain models. Brain 126:1092–1102

Townsend Dt, Portoghese PS, Brown DR (2004) Characterization of specific opioid binding sites in neural membranes from the myenteric plexus of porcine small intestine. J Pharmacol Exp Ther 308:385–393

Twillman RK, Long TD, Cathers TA, Mueller DW (1999) Treatment of painful skin ulcers with topical opioids. J Pain Symptom Manage 17:288–292

von Zastrow M (2004) A cell biologist's perspective on physiological adaptation to opiate drugs. Neuropharmacology 47 Suppl 1:286–292

Wang HL (2000) A cluster of Ser/Thr residues at the C-terminus of mu-opioid receptor is required for G protein-coupled receptor kinase 2-mediated desensitization. Neuropharmacology 39:353–363

Wang JB, Imai Y, Eppler CM, Gregor P, Spivak CE, Uhl GR (1993) mu opiate receptor: cDNA cloning and expression. Proc Natl Acad Sci U S A 90:10230–10234

Wang SC, Glaviano VV (1954) Locus of emetic action of morphine and hydergine in dogs. J Pharmacol Exp Ther 111:329–334

Watson CP, Babul N (1998) Efficacy of oxycodone in neuropathic pain: a randomized trial in postherpetic neuralgia. Neurology 50:1837–1841

Weil JV, McCullough RE, Kline JS, Sodal IE (1975) Diminished ventilatory response to hypoxia and hypercapnia after morphine in normal man. N Engl J Med 292:1103–1106

Weinberg DS, Inturrisi CE, Reidenberg B, Moulin DE, Nip TJ, Wallenstein S, Houde RW, Foley KM (1988) Sublingual absorption of selected opioid analgesics. Clin Pharmacol Ther 44:335–342

Weinger MB, Smith NT, Blasco TA, Koob GF (1991) Brain sites mediating opiate-induced muscle rigidity in the rat: methylnaloxonium mapping study. Brain Res 544:181–190

Whistler JL, Enquist J, Marley A, Fong J, Gladher F, Tsuruda P, Murray SR, von Zastrow M (2002) Modulation of postendocytic sorting of G protein-coupled receptors. Science 297:615–620

Whiteside GT, Harrison JE, Pearson MS, Chen Z, Fundytus ME, Rotshteyn Y, Turchin PI, Pomonis JD, Mark L, Walker K, Brogle KC (2004) DiPOA ([8-(3,3-diphenyl-propyl)-4-oxo-1-phenyl-1,3,8-triazaspiro[4.5]dec-3-yl]-acetic acid), a novel, systemically available, and peripherally restricted Mu opioid agonist with antihyperalgesic activity. II. In vivo pharmacological characterization in the rat. J Pharmacol Exp Ther 310:793–799

Zacny JP (2005) Differential effects of morphine and codeine on pupil size: dosing issues. Anesth Analg 100:598

Zadina JE, Hackler L, Ge LJ, Kastin AJ (1997) A potent and selective endogenous agonist for the mu-opiate receptor. Nature 386:499–502

Zech DF, Grond S, Lynch J, Hertel D, Lehmann KA (1995) Validation of World Health Organization Guidelines for cancer pain relief: a 10-year prospective study. Pain 63:65–76

Zhang P, Johnson PS, Zöllner C, Wang W, Wang Z, Montes AE, Seidleck BK, Blaschak CJ, Surratt CK (1999) Mutation of human mu opioid receptor extracellular "disulfide cysteine" residues alters ligand binding but does not prevent receptor targeting to the cell plasma membrane. Brain Res Mol Brain Res 72:195–204

Zöllner C, Shaqura MA, Bopaiah CP, Mousa S, Stein C, Schäfer M (2003) Painful inflammation-induced increase in mu-opioid receptor binding and G-protein coupling in primary afferent neurons. Mol Pharmacol 64:202–210

HEP (2006) 177:65–93
© Springer-Verlag Berlin Heidelberg 2006

Antipyretic Analgesics: Nonsteroidal Antiinflammatory Drugs, Selective COX-2 Inhibitors, Paracetamol and Pyrazolinones

B. Hinz (✉) · K. Brune

Department of Experimental and Clinical Pharmacology and Toxicology, Friedrich Alexander University Erlangen-Nuremberg, Fahrstrasse 17, 91054 Erlangen, Germany
hinz@pharmakologie.uni-erlangen.de

1	Mode of Action of Antipyretic Analgesics	66
1.1	Inhibition of Cyclooxygenase Enzymes	66
1.2	Impact of Biodistribution on Pharmacological Effects of Antipyretic Analgesics	68
1.3	Mechanisms of Hyperalgesia	68
2	Acidic Antipyretic Analgesics	72
2.1	NSAIDs with Low Potency and Short Elimination Half-Life	72
2.2	NSAIDs with High Potency and Short Elimination Half-Life	76
2.3	NSAIDs with Intermediate Potency and Intermediate Elimination Half-Life . .	76
2.4	NSAIDs with High Potency and Long Elimination Half-Life	77
2.5	Compounds of Special Interest	77
3	Non-acidic Antipyretic Analgesics	78
3.1	Aniline Derivatives	78
3.2	Pyrazolinone Derivatives	80
4	Selective COX-2 Inhibitors	81
4.1	Definition and Structural Basis of COX-2 Selectivity	81
4.2	Comparison of the Pharmacokinetics of Different Selective COX-2 Inhibitors .	82
4.3	Gastrointestinal Safety Profile of Selective COX-2 Inhibitors	84
4.4	Cardiovascular Side Effects	84
5	Future Developments	87
References	. . . .	87

Abstract Antipyretic analgesics are a group of heterogeneous substances including acidic (nonsteroidal antiinflammatory drugs, NSAIDs) and nonacidic (paracetamol, pyrazolinones) drugs. Moreover, various selective cyclooxygenase-2 (COX-2) inhibitors with improved gastrointestinal tolerability as compared with conventional NSAIDs have been established for symptomatic pain treatment in recent years. The present review summarizes the pharmacology of all of these drugs with particular emphasis on their rational use based on the diverse pharmacokinetic characteristics and adverse drug reaction profiles. Referring to the current debate, potential mechanisms underlying cardiovascular side effects associated with long-term use of COX inhibitors are discussed.

Keywords Nonsteroidal antiinflammatory drugs · Selective cyclooxygenase-2 inhibitors · Paracetamol · Pyrazolinones · Pharmacokinetics · Mechanisms of hyperalgesia

1
Mode of Action of Antipyretic Analgesics

1.1
Inhibition of Cyclooxygenase Enzymes

In 1971, Vane showed that the antiinflammatory action of nonsteroidal antiinflammatory drugs (NSAIDs) rests in their ability to inhibit the activity of the cyclooxygenase (COX) enzyme, which in turn results in a diminished synthesis of
proinflammatory prostaglandins (Vane 1971). This action is considered not the
sole but a major factor of the mode of action of NSAIDs. The pathway leading to
the generation of prostaglandins has been elucidated in detail. Within this process, the COX enzyme (also referred to as prostaglandin H synthase) catalyzes
the first step of the synthesis of prostanoids by converting arachidonic acid into
prostaglandin H_2, which is the common substrate for specific prostaglandin
synthases. The enzyme is bifunctional, with fatty-acid COX activity (catalyzing the conversion of arachidonic acid to prostaglandin G_2) and prostaglandin
hydroperoxidase activity (catalyzing the conversion of prostaglandin G_2 to
prostaglandin H_2; Fig. 1).

In the early 1990s, COX was demonstrated to exist as two distinct isoforms (Masferrer et al. 1990; Xie et al. 1991). COX-1 is constitutively expressed as a "housekeeping" enzyme in nearly all tissues, and mediates physiological responses (e.g., cytoprotection of the stomach, platelet aggregation).
COX-2 expressed by cells that are involved in inflammation (e.g., macrophages,
monocytes, synoviocytes) has emerged as the isoform that is primarily responsible for the synthesis of prostanoids involved in pathological processes,
such as acute and chronic inflammatory states. The expression of the COX-2
enzyme is regulated by a broad spectrum of other mediators involved in
inflammation. Accordingly, glucocorticoids and antiinflammatory cytokines
(interleukin-4, -10, -13) have been reported to inhibit the expression of the
COX-2 isoenzyme (Masferrer et al. 1990; Onoe et al. 1996; Niiro et al. 1997). On
the other hand, products of the COX-2 pathway [e.g., prostaglandin $_2$ by virtue
of its second messenger cyclic AMP (cAMP)] may exert a positive feedback
action on the expression of its biosynthesizing enzyme in the inflamed tissue
(Nantel et al. 1999) as well as in numerous cell types (Hinz et al. 2000a, b,
2005b; Maldve et al. 2000). Likewise, the arachidonic acid derivative and endocannabinoid anandamide has recently been shown to elicit COX-2 expression
via de novo synthesis of ceramide (Ramer et al. 2003; Hinz et al. 2004).

All conventional NSAIDs interfere with the enzymatic activity of both COX-1 and COX-2 at therapeutic doses (Patrignani et al. 1997). Whereas many of the side effects of NSAIDs (e.g., gastrointestinal ulceration and bleeding, platelet dysfunctions) are due to a suppression of COX-1-derived prostanoids, inhibition of COX-2-derived prostanoids facilitates the antiinflammatory, analgesic, and antipyretic effects of NSAIDs. Consequently, the hypothesis that selective inhibition of COX-2 might have therapeutic actions similar to those of NSAIDs, but without causing the unwanted side effects, was the rationale for the development of selective COX-2 inhibitors. However, the simple concept of COX-2 being an exclusively proinflammatory and inducible enzyme cannot be sustained in the light of more recent experimental and clinical findings. Accordingly, COX-2 has also been shown to be expressed under basal conditions in organs including the ovary, uterus, brain, spinal cord, kidney, cartilage, bone and even the gut, suggesting that this isozyme may play a more complex physiological role than previously recognized (for review see Hinz and Brune 2002; Fig. 1). Moreover, during the past few years, evidence has increased to suggest that a constitutively expressed COX-2 may play a role in renal and cardiovascular functions which will be discussed later in detail (see Sect. 4.4).

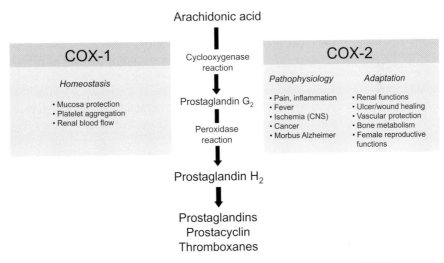

Fig. 1 Physiological and pathophysiological roles of COX-1 and COX-2. The COX-1 isozyme is expressed constitutively in most tissues and mediates housekeeping functions by producing prostaglandins. The COX-2 isoform is an inducible enzyme, which becomes expressed in inflammatory cells (e.g., macrophages, synoviocytes) after exposure to endotoxin, mitogens, or proinflammatory cytokines. COX-2 has been implicated in the pathophysiology of various inflammatory and mitogenic disorders. However, in some tissues (e.g., genital tract, bone, kidney, endothelial cells) COX-2 is already significantly expressed even in the absence of inflammation and appears to fulfill various physiological functions

1.2
Impact of Biodistribution on Pharmacological Effects
of Antipyretic Analgesics

Following the discovery that aspirin-like drugs exert their pharmacological action by suppressing the synthesis of prostaglandins, the question was asked why aspirin and its pharmacological relatives, the (acidic) NSAIDs, exerted antiinflammatory activity and analgesic effects, whereas the nonacidic drugs phenazone and paracetamol were analgesic only (Brune et al. 1974). It was speculated that all acidic antiinflammatory analgesics, which are highly bound to plasma proteins and show a similar degree of acidity (pK_a values between 3.5 and 5.5), should lead to a specific drug distribution within the body of man or animals (Fig. 2). In fact, high concentrations of these compounds are reached in blood stream, liver, spleen, and bone marrow (due to high protein binding and an open endothelial layer of the vasculature), but also in body compartments with acidic extracellular pH values (Brune et al. 1976). The latter type of compartments includes the inflamed tissue, the wall of the upper gastrointestinal tract and the collecting ducts of the kidneys. By contrast, paracetamol and phenazone, compounds with almost neutral pK_a values and a scarce binding to plasma proteins, are distributed homogeneously and quickly throughout the body due to their ability to penetrate barriers such as the blood–brain barrier easily (Brune et al. 1980). It is evident that the degree of prostaglandin synthesis inhibition depends on the potency of the drug and its local concentration.

On the other hand, the differential distribution of acidic and nonacidic antipyretic analgesics may explain why only the acidic compounds (NSAIDs) are antiinflammatory and cause acute side effects in the gastrointestinal tract (ulcerations), the blood stream (inhibition of platelet aggregation), and the kidney (fluid and sodium retention), whereas the nonacidic drugs are devoid of both antiinflammatory activity and gastric and (acute) renal toxicity. Finally, chronic inflammation of the upper respiratory tract (e.g., asthma, nasal polyps) leads to the accumulation of inflammatory prostaglandin-producing cells in the respiratory mucosa. Inhibition of COX appears to shift part of the metabolism of the prostaglandin precursor arachidonic acid to the production of leukotrienes which may induce pseudoallergic reactions (i.e., aspirin-induced asthma).

1.3
Mechanisms of Hyperalgesia

Inflammation causes an increased synthesis of COX-2-dependent prostaglandins, which sensitize peripheral nociceptor terminals and produce localized pain hypersensitivity. Prostaglandins regulate the sensitivity of so-called polymodal nociceptors that are present in nearly all tissues. A significant portion of these nociceptors cannot be easily activated by physiological stimuli such as mild pressure or some increase of temperature (Schaible and Schmidt 1988).

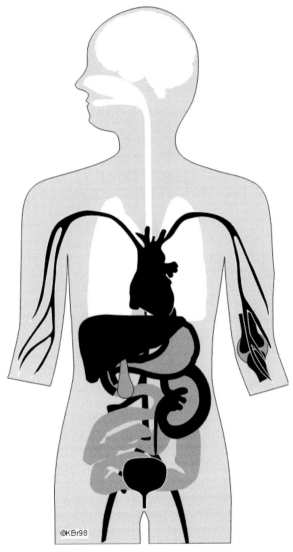

Fig. 2 Scheme of the distribution of acidic antipyretic analgesics in the human body (transposition of the data from animal experiments to human conditions). *Dark areas* indicate high concentrations of acidic antipyretic analgesics, i.e., stomach and upper wall of the gastrointestinal tract, blood, liver, bone marrow, spleen (not shown), and inflamed tissue (e.g., joints), as well as the kidney (cortex>medulla). Some acidic antipyretic analgesics are excreted in part unchanged in urine and achieve high concentration in this body fluid, others encounter enterohepatic circulation and are found in high concentrations as conjugates in the bile

However, following tissue trauma and subsequent release of prostaglandins, "silent" polymodal nociceptors become excitable to pressure, temperature changes, and tissue acidosis (Neugebauer et al. 1995). This process results in a phenomenon called hyperalgesia—in some instances allodynia.

Prostaglandin E_2 and other inflammatory mediators facilitate the activation of tetrodotoxin-resistant Na^+ channels in dorsal root ganglion neurons (Akopian et al. 1996; England et al. 1996; Gold et al. 1996). Compelling evidence indicates that small dorsal root ganglion neurons are the somata which give rise to thinly and unmyelinated C and Aδ nerve fibers, both conducting nociceptive stimuli. Increased opening of these Na^+ channels involves activation of the adenylyl cyclase enzyme and increases in cAMP possibly leading to protein kinase A-dependent phosphorylation of the channels. Meanwhile, two sensory neuron-specific tetrodotoxin-resistant sodium channel α-subunits, $Na_V1.8$ and $Na_V1.9$, have been characterized in dorsal root ganglia (Benn et al. 2001). Another important target of protein kinase A-mediated phosphorylation is the capsaicin receptor (transient receptor potential vanilloid 1, TRPV1), a nonselective cation channel of sensory neurons involved in the sensation of temperature and inflammatory pain (Lopshire and Nicol 1997; Caterina et al. 2000; Davis et al. 2000). TRPV1 responds to temperature above 40°C and to noxious stimuli including capsaicin, the pungent component of chili peppers, and extracellular acidification. On the basis of this mechanism, prostaglandins produced during inflammatory states may significantly increase the excitability of nociceptive nerve fibers, including reactivity to temperatures below 40°C (i.e., body temperature), thereby contributing to the activation of "sleeping" nociceptors and the development of burning pain. As such, it appears reasonable that at least a part of the peripheral antinociceptive action of acidic antipyretic analgesics arises from prevention of this peripheral sensitization.

Apart from sensitizing peripheral nociceptors, prostaglandins act in the central nervous system to produce central hyperalgesia. Experimental data suggest that both acidic and nonacidic COX inhibitors antagonize central hyperalgesia in the dorsal horn of the spinal cord by modulating the glutamatergic signal transfer from nociceptive C fibers to secondary neurons, which propagate the signals to the higher centers of the central nervous system. Some COX-2 is expressed constitutively in the dorsal horn of the spinal cord, and becomes upregulated briefly after a trauma, such as damage to a limb, in the corresponding sensory segments of the spinal cord (Beiche et al. 1996). The induction of spinal cord COX-2 expression may facilitate transmission of the nociceptive input. In line with a role of COX-2 in central pain perception, Smith et al. (1998) reported that selective COX-2 inhibition suppressed inflammation-induced prostaglandin levels in cerebrospinal fluid, whereas selective inhibition of COX-1 was inactive in this regard. These observations were substantiated by findings showing a widespread induction of COX-2 expression in spinal cord neurons and in other regions of the central nervous system following peripheral inflammation (Samad et al. 2001).

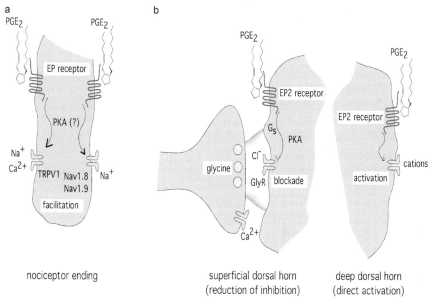

Fig. 3a, b Molecular mechanisms underlying peripheral and central hyperalgesia elicited by prostaglandin E_2 (adapted from Brune and Zeilhofer 2006). **a** In the periphery, prostaglandin E_2 increases excitability of nociceptor endings via cyclic AMP-protein kinase A-dependent activation of tetrodotoxin-resistant sodium channels ($Na_V1.8$, $Na_V1.9$) or the capsaicin receptor TRPV1 (nonselective cation channel). **b** The central component of inflammatory pain originates from a disinhibition of dorsal horn neurons, which are relieved from glycinergic neurotransmission by prostaglandin E_2. The latter activates EP_2 receptors thereby leading to a protein kinase A-dependent phosphorylation and inhibition of glycine receptors containing the $\alpha 3$ subunit (GlyR$\alpha 3$). Moreover, prostaglandin E_2 acting via EP_2 receptors has been shown to directly depolarize spinal neurons

Several mechanisms have been proposed to underlie the facilitatory action of prostaglandin E_2 on central pain sensation. Baba et al. (2001) showed that prostaglandin E_2 at relatively high concentrations directly depolarizes wide dynamic range neurons in the deep dorsal horn. More convincingly, prostaglandin E_2 at significantly lower concentrations reduces the inhibitory tone of the neurotransmitter glycine onto neurons in the superficial layers of the dorsal horn (Ahmadi et al. 2002) by phosphorylation of the specific glycine receptor subtype GlyR $\alpha 3$ (Harvey et al. 2004), thereby causing a disinhibition of spinal nociceptive transmission. In a recent study, the same group has identified PGE$_2$ receptors of the EP_2 receptor subtype as key signaling elements in spinal inflammatory hyperalgesia (Reinold et al. 2005), thus opening new avenues for the development of new analgesics. The current understanding of the molecular mechanisms underlying peripheral and central hyperalgesia elicited by prostaglandin E_2 are summarized in Fig. 3.

2
Acidic Antipyretic Analgesics

Based on the finding that aspirin at high doses (>3 g/day) not only inhibits fever and pain but also interferes with inflammation, Winter developed an assay to search for drugs with a similar profile of antiinflammatory activity (Winter et al. 1962). Amazingly, all substances that survived the test of experimental pharmacology and clinical trials turned out to be acids with a high degree of lipophilic-hydrophilic polarity, similar pK_a values and a high degree of plasma protein binding (for review see Brune and Lanz 1986; Hinz et al. 2000c). Suggestions for indications including treatment of rheumatoid diseases are listed in Table 1.

Apart from aspirin, all of these compounds differ in their potency, i.e., the single dose necessary to achieve a certain degree of effect ranges from a few milligrams (e.g., lornoxicam) to about 1 g (e.g., salicylic acid). They also differ in their pharmacokinetic characteristics, i.e., the speed of absorption (time to peak, t_{max}; which may also depend on the galenic formulation used), the maximal plasma concentrations (c_{max}), the elimination half-life ($t_{1/2}$), and the oral bioavailability. Interestingly, all traditional NSAIDs lack a relevant degree of COX-2 selectivity (Patrignani et al. 1997). This is surprising since they have all been selected on the basis of high antiinflammatory potency and low gastrotoxicity that depends on COX-1 inhibition. The key characteristics of the most important NSAIDs are compiled in Table 2 (most data are from Brune and Lanz 1985). This table also contains the data of aspirin which differs in many respects from the other NSAIDs and is therefore discussed at the end of this chapter in detail (see Sect. 2.5). Otherwise, the drugs can be categorized in four different groups that are discussed in the following sections.

2.1
NSAIDs with Low Potency and Short Elimination Half-Life

The drugs of this group are particularly useful for blocking occasional mild inflammatory pain. The prototype of this type of compounds is ibuprofen. Depending on its galenic formulation, fast or slow absorption of ibuprofen may be achieved. A fast absorption of ibuprofen was observed following administration of the respective lysine salt (Geisslinger et al. 1993). The bioavailability of ibuprofen is close to 100% and the elimination is always fast even in patients suffering from mild or severe impairment of liver or kidney function (Brune and Lanz 1985). Ibuprofen is used as single doses ranging from 200 mg to 1 g. A maximum dose of 3.2 g per day (United States) or 2.4 g (Europe) for rheumatoid arthritis is possible. At low doses ibuprofen appears particularly useful for the treatment of acute occasional inflammatory pain. High doses of ibuprofen may also be administered, although with less benefit, for the treatment of chronic rheumatic diseases. Remarkably, at high doses the otherwise harmless compound has been shown to result in an increased incidence of gastrointestinal side effects (Silverstein et al. 2000). In some countries ibuprofen is also

Table 1 Indications for antipyretic analgesics

Acidic antipyretic analgesics (antiinflammatory antipyretic analgesics, NSAIDs)[a]

	High dose	Middle dose	Low dose
Acute and chronic pain, produced by inflammation of different etiology			
Arthritis: chronic polyarthritis (rheumatoid arthritis), ankylosing spondylitis (Morbus Bechterew), acute gout (gout attack)	Diclofenac, indomethacin ibuprofen, piroxicam (phenylbutazone)[b]	Diclofenac, indomethacin ibuprofen, piroxicam (phenylbutazone)	No
Cancer pain (e.g. bone metastasis)	(Indomethacin)[c], diclofenac[c], ibuprofen[c], piroxicam[c]	(Indomethacin)[c], diclofenac[c], ibuprofen[c], piroxicam[c]	Aspirin[d], ibuprofen[c]
Active arthrosis (acute pain-inflammatory episodes)	No	Diclofenac, indomethacin, ibuprofen, piroxicam	Ibuprofen, ketoprofen
Myofascial pain syndromes (antipyretic analgesics are often prescribed but of limited value)	No	Diclofenac, ibuprofen, piroxicam	Ibuprofen, ketoprofen
Posttraumatic pain, swelling	No	(Indomethacin), diclofenac, ibuprofen	Aspirin[d], ibuprofen[c]
Postoperative pain, swelling	No	(Indomethacin), diclofenac, ibuprofen	Ibuprofen

Non-acidic antipyretic analgesics

	Pyrazolinones (high dose)	Pyrazolinones (low dose)	Anilines (high dose is toxic)
Acute pain and fever			
Spastic pain (colics)	Yes	Yes	No
Conditions associated with high fever	Yes	Yes	No
Cancer pain	Yes	Yes	Yes
Headache, migraine	No	Yes	Yes[f]
General disturbances associated with viral infections	No	Yes[e]	yes

[a]Dosage range of NSAIDs and example of monosubstances (but note dosage prescribed for each agent) [b]Indicated only in gout attacks [c]Compare the sequence staged scheme of WHO for cancer pain [d]Blood coagulation and renal function must be normal [e]If other analgesics and antipyretics are contraindicated, e.g. gastro–duodenal ulcer, blood coagulation disturbances, or asthma [f]In particular patients

Table 2 Physicochemical and pharmacological data of acidic antipyretic analgesics

Pharmacokinetic/chemical subclasses	pK_a	Binding to plasma proteins	Oral bio-availability	t_{max}[a]	$t_{1/2}$[b]	Single dose (maximal daily dose) for adults
Low potency/short elimination half-life						
Salicylates						
Aspirin	3.5	50%–70%	50% dose-dependent	15 min	15 min	0.05–1 g[c] (6 g)
Salicylic acid	3.0	80%–95% dose-dependent	80%–100%	0.5–2 h	2.5–4.5 h dose-dependent	0.5–1 g (6 g)
2-Arylpropionic acids						
Ibuprofen	4.4	99%	100%	0.5–2 h	2 h	200–800 mg (2.4 g)
Anthranilic acids						
Mefenamic acid	4.2	90%	70%	2–4 h	1–2 h	250–500 mg (1.5 g)
High potency/short elimination half-life						
2-Arylpropionic acids						
Flurbiprofen	4.2	>99%	No data	1.5–3 h	2.5–4(–8) h	50–100 mg (200 mg)
Ketoprofen	5.3	99%	90%	1–2 h	2–4 h	25–100 mg (200 mg)
Aryl-/heteroarylacetic acids						
Diclofenac	3.9	99.7%	50% dose-dependent	1–12 h[e] very variable	1–2 h	25–75 mg (150 mg)
Indomethacin	4.5	99%	100%	0.5–2 h	2–3(–11) h[d] very variable	25–75 mg (200 mg)
Oxicams						
Lornoxicam	4.7	99%	100%	0.5–2 h	4–10 h	4–12 mg (16 mg)

Table 2 continued

Pharmacokinetic/ chemical subclasses	pK_a	Binding to plasma proteins	Oral bio-availability	t_{max}[a]	$t_{1/2}$[b]	Single dose (maximal daily dose) for adults
Intermediate potency/intermediate elimination half-life						
Salicylates						
Diflunisal	3.3	98%–99%	80%–100%	2–3 h	8–12 h dose-dependent	250–500 mg (1 g)
2-Arylpropionic acids						
Naproxen	4.2	99%	90%–100%	2–4 h	12–15 h[d]	250–500 mg (1.25 g)
Arylacetic acids						
6-Methoxy-2-naphthyl-acetic acid (active metabolite of nabumetone)	4.2	99%	20%–50%	3–6 h	20–24 h	0.5–1 g (1.5 g)
High potency/long elimination half-life						
Oxicams						
Piroxicam	5.9	99%	100%	3–5 h	14–160 h[d]	20–40 mg; initial: 40 mg
Tenoxicam	5.3	99%	100%	0.5–2 h	25–175 h[d]	20–40 mg; initial: 40 mg
Meloxicam	4.08	99.5%	89%	7–8 h	20 h[e]	7.5–15 mg

[a]Time to reach maximum plasma concentration after oral administration [b]Terminal half-life of elimination [c]Single dose for inhibition of thrombocyte aggregation: 50–100 mg; single analgesic dose: 0.5–1 g [d]Enterohepatic circulation [e]Monolithic acid-resistant tablet or similar galenic form

administered as the pure S-enantiomer, which comprises the active entity of the racemic mixture in terms of COX inhibition. On the other hand, a substantial conversion of the less potent COX inhibitor R-ibuprofen (comprises 50% of the usual racemic mixture) into the active S-enantiomer has been observed following administration of the racemic mixture (Rudy et al. 1991). Other drugs of this group are salicylates and mefenamic acid. The latter does not appear to offer major advantages. By contrast, this and other fenamates are rather toxic at overdosage (central nervous system).

2.2
NSAIDs with High Potency and Short Elimination Half-Life

These drugs are predominantly prescribed for the treatment of rheumatic (arthritic) pain. The most widely used compound of this group is diclofenac, which appears to be less active on COX-1 as compared to COX-2 (Patrignani et al. 1997; Hinz et al. 2003). This is taken as a reason for the relatively low incidence of gastrointestinal side effects of diclofenac (Henry et al. 1996). The limitations of diclofenac result from its usual formulation (monolithic acid-resistant coated dragée or tablet). In fact, retention of such formulations in the stomach for hours or even days may cause retarded absorption of the active ingredient (Brune and Lanz 1985). Moreover, diclofenac has a considerable first-pass metabolism that causes its limited (about 50%) oral bioavailability. Consequently, a lack of therapeutic effect may require adaptation of the dosage or change of the drug. New formulations (microencapsulations, salts, etc.) remedy some of these deficits (Hinz et al. 2005a). The slightly higher incidence of liver toxicity associated with diclofenac may result from the high degree of first-pass metabolism, but other interpretations appear feasible. Recently, it has been demonstrated that pharmacologically relevant concentrations of diclofenac are generated through limited but sustained bioactivation following oral administration of aceclofenac (Hinz et al. 2003). As aceclofenac per se does not interfere with the COX enzymes, diclofenac seems to confer a major part of the pharmacological action of aceclofenac. Interestingly, metabolic generation of diclofenac after administration of a 100-mg dose of aceclofenac was associated with an apparently improved COX-2 selectivity as compared to a 75-mg dose of a sustained-release diclofenac formulation (Hinz et al. 2003).

This group contains further important drugs such as lornoxicam, flurbiprofen and indomethacin (very potent), but also ketoprofen and fenoprofen (less active). All of them show a high oral bioavailability and good effectiveness, but also a relatively high risk of unwanted drug effects (Henry et al. 1996).

2.3
NSAIDs with Intermediate Potency and Intermediate Elimination Half-Life

The third group is intermediate in potency and speed of elimination and comprises drugs such as diflunisal and naproxen. Because of its slow absorption, diflunisal is rarely used anymore.

2.4
NSAIDs with High Potency and Long Elimination Half-Life

The fourth group consists of the oxicams (meloxicam, piroxicam, and tenoxicam). These compounds are characterized by a high degree of enterohepatic circulation, slow metabolism, and slow elimination (Brune and Lanz 1985). Because of its long half-life (days), oxicams do not represent drugs of first choice for the treatment of acute pain of short duration. The main indication of the oxicams is inflammatory pain that persists for days, i.e., pain resulting from cancer (bone metastases) or chronic polyarthritis. The high potency and long persistence in the body may be the reason for the somewhat higher incidence of serious adverse drug effects in the gastrointestinal tract and in the kidney observed in the presence of these drugs (Henry et al. 1996).

2.5
Compounds of Special Interest

Aspirin, the prototype NSAID, deserves special discussion. This drug irreversibly inactivates both COX-1 (highly effective) and COX-2 (less effective) by acetylating an active-site serine. Consequently, this covalent modification interferes with the binding of arachidonic acid at the COX active site. Most cells compensate the enzyme loss due to acetylation by aspirin via de novo synthesis of this enzyme. However, as platelets are unable to generate fresh enzyme, a single dose of aspirin may suppress platelet COX-1-dependent thromboxane synthesis for the whole lifetime of thrombocytes (8–11 days) until new platelets are formed.

Following oral administration aspirin is substantially cleaved before, during, and shortly after absorption, to yield salicylic acid. Consequently, the oral bioavailability is low and the plasma half-life of aspirin is only about 15 min. Aspirin may be used as a solution (effervescent) or as a (lysine) salt, allowing very fast absorption, distribution, and pain relief. Aspirin may cause bleeding from existing ulcers due to its long-lasting antiplatelet effect and topical irritation of the gastrointestinal mucosa (Kimmey 2004). The inevitable irritation of the gastric mucosa may be acceptable in otherwise healthy patients. Aspirin should not be used in pregnant women (premature bleeding, closure of ductus arteriosus) or children before puberty (Reye's syndrome) in addition to the contraindications pertinent to all NSAIDs.

When low doses of aspirin ($\leq$100 mg) are administered, aspirin acetylates the COX-1 isozyme of platelets presystemically in the portal circulation before aspirin is deacetylated to salicylate in the liver. By contrast, COX-2-dependent synthesis of vasodilatory and antithrombotic prostacyclin by vascular endothelial cells outside the gut is not altered by low-dose aspirin. The reason for this phenomenon lies in the rapid cleavage of aspirin leaving little if any unmetabolized aspirin after primary liver passage. Thus, low-dose aspirin has its only indication in the prevention of thrombotic and embolic events. Previously, it has been shown that the concomitant administration of ibuprofen antagonizes the irreversible platelet inhibition induced by aspirin (Catella-Lawson et al. 2001). It has been suggested in this context that treatment with ibuprofen in patients with increased cardiovascular risk may limit the cardioprotective effects of aspirin. Another unresolved question concerns the use of low-dose aspirin together with other COX-2-selective or nonselective NSAIDs. In this context, it has been shown that the combination of low-dose aspirin with COX-2-selective inhibitors may abrogate the gastrointestinal-sparing effects of the latter compounds (Silverstein et al. 2000; Schnitzer et al. 2004; see Sect. 4.3).

Over the past three decades, the theory that suppression of prostaglandin biosynthesis accounts for the pharmacological actions of NSAIDs has been questioned by comparing the actions of salicylic acid and aspirin (for review see Weissmann 1993). Salicylate does not, unlike its acetylated derivative aspirin, inhibit COX-1 and COX-2 activity in vitro. On the other side, sodium salicylate has been demonstrated to be an effective inhibitor of prostaglandin formation in vivo at sites of inflammation and to be equally effective against arthritis as aspirin. From the data published by Kopp and Ghosh (1994) it appears that inhibition of the transcription factor nuclear factor (NF)-κB could be a mechanism by which salicylates exert their antiinflammatory action. However, relatively high concentrations of sodium salicylate (i.e., higher than that obtained after therapeutic dosing) were required to provide inhibition of NF-κB activation. On the other hand, pharmacological concentrations of salicylates have been shown to inhibit COX-2 expression in human umbilical vein endothelial cells and foreskin fibroblasts (Xu et al. 1999), pointing toward a possible (cell-specific) target of salicylic acid upstream to COX-2 enzyme activity. Furthermore, metabolites of salicylic acid have been shown to inhibit the COX-2-dependent synthesis of prostaglandins (Hinz et al. 2000d), suggesting that bioactivation may confer, at least in part, the capacity of salicylic acid to interfere with prostaglandin formation in vivo.

3
Non-acidic Antipyretic Analgesics

3.1
Aniline Derivatives

The main representative of the aniline derivatives is paracetamol (Table 3). This drug possesses only weak antiinflammatory but efficient antipyretic activity. The major advantage of paracetamol lies in its relative lack of serious side effects given that the dose limits are obeyed, although serious events can be observed with low doses, although rarely so (Bridger et al. 1998). A small proportion of paracetamol is metabolized to the highly toxic nucleophilic N-acetyl-benzoquinoneimine that is usually inactivated by reaction

Table 3 Physicochemical and pharmacological data of paracetamol and pyrazolinone derivatives

Chemical/ pharmacological class	Binding to plasma proteins	Oral bio-availability	t_{max}[a]	$t_{1/2}$[b]	Single dose (maximal daily dose) for adults
Aniline derivatives					
Paracetamol (acetaminophen)	5%–50% dose-dependent	70%–100% dose-dependent	0.5–1.5 h	1.5–2.5 h	0.5–1 g (4 g)
Pyrazolinone derivatives					
Phenazone	<10%	~100% dose-dependent	0.5–2 h	11–12 h	0.5–1 g (4 g)
Propyphenazone	~10%	~100% dose-dependent	0.5–1.5 h	1–2.5 h	0.5–1 g (4 g)
Metamizol-Na[c]	<20%	-	-	-	0.5–1 g (4 g)
4-Methylamino-phenazone[d]	58%	~100%	1–2 h	2–4 h	-
4-Aminophenazone[d]	48%	-	-	4–5.5 h	-

[a]Time to reach maximum plasma concentration after oral administration [b]Terminal half-life of elimination [c]Noraminopyrinemethansulfonate-Na, dipyrone [d]Metabolites of metamizol

with sulfhydryl groups in glutathione. However, following ingestion of large doses of paracetamol, hepatic glutathione is depleted, resulting in covalent binding of N-acetyl-benzoquinoneimine to DNA and structural proteins in parenchymal cells (e.g., in liver and kidney; for review see Seeff et al. 1986). Under these circumstances, dose-dependent, potentially fatal hepatic necrosis may occur. When detected early, overdosage can be antagonized within the first 12 h after intake of paracetamol by administration of N-acetylcysteine that regenerates detoxifying mechanisms by replenishing hepatic glutathione stores. Accordingly, paracetamol should not be given to patients with seriously impaired liver function.

Typical indications of paracetamol are fever and pain occurring in the context of viral infections. In addition, many patients with recurrent headache benefit from paracetamol and its low toxicity. Paracetamol is also used in children, but despite its somewhat lower toxicity in juvenile patients, fatalities due to involuntary overdosage have been reported. According to a recent update of the American College of Rheumatology (ACR) guidelines for osteoarthrosis, paracetamol remains first-line therapy because of its cost, efficacy, and safety profiles (Schnitzer 2002). In fact, paracetamol provides effective relief of pain for many patients with osteoarthrosis, and has been demonstrated to be safe in a wide range of populations, providing less severe and no gastro-toxic side effects as compared to NSAIDs (Brandt 2003). On the other hand, randomized trials have now demonstrated that NSAIDs and selective COX-2 inhibitors provide superior efficacy compared with paracetamol in patients with osteoarthrosis (Geba et al. 2002; Zhang et al. 2004).

In contrast to NSAIDs and selective COX-2 inhibitors, the analgesic and antipyretic mode of action of paracetamol is still a matter of debate. Evidence supporting a central analgesic mode of action has already been demonstrated by the finding that paracetamol may inhibit nociception-induced spinal prostaglandin synthesis (Muth-Selbach et al. 1999). A few years ago, paracetamol was claimed to inhibit a newly discovered COX isoform, derived from the same gene as COX-1 and referred to as COX-3 (Chandrasekharan et al. 2002). However, in this study COX-3 was only detected at relatively small amounts in the cerebral cortex of dogs. Moreover, studies indicating a pharmacologically different regulation of COX-3 as compared to the other two isoenzymes have been performed using canine COX-3 and murine COX-1 and -2 enzymes. In this context it is also noteworthy that COX-3 inhibition by acetaminophen was observed at concentrations above those inhibiting monocyte COX-2 in the human whole blood assay. Meanwhile, the existence of a full-length, catalytically active form of COX-3 in humans has been questioned by two independent groups (Dinchuk et al. 2003; Schwab et al. 2003).

A more plausible mode of action of the drug has been suggested on the basis of observations showing that paracetamol inhibits the COX enzymes by reducing the higher oxidation state of these proteins (Boutaud et al. 2002). In line with this finding, high levels of peroxides were shown to overcome the inhibitory effect of paracetamol on the COX enzymes in platelets and immune cells. As such, 12-hydroperoxyeicosatetraenoic acid, a major product of platelets, completely reversed the inhibitory action of paracetamol on COX-1. Likewise, addition of peroxides to interleukin-1-stimulated endothelial cells (as a model of a peroxide-enriched inflammatory tissue) abrogated COX-2 inhibition by paracetamol, whereas paracetamol inhibited COX-2 in these cells in the absence of peroxide at concentrations relevant to its antipyretic effect. Although the peroxide theory needs further confirmation, it may provide a plausible explanation of why paracetamol has only a slight effect on platelet function as well as little or no antiinflammatory effect in humans.

3.2
Pyrazolinone Derivatives

Following the discovery of phenazone 120 years ago, the pharmaceutical industry has tried to improve this compound in three ways: Phenazone was chemically modified to (1) create a more potent compound, (2) yield a water-soluble derivative to be given parenterally, and (3) produce a compound which is eliminated faster and more reliable than phenazone. The results of these attempts are the phenazone derivatives aminophenazone, dipyrone, and propyphenazone (Table 3). Aminophenazone is not in use anymore because it has been associated with formation of nitrosamines that may increase the risk of stomach cancer. The other two compounds differ from phenazone in their potency and elimination half-life, their water solubility (dipyrone is a watersoluble prodrug of methylaminophenazone), and their general toxicity (propyphenazone and dipyrone do not lead to the formation of nitrosamines in the acidic environment of the stomach). Phenazone, propyphenazone, and dipyrone (metamizol) are the predominantly used antipyretic analgesics in many countries (Latin America, many countries in Asia, Eastern and Central Europe). Dipyrone has been accused of causing agranulocytosis. Although there appears to be a statistically significant link, the incidence is extremely rare (1 case per million treatment periods; Kaufman et al. 1991; International Agranulocytosis and Aplastic Anemia Study 1986; Ibanez et al. 2005). Moreover, all antipyretic analgesics have also been claimed to cause Stevens–Johnson's syndrome and Lyell's syndrome, as well as shock reactions. New data indicate that the incidence of these events is in the same order of magnitude as with, e.g., penicillins (Roujeau et al 1995; Mockenhaupt et al. 1996; Anonymous 1998). All nonacidic phenazone derivatives lack antiinflammatory activity, and are devoid of gastrointestinal and (acute) renal toxicity. In contrast to paracetamol, dipyrone is safe even when given at overdosages. If one compares aspirin, paracetamol, and propyphenazone when used for the same indication (e.g., occasional headache), it is evident that aspirin is more dangerous than either propyphenazone or paracetamol.

4
Selective COX-2 Inhibitors
4.1
Definition and Structural Basis of COX-2 Selectivity

Selective inhibitors of the COX-2 enzyme, also referred to as coxibs, have been developed as substances with therapeutic actions similar to those of NSAIDs, but without causing gastrointestinal side effects. By definition, a substance may be regarded as a selective COX-2 inhibitor if it causes no clinically meaningful COX-1 inhibition at maximal therapeutic doses. Among the variety of available test systems, the ex vivo whole blood assay has emerged as the best method to estimate COX-2 selectivity in humans (Patrignani et al. 1997). X-ray crystallography of the three-dimensional structures of COX-1 and COX-2 has provided more insights into how COX-2 specificity is achieved. Within the hydrophobic channel of the COX enzyme, a single amino acid difference in position 523 (isoleucine in COX-1, valine in COX-2) has been detected that is critical for the COX-2 selectivity of several drugs. Accordingly, the smaller valine molecule in COX-2 gives access to a side pocket that has been proposed to be the binding site of COX-2 selective substances (Luong et al. 1996).

4.2
Comparison of the Pharmacokinetics of Different Selective COX-2 Inhibitors

Selective COX-2 inhibitors currently used are the sulfonamides celecoxib and parecoxib and the methylsulfone etoricoxib. Moreover, the phenylacetic acid derivative lumiracoxib is currently (August 2006) available in ten Latin American countries, Australia, New Zealand and Great Britain. Physicochemical and pharmacological data of these compounds as well as those of the COX-2 inhibitors recently withdrawn (rofecoxib and valdecoxib; see Sect. 4.4) are compiled in Table 4.

All selective COX-2 inhibitors are relatively lipophilic compounds. Whereas the sulfonamides and methylsulfones are nonacidic compounds, lumiracoxib is a phenylacetic acid derivative. Differences in physicochemical characteristics are reflected in different pharmacokinetic behavior. Accordingly, the volume of distribution of the nonacidic compounds is equal or above body weight, whereas that of lumiracoxib is, as with other acetic acid derivatives, around 15% of body weight. The nonacidic compounds distribute almost equally throughout the body with the exception of celecoxib, which is likely to be sequestered in body fat due to its extremely high lipophilicity. The acidic compound lumiracoxib apparently mimics diclofenac and indomethacin that reach high concentrations in the blood stream, kidney, liver, and inflamed tissue, but comparatively lower concentrations in other compartments. The physicochemical differences are also reflected in other pharmacokinetic parameters. As might be expected from its very high lipophilicity, the absorption of celecoxib is relatively slow and incomplete. The compound undergoes considerable first pass metabolization (20%–60% oral bioavailability) and its rate of elimination ($t_{1/2}$ ~6–12 h) appears to be highly variable (Werner et al. 2002, 2003). Etoricoxib encounters only slow metabolic elimination ($t_{1/2}$ ~20–26 h), while lumiracoxib is eliminated much faster with an elimination half-life of about 5 h. Indirect evidence suggests that all substances reach sufficiently high concentrations in the central nervous system to counter inflammatory pain by blocking COX-2 within about an hour. The fast absorption of etoricoxib appears to cause its fast onset of action. Moreover, all five compounds are eliminated predominantly by metabolization.

With the exception of rofecoxib, all COX-2 inhibitors undergo oxidative drug metabolism by cytochrome P450 (CYP) enzymes. Interestingly, celecoxib has recently been shown to inhibit the metabolism of the CYP2D6 substrate metoprolol, the most widely used β-blocker (Werner et al. 2003). This interaction is likely to occur as well with the concomitant administration of other CYP2D6 substrates, including sedatives, serotonin reuptake inhibitors, tricyclic antidepressants, and some neuroleptics. On the other hand, the interference of CYP3A4 by etoricoxib appears of minor importance given that CYP3A is inducible and many drugs metabolized by CYP3A are also substrates of other CYP enzymes.

Table 4 Physicochemical and pharmacological data of selective COX-2 inhibitors (data obtained from Brune and Hinz 2004). Despite withdrawal from the market, rofecoxib and valdecoxib are included for comparative reasons

	COX-1/ COX-2 ratio[a]	Binding to plasma proteins	V_d[b]	Oral bio-availability	t_{max}[c]	$t_{1/2}$[d]	Primary metabolism[e] (cytochrome P450 enzymes)	Single dose (maximal daily dose) for adults
Sulfonamides								
Celecoxib	30	97%	400 l	20%–60%	2–4 h	6–12 h	Oxidation (CYP2C9, 3A4)[f]	100–200 mg (400 mg) for osteoarthrosis and rheumatoid arthritis
Valdecoxib (parecoxib)[g]	61	98%	90 l	83%	2–4 h	6–10 h	Oxidation to hydroxyvaldecoxib (CYP2C9, 3A4)[f]	Valdecoxib was withdrawn in March 2005. Parecoxib (still marketed): 20–40 mg i.v./i.m. (80 mg) for short-term pain relief after surgery
Methylsulfons								
Etoricoxib	344	92%	120 l	100%	1 h	20–26 h	Oxidation to 6'-hydroxymethyletoricoxib (major role: CYP3A4; ancillary role: CYP2C9, 2D6, 1A2)	60 mg (60 mg) for osteoarthrosis 90 mg (90 mg) for rheumatoid arthritis 120 mg (120 mg) for acute gouty arthritis
Rofecoxib	272	87%	90 l	93%[h]	2–4 h	15–18 h	Cytosolic reductase[j]	Rofecoxib was withdrawn in September 2004
Arylacetic acid								
Lumiracoxib	700	99%	13 l	74%	1–3 h	2–6 h	Oxidation to hydroxylumiracoxib[k] (CYP2C9)	Not yet being marketed[l]

[a]Ratio of IC_{50} values (IC_{50} COX-1/IC_{50} COX-2) in the human whole blood assay [b]Volume of distribution [c]Time to reach maximum plasma concentration after oral administration [d]Terminal half-life of elimination [e]All metabolites are less active than the parent compound (except parecoxib) [f]Compounds may inhibit CYP2D6 [g]Parecoxib is the water soluble prodrug of valdecoxib releasing valdecoxib within about 15 min, t_{max}: 30 min [h]Less at not recommended dosage [i]Compound may inhibit CYP1A2 [k]In analogy to diclofenac, the metabolism of lumiracoxib involves probably also other CYP enzymes such as CYP2C8 or CYP2C19 [l]Lumiracoxib is currently (August 2006) available in ten Latin American countries, Australia, New Zealand and Great Britain. Intended doses are as follows: 100 mg (symptomatic relief of osteoarthritis); 400 mg (short-term relief of moderate to severe acute pain associated with primary dysmenorrhea, dental surgery, and orthopedic surgery)

On the basis of their diverse pharmacokinetic characteristics, a rational use of different selective COX-2 inhibitors in different clinical settings is recommended. Accordingly, the slow absorption and variable first pass metabolization of celecoxib should preclude this compound from the treatment of acute pain. By contrast, etoricoxib appears promising for this indication. However, final data are still lacking. This is even more the case with lumiracoxib. Based on experiences gathered with diclofenac, a structural analog, the administration of lumiracoxib in salt form to facilitate fast absorption appears promising for the treatment of acute pain.

4.3
Gastrointestinal Safety Profile of Selective COX-2 Inhibitors

The hypothesis that selective COX-2 inhibitors may provide an improved risk-benefit ratio in terms of gastrointestinal safety as compared with conventional NSAIDs was tested in three large phase III clinical trials on a total of 35,000 patients. In the Gastrointestinal Outcomes Research (VIGOR) study (Bombardier et al. 2000) and in the Therapeutic Arthritis Research and Gastrointestinal Event Trial (TARGET) (Schnitzer et al. 2004) rofecoxib and lumiracoxib were found to decrease the risk of confirmed gastrointestinal events (including ulcerations, bleedings, and perforations) associated with traditional NSAIDs by more than 50%. In the Celecoxib Long-term Arthritis Safety Study (CLASS), however, a significant beneficial effect of celecoxib was only evident when the definition of upper gastrointestinal endpoints was expanded to include symptomatic ulcers (Silverstein et al. 2000). Moreover, outcomes of the first 6 months were published instead of the complete 1-year data of this study. In addition, both the CLASS and TARGET studies have clearly shown that patients receiving low-dose aspirin for cardiovascular protection do not benefit from the gastrointestinal safety of these drugs.

Another interesting finding of the past few years was the observation that COX-2 may influence ulcer healing and the associated angiogenesis. In accord with this concept, COX-2 has previously been shown to be induced in tissue on the edges of ulcers (Mizuno et al. 1997). In animal studies selective COX-2 inhibitors have been demonstrated to retard ulcer healing (Schmassmann et al. 1998). Consequently, it is necessary to test whether effective ulcer healing occurs in patients with NSAID-associated ulcers switched to selective COX-2 inhibitors.

4.4
Cardiovascular Side Effects

Selective COX-2 inhibitors have been associated with an increased incidence of cardiovascular side effects. First data supporting a respective risk were published in the VIGOR study, where patients receiving rofecoxib had a significant fourfold increase in the incidence of myocardial infarctions, as compared with patients randomized to naproxen (Bombardier et al. 2000). There are several reasons for the fact that these results have not been considered sufficiently. Accordingly, in the CLASS and TARGET trials no statistically significant difference was noted in the incidence of cardiovascular events (cerebrovascular accident, myocardial infarction, angina) between celecoxib/lumiracoxib and standard NSAIDs (Silverstein et al. 2000; Farkouh et al. 2004). However, in the latter trials patients with osteoarthritis were included. By contrast, the VIGOR study was performed on patients with rheumatoid arthritis, a condition that has been associated with an enhanced rate of cardiovascular events. Moreover, about a quarter of the patients included in the CLASS and TARGET trials took aspirin as a cardioprotective agent, whereas the entry criteria for the VIGOR study precluded aspirin consumption.

Recently, long-term studies intended to find out whether selective COX-2 inhibitors may be used to prevent the formation of adenomatous colon polyps (adenomatous polyposis prevention study with rofecoxib: APPROVe; adenoma prevention with celecoxib: APC) or Alzheimer's disease (Alzheimer's Disease anti-inflammatory Prevention Trial: ADAPT) have shown that selective and nonselective COX inhibitors may increase the incidence of cardiac infarctions and other cardiovascular reactions (NIH 2004; Bresalier et al. 2005; Solomon et al. 2005). In these studies, the effect became fully evident only after treatment for more than $1\frac{1}{2}$ years in otherwise healthy patients. Moreover, in high-risk patients short-term treatment with valdecoxib/parecoxib was associated with an increased rate of severe thromboembolic events (Ott et al. 2003; Nussmeier et al. 2005). These observations had variable pharmacopolitical consequences including the withdrawal of rofecoxib (Vioxx) and valdecoxib (Bextra) from the market. Moreover, the outcome of these trials prompted regulatory bodies to request changes in the labeling of both selective and nonselective COX inhibitors, including those available for over-the-counter use (FDA 2005). Consequently, until proof of the opposite, all of these drugs are believed to go along with, at least in long-term use, an increased cardiovascular risk. To minimize this risk, the respective substances should be taken at the lowest effective dose for the shortest possible duration of treatment (European Agency for the Evaluation of Medicinal Products 2005a, b).

Scientifically these observations pose new questions: It has been assumed before that selective COX-2 inhibitors that do not inhibit platelet COX-1 might unfavorably alter the thromboxane/prostacyclin balance by inhibiting exclusively COX-2-dependent synthesis of vasoprotective prostacyclin in endothelial cells (Cheng et al. 2002). In fact, prostacyclin is a potent inhibitor of platelet aggregation, activation, and adhesion of leukocytes, and accumulation of cholesterol in vascular cells. Recent evidence, however, supports the view that disturbance of the thromboxane/prostacyclin balance cannot be the sole mechanism conferring the cardiovascular risk of COX-2 inhibitors. Accordingly, patients with coronary artery bypass grafting experienced severe cardiovascular events by valdecoxib/parecoxib, albeit apparently protected by low-dose aspirin (Ott et al. 2003; Nussmeier et al. 2005). Likewise, a subgroup analysis from the APC trial has demonstrated that aspirin may not abrogate the potential cardiovascular harm of celecoxib (Solomon et al. 2005). Moreover, given that in all long-term studies with coxibs and NSAIDs performed so far, an increased cardiovascular risk became evident after prolonged drug administration only, it appears feasible that a permanent COX-2 blockade may play a crucial role in the development of cardiovascular events. In line with this concept, COX-2-derived prostaglandins have been shown recently to upregulate the expression of the thrombin inhibitor thrombomodulin in human smooth muscle cells, thus providing a molecular basis for a hitherto unknown platelet-independent mechanism underlying the prothrombotic effects of both selective and nonselective COX-2 inhibitors (Rabausch et al. 2005). In this context it is also noteworthy that the traditional NSAID diclofenac, given as a retarded form, elicits a more pronounced inhibition of intravascular COX-2-dependent prostaglandin formation as compared to rofecoxib and celecoxib (Hinz et al. 2006). Finally, a recently published population-based nested case-control analysis has shown an increased risk of myocardial infarction associated with the current use of both selective (rofecoxib) and nonselective (diclofenac, ibuprofen) COX-2 inhibitors (Hippisley-Cox and Coupland 2005). Even though the methodology used in this study has been called in question, a potentially increased risk of traditional NSAIDs in eliciting myocardial infarctions warrants attention. Consequently, the cardiovascular safety of both selective COX-2 inhibitors and conventional NSAIDs should be reconsidered in future studies.

Although myocardial infarctions provide valuable data concerning cardiovascular safety of drugs, the cardiorenal profiles of NSAIDs and selective COX-2 inhibitors have also to be considered. As a matter of fact, the involvement of COX-2 in human renal function is supported by numerous clinical studies that showed that selective COX-2 inhibitors, similar to other NSAIDs, may cause peripheral edema, hypertension, and exacerbation of pre-existing hypertension by inhibiting water and salt excretion by the kidneys (Catella-Lawson et al. 1999; Whelton et al. 2000; Schwarz et al. 2000). These observations are of immense importance given that relatively small changes in blood pressure could have a significant impact on cardiovascular events. In patients with osteoarthritis, increases in systolic blood pressure of 1–5 mmHg have been associated with 7,100–35,700 additional ischemic heart disease and stroke events over 1 year (Singh et al. 2003). Likewise, the hypertension optimal treatment (HOT) study showed that diastolic blood pressure differences of +4 mmHg can lead to a 28% increase in myocardial infarctions (Hansson et al. 1998).

5
Future Developments

The available traditional antipyretic analgesics and selective COX-2 inhibitors still leave space for additional compounds. For acute pain a compound that is absorbed fast, fully bioavailable, and eliminated quickly (such as ibuprofen) might be of interest.

Inhibiting COX-1, COX-2, and 5-lipoxygenase (5-LOX) may be rewarding for the treatment of osteoarthrosis. The advantage of such compounds would be that they are not associated with alternative processing of arachidonic acid via the 5-LOX pathway. In fact, leukotrienes generated by 5-LOX may cause adhesion of neutrophils and vasoconstriction, resulting in ischemia and consequently mucosal lesions. A compound claimed to be endowed with such dual COX-/LOX-inhibitory properties is licofelone (ML3000) (Tries et al. 2002). However, clinical data supporting the claims are still scarce. Likewise, nitric oxide (NO)-releasing NSAIDs are widely discussed. They are hoped to protect the gastrointestinal tract by releasing vasodilatory NO and to produce the full therapeutic effects of, e.g., diclofenac or naproxen (Wallace 2002).

So far, hard clinical data are missing despite many years of research. It is also unclear how patients and physicians will solve the dosing problems of such compounds, which release two active ingredients (NO and NSAID) with different pharmacokinetic and toxicological properties. The microsomal prostaglandin E synthase I that is coexpressed with COX-2 under diverse inflammatory conditions may represent a potential target for treatment of inflammatory pain (Jakobsson et al. 1999). From the pharmacological point of view an inhibition of this enzyme would open the opportunity to inhibit the production of COX-2-dependent proinflammatory PGE_2 without a concomitant blockade of COX-2-dependent prostacyclin, which confers various protective actions in the cardiovascular and renal system. Finally, targeting of individual PG receptor subtypes may permit a separation of desired and unwanted effects of NSAIDs. Recently, blockade of the EP_2 receptor has attracted attention as a possible target for centrally acting, antihyperalgesic agents (Reinold et al. 2005).

References

Ahmadi S, Lippross S, Neuhuber WL, Zeilhofer HU (2002) PGE_2 selectively blocks inhibitory glycinergic neurotransmission onto rat superficial dorsal horn neurons. Nat Neurosci 5:34–40

Akopian AN, Sivilotti L, Wood JN (1996) A tetrodotoxin-resistant voltage-gated sodium channel expressed by sensory neurons. Nature 379:257–262

Anonymous (1998) An epidemiologic study of severe anaphylactic and anaphylactoid reactions among hospital patients: methods and overall risks. The International Collaborative Study of Severe Anaphylaxis. Epidemiology 9:141–146

Baba H, Kohno T, Moore KA, Woolf CJ (2001) Direct activation of rat spinal dorsal horn neurons by prostaglandin E_2. J Neurosci 21:1750–1756

Beiche F, Scheuerer S, Brune K, Geisslinger G, Goppelt-Struebe M (1996) Upregulation of cyclooxygenase-2 mRNA in the rat spinal cord following peripheral inflammation. FEBS Lett 390:165–169

Benn SC, Costigan M, Tate S, Fitzgerald M, Woolf CJ (2001) Developmental expression of the TTX-resistant voltage-gated sodium channels Nav1.8 (SNS) and Nav1.9 (SNS2) in primary sensory neurons. J Neurosci 21:6077–6085

Bombardier C, Laine L, Reicin A, Shapiro D, Burgos-Vargas R, Davis B, Day R, Ferraz MB, Hawkey CJ, Hochberg MC, Kvien TK, Schnitzer TJ (2000) Comparison of upper gastrointestinal toxicity of rofecoxib and naproxen in patients with rheumatoid arthritis. VIGOR Study Group. N Engl J Med 343:1520–1528

Boutaud O, Aronoff DM, Richardson JH, Marnett LJ, Oates JA (2002) Determinants of the cellular specificity of acetaminophen as an inhibitor of prostaglandin H_2 synthases. Proc Natl Acad Sci USA 99:7130–7135

Brandt K (2003) Paracetamol in the treatment of osteoarthritis pain. Drugs 63 Spec No 2:23–41

Bresalier RS, Sandler RS, Quan H, Bolognese JA, Oxenius B, Horgan K, Lines C, Riddell R, Morton D, Lanas A, Konstam MA, Baron JA (2005) Cardiovascular events associated with rofecoxib in a colorectal adenoma chemoprevention trial. N Engl J Med 352:1092–1102

Bridger S, Henderson K, Glucksman E, Ellis AJ, Henry JA, Williams R (1998) Deaths from low dose paracetamol poisoning. BMJ 316:1724–1725

Brune K (1974) How aspirin might work: a pharmacokinetic approach. Agents Actions 4:230–232

Brune K, Hinz B (2004) Selective cyclooxygenase-2 inhibitors: similarities and differences. Scand J Rheumatol 33:1–6

Brune K, Lanz R (1985) Pharmacokinetics of non-steroidal anti-inflammatory drugs. In: Bonta IL, Bray MA, Parnham MJ (eds) The pharmacology of inflammation. (Handbook of inflammation, vol 5) Elsevier Science, Amsterdam, pp 413–449

Brune K, Zeilhofer HU (2006) Antipyretic analgesics: basic aspects. In: Wall PD, Melzack R (eds) Textbook of pain. Elsevier, London

Brune K, Glatt M, Graf P (1976) Mechanism of action of anti-inflammatory drugs. Gen Pharmacol 7:27–33

Brune K, Rainsford KD, Schweitzer A (1980) Biodistribution of mild analgesics. Br J Clin Pharmacol 10 Suppl 2:279–284

Catella-Lawson F, McAdam B, Morrison BW, Kapoor S, Kujubu D, Antes L, Lasseter KC, Quan H, Gertz BJ, FitzGerald GA (1999) Effects of specific inhibition of cyclooxygenase-2 on sodium balance, hemodynamics, and vasoactive eicosanoids. J Pharmacol Exp Ther 289:735–741

Catella-Lawson F, Reilly MP, Kapoor SC, Cucchiara AJ, DeMarco S, Tournier B, Vyas SN, FitzGerald GA (2001) Cyclooxygenase inhibitors and the antiplatelet effects of aspirin. N Engl J Med 345:1809–1817

Caterina MJ, Leffler A, Malmberg AB, Martin WJ, Trafton J, Petersen-Zeitz KR, Koltzenburg M, Basbaum AI, Julius D (2000) Impaired nociception and pain sensation in mice lacking the capsaicin receptor. Science 288:306–313

Chandrasekharan NV, Dai H, Roos KL, Evanson NK, Tomsik J, Elton TS, Simmons DL (2002) COX-3, a cyclooxygenase-1 variant inhibited by acetaminophen and other analgesic/antipyretic drugs: cloning, structure, and expression. Proc Natl Acad Sci USA 99:13926–13931

Cheng Y, Austin SC, Rocca B, Koller BH, Coffman TM, Grosser T, Lawson JA, FitzGerald GA (2002) Role of prostacyclin in the cardiovascular response to thromboxane A_2. Science 296:539–541

Davis JB, Gray J, Gunthorpe MJ, Hatcher JP, Davey PT, Overend P, Harries MH, Latcham J, Clapham C, Atkinson K, Hughes SA, Rance K, Grau E, Harper AJ, Pugh PL, Rogers DC, Bingham S, Randall A, Sheardown SA (2000) Vanilloid receptor-1 is essential for inflammatory thermal hyperalgesia. Nature 405:183–187

Dinchuk JE, Liu RQ, Trzaskos JM (2003) COX-3: in the wrong frame in mind. Immunol Lett 86:121

England S, Bevan S, Docherty RJ (1996) PGE_2 modulates the tetrodotoxin-resistant sodium current in neonatal rat dorsal root ganglion neurones via the cyclic AMP-protein kinase A cascade. J Physiol (Lond) 495:429–440

European Agency for the Evaluation of Medicinal Products (2005a) Public statement: European medicines agency concludes action on COX-2 inhibitors. London, 27 June 2005

European Agency for the Evaluation of Medicinal Products (2005b) EMEA, press release: European Medicines Agency update on non-selective NSAIDs. London, 17 October 2005

Farkouh ME, Kirshner H, Harrington RA, Ruland S, Verheugt FW, Schnitzer TJ, Burmester GR, Mysler E, Hochberg MC, Doherty M, Ehrsam E, Gitton X, Krammer G, Mellein B, Gimona A, Matchaba P, Hawkey CJ, Chesebro JH, et al (2004) Comparison of lumiracoxib with naproxen and ibuprofen in the Therapeutic Arthritis Research and Gastrointestinal Event Trial (TARGET), cardiovascular outcomes: randomised controlled trial. Lancet 364:675–684

FDA (2006) FDA News: FDA announces series of changes to the class of marketed nonsteroidal anti-inflammatory drugs (NSAIDs). http://www.fda.gov/bbs/topics/news/2005/NEW01171.html. Cited 8 Apr 2006

Geba GP, Weaver AL, Polis AB, Dixon ME, Schnitzer TJ, et al (2002) Efficacy of rofecoxib, celecoxib, and acetaminophen in osteoarthritis of the knee: a randomized trial. JAMA 287:64–71

Geisslinger G, Menzel S, Wissel K, Brune K (1993) Single dose pharmacokinetics of different formulations of ibuprofen and aspirin. Drug Invest 5:238–242

Gold MS, Reichling DB, Shuster MJ, Levine JD (1996) Hyperalgesic agents increase a tetrodotoxin-resistant Na^+ current in nociceptors. Proc Natl Acad Sci USA 93:1108–1112

Hansson L, Zanchetti A, Carruthers SG, Dahlof B, Elmfeldt D, Julius S, Menard J, Rahn KH, Wedel H, Westerling S (1998) Effects of intensive blood-pressure lowering and low-dose aspirin in patients with hypertension: principal results of the Hypertension Optimal Treatment (HOT) randomised trial. HOT Study Group. Lancet 351:1755–1762

Harvey RJ, Depner UB, Wassle H, Ahmadi S, Heindl C, Reinold H, Smart TG, Harvey K, Schutz B, Abo-Salem OM, Zimmer A, Poisbeau P, Welzl H, Wolfer DP, Betz H, Zeilhofer HU, Muller U (2004) GlyR $\alpha 3$: an essential target for spinal PGE_2-mediated inflammatory pain sensitization. Science 304:884–887

Henry D, Lim LL, Garcia Rodriguez LA, Perez Gutthann S, Carson JL, Griffin M, Savage R, Logan R, Moride Y, Hawkey C, Hill S, Fries JT (1996) Variability in risk of gastrointestinal complications with individual non-steroidal anti-inflammatory drugs: results of a collaborative meta-analysis. Br Med J 312:1563–1566

Hinz B, Brune K (2002) Cyclooxygenase-2—ten years later. J Pharmacol Exp Ther 300: 367–375

Hinz B, Brune K, Pahl A (2000a) Cyclooxygenase-2 expression in lipopolysaccharide-stimulated human monocytes is modulated by cyclic AMP, prostaglandin E_2 and nonsteroidal anti-inflammatory drugs. Biochem Biophys Res Commun 278:790–796

Hinz B, Brune K, Pahl A (2000b) Prostaglandin E_2 up-regulates cyclooxygenase-2 expression in lipopolysaccharide-stimulated RAW 264.7 macrophages. Biochem Biophys Res Commun 272:744–748

Hinz B, Dorn CP, Shen TY, Brune K (2000c) Anti-inflammatory–antirheumatic drugs. McGuire JL (ed) Pharmaceuticals—classes, therapeutic agents, areas of application, vol 4. Wiley-VCH, Weinheim, pp 1671–1711

Hinz B, Kraus V, Pahl A, Brune K (2000d) Salicylate metabolites inhibit cyclooxygenase-2-dependent prostaglandin E_2 synthesis in murine macrophages. Biochem Biophys Res Commun 274:197–202

Hinz B, Rau T, Auge D, Werner U, Ramer R, Rietbrock S, Brune K (2003) Aceclofenac spares cyclooxygenase 1 as a result of limited but sustained biotransformation to diclofenac. Clin Pharmacol Ther 74:222–235

Hinz B, Ramer R, Eichele K, Weinzierl U, Brune K (2004) Upregulation of cyclooxygenase-2 expression is involved in R(+)-methanandamide-induced apoptotic death of human neuroglioma cells. Mol Pharmacol 66:1643–1651

Hinz B, Chevts J, Renner B, Wuttke H, Rau T, Schmidt A, Szelenyi I, Brune K, Werner U (2005a) Bioavailability of diclofenac potassium at low doses. Br J Clin Pharmacol 59: 80–84

Hinz B, Rösch S, Ramer R, Tamm E, Brune K (2005b) Latanoprost induces matrix metalloproteinase-1 expression in human non-pigmented ciliary epithelial cells through a cyclooxygenase-2-dependent mechanism. FASEB J 19:1929–1931

Hinz B, Dormann H, Brune K (2006) More pronounced inhibition of cyclooxygenase-2, increase of blood pressure and decrease of heart rate by treatment with diclofenac compared with celecoxib and rofecoxib. Arthritis Rheum 54:282–291

Hippisley-Cox J, Coupland C (2005) Risk of myocardial infarction in patients taking cyclooxygenase-2 inhibitors or conventional non-steroidal anti-inflammatory drugs: population based nested case-control analysis. BMJ 330:1366

Ibanez L, Vidal X, Ballarin E, Laporte JR (2005) Population-based drug-induced agranulocytosis. Arch Intern Med 165:869–874

International Agranulocytosis and Aplastic Anemia Study (1986) Risks of agranulocytosis and aplastic anemia: a first report of their relation to drug use with special reference to analgesics. JAMA 256:1749–1757

Jakobsson PJ, Thoren S, Morgenstern R, Samuelsson B (1999) Identification of human prostaglandin E synthase: a microsomal, glutathione-dependent, inducible enzyme, constituting a potent novel drug target. Proc Natl Acad Sci USA 96:7220–7225

Kaufman DW, Kelly JP, Levy M. Shapiro S (1991) The drug etiology of agranulocytosis an aplastic anemia. Monographs in epidemiology and biostatistics 18. Oxford University Press, London

Kimmey MB (2004) Cardioprotective effects and gastrointestinal risks of aspirin: maintaining the delicate balance. Am J Med 117 Suppl 5A:72S–78S

Kopp E, Ghosh S (1994) Inhibition of NF-κB by sodium salicylate and aspirin. Science 265:956–959

Lopshire JC, Nicol GD (1997) Activation and recovery of the PGE_2-mediated sensitization of the capsaicin response in rat sensory neurons. J Neurophysiol 78:3154–3164

Luong C, Miller A, Barnett J, Chow J, Ramesha C, Browner MF (1996) Flexibility of the NSAID binding site in the structure of human cyclooxygenase-2. Nat Struct Biol 3:927–933

Maldve RE, Kim Y, Muga SJ, Fischer SM (2000) Prostaglandin E_2 regulation of cyclooxygenase expression in keratinocytes is mediated via cyclic nucleotide-linked prostaglandin receptors. J Lipid Res 41:873–881

Masferrer JL, Zweifel BS, Seibert S, Needleman P (1990) Selective regulation of cellular cyclooxygenase by dexamethasone and endotoxin in mice. J Clin Invest 86:1375–1379

Mizuno H, Sakamoto C, Matsuda K, Wada K, Uchida T, Noguchi H, Akamatsu T, Kasuga M (1997) Induction of cyclooxygenase 2 in gastric mucosal lesions and its inhibition by the specific antagonist delays healing in mice. Gastroenterology 112:387–397

Mockenhaupt M, Schlingmann J, Schroeder W, Schoepf E (1996) Evaluation of non-steroidal anti-inflammatory drugs (NSAIDs) and muscle relaxants as risk factors for Stevens-Johnson syndrome (SJS) and toxic epidermal necrolysis (TEN). Pharmacoepidemiol Drug Saf 5:116

Muth-Selbach US, Tegeder I, Brune K, Geisslinger G (1999) Acetaminophen inhibits spinal prostaglandin E_2 release after peripheral noxious stimulation. Anesthesiology 91: 231–239

Nantel F, Denis D, Gordon R, Northey A, Cirino M, Metters KM, Chan CC (1999) Distribution and regulation of cyclooxygenase-2 in carrageenan-induced inflammation. Br J Pharmacol 128:853–859

Neugebauer V, Geisslinger G, Rümenapp P, Weiretter F, Szelenyi I, Brune K, Schaible HG (1995) Antinociceptive effects of R(−)- and S(+)-flurbiprofen on rat spinal dorsal horn neurons rendered hyperexcitable by an acute knee joint inflammation. J Pharmacol Exp Ther 275:618–628

NIH (2004) NIH News. Use of non-steroidal anti-inflammatory drugs suspended in large Alzheimer's disease prevention trial. http://www.nih.gov/news/pr/dec2004/od-20.htm. Cited 8 Apr 2006

Niiro H, Otsuka T, Izuhara K, Yamaoka K, Ohshima K, Tanabe T, Hara S, Nemoto Y, Tanaka Y, Nakashima H, Niho Y (1997) Regulation by interleukin-10 and interleukin-4 of cyclooxygenase-2 expression in human neutrophils. Blood 89:1621–1628

Nussmeier NA, Whelton AA, Brown MT, Langford RM, Hoeft A, Parlow JL, Boyce SW, Verburg KM (2005) Complications of the COX-2 inhibitors parecoxib and valdecoxib after cardiac surgery. N Engl J Med 352:1081–1091

Onoe Y, Miyaura C, Kaminakayashiki T, Nagai Y, Noguchi K, Chen QR, Seo H, Ohta H, Nozawa S, Kudo I, Suda T (1996) IL-13 and IL-4 inhibit bone resorption by suppressing cyclooxygenase-2-dependent prostaglandin synthesis in osteoblasts. J Immunol 156:758–764

Ott E, Nussmeier NA, Duke PC, Feneck RO, Alston RP, Snabes MC, Hubbard RC, Hsu PH, Saidman LJ, Mangano DT (2003) Efficacy and safety of the cyclooxygenase 2 inhibitors parecoxib and valdecoxib in patients undergoing coronary artery bypass surgery. J Thorac Cardiovasc Surg 125:1481–1492

Patrignani P, Panara MR, Sciulli MG, Santini G, Renda G, Patrono C (1997) Differential inhibition of human prostaglandin endoperoxide synthase-1 and -2 by nonsteroidal anti-inflammatory drugs. J Physiol Pharmacol 48:623–631

Rabausch K, Bretschneider E, Sarbia M, Meyer-Kirchrath J, Censarek P, Pape R, Fischer JW, Schror K, Weber AA (2005) Regulation of thrombomodulin expression in human vascular smooth muscle cells by COX-2-derived prostaglandins. Circ Res 96:e1–6

Ramer R, Weinzierl U, Schwind B, Brune K, Hinz B (2003) Ceramide is involved in R(+)-methanandamide-induced cyclooxygenase-2 expression in human neuroglioma cells. Mol Pharmacol 64:1189–1198

Reinold H, Ahmadi S, Depner UB, Layh B, Heindl C, Hamza M, Pahl A, Brune K, Narumiya S, Muller U, Zeilhofer HU (2005) Spinal inflammatory hyperalgesia is mediated by prostaglandin E receptors of the EP_2 subtype. J Clin Invest 115:673–679

Roujeau JC, Kelly JP, Naldi L, Rzany B, Stern RS, Anderson T, Auquier A, Bastuji-Garin S, Correia O, Locati F, Mockenhaupt M Paoletti C, Shapiro S, Sheir N, Schöpf E, Kaufman D (1995) Drug etiology of Stevens-Johnson syndrome and toxic epidermal necrolysis, first results from an international case-control study. N Engl J Med 333:1600–1609

Rudy AC, Knight PM, Brater DC, Hall SD (1991) Stereoselective metabolism of ibuprofen in humans: administration of R-, S- and racemic ibuprofen. J Pharmacol Exp Ther 259:1133–1139

Samad TA, Moore KA, Sapirstein A, Billet S, Allchorne A, Poole S, Bonventre JV, Woolf CJ (2001) Interleukin-1beta-mediated induction of Cox-2 in the CNS contributes to inflammatory pain hypersensitivity. Nature 410:471–475

Schaible HG, Schmidt RF (1988) Time course of mechanosensitivity changes in articular afferents during a developing experimental arthritis. J Neurophysiol 60:2180–2195

Schmassmann A, Peskar BM, Stettler C, Netzer P, Stroff T, Flogerzi B, Halter F (1998) Effects of inhibition of prostaglandin endoperoxide synthase-2 in chronic gastro-intestinal ulcer models in rats. Br J Pharmacol 123:795–804

Schnitzer TJ (2002) Update of ACR guidelines for osteoarthritis: role of the coxibs. J Pain Symptom Manage 23 Suppl 4:S24–S30

Schnitzer TJ, Burmester GR, Mysler E, Hochberg MC, Doherty M, Ehrsam E, Gitton X, Krammer G, Mellein B, Matchaba P, Gimona A, Hawkey CJ, et al (2004) Comparison of lumiracoxib with naproxen and ibuprofen in the Therapeutic Arthritis Research and Gastrointestinal Event Trial (TARGET), reduction in ulcer complications: randomised controlled trial. Lancet 364:665–674

Schwab JM, Beiter T, Linder JU, Laufer S, Schulz JE, Meyermann R, Schluesener HJ (2003) COX-3—a virtual pain target in humans? FASEB J 17:2174–2175

Schwartz JI, Vandormael K, Malice MP, Kalyani RN, Lasseter KC, Holmes GB, Gertz BJ, Gottesdiener KM, Laurenzi M, Redfern KJ, Brune K (2002) Comparison of rofecoxib, celecoxib, and naproxen on renal function in elderly subjects receiving a normal-salt diet. Clin Pharmacol Ther 72:50–61

Seeff LB, Cuccherini BA, Zimmerman HJ, Adler E, Benjamin SB (1986) Paracetamol hepatotoxicity in alcoholics. Ann Intern Med 104:399–404

Silverstein FE, Faich G, Goldstein JL, Simon LS, Pincus T, Whelton A, Makuch R, Eisen G, Agrawal NM, Stenson WF, Burr AM, Zhao WW, Kent JD, Lefkowith JB, Verburg KM, Geis GS (2000) Gastrointestinal toxicity with celecoxib vs nonsteroidal anti-inflammatory drugs for osteoarthritis and rheumatoid arthritis: the CLASS study: A randomized controlled trial. Celecoxib Long-term Arthritis Safety Study. JAMA 284:1247–1255

Singh G, Miller JD, Huse DM, Pettitt D, D'Agostino RB, Russell MW (2003) Consequences of increased systolic blood pressure in patients with osteoarthritis and rheumatoid arthritis. J Rheumatol 30:714–719

Smith CJ, Zhang Y, Koboldt CM, Muhammad J, Zweifel BS, Shaffer A, Talley JJ, Masferrer JL, Seibert K, Isakson PC (1998) Pharmacological analysis of cyclooxygenase-1 in inflammation. Proc Natl Acad Sci U S A 95:13313–13318

Solomon SD, McMurray JJ, Pfeffer MA, Wittes J, Fowler R, Finn P, Anderson WF, Zauber A, Hawk E, Bertagnolli M (2005) Cardiovascular risk associated with celecoxib in a clinical trial for colorectal adenoma prevention. N Engl J Med 352:1071–1080

Tries S, Neupert W, Laufer S (2002) The mechanism of action of the new antiinflammatory compound ML3000: inhibition of 5-LOX and COX-1/2. Inflamm Res 51:135–143

Vane JR (1971) Inhibition of prostaglandin synthesis as a mechanism of action of aspirin-like drugs. Nat New Biol 231:232–235

Wallace JL, Ignarro LJ, Fiorucci S (2002) Potential cardioprotective actions of NO-releasing aspirin. Nat Rev Drug Discov 1:375–382

Weissmann G (1993) Prostaglandins as modulators rather than mediators of inflammation. J Lipid Mediat 6:275–286

Werner U, Werner D, Pahl A, Mundkowski R, Gillich M, Brune K (2002) Investigation of the pharmacokinetics of celecoxib by liquid chromatography-mass spectrometry. Biomed Chromatogr 16:56–60

Werner U, Werner D, Rau T, Fromm MF, Hinz B, Brune K (2003) Celecoxib inhibits metabolism of cytochrome P450 2D6 substrate metoprolol in humans. Clin Pharmacol Ther 74:130–137

Whelton A, Maurath CJ, Verburg KM, Geis GS (2000) Renal safety and tolerability of celecoxib, a novel cyclooxygenase-2 inhibitor. Am J Ther 7:159–175

Winter CA, Risley EA, Nuss GW (1962) Carrageenin-induced edema in hind paw of the rat as an assay for anti-inflammatory drugs. Proc Soc Exp Biol Med 111:544–552

Xie W, Chipman JG, Robertson DL, Erikson RL, Simmons DL (1991) Expression of a mitogen-responsive gene encoding prostaglandin synthase is regulated by mRNA splicing. Proc Natl Acad Sci USA 88:2692–2696

Xu XM, Sansores-Garcia L, Chen XM, Matijevic-Aleksic N, Du M, Wu KK (1999) Suppression of inducible cyclooxygenase 2 gene transcription by aspirin and sodium salicylate. Proc Natl Acad Sci USA 96:5292–5297

Zhang W, Jones A, Doherty M (2004) Does paracetamol (acetaminophen) reduce the pain of osteoarthritis? A meta-analysis of randomised controlled trials. Ann Rheum Dis 63:901–907

HEP (2006) 177:95–127
© Springer-Verlag Berlin Heidelberg 2006

Local Anesthetics

F. Yanagidate · G. R. Strichartz (✉)

Pain Research Center, BWH/MRB611, 75 Francis Street, Boston MA, 02115-6110, USA
gstrichz@zeus.bwh.harvard.edu

1	Introduction	96
1.1	Mechanistic Overview	96
2	Molecular Targets of Local Anesthetics	97
2.1	Blockade of Action Potentials: The Classic Local Anesthetic Action	97
2.2	Binding of Local Anesthetics to Voltage-Gated Na^+ Channels	98
2.3	Local Anesthetic Binding to K^+ and Ca^{2+} Channels	99
2.4	G Protein-Coupled Receptors and Local Anesthetics	102
2.5	Inhibition of Protein Kinase A and Protein Kinase C	103
2.6	Transient Receptor Potential Channels and Local Anesthetics	106
3	Mechanisms of Spinal and Epidural Anesthesia	107
3.1	MAP Kinases and Pain Processing in the Spinal Cord	108
3.2	Presynaptic or Postsynaptic Sites for LA Inhibition	108
3.3	Neurotoxicity of Spinal Anesthetics	109
3.3.1	Local Anesthetics, MAP Kinases and Cell Death	111
3.3.2	Apoptosis and Necrosis	111
4	Intravenous Local Anesthetics and Neuropathic Pain	112
References	115

Abstract Local anesthetics are used broadly to prevent or reverse acute pain and treat symptoms of chronic pain. This chapter, on the analgesic aspects of local anesthetics, reviews their broad actions that affect many different molecular targets and disrupt their functions in pain processing. Application of local anesthetics to peripheral nerve primarily results in the blockade of propagating action potentials, through their inhibition of voltage-gated sodium channels. Such inhibition results from drug binding at a site in the channel's inner pore, accessible from the cytoplasmic opening. Binding of drug molecules to these channels depends on their conformation, with the drugs generally having a higher affinity for the open and inactivated channel states that are induced by membrane depolarization. As a result, the effective potency of these drugs for blocking impulses increases during high-frequency repetitive firing and also under slow depolarization, such as occurs at a region of nerve injury, which is often the locus for generation of abnormal, pain-related ectopic impulses. At distal and central terminals the inhibition of voltage-gated calcium channels by local anesthetics will suppress neurogenic inflammation and the release of neurotransmitters. Actions on receptors that contribute to nociceptive transduction, such as TRPV1 and the bradykinin B2 receptor, provide an independent mode of analgesia. In the spinal cord, where local anesthetics are present during epidural or intrathecal anesthesia, inhibition of inotropic receptors, such as those for glutamate, by local anesthetics further interferes with neuronal transmission. Activation of spinal cord mitogen-activated protein (MAP) kinases, which are essential for the hyperalgesia following injury or incision and occur in both neurons and glia, is inhibited by spinal local anesthetics. Many G protein-coupled receptors are susceptible to local anesthetics, with particular sensitivity of those coupled via the G_q α-subunit. Local anesthetics are also infused intravenously to yield plasma concentrations far below those that block normal action potentials, yet that are frequently effective at reversing neuropathic pain. Thus, local anesthetics modify a variety of neuronal membrane channels and receptors, leading to what is probably a synergistic mixture of analgesic mechanisms to achieve effective clinical analgesia.

Keywords Ion channels · Action potentials · Nociception · G protein-coupled receptors · MAP kinases

1
Introduction

Local anesthetics are widely used for the prevention and relief of both acute and chronic pain (Strichartz and Berde 2005). The reduction or abolition of acute pain from accidental or intentional trauma (surgery) is accomplished by delivery of local anesthetics to the skin by topical application or subcutaneous infiltration, to peripheral nerve by percutaneous injection, or to the neuraxis by administration into the epidural or intrathecal spaces (Gokin and Strichartz 1999). Chronic pain symptoms are also relieved, albeit mostly temporarily, by the "nerve blocking" procedures just described. In contrast, systemic local anesthetics, administered intravenously and to much lower plasma concentrations than those used for direct nerve block, also relieve many forms of neuropathic pain in humans and in animal models, and with a therapeutic benefit that often endures for weeks, months, or longer, far outlasting the presence of the drug in vivo (Boas et al. 1982; Mao and Chen 2000).

1.1
Mechanistic Overview

Whereas mechanisms for the nerve blocking actions of local anesthetics are relatively well understood, those that underlie the neuraxial block are probably more complex. The inhibition of neuronal voltage-gated sodium channels (VGSC) by direct binding of local anesthetics (Nau and Wang 2004) leads to failure in the generation or propagation of action potentials, the primary mechanisms for functional deficits during peripheral nerve blockade. After the delivery of local anesthetics to the epidural or intrathecal compartments, these drugs diffuse into the spinal cord where they can interact with a variety of other ion channels involved (1) in excitation/depolarization of presynaptic terminals, (2) in regulating release of neurotransmitters, and (3) with both pre- and postsynaptic receptor proteins for small neurotransmitters and neuropeptides (Gokin and Strichartz 1999). These receptors include both inotropic and metabotropic receptors, membrane macromolecules that are coupled to the activation of various intracellular signaling pathways using enzymes that themselves may be direct targets of local anesthetic action. Since clinically used local anesthetics are relatively impotent drugs, with inhibitory actions dependent on millimolar concentrations at their target molecule, and often have restricted access to their desired target site, they are used clinically at high enough concentrations that many different molecular targets are likely to be modified by them.

Like many "amphipathic" molecules, which contain both hydrophobic and hydrophilic—even ionized—regions, local anesthetics distribute into and have effects upon the dynamic properties of membranes (Lissi et al. 1990). Almost all of the recognized targets of local anesthetics are membrane-intrinsic or membrane-associated macromolecules, and the partitioning within and permeation through biomembranes is a feature of local anesthetics that is essential for their fundamental actions and also governs their clinical effectiveness (de Paula and Schreier 1995).

In this chapter we will describe the various mechanisms and molecular and cellular targets for local anesthetics during neural blockade, as well present the phenomenon of and speculate on mechanisms for long-term relief of chronic pain by intravenous local anesthetics. Unlike the acute nerve-blocking actions of local anesthetics, the mechanisms underlying the long-term effects of intravenous drugs to relieve chronic pain symptoms remain a mystery. We will also consider the long-held possibility of using certain naturally occurring toxins to effect analgesia by potent and specific binding to single classes of ion channels.

Finally, we will examine recently described nontraditional actions of local anesthetics, particularly their antiinflammatory effects, and relate the known mechanisms in neuronal tissues to those on immune cell functions.

2
Molecular Targets of Local Anesthetics

2.1
Blockade of Action Potentials: The Classic Local Anesthetic Action

Action potentials are the hallmark of excitable membranes, and their occurrence is absolutely dependent on ion channels that open in response to depolarization and allow current to enter the cell. In most excitable membranes of nerve, skeletal, and cardiac cells, the major inward current that drives the fast depolarizing phase of the action potential is carried through VGSCs. In order to achieve the conditions for an action potential to occur, i.e., "threshold," the cell membrane must be adequately stimulated, depolarized sufficiently to open enough VGSCs to produce inward current that will overcome the outward current that flows through the K^+ and Cl^- channels that coexist in the membrane. The initial sources of these impulse-generating stimuli are physiological transducing events, such as occur at distal sensory endings, or postsynaptic "excitatory" receptors, such as occur in the CNS (spinal cord). Local circuit current from a depolarized membrane under an action potential flows to an unexcited adjacent region to stimulate it to threshold, accounting for the propagation of the depolarizing wave of the action potential along an axon. This mode of propagating stimulation has a higher "margin of safety" than the other stimulation modes, i.e., the current supplied by the adjacent excited membrane is about 5–10 times greater than that required to reach threshold. At any one of these locations, impulse-generating processes can be suppressed by local anesthetics to prevent or abolish action potentials. Corresponding to its higher margin of safety for conduction, propagating axonal action potentials are more resistant to treatments that block inward current than are, for example, the initial generation of action potentials at sensory endings. It therefore takes lower concentrations of local anesthetics to suppress the initiation of an impulse than those necessary to abolish that impulse once it has started propagating (Raymond 1992). Furthermore, the margin of safety for conduction is apparently greatest in nonmyelinated C-fibers (and in the smallest, i.e., slowest conducting, among these fibers) and is least in the small myelinated, A-delta and A-gamma fibers (Huang et al. 1997; Gokin et al. 2001). This accounts for the differential order of susceptibility to local anesthetics of axons documented directly, in vitro and in vivo (small myelinated>large myelinated>non-myelinated). These observations have been made by many experimentalists but are still challenged by the historical "size principle" that states that smaller fibers, regardless of micro-anatomy, are always more susceptible to local anesthetics than larger fibers, a principal extrapolated from very early observations on compound action potentials at a time before C-fibers had been identified (Raymond and Gissen 1987).

2.2
Binding of Local Anesthetics to Voltage-Gated Na$^+$ Channels

Blockade of action potentials relies on the inhibition of VGSCs. The regions of the VGSC that interact directly to bind local anesthetics have been identified, principally through site-directed mutation (Ragsdale et al. 1994; Wang et al. 2000, 2001). The picture that emerges is of a dynamically altered drug binding site that varies with the state of the channel. Resting closed channels have the lowest affinity. Inactivated closed channels are much higher in affinity, primarily because of a much slower dissociation rate (Chernoff 1990; Hille 1977), perhaps because the drug must escape from a sterically occluded channel, blocked by an "inactivation moiety" that closes the pore's cytoplasmic ending (Catterall 2000; Vedantham and Cannon 1999; Wang et al. 2004; Courtney and Strichartz 1987). Open channels also have a higher affinity, but bind the drugs much faster than inactivated channels do (Hille 1977; Chernoff 1990). One thermodynamic consequence of the differential binding affinity to different channel states is that the transitions between these states, the so-called "gating" of the channel, must be modified when local anesthetics are bound (Hille 1977; Balser et al. 1996).

Many of the amino acid side chains that appear to interact with the drug molecules are located around the cytoplasmic vestibule that forms a portal to the channel's narrow pore (Kondratiev and Tomaselli 2003; Ragsdale et al. 1994), although parts of the "inner pore domain," located deeper in the channel, also seem to influence binding (Sunami et al. 1997). Of the residues lining the vestibule, some are more influential in determining drug affinity for the resting state; others are more important for determining inactivation state binding (Li et al. 1999; Nau et al. 1999, 2003). From this we conclude that local anesthetic binding does not occur at a constant locus in the channel and, given the conformational flexibility of most local anesthetics, it is likely that they adjust their shape to fit the channel's altered conformations. The name that has been applied to this reciprocal adjustment of drug and channel during state-dependent binding is the "modulated receptor" (Hille 1977).

All VGSCs are composed of one large (ca. 180 kDa) α-subunit and 1 to 2 auxiliary β-subunits (Catterall 2000). The ion pore of the channel and the major gating machinery, including the loci for local anesthetic binding, are located on the α piece, although combination with β-subunits can influence the overall gating pattern and thus, through this modulation of state transitions, influence the state-dependent binding of these drugs (Wang et al. 1996; Wright et al. 1997, 1999). Each α-subunit carries four homologous domains, each domain contributing one segment of the channel's ion conducting pore and one part of the overall gating apparatus that couples membrane voltage to channel states. Each domain also contains regions that interact with local anesthetics, although it is unclear whether a tightly bound local anesthetic molecule simultaneously interacts with all four regions. Judging from their relatively low affinity, rarely having K_D values below 10 µM, and their weak stereoselectivitytency ratios rarely exceeding 5 (Lee-Son et al. 1992; Valenzuela et al. 1995; Brau et al. 2000; see review by Nau and Strichartz 2002), the fit of local anesthetics to VGSCs is apparently not very tight (Courtney and Strichartz 1987).

2.3
Local Anesthetic Binding to K$^+$ and Ca^{2+} Channels

There is much structural similarity among the voltage-gated, cation-selective ion channels (Yu et al. 2005). The charged transmembrane regions that act as "voltage-sensors," the hairpin segments that line the narrowest part of the pore to form the ion "selectivity filter," and several of the other transmembrane helices that support these critical functional regions are homologous structures among many of these ion channels. Not surprisingly, then, they also possess a similar pharmacology for drugs that interact with these regions, among which are the local anesthetics, although, in general, their affinity for these targets is less than that for the Na^+ channels.

Both the transient "A-type" and the more persistent "delayed rectifier" types of K^+ channels, both of which are activated by membrane depolarizations, are blocked by local anesthetics (Courtney and Kendig 1988; Castle 1990; Josephson 1988; Olschewski et al. 1998; Komai and McDowell 2001). The kinetics of the block are most consistent with high-affinity binding to the open state, and the mechanistic picture that accompanies these kinetics portrays one local anesthetic molecule entering an open channel's pore and occluding it, analogous to the mode for blocking open Na^+ channels (Castle 1990; Valenzuela et al. 1995). Classical "inward rectifier" K^+ channels are much less susceptible to local anesthetics (Castle 1990; Carmeliet et al. 1986), perhaps because they are not activated by voltage but instead may have a metal cation binding site in their pore that has few of the physicochemical properties that bind a local anesthetic, e.g., hydrophobicity. However, other K^+ channels that are not voltage-gated but are open at the resting potential are potently inhibited by local anesthetics (Brau et al. 1995; Olschewski et al. 1996; Kindler et al. 1999).

Voltage-gated Ca^{2+} channels also are blocked by local anesthetics (Palade and Almers 1985; Oyama et al. 1988; Guo et al. 1991; Sugiyama and Muteki 1994; Xiong and Strichartz 1998; Liu et al. 2001). Interestingly, in the case of the slowly inactivating L-type Ca^{2+} channels, the primary mode of block seems to be a promotion of the inactivated state (Carmeliet et al. 1986; Xiong and Strichartz 1998), like one of the actions of local anesthetics (LAs) on VGSCs and also like the dihydropyridine drugs, e.g., nifedipine, that are classical inhibitors of L-type channels. The LAs do not, however, bind at the dihydropyridine binding site on these channels (Hirota et al. 1997; Xiong and Strichartz 1998).

Pacemaker currents in neurons (and in cardiac muscle), I_h, carried by the hyperpolarization-activated, cyclic nucleotide-gated (HCN) class of channels which conduct Na^+ and K^+ about equally well, are LA sensitive too (Bischoff et al. 2003). Concentrations of bupivacaine and lidocaine to half block these channels, ca. 50 and 100 µM, respectively, are actually lower than those reported to block Na^+ channels in the same sensory neurons (Bischoff et al. 2003). Membrane-impermeant derivatives of local anesthetic—such as the permanently charged quaternary homolog of lidocaine, QX314—which block most cation channels from the intracellular direction, do not attenuate pacemaker currents when applied to the cell's exterior, suggesting that there is also an intracellular route to the local anesthetic binding site of these channels. Inasmuch as pacemaker channels are found in many neurons (Doan et al. 2004) and have been implicated as sources that drive the repetitive firing often associated with abnormal pain (Chaplan et al. 2003; Yao et al. 2003)—and because selective inhibitors of I_h delivered systemically are known to relieve certain neuropathic pain symptoms (Chaplan et al. 2003; Lee et al. 2005; cf. Raes et al. 1998)—their relative susceptibility to blockade by local anesthetics nominates them as likely targets for some of the clinical analgesic actions of these drugs.

The physiological, functional consequences of blocking these different channels will obviously depend on that channel's role in neural activity. Potassium channel block is often synergistic with the Na^+ channel blocking activity for effecting impulse blockade by local anesthetics (Drachman and Strichartz 1991). Blocking K^+ channels can depolarize the resting membrane and usually slows the repolarization of the action potential. In the absence of an accompanying Na^+ channel blockade by the drug, these actions will often enhance excitability, bringing the resting membrane closer to threshold and prolonging the duration of the action potential, an action that raises the margin of safety for impulse propagation and increases the likelihood of repetitive firing after a single stimulus (Raymond et al. 1990). When conjoined with the Na^+ channel blocking properties of local anesthetics, however, K^+ channel blockade has a remarkably synergistic action on action potentials. Both the steady depolarization of the resting potential and the prolonged depolarization of the action potential potentiate impulse blockade by increasing the presence of the open and inactivated Na^+ channels that bind LAs with high affinity. This overall effect illustrates an important pharmacological principle: the integrated actions of an agent that acts on several, physiologically coupled targets may differ from the action that would be predicted from the actions of that agent on the separate targets. Since the nervous system almost always utilizes plural ion channels and receptors in neural conduction and synaptic transmission (Hille 2001), the net effect of local anesthetics cannot always be predicted directly from their actions on only one of these targets.

Inhibition of the Ca^{2+} channels at nerve terminals by local anesthetics has dramatic physiological effects, disproportionally greater than the inhibition of action potentials through Na^+ channel blockade. Transmitter release from nerve terminals depends on the free cytosolic concentration of Ca^{2+} in the presynaptic ending, raised to the third power or higher. Therefore, if half the Ca^{2+} channels are blocked, the release of transmitter might be reduced to about 10% of the control value in drug-free conditions. By comparison, the margin of safety for impulse propagation is so large for most peripheral nerve axons that about 80% of the channels must be blocked before impulse conduction fails. These calculations are not intended to indicate the functional potency relationships for local anesthetics acting at different ion channels, but rather to emphasize the different forms of nonlinear relations between blockade of ion channels and the inhibition of the physiological functions to which they are coupled. Ultimately, it is these final physiological actions that are most directly related to analgesia, and the toxic side effects of local anesthetics.

2.4
G Protein-Coupled Receptors and Local Anesthetics

G proteins couple membrane receptors (GPCRs) to intracellular effectors and exist in various forms. Several different intracellular signaling pathways are affected by G proteins, some stimulated, some inhibited, and often converged upon by actions of plural receptors. For example, G proteins released from some GPCRs activate membrane-bound phospholipase C (PLC) that subsequently hydrolyzes the sugar moiety from the lipid phosphatidyl inositol, liberating inositol trisphosphate (IP$_3$) and diacylglycerol (DAG). In turn, IP$_3$ acts on "release channels" of the storage compartments inside cells to subsequently release Ca^{2+} into the intracellular domains. Ionized calcium, in turn, enhances or inhibits a number of cytoplasmic enzymes to acutely regulate cellular activity, and can regulate the long-term expression of cellular enzymes by binding to proteins that enter the nucleus and change cellular transcription. The other product of PLC activity, DAG, has a stimulating effect on protein kinase C (PKC) enzymes, many of which are also stimulated by the elevated cytoplasmic Ca^{2+}. Another major direct target of G protein activation is the enzyme that forms cyclic AMP (cAMP), adenylate cyclase (AC). Different G protein α-subunits will activate (G$_s$) or inhibit (G$_i$) adenylate cyclase, respectively increasing or decreasing the intracellular cAMP concentration (Hollmann et al. 2001).

In this complex scheme of multiple steps and interacting pathways local anesthetics may act at several molecular locations. There are some contradictory results of direct local anesthetic actions on specific GPCRs. Some caution should be applied, however, since many of these studies have been conducted on heterologous expression systems, such as *Xenopus* oocytes, where it is assumed that the enzymes that couple the GPCR to the measured endpoint are the same as those in mammalian cells expressing that particular GPCR. Local anesthetics inhibit certain GPCRs (e.g., LPA, TXA2, PAF, and m1 muscarinic receptors) expressed in *Xenopus* oocytes (Hollmann and Durieux 2000; Hollmann et al. 2000a, 2004; Honemann et al. 1999) but are ineffective on others, e.g., angiotensin receptor signaling (Nietgen et al. 1997). Although certain PLC-coupled GPCR activities are inhibited by local anesthetics, the actual release of Ca^{2+}, triggered by IP$_3$ that is liberated by phospholipase C (see above), is not affected by local anesthetics (Sullivan et al. 1999), indicating that the site(s) of LA action is located upstream of this segment of the pathway, at the receptor itself, or on the G protein, or at the interaction site in the complex of the two (Xiong et al. 1999).

For almost all the local anesthetic-sensitive GPCRs, the site of action can be located at the G protein:receptor interface. [In a minority of cases there appears to be an action at the extracellular surface of some receptors (Hollmann et al. 2000a), but these are very low-affinity interactions and we will not discuss them further here.] Durieux and colleagues have proposed that GPCRs linked to G$_q$ α-subunits are the ones distinctly sensitive to local anesthetics, based on the known G protein coupling of the susceptible pathways (Hollmann et al. 2001b, c, 2002). This hypothesis was confirmed by experiments where G_q was "knocked out" of a system with the accompanying loss of local anesthetic sensitivity of those coupled responses, while the pathways not coupled to G_q were unaffected (Hollmann et al. 2001b). In complementary experiments, introduction of G_q to cells, thus permitting this protein to couple to extant GPCRs, induced a sensitivity to local anesthetics that was not present before that manipulation (Hollmann et al. 2002). It is worth noting that the G protein coupling a particular GPCR to a specific pathway may differ among cells, and there may be multiple G proteins that can interact with one receptor, allowing for a diversity of sensitivities to local anesthetics. For example, substance P's neurokinin (NK)-1 receptors may be coupled to G_q or to G_{11} α-subunits (Macdonald et al. 1996). Cells with the first G protein will have substance P responses attenuated by local anesthetics (Li et al. 1995), cells with the second will be relatively insensitive. Interestingly, in one case $G\alpha_i$ protein function was enhanced by local anesthetics, apparently not by interaction with the coupled adenosine receptor but by a direct effect on the α_i G protein subunit (Benkwitz et al. 2003). The extent to which such activation occurs in general, and contributes to the overall inhibitory effect of local anesthetics, remains unexplored.

Acute pain is often accompanied by inflammation, and certain inflammatory processes are profoundly sensitive to local anesthetics via actions on GPCRs (Hollmann and Durieux 2000). In particular, the priming of neutrophils that is often critical for their rapid and vigorous response during inflammation (Condliffe et al. 1998) is suppressed by bupivacaine concentrations of ca. 10^{-8} M (Hollmann et al. 2001d; Fisher et al. 2001), far lower than the IC_{50}s for blocking ion channels (see Sects. 2.2 and 2.3 of this chapter, above). A second noteworthy behavior of this phenomenon is the very slow time course, taking hours to develop (Hollmann et al. 2004) compared to the several minutes required for inhibiting other GPCRs or the seconds for blocking ion channels (Oyama et al. 1998). One explanation for this very slow time-course is that the suppressed receptors are actually being removed from the plasma membrane—perhaps by some slow endocytotic process that is triggered or enhanced by the local anesthetic per se, or by some metabolic consequence, such as elevation of intracellular Ca^{2+}, that results from other actions of local anesthetics (see below, Sect. 3.3).

2.5
Inhibition of Protein Kinase A and Protein Kinase C

Many activated GPCRs cause acute cellular changes mediated by protein phosphorylation via specific protein kinases, a set of phospholipid-dependent enzymes, some of which are also dependent on calcium. Prominent among these are protein kinase A (PKA) and PKC, which are activated by separate pathways and are directed toward different protein substrates, although they may phosphorylate the same protein in interdependent ways (Cantrell et al. 2002; Cantrell and Catterall 2001). Other kinases, such as calmodulin-dependent kinase II, have also been identified as modulators of ion channels, but we will focus on PKA and PKC in this review as there are some data regarding their sensitivity to local anesthetics.

The PKC family is divided into three subgroups based on sequence homology and cofactor requirements: *classic-conventional* PKC isozymes (PKC-α, -βI, -βII, and -γ), which are Ca^{2+}-dependent and diacylglycerol (DAG)-stimulated kinases; *novel* isozymes (PKC-δ, -ε, -θ, and -η), which are Ca^{2+}-independent and DAG-stimulated kinases; and *atypical* PKC isozymes (PKC-ξ and λ), which are Ca^{2+}- and DAG-independent kinases (Newton 2003). Before stimulation, PKC is located almost exclusively in the cytosol, whereas its hydrophobic activators are present in the membrane. On binding a soluble G protein α-subunit, cytoplasmic PKC then translates to the plasma membrane where it associates with a lipid cofactor, i.e., phosphatidyl serine, and may subsequently modulate neuronal signal transduction by phosphorylation of several types of membrane proteins, including voltage-dependent channels.

There are many different isoenzymes of neuronal PKC, expressed in the brain and in the distal peripheral tissues and the dorsal horn of the spinal cord, that may be involved in pain transmission and in the modulation of nociceptor stimulation. In primary nociceptive neurons, the isozymes PKC-γ and -ε appear to be most important (Aley et al. 2000). They are implicated in the phosphorylation of a class of slow gating Na^+ channels (channels often resistant to inhibition by the classic blocker tetrodotoxin, thus termed "TTX-R," and comprising the channels $Na_v1.8$ and $Na_v1.9$; England et al. 1996; Cardenas et al. 1997; Gold et al. 1996, 1998; Wood et al. 2002; Rush and Waxman 2004; Baker et al. 2003; Baker 2005). Such TTX-R channels are selectively expressed in primary nociceptors (Elliott and Elliott 1993; Rush et al. 1998; Cummins et al. 1999; DibHajj et al. 1999) and contribute critically to increased nociceptive firing after inflammation or injury (Akopian et al. 1999; Porreca et al. 1999; Abdulla and Smith 2002; Roza et al. 2003; Black et al. 2004). Excitability changes after injury may have both rapid and slower components, however, resulting form different underlying processes, such as phosphorylation of existing channels, for the fast responses, and transcriptional regulation or redistribution of existing channels for the slower ones (Devor et al. 1993; Novakovic et al. 1998; Coward et al. 2001).

Several PKC-dependent pathways are suppressed by local anesthetics. One in vitro study assessed the effect of local anesthetics on a PKC-linked cascade of reactions and on the enzymatic activity of PKC itself, indicating that tetracaine and mepivacaine inhibited phosphatidylinositol hydrolysis, i.e., PLC action, an essential step in the activation of PKC (Irvine et al. 1978). Moreover, local anesthetics also inhibited purified PKC activity, possibly by competing with DAG or membrane phospholipid, and the lipid solubility of bupivacaine and mepivacaine correlated with their potency to inhibit PKC subtypes in vitro

(Uratsuji et al. 1985; Mikawa et al. 1990). Although some investigators have suggested that PKC-dependent pathways might have a role in the biochemical mechanism producing spinal anesthesia, there is no correlation between changes in PKC levels and either potency or lipid solubility of the anesthetics (Nivarthi et al. 1996). In immunohistochemical experiments, activation of the MAP kinase extracellular receptor activated kinase (ERK, see Sect. 3.1) in dorsal horn neurons of spinal cord by the PKC activator phorbol myristal acetate was insensitive to bupivacaine, although bupivacaine did inhibit the activation of ERK stimulated by several inotropic receptors (Yanagidate and Strichartz 2006). Such findings indicate that bupivacaine's action occurred neither at PKC itself nor at sites downstream toward ERK. The discrepancy in the results on purified PKC and the enzyme's effects in situ could be explained by a differential sensitivity of different PKC isozymes to local anesthetics or to drug sensitivities that depend on the cofactors for enzyme activation. Thus, particular PKC isozymes may be direct biochemical targets for local anesthetic action, but other sites of local anesthetics may be located along the upstream pathway that activates PKC.

cAMP-dependent protein kinase (PKA) is a major cellular participant in many neuronal functions, including modulation of ion channels (Gold et al. 1998a; Lopshire and Nicol 1998; Evans et al. 1999; Cantrell and Catterall 2001; Vijayaragavan et al. 2004; Yang and Gereau 2004; Matsumoto et al. 2005), and also in the maintenance of inflammatory pain (Aley et al. 1999). These actions of PKA usually increase neuronal excitability, sometimes through the modulation of subthreshold oscillations of membrane potential (Xing et al. 2003; see Amir et al. 1997), in keeping with the general activating role of cAMP in cellular functions. As a specific example in sensory systems, PKA contributes to the activation of ERK in dorsal horn neurons, where its effects are additive with those of PKC, indicating independent pathways (Kawasaki et al. 2004). Since ERK activation in spinal dorsal horn neurons is induced by nociceptive activity (Ji et al. 1999), the activation of spinal PKA is associated with pain signaling; other observations also implicate PKA in pain-related signaling in the peripheral and central nervous systems.

The cAMP–PKA pathway is a typical step in a neuronal second messenger pathway; binding of transmitter to receptor leads to the activation of a stimulatory G protein, G_s, which activates the enzyme adenylyl cyclase. The cyclase in turn catalyzes the conversion of ATP to cAMP. Four cAMP molecules bind to the two regulatory subunits of the cAMP-dependent protein kinase, liberating the two catalytic subunits, which are then free to phosphorylate specific substrate proteins that regulate several cellular response, often interacting in a physiologically synergistic manner (Schwartz and Kandel 2000). As with PKC-related activities, the steps leading to kinase activation as well as the enzyme's activity per se may be affected by local anesthetics.

There are, however, few studies of these effects. Local anesthetics have been reported to exert multiple actions on the catecholamine-sensitive adenylate cyclase system of frogs, thereby reducing its overall responsiveness to stimulation (Voeikov and Lefkowitz 1980). In contrast, bupivacaine had no effect on ERK activation induced by 8-Br-cAMP, a direct activator of PKA, in dorsal horn neurons in slices of spinal cord (Yanagidate and Strichartz 2006). These findings should be cautiously weighted, however, because the cAMP–PKA pathway is a complex nociceptive pathway, and the effects of LAs on different components of the overall pathway have not been established in general.

2.6
Transient Receptor Potential Channels and Local Anesthetics

Transient receptor potential (TRP) channels are widely distributed in mammalian tissue. The TRP family includes at least 20 related cation channels that are responsive to a range of chemical and physical stimuli (Clapham et al. 2001). The functions of TRP channels in sensory neurons include responding to painfully hot temperatures as well as to moderate warming and cooling and, perhaps, to noxious cold. Selectively expressed in many primary nociceptors, TRPV1 mediates the response to painful heat, to extracellular acidosis and to capsaicin, the pungent component in hot peppers (Caterina et al. 2000). TRPV1 is probably a tetramer that forms a nonspecific cation channel, depolarizing the cell by allowing influx of Na^+ and Ca^{2+} ions when it opens. The depolarization further activates other voltage-dependent channels, leading to an increase in excitability (lowering of threshold) for intermediate steady depolarizations or to a membrane that is strongly refractory to stimulation (i.e., a "depolarization block") for larger depolarizations. Entry of Ca^{2+} through the open TRPV1 channel can stimulate further increases in intracellular Ca^{2+}, e.g., via Ca^{2+}-induced Ca^{2+} release from intracellular stores. In addition, intracellular Ca^{2+} may be released in response to capsaicin that acts directly on membranes of the endoplasmic reticulum, an organelle that stores calcium and may contain TRPV1 channels (Karai et al. 2004). In distal terminals of skin, muscle, and joints and in central terminals in the dorsal horn of the spinal cord, activation of TRPV1 elevates intracellular Ca^{2+}, resulting in the release of glutamate and substance P from the primary nociceptor terminals and the subsequent activation of multiple ionotropic and metabotropic receptors on postsynaptic membranes. Some of these activations may have synergistic interactions, e.g., interactions between NK-1 receptors for substance P and N-methyl-D-aspartate (NMDA)-type glutamate receptors. These and other interactions may induce activation of *signal transduction pathways* in spinal neurons that have far-reaching acute and chronic actions (Ji and Strichartz 2004), likely important for central sensitization that contributes strongly to enduring pain from injury and inflammation.

Different local anesthetics appear to have different effects on TRPV1. For example, lidocaine and prilocaine suppress the capsaicin-induced increase in intracellular Ca^{2+} mediated by recombinant TRPV1 receptors (Hirota et al. 2003), and bupivacaine inhibits the capsaicin-induced current in isolated sensory neurons, although tetracaine actually enhances this current (Komai and Mc-Dowell 2005). The reasons underlying this difference are not known, and the sensitivity of other TRP channels to local anesthetics have not been investigated. Intracellular Ca^{2+} is elevated by many local anesthetics in several types of cells (Gold et al. 1998b; Johnson et al. 2002), very possibly through their ability to uncouple mitochondria and thereby release this organelle's stored Ca^{2+} into the cytoplasm (Chance et al. 1968, 1969). Consequently, a number of Ca^{2+}-dependent processes are stimulated by local anesthetics, including calmodulin-dependent reactions that turn on kinases and inactivate Ca^{2+} channels. Thus it is possible that part of the inhibition by local anesthetics of both TRPV1 receptors and other ion channels is due not to a direct action at those sites but through the recruitment of inhibitory pathways activated by such elevated Ca^{2+}.

Local anesthetics appear to have a potentiating effect on the long-lasting, impulse-inhibiting actions of vanilloids. Both in isolated nerves (Shin et al. 1994) and in rat sciatic nerve block in vivo (Kohane et al. 1999), partial reduction of action potentials by local anesthetics is furthered by the addition of capsaicin, possibly through the LA-induced elevation of intracellular Ca^{2+}, which is known to mediate the desensitization of TRPV1 receptors in sensory neurons (Cholewinski et al. 1993). Capsaicin is currently being used therapeutically for the relief of certain neuropathic pains (Rowbotham et al. 1995, 1996), and a related, high-potency vanilloid, resiniferatoxin, is being developed for analgesia via selective blockade of TRPV1-containing primary nociceptors (Kissin et al. 2002, 2005a, b). Both of these applications involve the coadministration of local anesthetics to block the generation of impulses during initial application. Interactions between local anesthetics and the vanilloid receptor are thereby clinically important as well as scientifically interesting.

3
Mechanisms of Spinal and Epidural Anesthesia

The mechanism by which local anesthetics block impulses in peripheral nerves through inhibition of voltage-gated Na^+ channel is well established. In contrast, the overall mechanism for spinal and epidural anesthesia is almost certainly more complex than simply the blockade of impulses in nerve roots, involving pre- and postsynaptic receptors as well as intracellular pathways (Butterworth and Strichartz 1990). Both epidural and spinal (intrathecal) delivery of local anesthetics results in their presence in the spinal cord, as well as in the spinal roots (Gokin and Strichartz 1999), allowing the possibility of altering both synaptic activity and impulse conduction and affecting the responses of cells contained within the spinal cord, including interneurons, astrocytes and microglia. At an even further level of resolution, local anesthetics can interact with membrane phospholipids and proteins and thereby affect various cellular activities. For example, local anesthetics can affect several subtypes of PKC (Mikawa et al. 1990; Nivarthi et al. 1996), PKA (Gordon et al. 1980), G proteins (Hagelüken et al. 1994), and the various receptors that activate them (Hitosugi et al. 1999). As noted above (Sect. 2.4 and 2.5), the effects of LAs on membrane-associated enzymes and second-messenger systems operating in the cytoplasm are extensive. One means of assessing the actions of local anesthetics on integrated responses in spinal cord, such as might occur during a spinal or epidural blockade, is to measure their effects on intracellular signal transduction pathways that are activated by many different inputs and thus report the overall "activation status" of cells in the spinal cord. This approach is described in the following section.

3.1
MAP Kinases and Pain Processing in the Spinal Cord

The mitogen-activated protein kinase (MAPK) enzymes are a family of serine-threonine protein kinases that are activated in response to many stimuli and play important roles in cellular signal transduction, both acutely by protein phosphorylation and chronically by affecting gene transcription. MAPKs were originally implicated in the regulation of mitosis, proliferation, differentiation, and survival of mammalian cells. ERKs 1 and 2 are the best-studied members of the MAPK family that transduce extracellular stimuli into intracellular responses. ERK activation in spinal dorsal horn neurons is driven by afferent activity of primary nociceptors (Ji et al. 1999). An increase in excitation in the superficial dorsal horn, caused by transmitters glutamate and substance P (Conn and Pin 1997), stimulates PKA and PKC, leading to the activation of ERK to pERK by its downstream phosphorylation, and subsequently to all those processes that follow ERK signaling. Elevation of cytoplasmic Ca^{2+} also appears essential for noxious stimulation-induced ERK activation (Lever et al. 2003). All the above-listed factors have been shown to enhance nociceptive processing in the spinal cord dorsal horn, one biochemical correlate of so-called "central sensitization" (Ji and Woolf 2001). Bupivacaine has been shown to suppress neuronal ERK activation in spinal cord slices by a variety of substances, including those that act directly on dorsal horn neurons, giving insight into potential mechanisms for spinal anesthesia.

3.2
Presynaptic or Postsynaptic Sites for LA Inhibition

Synaptic transmission in the spinal cord may be inhibited directly by LAs through the modification of postsynaptic receptors as well as the blockade of presynaptic calcium channels that must function to stimulate the release of transmitters (see Sect. 2.3, above). Bupivacaine can inhibit the elevation in dorsal horn neurons of pERK by excitatory ionotropic receptor agonists such as capsaicin, S-alpha-amino-3-hydroxy-5-methyl-4-isoxazolepropionic acid (AMPA)/kainate, and NMDA, but with no LA effects on ERK activation by GPCRs such as bradykinin, mGluR 1/5, and NK-1, by immunohistochemistry using spinal slices as assayed (Yanagidate and Strichartz 2006). Receptors for capsaicin, acting on the ligand-gated vanilloid-sensitive transient receptor potential channel, TRPV1, are exclusively located at presynaptic terminals of nociceptive afferents. Thus, bupivacaine almost certainly has presynaptic actions, blocking Na^+ channels, Ca^{2+} channels, and TRPV1 receptor channels. On the other hand, AMPA and NMDA are classically located on postsynaptic sites, but also can be found on presynaptic endings. Presynaptic NMDA autoreceptors appear to facilitate the release of substance P and glutamate in a positive-feedback network (Liu et al. 1997). In contrast, AMPA receptors have an excitatory postsynaptic action, but also a strong inhibitory presynaptic action on glutamate release from primary afferent terminals in the superficial dorsal horn (Lee et al. 2002). Therefore, the inhibitory effects of bupivacaine on NMDA-induced pERK might be at both pre- and postsynaptic sites and AMPA-induced pERK must be occurring predominantly through activation of postsynaptic receptors. Ionotropic glutamate receptors are known targets of local anesthetics (Nishizawa et al. 2002; Sugimoto et al. 2003). Other studies also showed the "presynaptic" actions of LAs to inhibit Ca^{2+} channels in dorsal root ganglion neurons, channels that are essential for the release of neurotransmitter during depolarization (Rane et al. 1987). Therefore, LAs will act at many locations to alter functions during spinal and epidural anesthesia, and any understanding of LA actions in the spinal cord should include their effects on a variety of ion channels, membrane-related enzymes, and intracellular second messenger pathways.

Local anesthetics at the neuraxis often provide analgesia synergistic with the actions of other drugs. Examples of the latter include Ca^{2+} channel blockers and opiates.

3.3
Neurotoxicity of Spinal Anesthetics

Toxic systemic reactions to local anesthetics primarily involve the CNS and the cardiovascular system. In general the CNS is more susceptible to the actions of systemic local anesthetics than the cardiovascular system. Thus, the dose and blood level of drug required to produce CNS toxicity, such as tinnitus and faintness, are usually lower than those resulting in cardiac rhythm abnormalities and the negative inotropy that is often followed by cardiovascular collapse (Strichartz and Berde 2005). There is little clinical evidence for functional losses indicative of local neurotoxicity after peripheral nerve block, but considerable data now document a range of neurological symptoms following intrathecal delivery of local anesthetics (Rigler at al. 1991; Schell et al. 1991).

The likelihood of LA spinal neurotoxicity seems to depend on both concentration and exposure time, particularly when lidocaine is injected into the subarachnoid space such that poor mixing with cerebrospinal fluid (CSF) leads to maldistribution and undiluted high local drug concentration (Rigler and Drasner 1991; Ross et al. 1992). The most probable mechanism for these events, which often manifest clinically as cauda equina syndrome, probably due to a loss of functions mediated by lower lumbar and sacral nerve roots, is an irreversible conduction block of these roots (Adams et al. 1974; Ready et al. 1985; Schell et al. 1991; Lambert and Hurley 1991). Exposure of isolated peripheral nerve to high concentrations of lidocaine acutely results in such irreversible blockade (Lambert et al. 1994; Bainton and Strichartz 1994) and also induces death of neurons isolated from rat dorsal root ganglia (Gold et al. 1998b; Johnson et al. 2002).

In vivo studies indicate that LA-induced neurotoxicity does not result from a blockade of voltage-gated Na^+ channels per se (Sakura et al. 1995) and that application of lidocaine to DRG neurons at concentrations greater than 10 mM caused neural death from a direct action of the compound itself, vs the vehicle or the method of administration (Gold et al. 1998b). Although some neuronal Ca^{2+} channels are inhibited by LAs (see Sect. 2.3, above), the lidocaine-induced increase in intracellular Ca^{2+} appears to be the mechanism of lidocaine-induced neuronal toxicity (Gold et al. 1998b; Johnson et al. 2002). Samples of human CSF taken 5 min after administration of a 5% ($\sim$200 mM) solution of lidocaine revealed a mean cerebrospinal drug concentration close to 16 mM (Van Zundert et al. 1996). Therefore, even minutes after dilution of the LA in the relatively large volume of the subarachnoid space, there is an intrathecal lidocaine concentration exceeding 10 mM, which has been proved to be neurotoxic on isolated axons exposed for an even briefer of time (Lambert et al. 1994; Bainton and Strichartz 1994).

Several clinical observations have also suggested that intrathecal local anesthetics, such as lidocaine, cause transient, reversible dysfunction (Rosen et al. 1983; Hampl et al. 1998; Freedman et al. 1998; Auroy et al. 1997; Pollock 2002). The neurological symptoms of this result, including numbness, paresthesias, and pain, often resolve after a day or two, and have been suggested to arise from inflammation of the nerve root, possibly due to perioperative posture (Warner et al. 2000), and appears to be much more frequent when lidocaine is used compared to other local anesthetics (Zaric et al. 2003). Although vasopressors contribute to these neurological symptoms (Sakura et al. 1997) and—together with the role of posture—suggest that ischemia, and possibly post-procedure renfusion, may induce inflammation as the cause of this pathology, no mechanism for these events has been tested.

3.3.1
Local Anesthetics, MAP Kinases and Cell Death

The MAPKs are a family of serine-threonine protein kinases (see Sect. 3.1, above) important for signal transduction from the cell surface to the nucleus, and they participate in the initiation and progression of cell death (Xia et al. 1995). In the nucleus the MAPK ERK phosphorylates transcription factors like Elk-1 and ATF-2, cellular markers for injured neurons. This signaling cascade mediates cellular responses to both growth factors and stress stimuli, and thus participates in cell growth and in cell death. The MAPK type called c-Jun N-terminal kinase (JNKs) includes several stress-activated protein kinases (p46-JUNK1-p54-JUNK2) that are particularly responsive to cellular stress stimuli (Kyriakis et al. 1995). In addition, p38 MAPK, another form that is activated by the specific MAPK-kinases MKK3 and MKK6, also regulates transcription factors such as ATF-2, Elk-1, and CHOP. Recent evidence suggests that many of these MAPKs are activated by cellular stress that is caused, directly or indirectly, by exposure to local anesthetics.

3.3.2
Apoptosis and Necrosis

The cytotoxicity of local anesthetics on different cell types could be caused by various factors. Cell death induced by chemical and physical stress has two forms, apoptosis and necrosis, which are defined by morphological and bio-chemical criteria. Apoptosis is characterized by cellular shrinkage, membrane bleeding, nuclear condensation, and internucleosomal DNA fragmentation (Wyllie et al. 1980). It has been reported that tetracaine-induced apoptosis of PC12 cells is mediated in a complex mode by mechanisms involving members of the MAPK family; ERK activation protects cells from death whereas JNK plays the opposite role (Xia et al. 1995; Kuan et al. 2003). An overload of cytoplasmic Ca^{2+}, rising as a result of activity-dependent or pathophysiological influx or from excessive release from intracellular organelles such as mitochondria, may damage cells by decreasing ERK phosphorylation or by elevating JNK's activity. Importantly the action of LA on cell survival does not involve voltage-gated Na^+ channels (or L-type Ca^{2+} channels, although there are other channels and pathways by which Ca^{2+} inside the cell can be modified; Xu et al. 2003), allowing the predominant therapeutic action of local anesthetics to be isolated from this most undesirable side effect. One in vitro study indicated that lidocaine neurotoxicity involves mitochondrial injury with activation of apoptotic pathways, which may or may not also involve MAPKs (Johnson et al. 2004). In contrast to apoptosis, necrosis is characterized by a rapid swelling of the cell and its subsequent lysis, with random degradation of DNA (Wyllie et al. 1980). Chloroprocaine has been shown to induce Schwann cell necrosis in rat peripheral nerve bundle exposed to this LA in vivo several days beforehand (Myers et al. 1986), and in cultured cells local anesthetics elevate cytoplasmic Ca^{2+} to toxic levels to induce plasma membrane lysis and death (necrosis; Joshi et al. 1999; Johnson et al. 2002).

Therefore, neurotoxicity from local anesthetics appears to be a complex, many-faceted process that may affect axons directly, and also have either direct or indirect (Wallerian degeneration) effects on glia, whether they be peripheral Schwann cells or spinal microglia and astrocytes. The latter two cell types are known to respond to peripheral and central nerve injury or inflammation with activation of different MAPK pathways. Therefore, to the extent that LAs induce acute cellular responses that mimic injury or inflammation, MAPK-mediated responses in neurons and glia may be involved in the overall pathological response.

4
Intravenous Local Anesthetics and Neuropathic Pain

Neuropathic pain arising from injury or disease is often effectively treated by intravenous administration of Na^+ channel blockers, including local anesthetics such as lidocaine (Abram and Yaksh 1994; Kastrup et al. 1987; Kalso et al. 1998; Amir et al. 2006). There are two remarkable features of this usage with regard to the traditional pharmacology of such drugs. First, extraordinarily low plasma concentrations are effective for relieving such pains (Chabal et al. 1989; Ferrante et al. 1996; Chaplan et al. 1995; Sinnott et al. 1999, 2000). Normal neurological functions, including nerve impulses measured electrophysiologically, are immune to such low concentrations of lidocaine (Devor et al. 1992; Chabal et al. 1989; Puig and Sorkin 1995). Regardless of whether the pain arises from disease, such as diabetic neuropathy, or from a previous nerve injury, analgesia occurs during infusions of lidocaine to 2–5 µg/ml free plasma concentration, corresponding to about 8–20 µM lidocaine, or even lower (Strichartz et al. 2002). Standard biophysical methods using a voltage-clamp to study Na^+ channels indicate that their IC_{50} for lidocaine inhibition in resting membranes (see Sect. 2.2, above) is about 200–250 µM (Brau et al. 1998, 2001; Oda et al. 2000). At the same time the local tissue concentrations that can block single action potentials at equilibrium in half of the sensory peripheral nerve axons in vivo are ca. 300 µM for the small myelinated Aδ-fibers, 400 µM for the large myelinated Aβ-fibers, and 800 µM for the small-diameter C-nociceptors (Huang et al. 1997; see notes on the size principle, above, Sect. 2.1). The phasic potentiation of action potential blockade by local anesthetics that occurs during repetitive stimulation can effectively increase the potency, but only by modest factors of approximately two- to five-fold (Gokin et al. 2001). For example, at a relatively low stimulation frequency, 1 Hz, lidocaine's IC_{50} for blocking individual impulses in Aβ-mechanoreceptors is about 350 µM, a value that drops to 250 µM when the fiber is stimulated at 200 Hz, well within its normal physiological firing range (Courtney and Strichartz 1987). None of these values even approaches the therapeutic plasma concentrations of less than 20 μM, leaving us to initially wonder whether these clinical actions result directly, or at all, from Na^+ channel blockade. Indeed, studies on intact animals suggest that a major site of lidocaine's actions may be in the brain (Pertovaara et al. 1996; Chen et al. 2004), and agents that cannot block Na^+ channels from the interstitial fluid (and that cross the blood–brain barrier very slowly) are nevertheless acutely effective at pain relief (Omana-Zapata et al. 1997; Chen et al. 2004).

Recent laboratory experiments, however, have begun to connect impulse blockade phenomena to therapeutic pain relief from systemic local anesthetics. It is known that after nerve injury the number of spontaneously active peripheral nerve fibers increases (Nordin et al. 1984; Kajander and Bennett 1992; Bennett 1994; Devor and Seltzer 1999; Liu et al. 2000) and that these spontaneous discharges often occur in rhythmic bursts that are superimposed on slow oscillations, primarily in medium diameter myelinated fibers (Amir et al. 1999, 2002). In order for such activity to occur, there must be elements of an inward, excitatory current that persist after a single impulse, sufficient to raise the (usually somewhat refractory) post-impulse membrane to threshold (Raymond et al. 1990). This current might come from an anomalous generator that has appeared in the nerve after injury (Black et al. 1999) or by a change in the phenotype of the recognized ion channels. Of the latter, there is evidence that certain Na^+ channels, particularly those that support a very slowly inactivating current, may be "upregulated" after injury (Dib-Hajj et al. 1999; Kerr et al. 2001; Black et al. 2004; Chung et al. 2003; Coggeshall et al. 2004; see Lai et al. 2003 for review). Certain K^+ channels may have reduced expression after nerve injury, and this will have a synergistic interaction with late Na^+ channel increases to promote repetitive firing and to lower threshold (Nashmi and Fehlings 2001; Yang et al. 2004). Under these conditions, action potentials can occur spontaneously. The possibility for repetitive firing is also greatly increased by expression of very slowly inactivating Na^+ channels, e.g., $Na_V1.3$ and $Na_V1.8$, which can maintain an inward current, drive a rebound depolarization, and thus induce impulses repetitively after a single stimulation (Lai et al. 2002; Gold et al. 2003; Kiernan et al. 2003). Voltage-clamp studies show that such Na^+ currents are remarkably sensitive to lidocaine, with effects occurring at the clinically therapeutic concentrations (Baker and Bostock 1997, 1998). It is also possible to experimentally change the gating of Na^+ channels that rapidly inactivate to ones that slowly inactivate by the binding of certain small peptide "toxins" isolated from scorpion venoms or the stinging organ of certain sea anemones (Ulbricht and Schmidtmayer 1981; Wang and Strichartz 1985). This acute action results in prolonged depolarizing plateaus on which repetitive impulses are superimposed after a single stimulus. What is noteworthy is that both the plateau and the repetitive firing are reversibly titrated in vitro by 5–30 μM lidocaine (Khodorova et al. 2001; Persaud and Strichartz 2002), suggesting an action that may occur in vivo during therapeutic treatment. Recall that, by contrast, propagating impulses in peripheral nerve require 0.3–1 mM for full blockade (see Sect. 2.1, above).

These repetitive action potentials are so much more susceptible to lidocaine than the "normal" propagated ones for two reasons. One is pharmacodynamic; the Na^+ channels that are essential for the formation of such abnormal impulse activity remain open for much of the time of the train of impulses, during and between actual spiking. Consequently there is a much longer time for high-affinity binding to the open channel states to occur (Grant et al. 1996, 2000; Hille 1977; Chernoff 1990), and many more channels are blocked than would occur with normally fast-inactivating channels. The second reason is "physiological"; the small inward Na^+ currents that sustain repetitive firing are just sufficient for this task, and the margin of safety is well below that for robustly propagated impulses. Recall that this margin is 5–10 for single action potentials in normal nerve; that is, 5–10 times more charge is delivered than is actually needed to bring the next unexcited region of the membrane to threshold and, correspondingly, about 75%–80% of the Na^+ channels must be inhibited to stop the action potential. In the membrane that supports repetitive firing, however, the net inward current is probably much smaller, the margin of safety might be 1.5 or 2, and inhibition of only 20% of these channels can block repetitive impulses. This latter factor alone accounts for about a tenfold difference in blocking potency for action potentials. Combined with the greater functional potency of local anesthetics binding to the persistently open channels, the overall potency for impulse blockade could imaginably be enhanced 50- to 200-fold, connecting the 10- to 20-µM lidocaine concentration for relief of neuropathic pain to the 300- to 1,000-µM concentration for blocking normal nerve impulses.

The second remarkable aspect of neuropathic pain relief by systemic local anesthetics is the unexpectedly long duration of that action. In both clinical trials and especially in animal models of nerve injury-induced mechanical or thermal hypernociception, the effects of a 30- to 60-min lidocaine infusion might last for several days, weeks, or even months (Chaplan et al. 1995; Sinnott et al. 1999). This is not a continuous reversal of pain, however, but one that shows several clearly separable phases (Araujo et al. 2003). Reversal of allodynia occurs when drug infusion ends, but allodynia is again relieved beginning hours later, peaking about 1 day later and then persisting for at least several weeks. Plasma levels of lidocaine fall to near zero within several hours after infusion ends, and the less active metabolic products do not last much longer (Kawai et al. 1985), obviating the likelihood that the persistent effect is from some long-dwelling drug. Experiments on isolated nerve after exposure to even higher lidocaine concentrations show a complete return to pre-drug electrical activity within an hour after washout has begun. Pain relief, it appears, is not due to the prolonged pharmacological blockade of ionic Na^+ channels. There may be other local anesthetic actions that alter neural injury responses, however, such as the inhibition of outgrowth of neurites (Hiruma et al. 1999) that are potential loci of hyperexcitability (Devor et al. 1993, 1999), inhibition of axonal transport (Lavoie et al. 1989; Kanai et al. 2001), or the destabilization of newly inserted channels within the plasma membrane (Novakovic et al. 1998; Coward et al. 2001; Gold et al. 2003). These actions thus tend to restore the channel population to its pre-injury state. At this writing, January 2006, these are untested speculations and the actual mechanisms of this intriguing effect await further investigation.

A third notable feature of the reversal of injury-induced allodynia by systemic lidocaine is the dependence of effectiveness on the treatment time after injury. Relatively early infusions given to rats just 2 days after nerve ligation show both the transient reversal phase during infusion and the persistent relief that develops later (Araujo et al. 2003). Allodynia that appears on the paw contralateral to the injured limb, which usually takes 4–5 days to manifest itself, is actually prevented by lidocaine infusion at post-injury day 2. When lidocaine is infused later, however, 7 days after the injury, the late phase of relief is present but cannot be sustained and disappears after several days, despite the robust degree of relief during the brief infusion at 7 days. The contralateral pain, having appeared by the time of the infusion, cannot be prevented but is also transiently suppressed by lidocaine treatment.

These findings in one animal model for neuropathic pain might be broadly generalized to clinical situations. Many types of chronic pain from injury or disease are responsive to systemic lidocaine, but not all patients are responsive, some receive no therapeutic benefit, and the duration of effect is also quite variable. Repeated lidocaine administration to the same plasma concentration in the same rats did not provide any incrementally accumulating relief; some rats had an almost complete reversal of allodynia whereas others were minimally responsive, despite the intentional genetic identity of these animals (Sinnott et al. 1999). Humans, on the other hand, often benefit with increased pain relief from each infusion in a series of treatments, usually spaced weeks apart. Tachyphylaxis to this treatment has not been clearly documented. Although neuropathic pain from nerve injury and from disease are both treatable by i.v. lidocaine, the conditions that optimize clinical pain relief from such inexpensive and generally safe treatments have not been systematically investigated, despite the broad use of this therapy. Hence, its profile of effectiveness in a range of animal models also deserves attention.

References

Abdulla FA, Smith PA (2002) Changes in Na(+) channel currents of rat dorsal root ganglion neurons following axotomy and axotomy-induced autotomy. J Neurophysiol 88: 2518–2529
Abram SE, Yaksh TL (1994) Systemic lidocaine blocks nerve injury-induced hyperalgesia and nociceptor-driven spinal sensitization in the rat. Anesthesiology 80:383–391

Adams HJ, Mastri AR, Eichollzer AW, Kilpatrick G (1974) Morphologic effects of intrathecal etidocaine and tetracaine on the rabbit spinal cord. Anesth Analg 53:994–998

Akopian AN, Souslova V, England S, Okuse K, Ogata N, Ure J, Smith A, Kerr BJ, McMahon SB, Boyce S, Hill R, Stanfa LC, Dickenson AH, Wood JH (1999) The tetrodotoxin-resistant sodium channel SNS has a specialized function in pain pathways. Nat Neurosci 2:541–548

Aley KO, Levine JD (1999) Role of protein kinase A in the maintenance of inflammatory pain. J Neurosci 19:2181–2186

Aley KO, Messing RO, Mochly-Rosen D, Levine JD (2000) Chronic hypersensitivity for inflammatory nociceptor sensitization mediated by the epsilon isozyme of protein kinase C. J Neurosci 20:4680–4685

Amir R, Devor M (1997) Spike-evoked suppression and burst patterning in dorsal root ganglion neurons. J Physiol (Lond) 501:183–196

Amir R, Michaelis M, Devor M (1999) Membrane potential oscillations in dorsal root ganglion neurons. Role in normal electrogenesis and neuropathic pain. J Neurosci 19: 8589–8596

Amir R, Michaelis M, Devor M (2002) Burst discharge in primary sensory neurons triggered by subthreshold oscillations, maintained by depolarizing after potentials. J Neurosci 22:1187–1198

Amir R, Argoff CE, Bennett GJ, Cummins TR, Durieux ME, Gerner P, Gold MS, Porreca F, Strichartz GR (2006) The role of sodium channels in chronic inflammatory and neuro-pathic pain. J Pain (in press)

Araujo MC, Sinnott CJ, Strichartz GR (2003) Multiple phases of relief from experimental mechanical allodynia by systemic lidocaine: responses to early and late infusions. Pain 103:21–29

Arner S, Lindblom U, Meyerson BA, Molander C (1990) Prolonged relief of neuralgia after regional anesthetic blocks. A call for further experimental and systematic clinical studies. Pain 43:287–297

Auroy Y, Narchi P, Messiah A, Litt L, Rouvier B, Samii K (1997) Serious complications related to regional anesthetic blocks. A call for further experimental and systematic clinical studies. Anesthesiology 87:479–486

Bainton CR, Strichartz GR (1994) Concentration dependence of lidocaine-induced irre-versible conduction loss in frog nerve. Anesthesiology 81:657–667

Baker MD (2005) Protein kinase C mediates up-regulation of tetrodotoxin-resistant, persis-tent Na+ current in rat mouse sensory neurones. J Physiol 567:851–867

Baker MD, Bostock H (1997) Low-threshold, persistent sodium current in rat large dorsal root ganglion neurons in culture. J Neurophysiol 77:1503–1513

Baker MD, Bostock H (1998) Inactivation of macroscopic late Na+ current and characteris-tics of unitary late Na+ currents in sensory neurons. J Neurophysiol 80:2538–2549

Baker MD, Chandra SY, Ding Y, Waxman SG, Wood JN (2003) GTP-induced tetrodotoxin-resistant Na+ current regulates excitability in mouse and rat small diameter sensory neurones. J Physiol 548:373–382

Balser JR, Nuss HB, Orias DW, Johns DC, Marban E, Tomaselli GF, Lawrence JH (1996) Local anesthetics as effectors of allosteric gating. Lidocaine effects on inactivation-deficient rat skeletal muscle Na channels. J Clin Invest 98:2874–2886

Benkwitz C, Garrison JC, Linden J, Durieux ME, Hollmann MW (2003) Lidocaine enhances Galphai protein function. Anesthesiology 99:1093–1101

Bennett GJ (1994) Neuropathic pain. In: Wall PD, Melzack R (eds) Textbook of pain, 3rd edn. Churchill Livingstone, Edinburgh, pp 201–224

Bischoff U, Brau ME, Vogel W, Hempelmann G, Olschewski A (2003) Local anesthetics block hyperpolarization-activated inward current in rat small dorsal root ganglion neurons. Br J Pharmacol 139:1273–81270

Black JA, Cummins TR, Plumpton C, Chen YH, Hormuzdiar W, Clare JJ, Waxman SG (1999) Upregulation of a silent sodium channel after peripheral, but not central, nerve injury in DRG neurons. J Neurophysiol 82:2776–2785

Black JA, Liu S, Tanaka M, Cummins TR, Waxman SG (2004) Changes in the expression of tetrodotoxin-sensitive sodium channels within dorsal root ganglia neurons in inflammatory pain. Pain 108:237–247

Boas RA, Covino BG, Shahnarian A (1982) Analgesic responses to i.v. lignocaine. Br J Anaesth 54:501–504

Brau ME, Branitzki P, Olschewski A, Vogel W, Hempelmann G (1995) Block of neuronal tetrodotoxin-resistant Na+ currents by stereoisomers of piperidine local anesthetics. Anesth Analg 91:1499–1505

Brau ME, Vogel W, Hempelmann G (1998) Fundamental properties of local anesthetics: half-maximal blocking concentrations for tonic block of Na+ and K+ channels in peripheral nerve. Anesth Analg 87:885–889

Brau ME, Dreimann M, Olschewski A, Vogel W, Hempelmann G (2001) Effect of drugs used for neuropathic pain management on tetrodotoxin-resistant Na(+) currents in rat sensory neurons. Anesthesiology 94:137–144

Butterworth JF, Strichartz GR (1990) Molecular mechanisms of local anesthesia: a review. Anesthesiology 72:711–734

Cantrell AR, Catterall WA (2001) Neuromodulation of Na+ channels: an unexpected form of cellular plasticity. Nat Rev Neurosci 2:397–407

Cantrell AR, Tibbs VC, Yu FH, Murphy BJ, Sharp EM, Qu Y, Catterall WA, Scheuer T (2002) Molecular mechanism of convergent regulation of brain Na+ channels by protein kinase C and protein kinase A anchored to AKAP-15. Mol Cell Neurosci 21:63–80

Cardenas CG, Del Mar LP, Cooper BY, Scroggs RS (1997) 5HT4 receptors couple positively to tetrodotoxin-insensitive sodium channels in a subpopulation of capsaicin-sensitive rat sensory neurons. J Neurosci 17:7181–7189

Carmeliet E, Morad M, Van der Heyden G (1986) Electrophysical effects of tetracaine in single guinea-pig ventricular myocytes. J Physiol 376:143–161

Castle NA (1990) Bupivacaine inhibits the transient outward K+ current but not the inward rectifier in rat ventricular myocytes. J Pharmacol Exp Ther 255:1038–1046

Caterina MJ, Leffler A, Malmaberg AB, et al (2000) Impaired nociception and pain sensation in mice lacking the capsaicin receptor. Science 288:306–313

Catterall WA (2000) From ionic currents to molecular mechanisms: the structure and function of voltage-gated sodium channels. Neuron 26:13–25

Chabal C, Russell LC, Burchiel KJ (1989) The effect of intravenous lidocaine, tocainide, and mexiletine on spontaneously active fibers originating in rat sciatic neuromas. Pain 38:333–338

Chance B, Mela L, Harris EJ (1968) Interaction of ion movements and local anesthetics in mitochondrial membranes. Fed Proc 27:902–906

Chance B, Azzi A, Mela L, Radda G, Vainio H (1969) Local anesthetic induced changes of a membrane-bound fluorochrome A link between ion uptake and membrane structure. FEBS Lett 3:10–13

Chaplan SR, Bach FW, Shafer SL, Yaksh TL (1995) Prolonged alleviation of tactile allodynia by intravenous lidocaine in neuropathic rats. Anesthesiology 83:775–785

Chaplan SR, Guo HQ, Lee DH, Luo L, Liu C, Kuei C, Velumain AA, Butler MP, Brown SM, Dubin AE (2003) Neuronal hyperpolarization-activated pacemaker channels drive neuropathic pain. J Neurosci 23:1169–1178

Chen Q, King T, Vanderah TW, Ossipov MH, Malan TP, Lai J, Porreca F (2004) Differential blockade of nerve injury-induced thermal and tactile hypersensitivity by systemically administered brain-penetrating and peripherally restricted local anesthetics. J Pain 5:281–289

Chernoff DM (1990) Kinetic analysis of phasic inhibition of neuronal sodium currents by lidocaine and bupivacaine. Biophys J 58:53–68

Cholewinski A, Burgess GM, Bevan S (1993) The role of calcium in capsaicin-induced desensitization in rat cultured dorsal root ganglion neurons. Neuroscience 44: 1015–1023

Chung JM, Dib-Hajj SD, Lawson SN (2003) Sodium channel subtypes and neuropathic pain. In: Dostrovsky JO, Carr DB, Koltzenburg M (eds) Proceedings of the 10th World Congress on Pain, Progress in Pain Research and Management, vol 24. IASP Press, Seattle, pp 99–114

Clapham DE, Runnels LW, Strubing C (2001) The TRP ion channel family. Nat Rev Neurosci 2:387–396

Coggeshall RE, Tate S, Carlton SM (2004) Differential expression of tetrodotoxin-resistant sodium channels Nav1.8 and Nav1.9 in normal and inflamed rats. Neurosci Lett 355: 45–48

Condliffe AM, Kitchen E, Chilvers ER (1998) Neutrophil priming: pathophysiological consequences and underlying mechanisms. Clin Sci (Lond) 94:461–471

Conn PJ, Pin JP (1997) Pharmacology and functions of metabotropic glutamate receptors. Annu Rev Pharmacol Toxicol 37:205–237

Courtney KR, Kendig JJ (1988) Bupivacaine is an effective potassium channel blocker in heart. Biochim Biophys Acta 999:163–166

Courtney KR, Strichartz GR (1987) Structural elements which determine local anesthetic activity. In: Strichartz GR (ed) Local anesthetics. (Handbook of experimental pharmacology, vol 81) Springer-Verlag, Berlin Heidelberg New York, pp 53–94

Coward K, Mosahebi A, Plumpton C, Facer P, Birch R, Tate S, Bountra C, Terenghi G, Anand P (2001) Immunolocalisation of sodium channel NaG in the intact and injured human peripheral nervous system. J Anat 198:175–180

Cummins TR, Dib-Hajj SD, Black JA, Akopian AN, Wood JN, Waxman SG (1999) A novel persistent tetrodotoxin-resistant sodium current in SNS-null and wild-type small primary sensory neurons. J Neurosci 19:RC43

de Paula S, Schreier S (1995) Use of a novel method for determination of partition coefficients to compare the effect of a local anesthetics on membrane structure. Biochim Biophys Acta 1240:25–33

Devor M, Seltzer Z (1999) Pathophysiology of damaged nerves in relation to chronic pain. In: Wall PD, Melzack R (eds) Textbook of pain, 4th edn. Churchill-Livingston, London, pp 129–164

Devor M, Wall PD, Catalan N (1992) Systemic lidocaine silences ectopic neuroma and DRG discharge without blocking nerve conduction. Pain 48:261–268

Devor M, Govrin-Lippman R, Angelides K (1993) Sodium channel immunolocalization in peripheral mammalian axons and changes following nerve injury and neuroma formation. J Neurosci 13:1976–1992

Dib-Hajj S, Fjell J, Cummins TR, Zheng Z, Fried K, LaMotte R, Black JA, Waxman SG (1999) Plasticity of sodium channel expression in DRG neurons in the chronic constriction injury model of neuropathic pain. Pain 83:591–600

Doan TN, Stephans K, Ramirez AN, Glazebrook PA, Andresen MC, Kunze DL (2004) Differential distribution and function of hyperpolarization-activated channels in sensory neurons and mechanosensitive fibers. J Neurosci 24:3335–3343

Drachman D, Strichartz GR (1991) Potassium channel blockers potentiate impulse inhibition by local anesthetics. Anesthesiology 75:1051–1061

Elliott AA, Elliott JR (1993) Characterization of TTX-sensitive and TTX-resistant sodium currents in small cells from adult rat dorsal root ganglia. J Physiol 463:39–56

England S, Bevan S, Docherty RJ (1996) PGE2 modulates the tetrodotoxin-resistant sodium current in neonatal rat dorsal root ganglion neurons via the cyclic AMP-protein kinase A cascade. J Physiol (Lond) 495:429–440

Evans AR, Vasko MR, Nicol GD (1999) The cAMP transduction cascade mediates the PGE2-induced inhibition potassium currents in rat sensory neurons. J Physiol 516:163–178

Ferrante FM, Paggiol J, Cherukuri S, Arthur GR (1996) The analgesic response to intravenous lidocaine in the treatment of neuropathic pain. Anesth Analg 82:91–97

Fischer LG, Bremer M, Coleman EJ, Conrad B, Krumm B, Gross A, Hollmann MW, Mandell G, Durieux ME (2001) Local anesthetics attenuate lysophosphatidic acid-induced priming in human neutrophils. Anesth Analg 92:1041–1047

Freedman JM, Li DK, Drasner K, et al (1998) Transient neurologic symptoms after spinal anesthesia: an epidemiologic study of 1,863 patients [erratum appears in Anesthesiology 1998 Dec:89(6):1614]. Anesthesiology 89:633–641

Gerner P, Mujtaba M, Sinnott CJ, Wang GK (2001) Amitriptyline versus bupivacaine in rat sciatic. nerve blockade. Anesthesiology 94:661–667

Gokin A, Strichartz G (1999) Local anesthetics acting on the spinal cord. Access, distribution, pharmacology and toxicology. In: Yaksh TL (ed) Spinal drug delivery: anatomy, kinetics and toxicology. Elsevier Science, New York, pp 477–501

Gokin AP, Philip B, Strichartz GR (2001) Preferential block of small myelinated sensory and motor fibers by lidocaine: in vivo electrophysiology in the rat sciatic nerve. Anesthesiology 95:1441–1454

Gold MS, Reichling DB, Shuster MJ, Levine JD (1996) Hyperalgesic agents increase a tetrodotoxin-resistant Na+ current in nociceptors. Proc Natl Acad Sci U S A 93:1108–1112

Gold MS, Levine JD, Correa AM (1998a) Modulation of TTX-R INa by PKC and PKA and their role in PG2-induced sensitization of rat sensory neurons in vitro. J Neurosci 18:10345–10355

Gold MS, Reichling DB, Shuster MJ, Levine JD (1998b) Lidocaine toxicity in primary afferent neurons from the rat. J Pharmacol Exp Ther 285:413–421

Gold MS, Weinrich D, Kim CS, Wang R, Treanor J, Porecca F, Lai J (2003) Redistribution of Na(V)1.8 in uninjured axons enables neuropathic pain. J Neurosci 23:158–166

Gordon LM, Dipple I, Sauerheber RD, Esgate MA, Houslay MD (1980) The selective effects of charged local anaesthetics on the glucagon- and fluoride-stimulated adenylate cyclase activity of rat-liver plasma membranes. J Supramol Struct 14:21–32

Grant AO, John JE, Nesterenko VV, Starmer CF, Moorman JR (1996) The role of inactivation in open-channel block of the sodium channel: studies with inactivation-deficient mutant channels. Mol Pharmacol 50:1643–1650

Guo X, Castle NA, Chernoff DM, Strichartz GR (1991) Comparative inhibition of voltage gated cation channels by anesthetics. Ann N Y Acad Sci 625:181–199

Hagelüken A, Grünbaum L, Nürnberg B, Harhammer R, Seifert R (1994) Lipophilic beta-adrenoceptor antagonists and local anesthetics are effective direct activators of G-proteins. Biochem Pharmacol 47:1789–1795

Hampl KF, Heinzmann-Wiedmer S, Luginbuehl I, Harms C, Seeberger M, Schneider MC, Drasner K (1998) Transient neurologic symptoms: after spinal anesthesia. A lower incidence of with prilocaine and bupivacaine that with lidocaine. Anesthesiology 88:629–633

Herzog RI, Cummins TR, Waxman SG (2001) Persistent TTX-resistant Na+ current affects resting potential and response to depolarization in simulated spinal sensory neurons. J Neurophysiol 86:1351–1364

Hille B (1977) Local anesthetics: hydrophilic and hydrophobic pathways for the drug-receptor reaction. J Gen Physiol 69:497–515

Hille B (2001) Ion channels of excitable membranes. Sinauer Associates, Sunderland

Hirota K, Browne T, Appadu BL, Lambert DG (1997) Do local anaesthetics interact with dihydropyridine binding sites on neuronal L-type Ca^{2+} channels? Br J Anaesth 78: 185–188

Hirota K, Smart D, Lambert DG (2003) The effects of local and intravenous anesthetics on recombinant rat VR1 vanilloid receptors. Anesth Analg 96:1656–1660

Hiruma H, Maruyama H, Simada ZB, Katakura T, Hoka S, Takenaka T, Kawakami T (1999) Lidocaine inhibits neurite growth in mouse dorsal root ganglion cells in culture. Acta Neurobiol Exp (Wars) 59:323–327

Hitosugi H, Kashiwazaki T, Ohsawa M, Kamei J (1999) Effects of mexiletine on algogenic mediator-induced nociceptive responses in mice. Methods Find Exp Clin Pharmacol 21:409–413

Hollman M, Durieux M (2000) Local anesthetics and the inflammatory response: a new therapeutic indication? Anesthesiology 93:858–875

Hollmann MW, Fischer LG, Byford AM, Durieux ME (2000) Local anesthetic inhibition of m1 muscarinic acetylcholine signaling. Anesthesiology 93:497–509

Hollmann MW, Difazio CA, Durieux ME (2001a) Ca-signaling G-protein-coupled receptors: a new site of local anesthetic action? Reg Anesth Pain Med 26:565–571

Hollmann MW, Wieczorek KS, Berger A, Durieux ME (2001b) Local anesthetic inhibition of G protein-coupled receptor signaling by interference with Galpha(q) protein function. Mol Pharmacol 59:294–301

Hollmann MW, Ritter CH, Henle P, de Klaver M, Kamatchi GL, Durieux ME (2001c) Inhibition of m3 muscarinic acetylcholine receptors by local anaesthetics. Br J Clin Pharmacol 133:207–216

Hollmann MW, Gross A, Jelacin N, Durieux ME (2001d) Local anesthetic effects on priming and activation of human neutrophils. Anesthesiology 95:113–122

Hollmann MW, McIntire WE, Garrison JC, Durieux ME (2002) Inhibition of mammalian Gq protein function by local anesthetics. Anesthesiology 97:1451–1457

Hollmann MW, Herroeder S, Kurz KS, Hoenmann CW, Struemper D, Hahnenkamp K, Durieux ME (2004) Time-dependent inhibition of G protein-coupled receptor signaling by local anesthetics. Anesthesiology 100:852–860

Honemann CW, Arledge JA, Podranski T, Aken HV, Durieux M (1999) Volatile and local anesthetics interfere with thromboxane A2 receptors recombinantly expressed in Xenopus oocytes. Adv Exp Med Biol 469:277–283

Huang JH, Thalhammer JG, Raymond SA, Strichartz GR (1997) Susceptibility to lidocaine of impulses in different somatosensory afferent fibers of rat sciatic nerve. J Pharmacol Exp Ther 292:802–811

Irvine RF, Hemington N, Dawson RM (1978) The hydrolysis of phosphatidylinositol by lysosomal enzymes of rat liver and brain. Biochem J 176:475–484

Ji RR, Strichartz G (2004) Cell signaling and the genesis of neuropathic pain. Sci STKE 2004:reE14

Ji RR, Woolf CJ (2001) Neuronal plasticity and signal transduction in nociceptive neurons: implications for the initiation and maintenance of pathological pain. Neurobiol Dis 8:1–10

Ji RR, Baba H, Brenner GJ, Woolf CJ (1999) Nociceptive-specific activation of ERK in spinal neurons contributes to pain hypersensitivity. Nat Neurosci 2:1114–1119

Johnson ME, Saenz JA, DaSilva AD, Uhl CB, Gores GJ (2002) Effect of local anesthetic on neuronal cytoplasmic calcium and plasma membrane lysis (necrosis) in a cell culture model. Anesthesiology 97:1466–1476

Johnson ME, Uhl CB, Spittler KH, Wang H, Gores GJ (2004) Mitochondrial injury and caspase activation by the local anesthetic lidocaine. Anesthesiology 101:1184–1194

Josephson IR (1988) Lidocaine blocks Na, Ca, and K currents in chick ventricular myocytes. J Mol Cell Cardiol 20:593–604

Joshi PG, Singh A, Ravichandra B (1999) High concentrations of tricyclic antidepressants increase intracellular Ca^{2+} in cultured neural cells. Neurochem Res 24:391–3988

Kajander KC, Bennett GJ (1992) Onset of a painful peripheral neuropathy in rat: a partial and differential deafferentation and spontaneous discharge in A beta and A delta primary afferent neurons. J Neurophysiol 68:734–744

Kalso E, Tramer MR, McQuay HJ, Morre RA (1998) Systemic local-anaesthetic-type drugs in chronic pain: a systematic review. Eur J Pain 2:3–14

Kanai A, Hiruma H, Katakura T, Sase S, Kawakami T, Hoka S (2001) Low-concentration lidocaine rapidly inhibits axonal transport in cultured mouse dorsal root ganglion neurons. Anesthesiology 95:675–680

Karai LJ, Russell JT, Iadrola MJ, Olah Z (2004) Vanilloid receptor 1 regulates multiple calcium compartments and contributes to Ca^{2+}-induced Ca^{2+} release in sensory neurons. J Biol Chem 279:16377–16387

Kastrup J, Petersen P, Dejgard A, Angelo HR, Hilsted J (1987) Intravenous lidocaine infusion—a new treatment of chronic painful diabetic neuropathy? Pain 28:69–75

Kawai R, Fujita S, Suzuki T (1985) Simultaneous quantitation of lidocaine and it four metabolites by high-performance liquid chromatography: application to studies on in vitro and in vivo metabolism of lidocaine in rats. J Pharm Sci 74:1219–1224

Kawasaki Y, Kohno T, Zhuang ZY, Brenner GJ, Wang H, Vandermeer C, Befort K, Woolf CJ, Ji RR (2004) Ionotropic and metabotropic receptors, protein kinase A, protein kinase C, and Src contribute to C-fiber-induced ERK activation and cAMP response element-binding protein phosphorylation in dorsal neurons, leading to central sensitization. J Neurosci 24:8310–8321

Kerr BJ, Souslova V, McMahon SB, Wood JN (2001) A role for the TTX-resistant sodium channel Nav 1.8 in NGF-induced hyperalgesia, but not neuropathic pain. Neuroreport 12:3077–3080

Khodorova A, Meissner K, Lee-Son S, Strichartz GR (2001) Lidocaine selectively blocks abnormal impulses arising from noninactivating Na channels. Muscle Nerve 24:634–647

Kiernan MC, Baker MD, Bostock H (2003) Characteristics of late Na(+) current in adult rat small sensory neurons. Neuroscience 119:653–660

Kindler CH, Yost CS, Gray AT (1999) Local anesthetic inhibition of baseline potassium channels with two pore domains in tandem. Anesthesiology 90:1092–1102

Kissin EY, Frietas CF, Kissin I (2005b) The effects of intraarticular resiniferatoxin in experimental knee-joint arthritis. Anesth Analg 101:1433–1439

Kissin I, Bright CA, Bradley EL (2002) Selective and long lasting neural blockade with resiniferatoxin prevents inflammatory pain and hypersensitivity. Anesth Analg 94: 1253–1258

Kissin I, Davison N, Bradley EL Jr (2005a) Perineural resiniferatoxin prevents hyperalgesia in a rat model of postoperative pain. Anesth Analg 100:774–780

Kohane DS, Kuang Y, Lu NT, Langer R, Strichartz GR, Berde CB (1999) Vanilloid receptor agonists potentiate the in vivo local anesthetic activity of percutaneously injected site 1 sodium channel blockers. Anesthesiology 90:524–534

Koltzenburg M, Torebjork HE, Wahren LK (1994) Nociceptor modulated central sensitization causes mechanical hyperalgesia in acute chemogenic and chronic neuropathic pain. Brain 117:579–591

Komai H, McDowell TS (2001) Local anesthetic inhibition of voltage-activated potassium currents in rat dorsal root ganglion neurons. Anesthesiology 94:1089–1095

Komai H, McDowell TS (2005) Differential effects of bupivacaine and tetracaine on capsaicin-induced currents in dorsal root ganglion neurons. Neurosci Lett 380:21–25

Kondratiev A, Tomaselli GF (2003) Altered gating and local anesthetic block mediated by residues in the l-S6 and ll-S6 transmembrane segments of voltage-dependent Na+ channels. Mol Pharmacol 64:741–752

Kuan CY, Whitmarsh AJ, Yang DD, Liao G, Schloemer AJ, Dong C, Bao J, Banasiak KJ, Haddad GG, Flavell RA, Davis RJ, Rakic P (2003) A critical role of neural specific JNK3 for ischemic apoptosis. Proc Natl Acad Sci USA 100:15184–15189

Kyriakis JM, Woodgett JR, Avruch J (1995) The stress-activated protein kinases. A novel ERK subfamily responsive to cellular stress and inflammatory cytokines. Ann N Y Acad Sci 766:303–319

Lai J, Gold MS, Kim CS, Bian D, Ossipov MH, Hunter JC, Porreca F (2002) Inhibitions of neuropathic pain by decreased expression of the tetrodotoxin-resistant sodium channel, NaV1.8. Pain 95:143–152

Lai J, Hunter JC, Porreca F (2003) The role of voltage-gated sodium channels in neuropathic pain. Curr Opin Neurobiol 13:291–297

Lambert DH, Hurley RJ (1991) Cauda equina syndrome and continuous spinal anesthesia. Anesth Analg 72:817–819

Lambert LA, Lambert DH, Strichartz GR (1994) Conduction block in isolated nerve by high concentrations local anesthetics. Anesthesiology 80:1082–1093

Lavoie PA, Khazen T, Filion PR (1989) Mechanisms of the inhibition of fast axonal transport by local anesthetics. Neuropharmacology 28:175–181

Lee CJ, Bardoni R, Tong CK, Engelman HS, Joseph DJ, Magherini PC, MacDermott AB (2002) Functional expression of AMPA receptors on central terminals of rat dorsal root ganglion neurons and presynaptic inhibition of glutamate release. Neuron 35:135–146

Lee DH, Chang L, Sorkin LS, Chaplan SR (2005) Hyperpolarization-activated, cation-nonselective, cyclic nucleotide-modulated channel blockade alleviates mechanical allodynia and suppresses ectopic discharge in spinal nerve ligated rats. J Pain 6:417–424

Lee-Son S, Wang GK, Concus A, Crill E, Strichartz G (1992) Stereoselective inhibition of neuronal sodium channels by local anesthetics: evidence for two sites of action? Anesthesiology 77:324–335

Lever IJ, Pezet S, McMahon SB, Malcangio M (2003) The signaling components of sensory fiber transmission involved in the activation of ERK MAP kinase in the mouse dorsal horn. Mol Cell Neurosci 24:259–270

Li HL, Galue A, Meadows L, Ragsdale DS (1999) A molecular basis for the different local anesthetic affinities of resting versus open and inactivated states of the sodium channel. Mol Pharmacol 55:134–141

Li YM, Wingrove DE, Too HP, Marnerakis M, Stimson ER, Strichartz GR, Maggio JE (1995) Local anesthetics inhibit substance P binding and evoked increases in intracellular CA2+. Anesthesiology 82:166–173

Lissi E, Bianconi ML, Amaral AT, de Paula E, Bianch LEB, Schreier S (1990) Methods for the determination of partition coefficients based on the effects of solutes upon membrane structure. Biochim Biophys Acta 1021:46–50

Liu BG, Zhuang XL, Li ST, Xu GH, Brull SJ, Zhang JM (2001) Effects of bupivacaine and ropivacaine on high-voltage-activated calcium currents of the dorsal horn neurons in. newborn rats. Anesthesiology 95:139–143

Liu H, Mantyh PW, Basbaum AI (1997) NMDA-receptor regulation of substance P release from primary afferent nociceptors. Nature 386:721–724

Lopshire JC, Nicol GD (1998) The cAMP transduction cascade mediates the prostaglandin E2 enhancement of the capsaicin-elicited current in rat sensory neurons: whole-cell and single-channel studies. J Neurosci 18:6081–6092

Macdonald SG, Duman JJ, Boyd ND (1996) Chemical cross-linking of the substance P (NK-1) receptor to the alpha subunits of the G proteins Gq and G11. Biochemistry 35:2909–2916

Mao J, Chen L (2000) Systemic lidocaine for neuropathic pain relief. Pain 87:7–17

Matsumoto S, Ikeda M, Yoshida S, Tanimoto T, Takeda M, Nasu M (2005) Prostaglandin E2-induced modification of tetrodotoxin-resistant Na+ currents involves activation of both EP2 and EP4 receptors in neonatal no dose ganglion neurones. Br J Clin Pharmacol 145:503–513

Mikawa K, Maekawa N, Hoshina H, Tanaka O, Shirakawa J, Goto R, Obara H, Kusunoki M (1990) Inhibitory effect of barbiturates and local anaesthetics on protein kinase C activation. J Int Med Res 18:153–160

Myers RR, Kalichman MW, Reisner LS, Powell HC (1986) Neurotoxicity of local anesthetics: altered perineurial permeability, edema and nerve fiber injury. Anesthesiology 64:29–35

Nashmi R, Fehlings MG (2001) Mechanisms of axonal dysfunction after spinal cord injury: with an emphasis on the role of voltage-gated potassium channels. Brain Res 38:165–191

Nau C, Strichartz GR (2002) Drug chirality in anesthesia. Anesthesiology 97:497–502

Nau C, Wang GK (2004) Topical review: interactions of local anesthetics with voltage-gated Na+ channels. J Membr Biol 201:1–8

Nau C, Wang SY, Strichartz GR, Wang GK (1999) Point mutations at N434 in D1-S6 of mu1 Na(+) channels modulate binding affinity and stereoselectivity of local anesthetic enantiomers. Mol Pharmacol 56:404–413

Nau C, Wang SY, Wang GK (2003) Point mutations at L1280 in Nav1.4 channel D3-s6 modulate binding affinity and stereoselectivity of bupivacaine enantiomers. Mol Pharmacol 63:1398–1406

Newton AC (2003) Regulation of the ABC kinases by phosphorylation: protein kinase C as a paradigm. Biochem J 370:361–371

Nietgen GW, Chan CK, Durieux ME (1997) Inhibition of lysophosphatidate signaling by lidocaine and bupivacaine. Anesthesiology 86:1112–1119

Nishizawa N, Shirasaki T, Nakao S, Matsuda H, Shingu K (2002) The inhibition of the N-methyl-d-aspartate receptor channel by local anesthetics in mouse CA1 pyramidal neurons. Anesth Analg 94:325–330

Nivarthi RN, Grant GJ, Turndorf H, Bansinath M (1996) Spinal anesthesia by local anesthetics stimulates the enzyme protein kinase C and induces the expression of an immediate early oncogene, c-Fos. Anesth Analg 83:542–547

Nordin M, Nystrom B, Wallin U, Hagbarth KE (1984) Ectopic sensory discharges and paresthesiae in patients with disorders of peripheral nerves, dorsal roots and dorsal columns. Pain 20:231–245

Novakovic SD, Tzoumaka E, McGivern JG, Haraguchi M, Sangameswaran L, Gogas KR, Eglen RM, Hunter JC (1998) Distribution of the tetrodotoxin-resistant sodium channel PN3 in rat sensory neurons in normal and neuropathic conditions. J Neurosci 18: 2174–2187

Oda A, Ohashi H, Komori S, Lida H, Dohi S (2000) Characteristics of ropivacaine block of Na+ channels in rat dorsal root ganglion neurons. Anesth Analg 91:1213–1220

Olschewski A, Brau ME, Olsechewki H, Hempelmann G, Vogel W (1996) ATP-dependent potassium channel in rat cardiomyocytes is blocked by lidocaine. Possible impact on the antiarrhythmic action of lidocaine. Circulation 93:656–659

Olschewski A, Hempelmann G, Vogel W, Safronov RV (1998) Blockade of Na+ and K+ currents by local anesthetics in the dorsal horn neurons of the spinal cord. Anesthesiology 88:172–179

Omana-Zapata I, Khabbaz MA, Hunter JC, Bley KR (1997) QX-314 inhibits ectopic nerve activity associated with neuropathic pain. Brain Res 771:228–237

Oyama Y, Sadoshima JI, Tokutomi N, Akaik N (1988) Some properties of inhibitory action of lidocaine on the Ca^{2+} current of single isolated frog sensory neurons. Brain Res 442:223–228

Palade PT, Almers W (1985) Slow calcium and potassium currents in frog skeletal muscle: their relationship and pharmacologic properties. Pflugers Arch 405:91–101

Persaud N, Strichartz GR (2002) Micromolar lidocaine selectively blocks propagating ectopic impulses at a distance from their site of origin. Pain 99:333–340

Pertovaara A, Wei H, Hamalainen MM (1996) Lidocaine in the rostroventromedial medulla and the periaqueductal gray attenuates allodynia in neuropathic rats. Neurosci Lett 218:127–130

Pollock JE (2002) Transient neurologic symptoms: etiology risk factors, and management. Reg Anesth Pain Med 27:581–586

Porreca F, Lai J, Bian D, Wegert S, Ossipov MH, Eglen RM, Kassotakis L, Novakovic S, Rabert DK, Sangameswaran L, Hunter JC (1999) A comparison of the potential role of the tetrodotoxin-insensitive sodium channels, PN3/SNS and NaN/SNS2, in rat models of chronic pain. Proc Natl Acad Sci USA 96:7640–7644

Puig S, Sorkin LS (1995) Formalin-evoked activity in identified primary afferent fibers: systemic lidocaine suppresses phase-2 activity. Pain 64:345–355

Raes A, Van de Vijver G, Goethals M, VanBoggart PP (1998) Use-dependent block of Ih in mouse dorsal root ganglion neurons by sinus node inhibitors. Br J Pharmacol 125:741–750

Ragsdale DS, McPhee JC, Scheuer T, Catterall WA (1994) Molecular determinants of state-dependent block of Na+ channels by local anesthetics. Science 265:1724–1728

Rane SG, Holz GG, Dunlap K (1987) Dihydropyridine inhibition of neuronal calcium current and substance P release. Pflugers Arch 409:361–366

Raymond SA (1992) Subblocking concentration of local anesthetics: effects on impulse generation and conduction in single myelinated sciatic nerve axons in frog. Anesth Analg 75:906–921

Raymond SA, Gissen AJ (1987) Mechanisms of differential nerve block. In: Strichartz GR (ed) Local anesthetics. (Handbook of experimental pharmacology, vol 81) Springer-Verlag, Berlin Heidelberg New York, pp 95–164

Raymond SA, Thalhammer JG, Strichartz GR (1990) Neuronal excitability: endogenous and exogenous modulation. In: Dimitrijevic MR, Wall PU, Lindblom U (eds) Altered sensation and pain: recent achievements in restorative neurology 3. S Karger, Basel, pp 112–127

Ready LB, Plumer MH, Haschke RH, Austin E, Sumi SM (1985) Neurotoxicity of intrathecal local anesthetics in rabbits. Anesthesiology 63:364–470

Rigler ML, Drasner K (1991) Distribution of catheter-injected local anesthetic in a model of the. subarachnoid space. Anesthesiology 75:684–692

Rigler ML, Drasner K, Drejecie TC, Yelich SJ, Scholnick FT, DeFonters J, Bohner D (1991) Cauda equine syndrome after continuous spinal anesthesia. Anesth Analg 72:275–281

Rosen MA, Baysinger CL, Shnider SM, Dailey PA, Norton M, Curtis JD, Collins M, Davis RL (1983) Evaluation of neurotoxicity after subarachnoid injection of large volumes of local anesthetic solutions. Anesth Analg 62:802–808

Ross BK, Coda B, Heath CH (1992) Local anesthetic distribution in a spinal model: a possible mechanism of neurologic injury after continuous spinal anesthesia. Reg Anesth 17:69–77

Rowbotham MC, Davies PS, Fields HL (1995) Topical lidocaine gel relieves postherpetic neuralgia. Ann Neurol 37:246–253

Rowbotham MC, Davies PS, Verkempinck C, Galer BS (1996) Lidocaine patch: double-blind controlled study of a new treatment method for post-herpetic neuralgia. Pain 65:39–44

Roza C, Laird JMA, Souslova V, Wood JN, Cervero F (2003) The tetrodotoxin-resistant Na+ channel Nav1.8 is essential for the expression of spontaneous activity in damaged sensory axons of mice. J Physiol (Lond) 550:921–926

Rush AM, Waxman SG (2004) PGE2 increases the tetrodotoxin-resistant Nav 1.9 sodium current in mouse DRG neurons via G-proteins. Brain Res 1023:345–364

Rush AM, Bräu ME, Elliott AA, Elliott JR (1998) Electrophysiological properties of sodium current subtypes in small cells from adult rat dorsal root ganglia. J Physiol 5113:771–789

Sakura S, Bollen AW, Cirales R, Drasner K (1995) Local anesthetic neurotoxicity does not result from blockade of voltage-gated sodium channels. Anesth Analg 81:338–346

Sakura S, Sumi M, Sakaguchi Y, Saito Y, Kosaka Y, Drasner K (1997) The addition of phenylephrine contributes to the development of transient neurologic symptoms after spinal anesthesia with 05% tetracaine. Anesthesiology 87:771–778

Schell RM, Brauer FS, Cole DJ, Applegate RL 2nd (1991) Persistent sacral nerve root deficits after continuous spinal anaesthesia. Can J Anaesth 38:908–911

Schwartz JH, Kandel ER (2000) Modulation of synaptic transmission. In: Kandel ER, Schwartz JH, Jessell TM (eds) Second messengers, principles of neural Science, 4th edn. Elsevier Science, New York, pp 229–252

Shin HC, Park HJ, Raymond SA, Strichartz GR (1994) Potentiation by capsaicin of lidocaine's tonic impulse block in isolated rat sciatic nerve. Neurosci Lett 174:14–16

Sinnott CJ, Garfield JM, Strichartz GR (1999) Differential efficacy of intravenous lidocaine in alleviating ipsilateral versus contralateral neuropathic pain in the rat. Pain 80:521–531

Sinnott CJ, Garfield JM, Zeitlin A, Teo S, Wu M, Chen J, Shafer SL, Strichartz GR (2000) Enantioselective relief of neuropathic pain by systemic mexiletine in the rat. J Pain 2:128–137

Strichartz GR, Berde CB (2005) Local anesthetics. In: Miller RD (ed) Miller's anesthesia. Elsevier, Philadelphia, pp 573–603

Strichartz GR, Zhou Z, Sinnott C, Khodorova A (2002) Therapeutic concentrations of local anaesthetics unveil the potential role of sodium channels in neuropathic pain. In: Bock G, Goode JA (eds) Sodium channels and neuronal hyperexcitability (Novartis Foundation Symposium 241). Wiley, Chichester, pp 189–205

Sugimoto M, Uchida I, Mashimo T (2003) Local anaesthetics have different mechanisms and sites of action at the recombinant N-methyl-d-aspartate (NMDA) receptors. Br J Pharmacol 138:876–882

Sugiyama K, Muteki T (1994) Local anesthetics depress the calcium current of rat sensory neurons in culture. Anesthesiology 80:1369–1378

Sullivan LM, Honemann CW, Arledge JA, Durieux ME (1999) Synergistic inhibition of lysophosphatidic acid signaling by charged and uncharged local anesthetics. Anesth Analg 88:1117–1124

Sunami A, Dudley SC, Fozzard HA (1997) Sodium channel selectivity filter regulates antiarrhythmic drug binding. Proc Natl Acad Sci USA 94:14126–14131

Tu H, Deng L, Sun Q, Yao L, Han JS, Wan Y (2004) Hyperpolarization-activated, cyclic nucleotide-gated cation channels: roles in the differential electrophysiological properties of rat primary afferent neurons. J Neurosci Res 76:713–722

Ulbricht W, Schmidtmayer J (1981) Modification of sodium channels in myelinated nerve by anemonia sulcata toxin II. J Physiol 77:1103–1111

Uratsuji Y, Nakanishi H, Takeyama Y, Kishimoto A, Nishizuka Y (1985) Activation of cellular protein kinase C and mode of inhibitory action of phospholipid-interacting compounds. Biochem Biophys Res Commun 130:654–661

Valenzuela C, Delpón E, Tamkun MM, Tamargo J, Snyders DJ (1995) Stereoselective block of a human cardiac potassium channel (Kv1.5) by bupivacaine enantiomers. Biophys J 69:418–427

Van Zundert AA, Grouls Rj, Korsten HH, Lambert DH (1996) Spinal anesthesia. Volume or concentration—what matters? Reg Anesth 21:112–118

Vedantham V, Cannon SC (1999) The position of the fast inactivation gate during lidocaine block of voltage-gated N+ channels. J Gen Physiol 113:7–16

Vijayaragavan K, Boutjdir M, Chahine M (2004) Modulaton of Nav1.7 and Nav1.8 peripheral nerve sodium channels by protein kinase and protein kinase C. J Neurophysiol 91:1556–1569

Voeikov VL, Lefkowitz RJ (1980) Effects of local anesthetics on guanyl nucleotide modulation of the catecholamine-sensitive adenylate cyclase system and on beta-adrenergic receptors. Biochim Biophys Acta 629:266–281

Wang DW, Nie L, George AL Jr, Bennett PB (1996) Distinct local anesthetic affinities in Na+ channel subtypes. Biophys J 70:1700–1708

Wang G, Russell G, Wang SY (2004) Mexiletine block of wild-type and inactivation-deficient human skeletal muscle in hNav1.4 Na+ channels. J Physiol 554:621–633

Wang GK, Strichartz GR (1985) Kinetic analysis of the action of Leiurus scorpion toxin on ionic currents in myelinated nerve. J Gen Physiol 86:739–762

Wang SY, Nau C, Wang GK (2000) Residues in Na(+) channel D3-S6 segment modulate both batrachotoxin and local anesthetic affinities. Biophys J 79:1379–1387

Wang SY, Barile M, Wang GK (2001) Disparate role of Na(+) channel D22-S6 residues in batrachotoxin and local anesthetic affinities. Mol Pharmacol 59:1100–1107

Warner MA, Warner DO, Harper CM, Schroeder DR, Maxson PM (2000) Lower extremity neuropathies associated with lithotomy positions. Anesthesiology 93:938–942

Wood JN, Akopian AN, Baker M, Ding Y, Goghegan F, Nassar M, Malik-Hall M, Okuse K, Poon L, Ravenall S, Sukumaran M, Souslova, V (2002) Sodium channels in primary sensory neurons: relationship to pain states. In: Bock G, Goode JA (eds) Sodium channels and neuronal hyperexcitability. Wiley and sons, Chichester, pp 159–168

Wright SN, Wang SY, Kallen RG, Wang GK (1997) Differences in steady-state inactivation between Na channel isoforms affect local anesthetic binding affinity. Biophys J 73:779–788

Wright SN, Wang SY, Xiao YF, Wang GK (1999) State-dependent cocaine block of sodium channel isoforms, chimeras, and channels coexpressed with the beta1 subunit. Biophys J 76:233–245

Wyllie AH, Kerr JF, Currie AR (1980) Cell death: the significance of apoptosis. Int Rev Cytol 68:251–306

Xia Z, Dickens M, Raingeaud J, Davis RJ, Greenberg ME (1995) Opposing effects of ERK and JNK-p38 MAP kinases on apoptosis. Science 270:1326–1331

Xing JL, Hu SJ, Jian z, Duan JH (2003) Subthreshold membrane potential oscillation mediates the excitatory effect of norepinephrine in chronically compressed dorsal root ganglion neurons in the rat. Pain 1051:177–183

Xiong Z, Strichartz GR (1998) Inhibition by local anesthetics of calcium channels in rat anterior pituitary cells. Eur J Clin Pharmacol 363:81–90

Xiong Z, Bukusoglu C, Strichartz GR (1999) Local anesthetics inhibit the G protein-mediated modulation of K+ and Ca++ currents in anterior pituitary cells. Mol Pharmacol 55: 150–158

Xu F, Garavito-Aguilar Z, Recio-Pinto E, Zhang J, Blanck TJ (2003) Local anesthetics modulate neuronal calcium signaling through multiple sites of action. Br J Pharmacol 139:1273–1280

Yanagidate F, Strichartz GR (2006) Bupivacaine inhibits activation of neuronal spinal extracellular receptor activated kinase through selective effects on ionotropic receptors. Anesthesiology 104:805–814

Yang D, Gereau RW (2004) Group II metabotropic glutamate receptors inhibit cAMP-dependent protein kinase-mediated enhancement of tetrodotoxin-resistant sodium currents in mouse dorsal root ganglion neurons. Neurosci Lett 357:159–162

Yang EK, Takimoto K, Hayashi Y, de Groat WC, Yoshimura N (2004) Altered expression of potassium channel subunit mRNA and alpha-dendrotoxin sensitivity of potassium currents in rat dorsal root ganglion neurons after axotomy. Neuroscience 123:867–874

Yao H, Donnelly DF, Ma C, Lamotte RH (2003) Upregulation of the hyperpolarization-activated cation current after chronic compression of the dorsal root ganglion. J Neurosci 23:2069–2074

Yu FH, Yarov-Yarovoy V, Gutman GA, Catterall WA (2005) Overview of molecular relationships in the voltage-gated ion channel superfamily. Pharmacol Rev 57:387–395

Zaric D, Christiansen C, Pace NL, Punjasawadwong Y (2003) Transient neurologic symptoms (TNS) following spinal anaesthesia with lidocaine versus other local anesthetics. Cochrane Database System Rev CD003006

HEP (2006) 177:129–143

Serotonin Receptor Ligands: Treatments of Acute Migraine and Cluster Headache

P. J. Goadsby

Institute of Neurology, Queen Square, London WC1N 3BG, UK
peterg@ion.ucl.ac.uk

1	The Trigeminovascular System	130
1.1	Modelling the Trigeminovascular System	130
2	Triptans, 5-HT$_{1B/1D}$ Receptor Agonists: Peripheral Pharmacology	132
2.1	Plasma Protein Extravasation	132
2.1.1	Sensitisation and Migraine	132
3	Triptans, 5-HT$_{1B/1D}$ Receptor Agonists: Central Pharmacology	133
3.1	The Trigeminocervical Complex	133
3.2	Higher Order Processing	134
3.2.1	Thalamus	134
3.2.2	Activation of Modulatory Regions	135
4	Non-triptan Serotonergic Strategies	135
4.1	5-HT$_{1F}$ Receptor Agonists	135
4.2	5-HT$_{1D}$ Receptors	136
5	Conclusion	136
References		137

Abstract Fuelled by the development of the serotonin 5-HT$_{1B/1D}$ receptor agonists, the triptans, the last 15 years has seen an explosion of interest in the treatment of acute migraine and cluster headache. Sumatriptan was the first of these agonists, and it launched a wave of therapeutic advances. These medicines are effective and safe. Triptans were developed as cranial vasoconstrictors to mimic the desirable effects of serotonin, while avoiding its side-effects. It has subsequently been shown that the triptans' major action is neuronal, with both peripheral and central trigeminal inhibitory effects, as well as actions in the thalamus and at central modulatory sites, such as the periaqueductal grey matter. Further refinements may be possible as the 5-HT$_{1D}$ and 5-HT$_{1F}$ receptor agonists are explored. Serotonin receptor pharmacology has contributed much to the better management of patients with primary headache disorders.

Keywords Triptans · Trigeminovascular · Migraine · Cluster headache

The last 15 years has seen an explosion of interest in the treatment of acute migraine. The description of serotonin 5-HT$_{1B/1D}$ receptor agonists, triptans (Goadsby 2000), as acute anti-migraine compounds (Doenicke et al. 1987), and the subsequent validation of sumatriptan (Doenicke et al. 1988) launched a wave of therapeutic advances. Many countries now have a triptan available and some have up to seven. These medicines are safe (Dodick et al. 2004) and effective (Ferrari et al. 2001); they have done much good both for patients and for the headache field more broadly.

Triptans were developed as cranial vasoconstrictors to mimic the desirable effects of serotonin (Kimball et al. 1960; Lance et al. 1967), while avoiding its side-effects (Humphrey et al. 1990). The developmental rationale (Humphrey et al. 1990) was based on clinical data, i.e. that of serotonin and methysergide (Lance et al. 1963), and a pre-clinical rationale of cranial vasoconstriction, specifically selective constriction of arteriovenous anastomoses (Johnston and Saxena 1978). However, as the 1990s unfolded, views on migraine have changed. It is now generally accepted that migraine is a disorder of brain (Goadsby et al. 2002), with neurovascular changes being secondary to brain activity. I will review here the models used for triptan development, explore the specific pharmacology and experimental data regarding triptans, using a largely neuroanatomical approach (Table 1), and then review the possibility for even more specific 5-HT ligands in migraine.

1
The Trigeminovascular System

The brain itself is largely insensate and, with some exceptions (Raskin et al. 1987; Veloso et al. 1998), does not seem to produce headache when stimulated (Wolff 1948). The pain-producing innervation of the intracranial contents is largely supplied by branches of the ophthalmic (first) division of the trigeminal nerve (Penfield 1932a, b, 1934; Penfield and McNaughton 1940; Feindel et al. 1960; McNaughton 1966). The crucial structures that produce pain seem to be the dura mater and the large intracranial blood vessels (Wolff 1948). Electrical stimulation of large venous sinuses, such as the superior sagittal sinus (SSS), will produce pain (Ray and Wolff 1940) although, remarkably, mechanical stimulation is much less likely to do so (Wolff 1948). Because these structures— dura mater and dural/large intracranial vessels—are pain-producing, they have been used to model trigeminovascular nociception (Edvinsson 1999), thus helping us make predictions concerning new anti-migraine compounds.

1.1
Modelling the Trigeminovascular System

Several approaches are used to model the trigeminovascular system. One can look at pre- and post-junctional targets peripherally, i.e. the nerve-vessel inter-

Table 1 Neuroanatomical processing of intracranial nociceptive activation

	Structure	Comments
Target innervation:		
• Cranial vessels	Ophthalmic branch of trigeminal nerve	
• Dura mater		
1st	Trigeminal ganglion	Middle cranial fossa
2nd	Trigeminal nucleus (quintothalamic tract)	Trigeminal n. caudalis and C_1/C_2 dorsal horns[a]
3rd	Thalamus	Ventrobasal complex[a]
		Medial n. of posterior group
		Intralaminar complex
Modulatory	Midbrain	Periaqueductal grey matter (PAG)[a]
	Hypothalamus	?
Final	Cortex	• Insulae
		• Frontal cortex
		• Anterior cingulate cortex
		• Basal ganglia

[a]Central nervous system sites where serotonin $5\text{-}HT_{1B/1D}$ receptor agonists modulate trigeminovascular nociceptive processing

face, or pre- and post-synaptic targets centrally, i.e. the second order neuron interface (De Vries et al. 1999; Goadsby and Kaube 2000). The first model for post-junctional craniovascular targets was the arteriovenous anastomoses (Saxena and De Boer 1991), which at the time were considered as a target independent of the trigeminal nerve as such. Interestingly, a pre-junctional action for ergotamine is not a new concept (Saxena and Cairo-Rawlins 1979). Subsequently, the plasma-protein extravasation model was developed (Markowitz et al. 1987) and used to explore anti-migraine compounds (Markowitz et al. 1988). The intravital model of Williamson and Hargreaves (Williamson et al. 1997) studies both pre- and post-junctional effects of compounds and has been very useful in evaluating new receptor targets. At the other end of the trigeminovascular neuron one can study pre-synaptic and post-synaptic events in the trigeminocervical complex to begin to infer possible brain effects of anti-migraine compounds (Kaube et al. 1992). These approaches have all been exploited to characterise the effects of various transmitters on the trigeminovascular system, particularly the pre-junctional/pre-synaptic effects that may be a crucial part of the action of these compounds.

2
Triptans, 5-HT$_{1B/1D}$ Receptor Agonists: Peripheral Pharmacology

2.1
Plasma Protein Extravasation

Moskowitz (1990) has provided a series of experiments to suggest that the pain of migraine may be a form of sterile neurogenic inflammation. Although many aspects of this view seem clinically implausible, the model system has been helpful in understanding some aspects of trigeminovascular pharmacology. Neurogenic plasma extravasation can be seen during electrical stimulation of the trigeminal ganglion in the rat (Markowitz et al. 1987). Plasma extravasation can be blocked by ergot alkaloids, indomethacin, acetylsalicylic acid, and the serotonin-5-HT$_{1B/1D}$ agonist, sumatriptan (Moskowitz and Cutrer 1993). The pharmacology of abortive anti-migraine drugs has been reviewed in detail (Cutrer et al. 1997). In addition, there are structural changes in the dura mater that are observed after trigeminal ganglion stimulation. These include mast cell degranulation and changes in post-capillary venules including platelet aggregation (Dimitriadou et al. 1991, 1992). While it is generally accepted that such changes, and particularly the initiation of a sterile inflammatory response, would cause pain (Strassman et al. 1996; Burstein et al. 1998), it is not clear whether this is sufficient of itself or requires other stimulators or promoters. Preclinical studies suggest that cortical spreading depression may be a sufficient stimulus to activate trigeminal neurons (Bolay et al. 2002), although this has been a controversial area (Moskowitz et al. 1993; Ingvardsen et al. 1997, 1998; Ebersberger et al. 2001; Goadsby 2001).

Although plasma extravasation in the retina, which is blocked by sumatriptan, can be seen after trigeminal ganglion stimulation in experimental animals, no changes are seen with retinal angiography during acute attacks of migraine or cluster headache (May et al. 1998b). A limitation of this study was the probable sampling of both retina and choroid elements in rat, given that choroidal vessels have fenestrated capillaries (Steuer et al. 2004). Clearly, however, blockade of neurogenic plasma protein extravasation is not completely predictive of anti-migraine efficacy in humans as evidenced by the failure in clinical trials of substance P, neurokinin-1 antagonists (Goldstein et al. 1997; Connor et al. 1998; Norman et al. 1998; Diener and The RPR100893 Study Group 2003), specific blockers of dural plasma protein extravasation (PPE) [CP122,288 (Roon et al. 1997) and 4991w93 (Earl et al. 1999)], an endothelin antagonist (May et al. 1996) and a neurosteroid (Data et al. 1998).

2.1.1
Sensitisation and Migraine

While it is highly doubtful that there is a significant sterile inflammatory response in the dura mater during migraine, it is clear that some form of sensitisation takes place during migraine, since allodynia is common. About two-thirds of patients complain of pain from non-noxious stimuli (Selby and Lance 1960; Burstein et al. 2000a,b). Sensitisation in migraine may be peripheral with local release of inflammatory markers, which would certainly activate trigeminal nociceptors (Strassman et al. 1996). More likely in migraine there is a form of central sensitisation—which may be classical central sensitisation (Burstein et al. 1998)—or a form of disinhibitory sensitisation with dysfunction of descending modulatory pathways (Knight et al. 2002). Just as dihydroergotamine (DHE) can block trigeminovascular nociceptive transmission (Hoskin et al. 1996), probably at least by a local effect in the trigeminocervical complex (Lambert et al. 1992; Storer and Goadsby 1997), DHE can block central sensitisation associated with dural stimulation by an inflammatory soup (Pozo-Rosich and Oshinsky 2005).

3
Triptans, 5-HT$_{1B/1D}$ Receptor Agonists: Central Pharmacology

3.1
The Trigeminocervical Complex

Fos immunohistochemistry is a method for looking at activated cells by plotting the expression of Fos protein (Morgan and Curran 1991). After meningeal irritation with blood, Fos expression is noted in the trigeminal nucleus caudalis (Nozaki et al. 1992), while after stimulation of the superior sagittal sinus, Fos-like immunoreactivity is seen in the trigeminal nucleus caudalis and in the dorsal horn at the C_1 and C_2 levels in the cat (Kaube et al. 1993c) and monkey (Goadsby and Hoskin 1997; Hoskin et al. 1999). These latter findings are in accordance with similar data using 2-deoxyglucose measurements with superior sagittal sinus stimulation (Goadsby and Zagami 1991). Similarly, stimulation of a branch of C_2, the greater occipital nerve, increases metabolic activity in the same regions, i.e. trigeminal nucleus caudalis and $C_{1/2}$ dorsal horn (Goadsby et al. 1997). In experimental animals one can record directly from trigeminal neurons with both supratentorial trigeminal input and input from the greater occipital nerve, a branch of the C_2 dorsal root (Bartsch and Goadsby 2002). Stimulation of the greater occipital nerve for 5 min results in substantial increases in responses to supratentorial dural stimulation, which can last for over an hour (Bartsch and Goadsby 2002). Conversely, stimulation of the middle meningeal artery dura mater with the C-fibre irritant mustard oil sensitises responses to occipital muscle stimulation (Bartsch and Goadsby 2003). Taken together these data suggest convergence of cervical and ophthalmic inputs at the level of the second order neuron. Moreover, stimulation of a lateralised structure, the middle meningeal artery, produces Fos expression bilaterally in both cat and monkey brain (Hoskin et al. 1999). This group of neurons from the superficial laminae of trigeminal nucleus caudalis and $C_{1/2}$ dorsal horns should be regarded functionally as the *trigeminocervical* complex.

These data demonstrate that trigeminovascular nociceptive information comes by way of the most caudal cells. This concept provides an anatomical explanation for the referral of pain to the back of the head in migraine. Moreover, experimental pharmacological evidence suggests that some abortive anti-migraine drugs, such as, ergot derivatives (Lambert et al. 1992; Hoskin et al. 1996), acetylsalicylic acid (Kaube et al. 1993b), sumatriptan (Kaube et al. 1993a; Levy et al. 2004), eletriptan (Goadsby and Hoskin 1999; Lambert et al. 2002), naratriptan (Goadsby and Knight 1997; Cumberbatch et al. 1998), rizatriptan (Cumberbatch et al. 1997) and zolmitriptan (Goadsby and Hoskin 1996) can have actions at these second order neurons that reduce cell activity and suggest a further possible site for therapeutic intervention in migraine. This action can be dissected out to involve each of the $5\text{-}HT_{1B}$, $5\text{-}HT_{1D}$ and $5\text{-}HT_{1F}$ receptor subtypes (Goadsby and Classey 2003), and are consistent with the localisation of these receptors on peptidergic nociceptors (Potrebic et al. 2003). Interestingly, triptans also influence the calcitonin gene-related peptide (CGRP) promoter (Durham et al. 1997) and regulate CGRP secretion from neurons in culture (Durham and Russo 1999). Furthermore, the demonstration that some part of this action is post-synaptic with either $5\text{-}HT_{1B}$ or $5\text{-}HT_{1D}$ receptors located non-presynaptically (Goadsby et al. 2001; Maneesi et al. 2004) offers a prospect of highly anatomically localised treatment options.

3.2
Higher Order Processing

Following transmission in the caudal brain stem and high cervical spinal cord information is relayed rostrally. Given that triptan receptors are found at every level of the peripheral neuraxis from trigeminal ganglion to cervical, thoracic, lumbar and sacral sensory ganglia (Classey et al. 2002), another explanation needs to be found to explain the particular specificity of triptans to primary neurovascular headache, such as migraine (Ferrari et al. 2002) and cluster headache (Matharu and Goadsby 2004), but not, for example, atypical facial pain (Harrison et al. 1997) or even tension-type headache (Lipton et al. 2000).

3.2.1
Thalamus

Processing of vascular nociceptive signals in the thalamus occurs in the ventroposteromedial (VPM) thalamus, medial nucleus of the posterior complex and the intralaminar thalamus (Zagami and Goadsby 1991). Zagami (1991) has shown by application of capsaicin to the superior sagittal sinus that trigeminal projections with a high degree of nociceptive input are processed in neurons particularly in the VPM thalamus and in its ventral periphery. These neurons in the VPM can be modulated by activation of γ-aminobutyric acid $(GABA)_A$ inhibitory receptors (Shields et al. 2003), and perhaps with more direct clinical relevance by propranolol though a β_1-adrenoceptor mechanism (Shields and Goadsby 2005). Remarkably, triptans through $5\text{-}HT_{1B/1D}$ mechanisms can also inhibit VPM neurons locally, as demonstrated by microiontophoretic application (Shields and Goadsby 2004), suggesting a hitherto unconsidered locus of action for triptans in acute migraine. Human imaging studies have confirmed activation of thalamus contralateral to pain in acute migraine (Bahra et al. 2001; Afridi et al. 2005), cluster headache (May et al. 1998a) and in SUNCT (short-lasting unilateral neuralgiform headache with conjunctival injection and tearing) (May et al. 1999; Cohen et al. 2004).

3.2.2
Activation of Modulatory Regions

Stimulation of nociceptive afferents by stimulation of the superior sagittal sinus in the cat activates neurons in the ventrolateral periaqueductal grey matter (PAG) (Hoskin et al. 2001). PAG activation in turn feeds back to the trigeminocervical complex with an inhibitory influence (Knight and Goadsby 2001; Knight et al. 2003). PAG is clearly included in the area of activation seen in positron emission tomography (PET) studies in migraineurs (Weiller et al. 1995). Local injection of the triptan naratriptan into the ventrolateral PAG inhibits nociceptive activation from intracranial afferents, while not altering processing of afferent signals from facial stimuli (Bartsch et al. 2004). Given the remarkable *functionotopic* specificity of central pain modulatory systems (Benedetti et al. 1999), it seems plausible that the clinical specificity of the triptans resides in the central sites of action.

4
Non-triptan Serotonergic Strategies

Following the success of the triptans and based upon the fact that all of the triptans are $5\text{-}HT_{1D}$ receptor agonists and many are $5\text{-}HT_{1F}$ receptor agonists (Goadsby 2000), specific agonists have been developed and tested at these targets.

4.1
5-HT₁F Receptor Agonists

The $5\text{-}HT_{1F}$ receptor (Adham et al. 1993) may be a target for anti-migraine treatments (Branchek and Archa 1997). The potent, specific $5HT_{1F}$ agonist LY334,370 has been developed (Phebus et al. 1997) and shown to block neurogenic plasma protein extravasation in the rat dura mater (Johnson et al. 1997),

consistent with early molecular studies (Wainscott et al. 1998). Activation of
$5-HT_{1F}$ receptors does not seem to have vascular effects (Cohen and Schenck
1999; Razzaque et al. 1999). LY334,370 is effective in acute migraine, albeit at
doses with some central nervous system side-effects (Goldstein et al. 2001). No
cardiovascular problems were seen in these studies (Goldstein et al. 2001), but
unfortunately development has stopped because of a toxicity problem in dog.
$5-HT_{1F}$ receptors are found in the trigeminal nucleus (Waeber and Moskowitz
1995; Pascual et al. 1996; Castro et al. 1997; Fugelli et al. 1997) and trigeminal
ganglion (Bouchelet et al. 1996). $5-HT_{1F}$ receptor activation is inhibitory in the
trigeminal nucleus in rat (Mitsikostas et al. 1999) and cat (Goadsby and Classey
2003). Most recently it has been shown using electron microscopy (EM) that
there are pre- and post-synaptic $5-HT_{1F}$ receptors in the trigeminal nucleus
of cat (Maneesi et al. 2004), so it is clear that the $5-HT_{1F}$ receptor is a putative
pre-junctional/pre-synaptic target in migraine.

4.2
5-HT$_{1D}$ Receptors

$5-HT_{1D}$ receptor agonists are potent inhibitors of neurogenic dural plasma protein extravasation (Waeber et al. 1997) and have no vascular effects. Specific
potent $5-HT_{1D}$ agonists have been developed by taking advantage of similarities
between human and non-human primate $5-HT_{1B}$ and $5-HT_{1D}$ receptors (Pregenzer et al. 1997). One compound that went into clinical studies, PNU 142633,
was ineffective (Gomez-Mancilla et al. 2001), although it was a relatively weak
agonist when compared to sumatriptan in *in vitro* studies (Pregenzer et al.
1999), and was poorly brain penetrant. This compound was developed using
gorilla receptors (McCall et al. 2002). It must, therefore, be asked whether this
was the correct compound to test the $5-HT_{1D}$ hypothesis. It is perhaps more
remarkable that there were no complaints of adverse events of a cardiovascular nature in the placebo group, with cardiovascular adverse events, including
chest pain, in the PNU 142633-treated group (Fleishaker et al. 1999). It would
be very important to show conclusively that some part of the triptan group's
chest symptoms were non-vascular, as these data suggest. A further study with
a more potent, preferably brain penetrant, agonist would clarify this situation
enormously and is clearly warranted.

5
Conclusion

Serotonin receptor ligands have provided effective treatments of both migraine
and cluster headache, and in doing so have launched a wave of interest in
primary headache syndromes. Patients have benefited and neuroscientists
and pharmacologists have seen their efforts translate to better management

of a group of important and disabling medical conditions. The future offers the promise of even further advances and thus a bright future for serotonin pharmacology and for patients.

Acknowledgements The work of the author has been supported by the Wellcome Trust.

References

Adham N, Kao HT, Schechter LE, Bard J, Olsen M, Urquhart D, Durkin M, Hartig PR, Weinshank RL, Branchek TA (1993) Cloning of another human serotonin receptor (5-HT1F): a fifth 5-HT1 receptor subtype coupled to the inhibition of adenylate cyclase. Proc Natl Acad Sci U S A 90:408–412

Afridi S, Giffin NJ, Kaube H, Friston KJ, Ward NS, Frackowiak RSJ, Goadsby PJ (2005) A positron emission tomographic study in spontaneous migraine. Arch Neurol 62: 1270–1275

Bahra A, Matharu MS, Buchel C, Frackowiak RSJ, Goadsby PJ (2001) Brainstem activation specific to migraine headache. Lancet 357:1016–1017

Bartsch T, Goadsby PJ (2002) Stimulation of the greater occipital nerve induces increased central excitability of dural afferent input. Brain 125:1496–1509

Bartsch T, Goadsby PJ (2003) Increased responses in trigeminocervical nociceptive neurones to cervical input after stimulation of the dura mater. Brain 126:1801–1813

Bartsch T, Knight YE, Goadsby PJ (2004) Activation of 5-HT1B/1D receptors in the periaqueductal grey inhibits meningeal nociception. Ann Neurol 56:371–381

Benedetti F, Arduino C, Amanzio M (1999) Somatotopic activation of opioid systems by target-directed expectations of analgesia. J Neurosci 19:3639–3648

Bolay H, Reuter U, Dunn AK, Huang Z, Boas DA, Moskowitz MA (2002) Intrinsic brain activity triggers trigeminal meningeal afferents in a migraine model. Nat Med 8:136–142

Bouchelet I, Cohen Z, Case B, Hamel E (1996) Differential expression of sumatriptan-sensitive 5-hydroxytryptamine receptors in human trigeminal ganglia and cerebral blood vessels. Mol Pharmacol 50:219–223

Branchek T, Archa JE (1997) Recent advances in migraine therapy. In: Robertson DW (ed) Central nervous system disease. Academic Press, San Diego, pp 1–10

Burstein R, Yamamura H, Malick A, Strassman AM (1998) Chemical stimulation of the intracranial dura induces enhanced responses to facial stimulation in brain stem trigeminal neurons. J Neurophysiol 79:964–982

Burstein R, Cutrer MF, Yarnitsky D (2000a) The development of cutaneous allodynia during a migraine attack. Brain 123:1703–1709

Burstein R, Yarnitsky D, Goor-Aryeh I, Ransil BJ, Bajwa ZH (2000b) An association between migraine and cutaneous allodynia. Ann Neurol 47:614–624

Castro ME, Pascual J, Romon T, del Arco C, del Olmo E, Pazos A (1997) Differential distribution of [3H]sumatriptan binding sites (5-HT1B, 5-HT1D and 5-HT1F receptors) in human brain: focus on brainstem and spinal cord. Neuropharmacology 36:535–542

Classey JD, Bartsch T, Goadsby PJ (2002) Immunohistochemical examination of 5HT1B, 5HT1D and 5HT1F receptor expression in rat trigeminal ganglion (TRG) and dorsal root ganglia (DRG) neurons. Cephalalgia 22:595–596

Cohen AS, Matharu MS, Kalisch R, Friston K, Goadsby PJ (2004) Functional MRI in SUNCT shows differential hypothalamic activation with increasing pain. Cephalalgia 24: 1098–1099

Cohen ML, Schenck K (1999) 5-Hydroxytryptamine(1F) receptors do not participate in vasoconstriction: lack of vasoconstriction to LY344864, a selective serotonin(1F) receptor agonist in rabbit saphenous vein. J Pharmacol Exp Ther 290:935–939

Connor HE, Bertin L, Gillies S, Beattie DT, Ward P, The GR205171 Clinical Study Group (1998) Clinical evaluation of a novel, potent, CNS penetrating NK1 receptor antagonist in the acute treatment of migraine. Cephalalgia 18:392

Cumberbatch MJ, Hill RG, Hargreaves RJ (1997) Rizatriptan has central antinociceptive effects against durally evoked responses. Eur J Pharmacol 328:37–40

Cumberbatch MJ, Hill RG, Hargreaves RJ (1998) Differential effects of the 5HT1B/1D receptor agonist naratriptan on trigeminal versus spinal nociceptive responses. Cephalalgia 18:659–664

Cutrer FM, Limmroth V, Waeber C, Yu X, Moskowitz MA (1997) New targets for antimigraine drug development. In: Goadsby PJ, Silberstein SD (eds) Headache. Butterworth-Heinemann, Philadelphia, pp 59–72

Data J, Britch K, Westergaard N, Weihnuller F, Harris S, Swarz H, Silberstein S, Goldstein J, Ryan R, Saper J, Londborg P, Winner P, Klapper J (1998) A double-blind study of ganaxolone in the acute treatment of migraine headaches with or without an aura in premenopausal females. Headache 38:380

De Vries P, Villalon CM, Saxena PR (1999) Pharmacological aspects of experimental headache models in relation to acute antimigraine therapy. Eur J Pharmacol 375:61–74

Diener HC, The RPR100893 Study Group (2003) RPR100893, a substance-P antagonist, is not effective in the treatment of migraine attacks. Cephalalgia 23:183–185

Dimitriadou V, Buzzi MG, Moskowitz MA, Theoharides TC (1991) Trigeminal sensory fiber stimulation induces morphological changes reflecting secretion in rat dura mater mast cells. Neuroscience 44:97–112

Dimitriadou V, Buzzi MG, Theoharides TC, Moskowitz MA (1992) Ultrastructural evidence for neurogenically mediated changes in blood vessels of the rat dura mater and tongue following antidromic trigeminal stimulation. Neuroscience 48:187–203

Dodick D, Lipton RB, Martin V, Papademetriou V, Rosamond W, MaassenVanDenBrink A, Loutfi H, Welch KM, Goadsby PJ, Hahn S, Hutchinson S, Matchar D, Silberstein S, Smith TR, Purdy RA, Saiers J (2004) Consensus statement: cardiovascular safety profile of triptans (5-HT1B/1D agonists) in the acute treatment of migraine. Headache 44:414–425

Doenicke A, Siegel E, Hadoke M, Perrin VL (1987) Initial clinical study of AH25086B (5-HT1-like agonist) in the acute treatment of migraine. Cephalalgia 7:437–438

Doenicke A, Brand J, Perrin VL (1988) Possible benefit of GR43175, a novel 5-HT1-like receptor agonist, for the acute treatment of severe migraine. Lancet 1:1309–1311

Durham PL, Russo AF (1999) Regulation of calcitonin gene-related peptide secretion by a serotonergic antimigraine drug. J Neurosci 19:3423–3429

Durham PL, Sharma RV, Russo AF (1997) Repression of the calcitonin gene-related peptide promoter by 5-HT1 receptor activation. J Neurosci 17:9545–9553

Earl NL, McDonald SA, Lowy MT, 4991W93 Investigator Group (1999) Efficacy and tolerability of the neurogenic inflammation inhibitor, 4991W93, in the acute treatment of migraine. Cephalalgia 19:357

Ebersberger A, Schaible HG, Averbeck B, Richter F (2001) Is there a correlation between spreading depression, neurogenic inflammation, and nociception that might cause migraine headache? Ann Neurol 49:7–13

Edvinsson L (1999) Experimental headache models in animals and man. Martin Dunitz, London

Feindel W, Penfield W, McNaughton F (1960) The tentorial nerves and localization of intracranial pain in man. Neurology 10:555–563

Ferrari MD, Roon KI, Lipton RB, Goadsby PJ (2001) Oral triptans (serotonin, 5-HT1B/1D agonists) in acute migraine treatment: a meta-analysis of 53 trials. Lancet 358:1668–1675

Ferrari MD, Goadsby PJ, Roon KI, Lipton RB (2002) Triptans (serotonin, 5-HT1B/1D agonists) in migraine: detailed results and methods of a meta-analysis of 53 trials. Cephalalgia 22:633–658

Fleishaker JC, Pearson LK, Knuth DW, GomezMancilla B, Francom SF, McIntosh MJ, Freestone S, Azie NE (1999) Pharmacokinetics and tolerability of a novel 5-HT1D agonist, PNU-142633F. Int J Clin Pharmacol Ther 37:487–492

Fugelli A, Moret C, Fillion G (1997) Autoradiographic localization of 5-HT1E and 5-HT1F binding sites in rat brain: effect of serotonergic lesioning. J Recept Signal Transduct Res 17:631–645

Goadsby PJ (2000) The pharmacology of headache. Prog Neurobiol 62:509–525

Goadsby PJ (2001) Migraine, aura and cortical spreading depression: why are we still talking about it? Ann Neurol 49:4–6

Goadsby PJ, Classey JD (2003) Evidence for 5-HT1B, 5-HT1D and 5-HT1F receptor inhibitory effects on trigeminal neurons with craniovascular input. Neuroscience 122:491–498

Goadsby PJ, Hoskin KL (1996) Inhibition of trigeminal neurons by intravenous administration of the serotonin (5HT)1B/D receptor agonist zolmitriptan (311C90): are brain stem sites a therapeutic target in migraine? Pain 67:355–359

Goadsby PJ, Hoskin KL (1997) The distribution of trigeminovascular afferents in the nonhuman primate brain Macaca nemestrina: a c-fos immunocytochemical study. J Anat 190:367–375

Goadsby PJ, Hoskin KL (1999) Differential effects of low dose CP122,288 and eletriptan on fos expression due to stimulation of the superior sagittal sinus in cat. Pain 82:15–22

Goadsby PJ, Kaube H (2000) Animal models of headache. In: Olesen J, Tfelt-Hansen P, Welch KMA (eds) The headaches. Lippincott Williams and Wilkins, Philadelphia, pp 195–202

Goadsby PJ, Knight YE (1997) Inhibition of trigeminal neurons after intravenous administration of naratriptan through an action at the serotonin (5HT1B/1D) receptors. Br J Pharmacol 122:918–922

Goadsby PJ, Zagami AS (1991) Stimulation of the superior sagittal sinus increases metabolic activity and blood flow in certain regions of the brainstem and upper cervical spinal cord of the cat. Brain 114:1001–1011

Goadsby PJ, Hoskin KL, Knight YE (1997) Stimulation of the greater occipital nerve increases metabolic activity in the trigeminal nucleus caudalis and cervical dorsal horn of the cat. Pain 73:23–28

Goadsby PJ, Akerman S, Storer RJ (2001) Evidence for postjunctional serotonin (5-HT1) receptors in the trigeminocervical complex. Ann Neurol 50:804–807

Goadsby PJ, Lipton RB, Ferrari MD (2002) Migraine—current understanding and treatment. N Engl J Med 346:257–270

Goldstein DJ, Wang O, Saper JR, Stoltz R, Silberstein SD, Mathew NT (1997) Ineffectiveness of neurokinin-1 antagonist in acute migraine: a crossover study. Cephalalgia 17:785–790

Goldstein DJ, Roon KI, Offen WW, Ramadan NM, Phebus LA, Johnson KW, Schaus JM, Ferrari MD (2001) Selective serotonin 1F [5-HT(1F)] receptor agonist LY334370 for acute migraine: a randomised controlled trial. Lancet 358:1230–1234

Gomez-Mancilla B, Cutler NR, Leibowitz MT, Spierings ELH, Klapper JA, Diamond S, Goldstein J, Smith T, Couch JR, Fleishaker J, Azie N, Blunt DE (2001) Safety and efficacy of PNU-142633, a selective 5-HT1D agonist, in patients with acute migraine. Cephalalgia 21:727–732

Harrison SD, Balawi SA, Feinmann C, Harris M (1997) Atypical facial pain: a double-blind placebo-controlled crossover pilot study of subcutaneous sumatriptan. Eur Neuropsychopharmacol 7:83–88

Hoskin KL, Kaube H, Goadsby PJ (1996) Central activation of the trigeminovascular pathway in the cat is inhibited by dihydroergotamine. A c-Fos and electrophysiology study. Brain 119:249–256

Hoskin KL, Zagami A, Goadsby PJ (1999) Stimulation of the middle meningeal artery leads to Fos expression in the trigeminocervical nucleus: a comparative study of monkey and cat. J Anat 194:579–588

Hoskin KL, Bulmer DCE, Lasalandra M, Jonkman A, Goadsby PJ (2001) Fos expression in the midbrain periaqueductal grey after trigeminovascular stimulation. J Anat 197:29–35

Humphrey PPA, Feniuk W, Perren MJ, Beresford IJM, Skingle M, Whalley ET (1990) Serotonin and migraine. Ann NY Acad Sci 600:587–598

Ingvardsen BK, Laursen H, Olsen UB, Hansen AJ (1997) Possible mechanism of c-fos expression in trigeminal nucleus caudalis following spreading depression. Pain 72: 407–415

Ingvardsen BK, Laursen H, Olsen UB, Hansen AJ (1998) Comment on Ingvardsen et al., Pain 72 (1997) 407–415—reply to Moskowitz et al. Pain 76:266–267

Johnson KW, Schaus JM, Durkin MM, Audia JE, Kaldor SW, Flaugh ME, Adham N, Zgombick JM, Cohen ML, Branchek TA, Phebus LA (1997) 5-HT1F receptor agonists inhibit neurogenic dural inflammation in guinea pigs. NeuroReport 8:2237–2240

Johnston BM, Saxena PR (1978) The effect of ergotamine on tissue blood flow and the arteriovenous shunting of radioactive microspheres in the head. Br J Pharmacol 63: 541–549

Kaube H, Hoskin KL, Goadsby PJ (1992) Activation of the trigeminovascular system by mechanical distension of the superior sagittal sinus in the cat. Cephalalgia 12:133–136

Kaube H, Hoskin KL, Goadsby PJ (1993a) Inhibition by sumatriptan of central trigeminal neurones only after blood-brain barrier disruption. Br J Pharmacol 109:788–792

Kaube H, Hoskin KL, Goadsby PJ (1993b) Intravenous acetylsalicylic acid inhibits central trigeminal neurons in the dorsal horn of the upper cervical spinal cord in the cat. Headache 33:541–550

Kaube H, Keay KA, Hoskin KL, Bandler R, Goadsby PJ (1993c) Expression of c-Fos-like immunoreactivity in the caudal medulla and upper cervical cord following stimulation of the superior sagittal sinus in the cat. Brain Res 629:95–102

Kimball RW, Friedman AP, Vallejo E (1960) Effect of serotonin in migraine patients. Neurology 10:107–111

Knight YE, Goadsby PJ (2001) The periaqueductal gray matter modulates trigeminovascular input: a role in migraine? Neuroscience 106:793–800

Knight YE, Bartsch T, Kaube H, Goadsby PJ (2002) P/Q-type calcium channel blockade in the PAG facilitates trigeminal nociception: a functional genetic link for migraine? J Neurosci 22:1–6

Knight YE, Bartsch T, Goadsby PJ (2003) Trigeminal antinociception induced by bicuculline in the periaqueductal grey (PAG) is not affected by PAG P/Q-type calcium channel blockade in rat. Neurosci Lett 336:113–116

Lambert GA, Lowy AJ, Boers P, Angus-Leppan H, Zagami A (1992) The spinal cord processing of input from the superior sagittal sinus: pathway and modulation by ergot alkaloids. Brain Res 597:321–330

Lambert GA, Boers PM, Hoskin KL, Donaldson C, Zagami AS (2002) Suppression by eletriptan of the activation of trigeminovascular sensory neurons by glyceryl trinitrate. Brain Res 953:181–188

Lance JW, Fine RD, Curran DA (1963) An evaluation of methysergide in the prevention of migraine and other vascular headache. Med J Aust 1:814–818

Lance JW, Anthony M, Hinterberger H (1967) The control of cranial arteries by humoral mechanisms and its relation to the migraine syndrome. Headache 7:93–102

Levy D, Jakubowski M, Burstein R (2004) Disruption of communication between peripheral and central trigeminovascular neurons mediates the antimigraine action of 5HT 1B/1D receptor agonists. Proc Natl Acad Sci U S A 101:4274–4279

Lipton RB, Stewart WF, Cady R, Hall C, O'Quinn S, Kuhn T, Gutterman D (2000) Sumatriptan for the range of headaches in migraine sufferers: results of the Spectrum Study. Headache 40:783–791

Maneesi S, Akerman S, Lasalandra MP, Classey JD, Goadsby PJ (2004) Electron microscopic demonstration of pre- and postsynaptic 5-HT1D and 5-HT1F receptor immunoreactivity (IR) in the rat trigeminocervical complex (TCC) new therapeutic possibilities for the triptans. Cephalalgia 24:148

Markowitz S, Saito K, Moskowitz MA (1987) Neurogenically mediated leakage of plasma proteins occurs from blood vessels in dura mater but not brain. J Neurosci 7:4129–4136

Markowitz S, Saito K, Moskowitz MA (1988) Neurogenically mediated plasma extravasation in dura mater: effect of ergot alkaloids. A possible mechanism of action in vascular headache. Cephalalgia 8:83–91

Matharu MS, Goadsby PJ (2004) Cluster headache: a review with a focus on emerging therapies. Expert Rev Neurother 4:895–907

May A, Gijsman HJ, Wallnoefer A, Jones R, Diener HC, Ferrari MD (1996) Endothelin antagonist bosentan blocks neurogenic inflammation, but is not effective in aborting migraine attacks. Pain 67:375–378

May A, Bahra A, Buchel C, Frackowiak RSJ, Goadsby PJ (1998a) Hypothalamic activation in cluster headache attacks. Lancet 352:275–278

May A, Shepheard S, Wessing A, Hargreaves RJ, Goadsby PJ, Diener HC (1998b) Retinal plasma extravasation can be evoked by trigeminal stimulation in rat but does not occur during migraine attacks. Brain 121:1231–1237

May A, Bahra A, Buchel C, Turner R, Goadsby PJ (1999) Functional MRI in spontaneous attacks of SUNCT: short-lasting neuralgiform headache with conjunctival injection and tearing. Ann Neurol 46:791–793

McCall RB, Huff R, Chio CL, TenBrink R, Bergh CL, Ennis MD, Ghazal NB, Hoffman RL, Meisheri K, Higdon NR, Hall E (2002) Preclinical studies characterizing the anti-migraine and cardiovascular effects of the selective 5-HT 1D receptor agonist PNU-142633. Cephalalgia 22:799–806

McNaughton FL (1966) The innervation of the intracranial blood vessels and the dural sinuses. In: Cobb S, Frantz AM, Penfield W, Riley HA (eds) The circulation of the brain and spinal cord. Hafner Publishing, New York, pp 178–200

Mitsikostas DD, Sanchez del Rio M, Moskowitz MA, Waeber C (1999) Both 5-HT1B and 5-HT1F receptors modulate c-fos expression within rat trigeminal nucleus caudalis. Eur J Pharmacol 369:271–277

Morgan JI, Curran T (1991) Stimulus-transcription coupling in the nervous system: involvement of the inducible proto-oncogenes fos and jun. Annu Rev Neurosci 14:421–451

Moskowitz MA (1990) Basic mechanisms in vascular headache. Neurol Clin 8:801–815

Moskowitz MA, Cutrer FM (1993) Sumatriptan: a receptor-targeted treatment for migraine. Annu Rev Med 44:145–154

Moskowitz MA, Nozaki K, Kraig RP (1993) Neocortical spreading depression provokes the expression of C-fos protein-like immunoreactivity within the trigeminal nucleus caudalis via trigeminovascular mechanisms. J Neurosci 13:1167–1177

Norman B, Panebianco D, Block GA (1998) A placebo-controlled, in-clinic study to explore the preliminary safety and efficacy of intravenous L-758,298 (a prodrug of the NK1 receptor antagonist L-754,030) in the acute treatment of migraine. Cephalalgia 18:407

Nozaki K, Boccalini P, Moskowitz MA (1992) Expression of c-fos-like immunoreactivity in brainstem after meningeal irritation by blood in the subarachnoid space. Neuroscience 49:669–680

Pascual J, Arco Cd, Romon T, Olmo Cd, Pazos A (1996) [3H] Sumatriptan binding sites in human brain: regional-dependent labelling of 5HT1D and 5HT1F receptors. Eur J Pharmacol 295:271–274

Penfield W (1932a) Intracerebral vascular nerves. AMA Arch Neurol Psychiatry 27:30–44

Penfield W (1932b) Operative treatment of migraine and observations on the mechanism of vascular pain. Trans Am Acad Ophthalmol Otolaryngol III:1–16

Penfield W (1934) A contribution to the mechanism of intracranial pain. Proc Assoc Res Nerv Mental Dis 15:399–415

Penfield W, McNaughton FL (1940) Dural headache and the innervation of the dura mater. AMA Arch Neurol Psychiatry 44:43–75

Phebus LA, Johnson KW, Zgombick JM, Gilbert PJ, Van Belle K, Mancuso V, Nelson DLG, Calligaro DO, Kiefer AD, Branchek TA, Flaugh ME (1997) Characterization of LY334370 as a pharmacological tool to study 5HT1F receptors—binding affinities, brain penetration and activity in the neurogenic dural inflammation model of migraine. Life Sci 61: 2117–2126

Potrebic S, Ahan AH, Skinner K, Fields HL, Basbaum AI (2003) Peptidergic nociceptors of both trigeminal and dorsal root ganglia express serotonin 1D receptors: implications for the selective antimigraine action of triptans. J Neurosci 23:10988–10997

Pozo-Rosich P, Oshinsky M (2005) Effect of dihydroergotamine (DHE) on central sensitisation of neurons in the trigeminal nucleus caudalis. Neurology 64:A151

Pregenzer JF, Alberts GL, Block JH, Slightom JL, Im WB (1997) Characterisation of ligand binding properties of the 5-HT1D receptors cloned from chimpanzee, gorilla and rhesus monkey in comparison with those from the human and guinea pig receptors. Neurosci Lett 235:117–120

Pregenzer JF, Alberts GL, Im WB, Slightom JL, Ennis MD, Hoffman RL, Ghazal NB, Ten-Brink RE (1999) Differential pharmacology between the guinea-pig and the gorilla 5-HT1D receptor as probed with isochromans (5-HT1D-selective ligands). Br J Pharmacol 127:468–472

Raskin NH, Hosobuchi Y, Lamb S (1987) Headache may arise from perturbation of brain. Headache 27:416–420

Ray BS, Wolff HG (1940) Experimental studies on headache. Pain sensitive structures of the head and their significance in headache. Arch Surg 41:813–856

Razzaque Z, Heald MA, Pickard JD, Maskell L, Beer MS, Hill RG, Longmore J (1999) Vasoconstriction in human isolated middle meningeal arteries: determining the contribution of 5-HT1B- and 5-HT1F-receptor activation. Br J Clin Pharmacol 47:75–82

Roon K, Diener HC, Ellis P, Hettiarachchi J, Poole P, Christiansen I, Ferrari MD, Olesen J (1997) CP-122,288 blocks neurogenic inflammation, but is not effective in aborting migraine attacks: results of two controlled clinical studies. Cephalalgia 17:245

Saxena PR, Cairo-Rawlins WI (1979) Presynaptic inhibition by ergotamine of the responses to cardioaccelerator nerve stimulations in the cat. Eur J Pharmacol 58:305–312

Saxena PR, De Boer MO (1991) Pharmacology of antimigraine drugs. J Neurol 238:S28–S35

Selby G, Lance JW (1960) Observations on 500 cases of migraine and allied vascular headache. J Neurol Neurosurg Psychiatry 23:23–32

Shields KG, Goadsby PJ (2004) Naratriptan modulates trigeminovascular nociceptive transmission in the ventroposteromedial (VPM) thalamic nucleus of the rat. Cephalalgia 24:1098

Shields KG, Goadsby PJ (2005) Propranolol modulates trigeminovascular responses in thalamic ventroposteromedial nucleus: a role in migraine? Brain 128:86–97

Shields KG, Kaube H, Goadsby PJ (2003) GABA receptors modulate trigeminovascular nociceptive transmission in the ventroposteromedial (VPM) thalamic nucleus of the rat. Cephalalgia 23:728

Steuer H, Jaworski A, Stoll D, Schlosshauer B (2004) In vitro model of the outer blood-retina barrier. Brain Res Brain Res Protoc 13:26–36

Storer RJ, Goadsby PJ (1997) Microiontophoretic application of serotonin (5HT)1B/1D agonists inhibits trigeminal cell firing in the cat. Brain 120:2171–2177

Strassman AM, Raymond SA, Burstein R (1996) Sensitization of meningeal sensory neurons and the origin of headaches. Nature 384:560–563

Veloso F, Kumar K, Toth C (1998) Headache secondary to deep brain implantation. Headache 38:507–515

Waeber C, Moskowitz MA (1995) [3H]Sumatriptan labels both 5-HT1D and 5HT1F receptor bindings sites in the guinea pig brain: an autoradiographic study. Naunyn Schmiedebergs Arch Pharmacol 352:263–275

Waeber C, Cutrer FM, Yu XJ, Moskowitz MA (1997) The selective 5HT1D receptor agonist U-109291 blocks dural plasma extravasation and c-fos expression in the trigeminal nucleus caudalis. Cephalalgia 17:401

Wainscott DB, Johnson KW, Phebus LA, Schaus JM, Nelson DL (1998) Human 5-HT1F receptor-stimulated [S-35]GTP gamma S binding: correlation with inhibition of guinea pig dural plasma protein extravasation. Eur J Pharmacol 352:117–124

Weiller C, May A, Limmroth V, Juptner M, Kaube H, Schayck RV, Coenen HH, Diener HC (1995) Brain stem activation in spontaneous human migraine attacks. Nat Med 1:658–660

Williamson DJ, Hargreaves RJ, Hill RG, Shepheard SL (1997) Sumatriptan inhibits neurogenic vasodilation of dural blood vessels in the anaesthetized rat—intravital microscope studies. Cephalalgia 17:525–531

Wolff HG (1948) Headache and other head pain. Oxford University Press, New York

Zagami AS, Goadsby PJ (1991) Stimulation of the superior sagittal sinus increases metabolic activity in cat thalamus. In: Rose FC (ed) New advances in headache research: 2. Smith-Gordon, London, pp 169–171

Zagami AS, Lambert GA (1991) Craniovascular application of capsaicin activates nociceptive thalamic neurons in the cat. Neurosci Lett 121:187–190

HEP (2006) 177:145–177
© Springer-Verlag Berlin Heidelberg 2006

Anti-convulsants and Anti-depressants

A. H. Dickenson (✉) · J. Ghandehari

Dept. Pharmacology, University College London, Gower Street, London WC1E 6BT, UK
anthony.dickenson@ucl.ac.uk

1	Introduction	146
2	Anti-convulsants	148
2.1	Mode of Action	148
2.1.1	Phenytoin	150
2.1.2	Carbamazepine and Oxcarbazepine	151
2.1.3	Valproic Acid	153
2.1.4	Lamotrigine	155
2.1.5	Topiramate	157
2.1.6	Gabapentin	158
2.1.7	Ethosuximide	162
3	Anti-depressants	163
3.1	Mode of Action	163
4	Classical Anti-depressants	166
5	Conclusion	170
	References	171

Abstract Damage to a nerve should only lead to sensory loss. While this is common, the incidence of spontaneous pain, allodynia and hyperalgesia indicate marked changes in the nervous system that are possible compensations for the loss of normal function that arises from the sensory loss. Neuropathic pain arises from changes in the damaged nerve which then alter function in the spinal cord and the brain and lead to plasticity in areas adjacent to those directly influenced by the neuropathy. The peripheral changes drive central compensations so that the mechanisms involved are multiple and located at a number of sites. Nerve damage increases the excitability of both the damaged and undamaged nerve fibres, neuromas and the cell bodies in the dorsal root ganglion. These peripheral changes are substrates for the ongoing pain and the efficacy of excitability blockers such as carbamazepine, lamotrigine and mexiletine, all anti-convulsants. A better understanding of ion channels at the sites of injury has shown important roles of particular sodium, potassium and calcium channels in the genesis of neuropathic pain. Within the spinal cord, increases in the activity of calcium channels and the receptors for glutamate, especially the N-methyl-D-aspartate (NMDA) receptor, trigger wind-up and central hyperexcitability. Increases in transmitter release, neuronal excitability and receptive field size result from the damage to the peripheral nerves. Ketamine and gabapentin/pregabalin, again with anti-convulsant activity, may interact with these mechanisms. Ketamine acts on central spinal mechanisms of excitability whereas gabapentin acts on a subunit of calcium channels that is responsible for the release of pain transmitters into the spinal cord. In addition to these spinal mechanisms of hyperexcitability, spinal cells participate in a spinal–supraspinal loop that involves parts of the brain involved in affective responses to pain but also engages descending excitatory and inhibitory systems that use the monoamines. These pathways become more active after nerve injury and are the site of action of anti-depressants. This chapter reviews the evidence and mechanisms of drugs, both anti-depressants and anti-convulsants, that are believed to be effective in pain control, with a major emphasis on the neuropathic state.

Keywords Neuropathic pain · Anti-depressants · Anti-convulsants · Ion channels · Monoamines

1
Introduction

Neuropathic pain is caused by injury, disease or dysfunction to the peripheral or central nervous system (Tremont-Lukats et al. 2000). The development and maintenance of chronic pain due to nerve injury is characterized by damage to the nervous system which in turn leads to changes at peripheral and central levels that ultimately cause neuronal hyper-excitability (Dickenson et al. 2002). This neuronal hyper-excitability in neurons without their normal pattern input seems to be a common mechanism present in the pathophysiology associated with neuropathic pain states. A heterogeneous group of pain conditions such as painful diabetic neuropathy, trigeminal neuralgia (TN), human immunodeficiency virus (HIV)-associated painful neuropathy, mixed neuropathic pain syndromes, phantom limb pain, Guillain-Barré syndrome, and acute and chronic pain from spinal cord injury are characterized by lesions or dysfunction of the normal sensory pathways and may be referred to as neuropathic pains. The two most common neuropathic pain states are post-herpetic neuralgia (PHN) and painful diabetic neuropathy (Jensen et al. 2001a; Gordon and Love 2004). Neuropathic pain states have clinical manifestations such as the delayed onset of pain after nervous system lesion, pain in the area of sensory loss, increased sensory response to supra-threshold stimulus, increase of the peripheral areas from where a central neuron can be activated, and recruitment of previous non-responding nociceptive neurons (Tremont-Lukats et al. 2000; Jensen 2001). In neuropathic pain the nervous system adapts both morphologically and functionally to external stimuli, causing an onset and continuance of pain symptoms. Both animal and human models of neuropathic pain have been studied to understand this neuroplasticity in terms of its biochemistry and pathophysiology (Tremont-Lukats et al. 2000). Basic science research has contributed to the knowledge of pain processes as well as the molecular and neuronal bases for neuroplasticity associated with neuropathic pain. Research and discovery of a number of pain targets have made it possible to modulate the neuronal hyper-excitability that exists in neuropathic pain states. Furthermore, basic science research suggests that the changes in neuronal responsiveness appear to be partly time and intensity dependent but with minimal dependence on aetiology. Unfortunately, this increase in knowledge from basic science has not yet resulted in a proportional improvement in the clinical ability to treat chronic pain. Chronic unrelieved pain is a common problem in many patients, and the newest treatments have not resulted in significantly better outcomes (Jensen et al. 2001b).

The drugs used to treat neuropathic pain act to modulate N-methyl-D-aspartate (NMDA) receptors, sodium or calcium channels, the process of reuptake of monoamines [noradrenaline (NA) or serotonin (5-hydroxytryptamine, 5HT)], opioid receptors, and other cell processes (Gordon and Love 2004; Dickenson et al. 2002).

The management of neuropathic pain is complex and requires an understanding that multiple mechanisms may be responsible for single symptoms and single mechanisms may be responsible for multiple symptoms in both the central and peripheral nervous systems (Gordon and Love 2004).

The role of anti-depressants and anti-convulsants in the therapy of neuropathic pain is clear from not only clinical studies but from meta-analyses of the published data where the numbers needed to treat (NNTs) for these drug classes are similar, about 3. Nevertheless, the initial use of compounds in these classes was pragmatic and not based on any clear mechanistic basis. Indeed, part of the basis for the use of anti-depressants for pain was the recognition of depression as a treatable co-morbidity with pain. Now it is clear that the mood changes are independent of the ability of these drugs to reduce pain and often the doses and time course differ as well. The anti-depressant drugs include the old tricyclic anti-depressants (TCAs) and imipramine as well as the newer selective serotonin reuptake inhibitors (SSRIs) and the latest balanced serotonin/NA reuptake inhibitors (SNRIs). The anti-convulsants had a more rational basis in that epilepsy and pain share the common characteristic of arising from excessive activity in neuronal circuits but still had no mechanistic basis. Within this class the main drugs are excitability blockers such as carbamazepine (CBZ) and lamotrigine and what have now been termed $\alpha_2\delta$ ligands, gabapentin (GBP) and pregabalin (PGB). Over the years the use of animal models of pain from nerve injury has enabled a basis for the use of both drug classes to be determined. However, their modes of action are very different, which lends credence to the concept that multiple co-existing mechanisms are at play in neuropathic states that generate common symptoms and common treatments (Hansson and Dickenson 2005). Some advocate the use of a mechanism-based classification scheme as an attractive approach to the study of neuropathic pain because it provides a framework for pharmacological therapy in neuropathic pain (Jensen et al. 2001a). Unfortunately, there exists a large gap in our body of knowledge in regards to both the mechanisms involved in the pathophysiology of neuropathic pain states as well as with the pharmacotherapy of neuropathic pain, rendering this approach theoretically appealing but practically daunting.

On this basis we will review the evidence on how and why anti-depressants and anti-convulsants work in pain from nerve injury.

2
Anti-convulsants

2.1
Mode of Action

As mentioned above, the peripheral and central changes resulting from nerve injury account for the mechanisms of action of anti-convulsant drug therapies in neuropathic pain (Hansson and Dickenson 2005). The anti-epileptic drugs (AEDs) act by decreasing excitation by blocking sodium or calcium channels or by increasing inhibition via γ-aminobutyric acid (GABA) function. Other drugs used to treat neuropathic pain, such as ketamine, act by decreasing excitation via NMDA receptor antagonism (Dickenson et al. 2002).

Peripheral pain and central neuropathic pain are both marked by a neuronal hyper-excitability in damaged areas of the nervous system (Suzuki and Dickenson 2000). This hyper-excitability and its resultant molecular changes in neuropathic pain have common features with the cellular changes in some forms of epilepsy (Jensen 2002). This similar pathophysiology of neuropathic pain and some epilepsy models promotes the use and study of anti-convulsant drugs in the symptomatic management of neuropathic pain states (Tremont-Lukats et al. 2000; Backonja 2000).

In peripheral neuropathic pain an increased and novel expression of sodium channels, increased activity at glutamate receptor sites, modulation in GABAergic inhibition, and a change in calcium current contributes to the damaged nerve increased activity and pathological spontaneous activity. The allodynia and spontaneous pain associated with central pain are also explained by neuronal hyper-excitability. These neuropathic changes occur at the level of the peripheral nociceptor, in dorsal root ganglia, in the dorsal horn of the spinal cord and in the brain (Jensen 2002). The existence of certain sodium channels that are selectively located in small peripheral fibres and the re-emergence of other channels may allow for better therapy in the future (see chapter by J.N. Wood, this volume).

Anti-convulsants with proven efficacy in neuropathic pain are predominantly GBP and PGB or the excitability blockers or membrane stabilizers. These drugs that act to block sodium channels attenuate neuronal excitability. Given the important role of sodium channels at and around the site of injury in the peripheral fibres, it is likely that a main component of their actions are to reduce peripheral nerve firing, either ectopic or evoked. However, given the ubiquity of these channels, effects within the CNS are likely, given that this latter action underlies their anti-convulsant effects. The peripheral action is supported by the ability of lignocaine patches to be effective in animal and human psychophysical approaches.

GBP and PGB are yet again examples of drugs designed for one therapeutic area (epilepsy) that have been shown to be additionally highly effective in pain. The original idea was that these drugs should have actions on GABA function, a rational basis that subsequently was found not to be their mode of action. There were animal data that showed these compounds were effective in animal models of pain, with the first data being in inflammatory states, soon followed by evidence in rodent models of nerve injury, clinical trials and a licence for this therapeutic use. In parallel, it emerged that these compounds interacted with calcium channels, binding to the accessory $\alpha_2\delta$ protein. Given the key roles of calcium channels in triggering the release of transmitters at synapses, this action is logical. What is less clear is how these compounds interact with a target common to all calcium channels in the body, yet produce selective effects on pain, although also having anti-convulsant, anxiolytic and sleep-promoting actions. It would be predicted that actions on calcium channels would reduce function at all synapses in the peripheral and central nervous systems, as well as those on cardiovascular and smooth muscle systems. However, there are up-regulations of both particular calcium channels after nerve injury and inflammation as well as the $\alpha_2\delta$ binding site that may impart a state-dependency on the actions of these drugs (Luo et al. 2001, 2002; Dickenson et al. 2002). Further, the descending facilitatory 5HT3 system is permissive for the actions of these compounds. Thus the drugs appear to produce their selective actions on pathophysiological pain states when their target channels and descending facilitatory systems are altered by the pain state. This allows rather selective actions, but in animals—and now in humans—their actions are not limited to peripheral neuropathic pain but comprise other pain models that include hyper-excitability such as chemical trauma, spinal cord injury and cancer-induced bone pain (Hansson and Dickenson 2005).

Central neuropathic pain (CP) following lesions of the CNS that result in neuronal hyper-excitability may also be treated with some anti-convulsants. First-generation anti-convulsant drugs such as phenytoin, benzodiazepines, valproate and CBZ and second-generation anti-convulsant drugs such as lamotrigine, GBP and topiramate are used to treat CP syndromes. According to Finnerup et al. (2002), few randomized controlled trials of CP had been published. Also, lamotrigine was the first choice in anti-convulsant treatment for CP, followed by GBP or CBZ/oxcarbazepine, which are considered to be as effective as amitriptyline, the anti-depressant (Finnerup et al. 2002). McQuay et al. (1995) performed a systematic review of anti-convulsant drugs for both effectiveness and adverse effects in the management of pain. Later, Wiffen et al. (2000) updated this review and support the findings of McQuay et al. (1995). The numbers listed here are from Wiffen et al. (2000).

Overall, treatment of diabetic neuropathy with anti-convulsants has a combined NNT of 3 for effectiveness, 2.5 for adverse effects and 20 for severe effects. Anti-convulsant combined effect in migraine prophylaxis has an NNT of 2.4 for effectiveness, 2.4 for adverse effects and 39 for severe effects (Wiffen et al. 2000c).

The burst activity associated with pain that corresponds to the phenomenon of hyper-excitability and increased baseline sensitivity of primary sensory neurons after nerve injury seems to be initiated by a change in sodium channel expression in dorsal root ganglion (DRG) neurons. However, roughly a dozen distinct sodium channels encoded by different genes are known. Abnormal accumulations of sodium channels are observable at the tips of injured axons; specifically, Waxman (1999) observes dramatic alterations in sodium channel expression in DRG neurons following axonal injury and demonstrates a down-regulation of SNS/PN3 and NaN sodium channel genes and up-regulation of the usually silent type III sodium channel gene. Spontaneous firing or firing at inappropriately high frequencies is observable in DRG neurons—which includes nociceptive cells—in electrophysiological studies demonstrating that altered expression of sodium channels plays a role in the pathophysiology of pain (Waxman 1999; Suzuki and Dickenson 2000).

2.1.1
Phenytoin

Historically, the sodium channel blocker phenytoin was the first anti-convulsant used to treat neuropathic pain when Bergouignan successfully used this drug to treat patients with neuropathic pain caused by TN (see Backonja 2000). The analgesic activity of phenytoin is due to an inhibition of voltage gated Na^+ channels, which limits the repetitive firing associated with neuropathic pain (Sindrup and Jensen 1999; Dickenson et al. 2002), as well as an upstream inhibition of presynaptic glutamate release (David et al. 1985). Furthermore, an early basic science report that phenytoin causes a reduction of autotomy in rats with dorsal rhizotomy (Duckrow and Taub 1977) forms a basis for its use to treat neuropathic pain.

In clinical trial, however, a small randomized, double-blind, placebo-controlled, cross-over trial by Saudek et al. (1977) of phenytoin in diabetic neuropathy shows no significant improvement in pain score with the use of this drug. It is noteworthy that, in this study, diabetic patients treated with phenytoin experienced an increased blood glucose level and also an increase in undesirable side-effects. A contradictory report showed successful symptom treatment of neuropathic pain with phenytoin; Chadda and Mathur (1978) published a randomized, double-blind, placebo-controlled, cross-over trial of phenytoin in diabetic neuropathy that found this drug to be effective when compared to placebo with an NNT of 2.1. Tremont-Lukats et al. (2000) attribute this discrepancy to possible differences in sample size, duration of follow-up time, and low statistical power, which may contribute to a lack of detection of differences between phenytoin and placebo. According to Backonja (2000) there was no evidence in clinical trials for phenytoin's efficacy in treatment of neuropathic pain. However, a randomized, double-blinded, placebo-controlled, cross-over study by McCleane et al. (2003) shows that i.v. administration of 15 mg/kg phenytoin provides an analgesic effect that lasts longer than the infusion time as well as the plasma half-life of the drug in acute flare-ups associated with neuropathic pain. This study demonstrates that i.v. phenytoin causes significant reduction in burning pain, shooting pain, sensitivity, numbness and overall pain throughout the infusion period. Furthermore, this study shows depression of overall pain lasting for 1 day, depression of sensitivity lasting for 2 days, and depression in shooting pain lasting for 4 days after infusion.

Phenytoin is a first generation anti-convulsant that is used in the treatment of CP caused by lesions of the CNS which result in neuronal hyper-excitability (Finnerup et al. 2002). The side-effects of phenytoin such as sedation and motor disturbances limit its use in the treatment of chronic neuropathic pain. Nevertheless, this drug's availability for intravenous infusion makes it an appropriate choice for treatment of acute attacks associated with neuropathic pain (Jensen 2002).

2.1.2
Carbamazepine and Oxcarbazepine

The first anti-convulsant to be studied in clinical trials was CBZ. The drug causes a decreased conductance in Na^+ channels, inhibits ectopic discharges and has been shown to treat neuropathic pain in TN, painful diabetic neuropathy and PHN (Backonja 2000; Tremont-Lukats et al. 2000).

Optimal pharmacotherapy for epilepsy as well as for neuropathic pain requires that spontaneous activity is suppressed without interference with normal nerve conductance. CBZ blocks the spontaneous activity of the A-δ and C fibres responsible for pain and abnormal nerve conductance via frequency-dependent inhibition of sodium currents (Tanelian and Brose 1991; Suzuki and Dickenson 2000; Dickenson et al. 2002).

Rush and Elliott (1997) studied CBZ and phenytoin's effects on a heterogeneous population of Na^+ channels in patch-clamped small cells from adult rat dorsal horn ganglia to show that TTX-R Na^+ currents are inhibited by these anti-convulsant agents used as pain therapy. Future development of modality-specific treatment may be aided with the knowledge that different Na^+ channels possess distinct activation profiles (Suzuki and Dickenson 2000).

The basic science research conduced by Fox et al. (2003) gives supporting evidence that the anti-convulsant CBZ and oxcarbazepine (as well as lamotrigine and GBP) are effective in treating mechanical hyperalgesia and tactile allodynia in an animal model of neuropathic pain. The side-effect profile of oxcarbazepine is improved compared to existing therapies. These data give support for the use of these AEDs in the clinical treatment of neuropathic pain. Specifically, this study examines the effects of oxcarbazepine and the other AEDs in rat and guinea-pig models of neuropathic pain. The results of these drugs varied between the rat model and the guinea-pig model of neuropathic pain induced by partial sciatic nerve ligation. Oxcarbazepine and CBZ had no effect on mechanical hyperalgesia or tactile allodynia in the rat following drug administration. However, in the guinea-pig with the same model of neuropathic pain used in the rat, a 90% depression of mechanical hyperalgesia with oxcarbazepine and CBZ is seen. Also, a similar drop in mechanical hyperalgesia is observed solely in the guinea-pig pain model with the active human metabolite of oxcarbazepine, monohydroxy derivative (Fox et al. 2003).

Today, CBZ is the treatment of choice for TN as studied in three placebo-controlled trials (Campbell et al. 1966; Nicol 1969; Killian and Fromm 1968). CBZ has an NNT of 2.6 in TN (Wiffen et al. 2000; Jensen 2002). Second line drugs used to treat this neuropathic pain condition are phenytoin, baclofen, clonazepam and sodium valproate (Perkin 1999).

CBZ produces significant pain reduction in patients suffering from painful diabetic neuropathy with an NNT of 3.3 based on a study by Rull et al. (Rull et al. 1969; McQuay et al. 1995). A 15-patient, double-blind, 3-phase, cross-over, placebo-controlled trial by Leijon and Boivie (1989) studied the effect on central post-stroke pain (CPSP) of amitriptyline and CBZ. Compared to amitriptyline, CBZ was less effective in the treatment of CPSP and not statistically different when compared to placebo (Leijon and Boivie 1989). The small number of patients studied could account for the results of this study.

The number needed to harm (NNH) for CBZ is 3.4 for minor side-effects and NNH of 24 for severe effects. The common side-effects of CBZ are drowsiness, diplopia, blurred vision, nausea and vomiting. In treatment of the elderly population with this drug, one must be aware of possible cardiac disease, water retention, decreased osmolality and hyponatremia complications (Wiffen et al. 2000; Jensen 2002).

The second-generation AED, oxcarbazepine, the dihydro-ketone analogue of CBZ, provides significant analgesia in TN, painful diabetic neuropathy and many other neuropathic pain conditions refractory to other AEDs like CBZ and GBP. The documented effects of oxcarbazepine in neuropathic pain as well as its improved safety profile and low side-effects suggest that this drug should be considered as a treatment therapy for neuropathic pain (Carrazana and Mikoshiba 2003).

CBZ, oxcarbazepine and the dihydro-monohydroxy analogue of CBZ were examined by Farago et al. (1987) in 13 patients suffering from TN. Both analogues reduced the pain or symptoms associated with TN in all patients. The effective dose was between 10 and 20 mg/kg in most patients. These analogues can be dispensed at higher doses than CBZ because adverse effects such as dizziness and ataxia occur much less often with them (Farago 1987).

Zakrzewska et al. (1997) examined the effect of oxcarbazepine in six patients with TN who were unsuccessfully treated with CBZ. This study finds that oxcarbazepine has therapeutic effect in pain control of TN with no significant side-effects.

Oxcarbazepine has a distinct pharmacokinetic profile from oxcarbazepine. Oxcarbazepine is rapidly reduced to 10,11-dihydro-10-hydroxy-carbamazepine, its active metabolite; neither oxcarbazepine nor its active metabolite induce hepatic oxidative metabolism with the exception of the P450IIIA isozyme of the cytochrome P450 family. Due to hyponatraemia observed in some patients, fluid restriction may be advisable in some epileptic patients in order to reduce the risk of precipitating seizures secondary to low serum sodium. This drug appears to be a suitable substitute for CBZ in patients who do not tolerate CBZ or suffer from significant drug interactions (Grant and Faulds 1992).

The FDA approved oxcarbazepine in 2000 for add-on treatment of partial seizures in adults. This anti-convulsant is a membrane stabilizer and acts as a weak hepatic inducer without auto-induction. Like CBZ, oxcarbazepine acts to treat TN with comparable efficacy and less side-effects. In comparison to CBZ, this newer AED has no hepatotoxicity or bone marrow suppression. The side-effect profile includes nausea, vomiting or dizziness, skin rash and oedema. Oxcarbazepine may be used to treat refractory neuropathic pain (Royal 2001).

In summary, as the first anti-convulsant drugs to be tested in controlled clinical trials, CBZ and phenytoin have proved to act effectively to relieve painful diabetic neuropathy and paroxysmal attacks associated with TN. CBZ, oxcarbazepine and lamotrigine have replaced phenytoin because of its complicated pharmacokinetic profile and undesired side-effects.

Oxcarbazepine has a side-effect profile that is better tolerated than that of CBZ. Thus, oxcarbazepine has become the drug of choice to treat TN in many Western countries (Jensen 2002). At present, there is no explanation of why drugs that have actions on sodium channels have proven efficacy in TNs rather than a broad action on pain from other areas of the body.

2.1.3
Valproic Acid

Valproic acid has a wide range of clinical uses today due to its multiple mechanisms of action. It has often been suggested that valproic acid acts by a combination of several different mechanisms because of its wide range of therapy uses such as its use in different seizure types, bipolar and schizo-affective disorders, neuropathic pain and prophylactic treatment of migraine (Loscher 1999; Johannessen 2000). The first studies on use of valproic acid to treat neuropathic pain appeared in the early 1980s; this drug caused a reduction of pain in 50%–80% of patients with TN (Peiris et al. 1980; Savitskaya 1980; Tremont-Lukats et al. 2000). Similar to other first-generation anti-convulsant drugs such as phenytoin and CBZ, valproic acid is used to treat central neuropathic pain (Finnerup et al. 2002).

Preclinical animal models of seizures or epilepsy also reflect the wide range of therapeutic effects of valproate. Evidence shows that valproic acid increases GABA synthesis and release in the central nervous system (Dickenson et al. 2002), thus potentiating GABAergic functions (Lee et al. 1995; Loscher 1999).

Moreover, valproic acid prolongs the repolarization phase of voltage-sensitive sodium channels and modulates TCA cycle enzymes including succinate semialdehyde dehydrogenase (SSA-DH), GABA transaminase (GABA-T), and α-ketoglutarate dehydrogenase, thus affecting cerebral metabolism (Johannessen 2000; Tremont-Lukats et al. 2000; Jensen 2002). In vitro studies show valproic acid as a potent inhibitor of SSA-DH. Also, only high concentrations of this drug inhibit GABA-T in brain homogenates, and there is possible inhibition of α-ketoglutarate dehydrogenase of the TCA cycle. It has been thought that the GABA-mediated action of valproate is responsible for its use in neuropathic pain. The effect of the drug on excitatory neurotransmission and on excitatory membranes is likely a result of its mechanisms in 'mood-stabilizing' and in its use in migraine prophylaxis (Johannessen 2000; Johannessen and Johannessen 2003). Valproic acid seems to reduce γ-hydroxybutyric acid release and alters neuronal excitation which is induced by NMDA-type glutamate receptors. Additionally, valproic acid acts with direct effects on excitable membranes. Loscher (1999) has stated that microdialysis data support an alteration in dopaminergic and serotonergic function due to valproic acid. It is noteworthy that valproic acid is metabolized into many pharmacologically active compounds. However, the low concentration levels in the plasma and brain makes it unlikely that they have a significant role in the anti-convulsant or toxic effects of valproic acid (Loscher 1999).

After four decades of investigation of the mechanisms of action of one of the most widely used anti-epileptic drugs, the cellular mechanisms of valproic acid on synaptic physiology remain unclear. Martin et al. (2004) examined valproic acid's effects on synaptic transmission using the in vitro rat hippocampal slice technique. Results from this study suggest that the effects of valproate are caused in part by a decrease in excitatory synaptic activity by modulation of postsynaptic non-NMDA receptors while leaving synaptic inhibition unchanged (Martin and Pozo 2004).

Hardy et al. (2001) conducted a phase II study of sodium valproate for cancer-related neuropathic pain. Response to the drug was defined as a decrease in pain score without increased need for analgesic medications. This study's response rate for average pain at day 15 is 55.6%. However, this study has a large variability in response rates, depending on the mode of analysis (Hardy et al. 2001).

Unfortunately, in a randomized, double-blind, placebo-controlled, crossover clinical study, valproic acid had no significant effect when compared with placebo in painful polyneuropathy (Otto et al. 2004). Furthermore, sodium valproate is found to have no analgesic effect in the only placebo-controlled study of acute pain (Wiffen et al. 2000). As it stands, the current literature is unable to explain the precise role of valproic acid in the symptom management of neuropathic pain, and further studies are needed to examine this drug's role in peripheral neuropathic pain disorders such as painful diabetic neuropathy (Tremont-Lukats et al. 2000).

2.1.4
Lamotrigine

Early clinical reports that lamotrigine, a voltage-activated sodium channel blocker as well as a potential calcium channel blocker, confers beneficial therapeutic effects in central pain have prompted studies of use of this drug in the treatment of neuropathic pain (Canavero and Bonicalzi 1996).

An in vitro study by Cheung et al. (1992) suggests a direct interaction of lamotrigine with voltage-activated sodium channels which results in a block of sustained repetitive firing of sodium-dependent action potentials in cultured neurons from mouse spinal cord, as well as an inhibition of sodium channel binding in rat brain synaptosomes. This voltage-activated sodium channel blocker dampens the ectopic discharges in the peripheral nervous system associated with neuropathic pain in a use-dependent manner. Lamotrigine acts by decreasing the increased neuronal excitability of afferent fibres and also by acting at the synaptic contacts of these fibres with the spinal cord (Blackburn-Munro and Fleetwood-Walker 1999; Dickenson et al. 2002; Jensen 2002).

Blackburn-Munro and Fleetwood-Walker (1999) examined the mechanism of action of lamotrigine on the sodium channel auxiliary subunits β_1 and β_2 in the spinal cord of neuropathic rats. It is known that Na^+ channels are composed of a main subunit which can vary and two supporting subunits $\beta1$ and $\beta2$. These two β-subunits act to modulate the rate of channel activation and inactivation as well as to modify α-subunit density within the plasma membrane. In a chronic constrictive nerve injury model, Blackburn-Munro and Fleetwood-Walker (1999) show that β_1 messenger RNA (mRNA) levels increase with a corresponding decrease in β_2 mRNA levels in laminae I and II on the ipsilateral side of the cord relative to β levels in the contralateral side of the cord. This study suggests that the altered excitability of the central neurons associated with neuropathic pain may be partly explained by altered expression of β Na^+ channel subunit types (Blackburn-Munro and Fleetwood-Walker 1999; Blackburn-Munro et al. 2001). It also showed that the opioid/cholecystokinin pathway is not involved in lamotrigine's anti-nociceptive effects (Blackburn-Munro et al. 2001). It follows that lamotrigine inhibits the neuronal release of glutamate indirectly by blocking sodium channels (Klamt 1998).

Furthermore, lamotrigine is claimed to act to modulate central sensitization via high-threshold N-type calcium channels, although this is unlikely to be a major primary action of the drug (Gordon and Love 2004).

Early in vivo studies support the use of lamotrigine in the treatment of neuropathic pain. Hunter et al. (1997) have reported that lamotrigine reverses cold allodynia 1 h post dose in a chronic constriction injury rat model of neuropathic pain. Erichsen et al. (2003) have shown that lamotrigine significantly modulates mechanical hyperalgesia in a rat spared nerve injury model. However, lamotrigine had no effect on mechanical or cold allodynia in either a photo-chemically induced model of nerve injury (Gazelius) or in a spared nerve injury model (Erichsen et al. 2003).

A study by Christensen et al. (2001) comparing GBP and lamotrigine in a rat model of trigeminal neuropathic pain found that repeated GBP but not lamotrigine partially alleviates the mechanical allodynia associated with trigeminal neuropathic pain states. Single doses of either GBP or lamotrigine produced no effect on the mechanical allodynia-like behaviour in this study (Christensen et al. 2001). However, another study shows lamotrigine has an analgesic effect in both short- and long-term models of hyperalgesia in rats. In a chronic constriction injury neuropathic model of hyperalgesia as well as a diabetic neuropathic model induced by streptozotocin, Klamt (1998) found that intrathecal lamotrigine has a spinal, dose-dependent, long-lasting hyperalgesic effect.

Many randomized, controlled trials show lamotrigine to act as an effective treatment of neuropathic pain (Zakrzewska et al. 1997; Simpson et al. 2000; Eisenberg et al. 2001; Simpson et al. 2003). To treat the pain associated with TN, lamotrigine has been found to have an NNT of 2.1 (Zakrzewska and Patsalos 2002).

Simpson et al. (2000) initially studied the effect of lamotrigine for the treatment of painful HIV-associated distal sensory polyneuropathy (DSP) in a randomized, double-blind, placebo-controlled study with titration of drug. Of 42 patients, 13 did not complete the study, with 5 of these drop-outs due to the side-effect of rash. This rash showed a greater frequency in this study than in epilepsy studies. This initial study indicates lamotrigine for treatment in pain associated with HIV-related DSP (Simpson et al. 2000). Later, Simpson et al. (2003) performed a randomized, double-blind, pharmacological study of patients with HIV-associated DSP. HIV-associated neuropathic pain patients receiving concurrent lamotrigine treatment with anti-retroviral therapy showed improvement in the slope of the change in Gracely Pain Scale score for average pain as compared to placebo. Also, no measurable difference from baseline in Gracely Pain Scale score for average pain vs placebo patients with DSP was observed. Although further research is needed to understand the differences between HIV patients receiving ART and those not receiving ART, Simpson et al. (2003) have demonstrated that lamotrigine is well-tolerated and effective in the treatment of HIV-associated neuropathic pain in patients using ART (Simpson et al. 2003).

Eisenberg et al. (2001) conclude that the therapeutic use of lamotrigine in pain control of diabetic neuropathy is effective and safe (Eisenberg et al. 2001). Although these studies show lamotrigine to act effectively in neuropathic pain treatment, there is controversy surrounding the use of lamotrigine in these pain disorders. There are also studies that have produced negative results (Tremont-Lukats et al. 2000; McCleane 1999; Petersen et al. 2003; Wallace et al. 2004). A randomized, double-blind, placebo-controlled study examining lamotrigine in the treatment of 100 patients with neuropathic pain by McCleane (1999) finds that lamotrigine has no analgesic effect at a dose administration increasing to 200 mg (McCleane 1999).

A randomized, double-blind, placebo-controlled study by Petersen et al. (2003) concludes that oral lamotrigine (400 mg) does not reduce secondary hyperalgesia or acute thermal nociception. Also, lamotrigine has no hyperalgesic effect in an intradermal capsaicin-induced hyperalgesia model, according to a placebo-controlled, randomized, double-blind study by Wallace (2004). These studies further add to the disparities in the reported effects of sodium channel blockers on preclinical models of cutaneous hyperalgesia or the clinical effects of lamotrigine in neuropathic pain. The lack of effect of lamotrigine in human experimental pain may be due to nerve injury associated irregularities that have not yet been replicated in healthy human volunteers. Further well-designed studies are necessary to better define the role of lamotrigine as a drug in the treatment regime of neuropathic pain (Petersen et al. 2003; Tremont-Lukats et al. 2000; Wallace et al. 2004).

The most common side-effects of lamotrigine are dizziness, unsteadiness and drowsiness (Ahmad and Goucke 2002; Jensen 2002). Furthermore, the side-effect profile of lamotrigine requires slow titration of the drug due to possible severe rash and the possibly fatal epidermal necrosis Steven–Johnson syndrome (Gordon and Love 2004).

2.1.5
Topiramate

The second generation anti-epileptic drug topiramate may be used to treat central neuropathic pain (Finnerup et al. 2002). Topiramate has a research history similar to phenytoin and CBZ in that its use to treat neuropathic pain in humans preceded its systematic research in animals models of pain (Tremont-Lukats et al. 2000).

There are five known mechanisms by which topiramate acts to affect neuronal transmission: a dose-dependant inhibition of voltage-gated sodium ion channels, potentiation of the action of $GABA_A$ receptors and thus GABA-medicated chloride ion flow, blocking of excitatory glutamate neurotransmission, modulation of L-type voltage-gated calcium channels, and a weak inhibition on carbonic anhydrase isozymes II and IV. The latter of these mechanisms of action may be responsible for the adverse effects of this drug, including perioral and digital paresthesias and nephrolithiasis. It is worth mentioning that all five of the known mechanisms of action of topiramate are regulated by protein phosphorylation (Chong and Libretto 2003). Like CBZ and GBP,

Topiramate modulates intracortical excitability via selective interactions on excitatory interneurons (Inghilleri et al. 2004). With the several mechanisms of action of this drug, topiramate should act to inhibit many of the known and assumed mechanisms involved in the pathophysiology of neuropathic pain. Jensen (2002) and Wieczorkiewicz-Plaza et al. (2004) have shown that chronic administration of topiramate significantly reduces mechanical sensitivity and also the time course of allodynia in the rat Seltzer mononeuropathy model (Wieczorkiewicz-Plaza et al. 2004). Using two neuropathic pain models, a unilateral chronic constrictive injury (CCI) and a crush lesion of the sciatic nerve, moderate anti-hyperalgesic effects of topiramate were seen. Topiramate attenuates mechanical hyperalgesia and cold allodynia in the CCI model of neuropathic pain; it also attenuates thermal hyperalgesia and reduces cold allodynia at both the early and late phase of observation (Bischofs et al. 2004).

There is limited clinical documentation concerning the role of topiramate in the treatment of neuropathic pain. Potter et al. (1998) report a non-blind trial including many neuropathic pain conditions, with the exception of painful diabetic neuropathy, that finds significantly improved pain scores in patients treated with topiramate as compared to pretreatment scores.

Currently, topiramate does not seem to have a beneficial effect in the treatment of painful diabetic neuropathy: findings from three double-blind placebo-controlled trials do not find significant difference in topiramate and placebo in reduction of pain scores in patients with painful diabetic polyneuropathy. However, possible design features of these studies may explain a lack of adequate sensitivity to differentiate successful treatments from placebo (Thienel et al. 2004).

Topiramate exhibits adverse effects including dizziness, fatigue, ataxia, confusion, somnolence, nephrolithiasis, paraesthesia and weight loss (Glauser 1999).

2.1.6
Gabapentin

GBP, with a favourable side-effect profile, has proved to be quite effective in the treatment of neuropathic pain and is effective as add-on therapy for epilepsy (Maneuf et al. 2003). Specifically, GBP is an effective treatment for the pain associated with painful diabetic neuropathy, mixed neuropathies, PHN, phantom limb pain, Guillain-Barré syndrome and both acute and chronic pain associated with spinal cord injury (Tremont-Lukats et al. 2000; Jensen 2002; Dworkin et al. 2003). Furthermore, there have been positive studies of the effects of GBP in painful HIV-related peripheral neuropathy (La Spina et al. 2001) and neuropathic pain associated with cancer (Caraceni et al. 1999).

Currently, GBP has become the first choice of treatment in neuropathic pain due to positive results from many clinical trials, as well as its effectiveness in ameliorating symptoms of thermo-allodynia, thermal hyperalgesia, mechanical allodynia and mechanical hyperalgesia in animal models (Backonja 2000; Levendoglu et al. 2004; Taylor 1997; Field et al. 1999; Maneuf et al. 2003; Dickenson et al. 2002).

GBP was originally designed as an anti-convulsant GABA mimetic capable of crossing the blood–brain barrier. There is now consensus that GBP is not a GABA mimetic (Maneuf et al. 2003). It is now known that GBP acts by increasing inhibitions not via an increased GABA synthesis, or any direct non-NMDA receptor antagonism, but by decreasing release of excitatory neurotransmitters through binding to the $\alpha_2\delta$ subunit of voltage-dependent calcium channels (VDCCs), a binding site expressed in high density within the peripheral and central nervous systems (Gee et al. 1996; Maneuf et al. 2003; Bennett and Simpson 2004; Marais et al. 2001; Luo et al. 2001; Matthews and Dickenson 2001). Treatment of neuropathic pain with GBP can modulate central sensitization by interacting with high-threshold (likely to be predominantly N-type due to a large body of evidence for a major role of these in animal models of nerve injury) calcium channels (Matthews and Dickenson 2001; Finnerup et al. 2002; Sutton et al. 2002; Gordon and Love 2004; Dickenson et al. 2002).

Sutton et al. (2002) were the first to show the direct inhibition of voltage-gated Ca^{2+} channels by GBP in DRG neurons, illustrating a potential mechanism for this drug to modulate spinal anti-nociception. This group uses specific Ca^{2+} channel antagonists to study N-, L- and P/Q-type Ca^{2+} channels and show that GBP acts via inhibition of N-type Ca^{2+} channels. GBP acts to reduce a non-activating component of whole-cell current that is activated at comparatively depolarized potentials (Sutton et al. 2002). Using fura-2 based fluorescence Ca^{2+} imaging and whole cell patch clamp techniques, this group shows that GBP causes voltage-dependent Ca^{2+} current inhibition, a significant reduction of duration for 50% of the maximum response (W50), and a total Ca^{2+} influx by 25%–30%. A dramatic decrease in current with the neutral amino acid L-isoleucine and a lack of effect in the presence of saclofen (200 µM), a GABA(B) antagonist, further exemplifies that GBP acts directly on the $\alpha_2\delta$ subunit of the Ca^{2+} channel. Interestingly, GBP is the first pharmacological agent known to interact with an $\alpha_2\delta$ subunit of a voltage-dependent Ca^{2+} (Gee et al. 1996; Sutton et al. 2002). This is an auxiliary protein that modulates high-voltage activated calcium channels. Three $\alpha_2\delta$ subunits are known: $\alpha_2\delta$-1, $\alpha_2\delta$-2 and $\alpha_2\delta$-3. Each $\alpha_2\delta$ subunit is highly N-glycosylated with almost 30 kDa consisting of oligosaccharides with a large α_2 protein and a smaller δ protein. According to Marais et al. (2001), $\alpha_2\delta$-1 is detectable in all mouse tissue studied, $\alpha_2\delta$-2 is found in high levels in mouse brain and heart tissue and $\alpha_2\delta$-3 is observable only in mouse brain tissue. This study finds a high affinity for $\alpha_2\delta$-1 to bind to GBP with a K_d of 59 nM and $\alpha_2\delta$-2 with a K^+_d of 153 nM. $\alpha_2\delta$-3 does not bind GBP (Marais et al. 2001).

It is well known that neuroplasticity after peripheral nerve injury contributes to neuropathic pain. Data from Luo et al. (2001) suggest that dorsal root ganglia $\alpha_2\delta$-1 regulation may contribute to the development of allodynia after peripheral nerve injury. In vitro studies show that GBP binds to the $\alpha_2\delta$-1 subunit of voltage-gated calcium channels. Gee et al. (1996), Sutton et al. (2002) and Luo et al. (2001) show a greater than 17-fold, time-dependant increase in $\alpha_2\delta$-1 subunit expression in DRGs ipsilateral to nerve injury in a rat neuropathic pain model of tight ligation of the left fifth and sixth lumbar spinal nerves characterized by GBP-sensitive tactile allodynia. $\alpha_2\delta$-1 subunit expression is also up-regulated in rats with unilateral sciatic nerve crush, but not in rats with dorsal rhizotomy, which suggests a peripheral origin of regulation of the subunit expression. $\alpha_2\delta$-1 subunit expression precedes the onset of allodynia and is reduced in rats recovering from tactile allodynia. The DRG $\alpha_2\delta$-1 regulation has been found by RNAse protection experiments to be regulated at the RNA level (Luo et al. 2001).

Luo et al. (2002) examined the up-regulation of calcium channel $\alpha_2\delta$-1 subunit in allodynic states occurring in different aetiologies to determine if a common mechanism is responsible in these allodynic states. Interestingly, of all allodynic states in this study, only the mechanical and diabetic neuropathies exhibit up-regulation of DRG and/or spinal cord $\alpha_2\delta$-1 subunits as well as GBP sensitivity. It follows that the regulation of the $\alpha_2\delta$-1 subunit in the DRG and spinal cord is specific for distinct neuropathies and is a possible explanation for GBP-sensitive allodynia (Lou 2002).

Dooley et al. (2000) use an in vitro superfusion model of stimulation-evoked neurotransmitter release using rat neocortical slices pre-labelled with [(3)H] norepinephrine [((3)H)NE] to examine the mechanism of action of GBP (Neurontin), PGB (Cl-1008, S-(+)-3-isobutylgaba), and its enantiomer R-(−)-3-isobutylgaba. This study finds that GBP and PGB act similarly to preferentially inhibit [((3)H)NE] release. Furthermore, longer slice exposure to GBP increased the inhibition caused by this drug (Dooley et al. 2000). However, this type of study, although showing a reduction in transmitter release, is likely to reflect actions in epilepsy rather than pain.

Hunter et al. (1997) compared GBP, lamotrigine and felbamate in acute and chronic pain models. All three drugs reverse cold allodynia. Interestingly, only GBP successfully treated tactile allodynia in the spinal nerve ligation model. The dosages at which these three drugs reversed allodynia were observed at levels that were too low to cause significant effect on acute nociceptive function or locomotor activity. It is noteworthy that only GBP reversed both cold and tactile allodynia. Fox et al. (2003) report that GBP shows little activity against mechanical hyperalgesia in both rat and guinea-pig models of neuropathic pain, induced by partial sciatic nerve ligation, after a single oral administration of (100 mg×kg^{-1}). Still, upon repetitive dosage of the drug, GBP reduced mechanical hyperalgesia by 70% in the rat and by 90% in the guinea-pig. There was, however, a significant dose-related depression of tactile allodynia in the rat following a single administration of GBP.

Jun et al. (1998) show that GBP, administered spinally, acts in a dose-dependent manner as an anti-hyperalgesic agent in a mild thermal injury model. $S(+)$-3-Isobutyl GABA produces a similar dose-dependent reversal of the hyperalgesia in this pain model. However, a large dose (300 μM) of the $R(-)$-3-isobutyl GABA does not produce the same hyperalgesia as GBP and its stereoisomer. The effect of these gabapentinoids is a selective modulation of spinal nociceptive processes that, clinically, are generated by persistent small afferent input generated by tissue injury (Jun and Yaksh 1998).

Clinically, Backonja and Glanzman (2003) found that, in the treatment of neuropathic pain in adults, GBP is effective and well tolerated at doses of 1,800 to 3,600 mg/day. Treatment should begin at 900 mg/day starting with 300 mg/day on day 1,600 mg/day on day two, and 900 mg/day on day three and additional titration to 1,800 mg/d for greater efficacy. However, some patients needed doses of GBP up to 3,600 mg/day. This study looked at the effective use of GBP to treat painful diabetic neuropathy, PHN and other neuropathic pain syndromes. Symptoms of allodynia, burning pain, shooting pain and hyperaesthesia were relieved with GBP (Backonja and Glanzman 2003). Furthermore, this drug has proved effective in the treatment of many neuropathic pain states in multiple large randomized controlled trials with a mean reduction in pain score of 2.05/11 is seen compared to 0.94/11 with a placebo. Approximately 30% of patients will have a greater than 50% pain relief with GBP (Bennett and Simpson 2004). In cancer pain, it is important to note that, due to synergy, response rates to GBP may be increased when administered with opioids (Bennett and Simpson 2004).

The pain and sleep problems associated with PHN are effectively treated with GBP therapy. Subsequently, mood and quality of life improve in PHN patients treated with GBP (Rowbotham et al. 1998).

Neuropathic pain related to spinal cord injury is refractory and current treatments are ineffective. In a study designed by Levendoglu et al. (2004) with 20 paraplegic patients, GBP reduced the intensity and the frequency of pain, improved quality of life ($p < 0.05$) and relieved all neuropathic pain descriptors with the exception of itchy, sensitive, dull and cold types. GBP may now be considered a first-line medication to treat chronic neuropathic pain in spinal cord injury patients (Levendoglu et al. 2004).

Mild to moderate adverse effects of GBP subside within about 10 days from the start of treatment (Backonja and Glanzman 2003). These adverse effects of GBP such as somnolence and dizziness are minor and may be experiences by about 30% of the patients (Bennett and Simpson 2004). The most common adverse effects observed are dizziness, somnolence, peripheral oedema, headache and dry mouth (Sabatowski et al. 2004).

PGB is an $\alpha_2\delta$ ligand with analgesic, anxiolytic and anti-convulsant activity. PGB effectively treats neuropathic pain associated with PHN, as seen in a 238-patient, multicentre, randomized, double-blind, placebo-controlled trial. Failure to respond to prior treatment for PHN with GBP at doses greater than or equal to 1,200 mg/day was part of the exclusion criteria for this study. Sabatowski et al. (2004) discuss end-point mean pain scores as significantly reduced in patients treated with PGB 150 mg/day or 300 mg/day as compared to placebo. By 1 week, efficacy of the drug was observed and maintained throughout the study. Furthermore, mean sleep interference scores were decreased at both doses by 1 week and health-related quality-of-life (HRQoL) measurements show improved mental health at both PGB doses. At 300 mg/day, body pain and vitality measurements were improved (Sabatowski et al. 2004).

Although the significance of the altered channel expression remains unclear, it was proposed to correlate with the development of tactile allodynia and relate to the injury-specific action of GBP (Luo et al. 2002). However, behavioural hyperalgesia can be observed as early as 1 day after injury (Kim 1997), whilst channel $\alpha_2\delta$-1 up-regulation is only evident after 7 days (Luo et al. 2001). Due to the ubiquitous nature of the channel $\alpha_2\delta$-1 subunit in all calcium channels, a pharmacological block of this subunit would be expected to result in significant side-effects; however, this clearly is not the case for GBP. It has therefore been unclear how GBP differentiates and targets physiological vs pathophysiological activation of VDCCs. Even in the absence of the altered subunit expression, GBP can exert anti-allodynic effects (Abe et al. 2002), providing further evidence that up-regulation is not the only determinant of full GBP efficacy. In normal animals with no nerve injury-induced changes, simply activating the 5HT3 receptor allowed GBP to inhibit—whereas block of the receptor or ablation of the neurokinin (NK)1-expressing neurons removed—the effectiveness of the drug after nerve injury. It would appear then that a channel $\alpha_2\delta$-1 up-regulation and 5HT3 receptor activation may both determine efficacy (Suzuki et al. 2005).

2.1.7
Ethosuximide

Although the role of high voltage-activated Ca^{2+} channels in nociception had been accepted as an important mechanism of pain transmission, Matthews and Dickenson (2001) were the first to show a possible role for low voltage-activated Ca^{2+} channels in the transmission of pain with a study of spinal ethosuximide in the Chung rodent model of neuropathy. In vivo electrophysiological examination of dorsal horn neurons show spinal ethosuximide exhibits dose-related inhibition of electrical, low-, and high-intensity mechanical and thermal evoked neuronal responses in this model of neuropathy (Matthews and Dickenson 2001). Later, Dogrul et al. (2003) showed that systemic ethosuximide produces a dose-dependent inhibition of tactile and thermal hypersensitivities in rats with spinal nerve ligation, which suggests that T-type calcium channels play a role in neuropathic pain states (Dogrul et al. 2003).

Flatters and Bennett (2004) show that ethosuximide almost completely inhibits mechanical allodynia and hyperalgesia caused by paclitaxel (Taxol), a chemotherapeutic used in the treatment of solid tumours. This study shows a dose-related consistent reversal of mechanical allodynia/hyperalgesia with ethosuximide. This study also shows that ethosuximide inhibits paclitaxel-induced cold allodynia and vincristine-induced mechanical allodynia and hyperalgesia. Neither morphine nor the NMDA receptor antagonist MK-801 produced a significant inhibition of mechanical allodynia or hyperalgesia.

3
Anti-depressants

3.1
Mode of Action

Pain-transmitting neurons are organized at three levels of the neuraxis: the midbrain, medulla and spinal cord. Pain-suppressing actions of neurons may be mediated partially by the endogenous opiate-like compounds endorphins. Neurons in the midbrain periaqueductal grey matter excite neurons in the rostral medulla. The medullary neurons, some of which contain serotonin, project to and inhibit trigeminal and spinal pain-transmitting neurons. Pain acts in a negative-feedback loop to inhibit pain transmission via this pain-suppression pathway (Basbaum and Fields 1978) but also in positive loops (Suzuki et al. 2005). The actions of the ant-depressants used in neuropathic pain are common in that they all block the re-uptake of the monoamines NA and serotonin; their differential effects on the synaptic levels of these modulatory transmitters varies from actions on both through to the SSRIs that are selective for serotonin (Millan 2002).

The first rational for the use of these agents came from early studies based on stimulation produced analgesia (SPA), largely mediated through midbrain and brainstem areas that projected to the spinal cord through descending pathways. Over the years, this was extended to show similar sites could support opioid analgesia and that monoamines, both serotonin and NA, were important in both SPA and opioid actions in the brainstem. Later it became clear that there are descending noradrenergic pathways from the brainstem that modulate spinal activity with a relatively universal inhibitory action, mediated through spinal α_2 adrenoceptors (Millan 2002). By contrast, the multitude of 5HT receptors suggested that this monoamine may play roles other than a simple inhibition of function.

There is now a great deal of evidence to suggest that the maintenance of chronic pain states, whether the result of nerve trauma or inflammation, is dependant to a large degree on descending pathways from the brainstem (Urban and Gebhart 1999; Monconduit et al. 2002; Porreca et al. 2002; Ren and Dubner 2002). While in the early stages the emphasis was on descending inhibitory pathways, it is now clear that descending facilitation is required for the full expression of chronic pain. Much of this research has focussed on the rostroventral medulla (RVM), an area that contains subsets of neurochemically distinct projection neurons some of which are serotonergic (5HT). Electrical stimulation of RVM results in inhibition or facilitation of spinal nociception, depending upon the intensity of the stimulus. Low-intensity stimulation tends to produce facilitation, and high intensity stimulation inhibition (Urban and Gebhart 1999; Fields 2004). Neurons in the RVM are able to code well for the intensity of noxious stimulus and have large receptive fields, covering most areas of the body. Stimulation of the RVM can enhance nociceptive and non-nociceptive input, and local anaesthetic block of the same area attenuates the mechanical hypersensitivity accompanying nerve injury. Based on responses to tail flick nocifensive behaviour, cells in the RVM have been classified into three groups: on, off and neutral. The off cells are thought to produce a tonic inhibition that is turned off by pain, but the finding of an increased cell discharge following prolonged noxious thermal stimulation led to the speculation that these cells facilitate nociception through activation of a descending pathway to the spinal cord. Destruction of ON-like cells abolished mechanical allodynia in the spinal nerve ligation (SNL) model of neuropathy (Porreca et al. 2001). RVM is in many ways seen as a relay between higher brain areas and the spinal cord and can be influenced by many areas of the brain involved in pain processing such as the periaqueductal grey (PAG), amygdala, and anterior cingulate and insular cortex. This is thought to allow the brain to make appropriate adjustments to nociceptive processing informed by environmental contingencies such as threat or recovery from injury (Fields 2004). Thus it is likely that the profile of anti-depressants in terms of their actions on NA and 5HT will lead to different functional effects on pain.

Over the past 4 years a general hypothesis concerning the regulation of spinal excitability and the control of chronic pain that builds upon previous work on both ascending and descending pathways has been proposed (Hunt 2000; Suzuki et al. 2002, 2004a). Essentially, starting from earlier observations, a key role of ascending pathways derived from a small group of neurons has been described. These neurons sit almost exclusively within laminae I and III of the dorsal horn of the spinal cord and:

– Express the substance P receptor (NK1) (Todd et al. 2000, 2002; Cheunsuang et al. 2002; Todd 2002)

– Are needed for both wind-up and long-term potentiation (LTP) of spinal neurons (Ikeda et al. 2003) following activation of nociceptive sensory afferents

– Project upon the brainstem particularly within areas that subsequently send information to the limbic system and somatosensory cortex (Gauriau and Bernard 2004).

Both neuropathic and inflammatory pain states are attenuated when this pathway is lesioned with a saporin-substance P conjugate applied intrathecally

(Nichols et al. 1999). The lamina I–III/NK1 pathway was essential for the generation of both 'wind-up' and LTP in deep dorsal horn neurons: both were lost following ablation of lamina I neurons, the coding of peripheral stimuli and properties of deep dorsal horn neurons in rats with neuropathic injury that increase considerably in terms of their increased response to innocuous stimuli and their enlarged receptive field sizes (Suzuki et al. 2002, 2004b). The link to the descending serotonergic pathway came from the observation that many of the effects of lamina I–III/NK1 lesions could be reproduced in part by either ablation of the descending serotonergic pathways or antagonism of the excitatory 5HT3 receptor with the selective 5HT3 receptor antagonist ondansetron given intrathecally over the dorsal horn.

We were also able to show that full activation of RVM serotonergic neurons did not occur following lamina I–III/NK1 ablation. Recent work has also indicated that local ablation of descending serotonergic pathways in the lumber spinal cord with 5,7 DHT can also severely attenuate the maintenance phase of both neuropathic and inflammatory pain states. Since this research, other work has begun to show some efficacy of ondansetron in clinical trials with chronic pain patients (McCleane et al. 2003) and so-called 'at level' pain that develops close to the site of a spinal cord transection has been ameliorated by reducing serotonergic function (Oatway et al. 2004).

There is compelling evidence to suggest that the ionotropic 5HT3 receptor mediates many of the pro-nociceptive effects of 5HT, although there is also evidence to suggest a role for 5HT2 receptors. Both are expressed by primary afferents and dorsal horn neurons mainly pre-synaptically (Miquel et al. 2002; Zeitz et al. 2002; Maxwell et al. 2003; Okamoto et al. 2005). The efficacy of the 5HT3 receptor antagonist ondansetron on at-level allodynia following cord damage in rat is thought to reflect sprouting of axotomized serotonergic axons at the site of lesion and increased release of 5HT (Oatway et al. 2004). Within the DRG, 5HT3R is found on a small proportion of CGRP-containing sensory neurons and in mouse expressed by an uncharacterized group of small-diameter myelinated and unmyelinated nociceptors (Miquel et al. 2002; Zeitz et al. 2002). The evidence strongly suggests a role for 5HT3 receptors and release of 5HT as essential for the maintenance of chronic pain states. However, consistent inhibitory effects of 5HT1 receptor activation have been reported in animals, and 5HT1B/D agonists have established roles in migraine. In the case of non-cranial pains, the 5HT1A receptor appears to be the key target for descending 5HT inhibitory actions (Millan 2002).

Noradrenergic inhibition mediated through α_2 receptors would therefore seem a key issue for effectiveness of anti-depressants in pain, since 5HT mechanisms can both enhance and inhibit pain.

Neuropathic pain is successfully treated with anti-depressant drugs. Of neuropathic pain patients treated with anti-depressants, 30% will achieve over 50% pain relief (McQuay et al. 1996). Anti-depressant anti-nociceptive action is independent of the presence of clinical depression (Clifford 1985). Although literature exists that shows that neither SSRIs nor TCAs seem to have superior anti-nociceptive effects to the other (see Mattia et al. 2002), older TCAs do exhibit superior anti-nociceptive effects to other anti-depressants when used in the treatment of chronic neuropathic pain (Mattia and Coluzzi 2003). Collins et al. (2000) found no data that would support the idea that SSRIs are better analgesics than older anti-depressants. According to Max, zimelidine and paroxetine, two SSRIs, have weak clinical effectiveness in the treatment of neuropathic pain (Max 1994). Clinically, there is no significant difference between TCAs. However, TCAs are significantly more effective than benzodiazepines according to three studies available for review. Imipramine, a TCA, is more effective than paroxetine, an SSRI, and mianserin, a tetracyclic anti-depressant (McQuay et al. 1996).

4
Classical Anti-depressants

The anti-nociceptive effects of anti-depressants require intact descending inhibitory bulbospinal pathways. A study by Ardid (1995) shows that the anti-nociceptive effects of clomipramine are suppressed only in the hindpaw ipsilateral to a unilateral lesion of the dorsolateral funiculus of the rat (Ardid et al. 1995). The effects of clomipramine, amitriptyline and desipramine were tested on a neuropathic pain model in rats induced by loosely tied ligatures around the common sciatic nerve. Acute injections of clomipramine, amitriptyline and desipramine caused pain relief. Chronic injections of these three TCAs resulted in pain relief as measured by a significant and progressive increase in vocalization threshold.

Sierralta et al. (1995) use p-chlorophenylalanine and α-methyltyrosine to examine the anti-depressant drugs clomipramine, zimelidine, imipramine and maprotiline in the acetic acid writhing test in mice. Each anti-depressant demonstrated an anti-nociceptive effect in this study. This study shows that critical levels of both 5-HT and NA are responsible for mediating the anti-nociceptive effects of anti-depressants on the writhing test in mice (Sierralta et al. 1995).

The streptozocin-induced diabetic rat is a model of chronic pain with signs of hyperalgesia and allodynia. The TCAs clomipramine, amitriptyline and desipramine, as well as clonidine, an α-adrenergic stimulating agent, were studied in this pain model to show that noradrenergic drugs seem to be the most active of these drugs that act on monoaminergic transmission to cause pain relief (Courteix et al. 1994).

Fishbain et al. (2000) conducted a review of 22 controlled animal studies and 5 double-blind placebo-controlled studies that examined anti-depressants in various pain models. This group found that anti-depressants that attenuate both serotonin and norepinephrine levels have greater anti-nociceptive activity than anti-depressants that solely act to modulate the NA levels. Furthermore, anti-depressants that act solely to modulate serotonin levels have weaker anti-nociceptive properties than the two previously mentioned classes of anti-depressants (Fishbain et al. 2000). Bomholt (2005) in a study of various anti-depressants in the chronic constriction injury rat model of neuropathic pain suggests that anti-depressant drugs that act on both serotonin and NA levels have greater anti-nociceptive effects than SSRIs (Bomholt et al. 2005). The anti-depressants amitriptyline, duloxetine, mirtazapine and citalopram were able to attenuate thermal hyperalgesia in the chronic constriction injury rat model of neuropathic pain. Interestingly, only amitriptyline, a TCA, and duloxetine, a dual serotonin-norepinephrine reuptake inhibitor, fully reversed thermal hypersensitivity. Amitriptyline, duloxetine and mirtazapine, a noradrenergic and specific serotoninergic anti-depressant (NaSSA) caused a significant reduction of mechanical hyperalgesia, whereas citalopram, an SSRI, was ineffective in attenuating mechanical hyperalgesia. Mechanical allodynia was not affected by any of these four anti-depressants (Bomholt et al. 2005).

Which receptors underlie the effects of the increased levels of monoamines in synapses as a result of their primary action on uptake mechanisms? Mico (1997) provides supporting evidence that β-adrenoceptors play a role in the analgesic effect of desipramine and nortriptyline. However, only the β_1 adrenergic receptor is involved when the painful stimulus is chemical, as tested by the non-neuropathic acetic acid and formalin tests (Mico et al. 1997). However, these are not neuropathic states, and further studies that show α-adrenoceptors play a role in the physiology of pain transmission. Anti-depressant antinociception is mediated by α_2-adrenoceptors, and not α_1-adrenoceptors, and not only by drugs that act by re-uptake inhibition of NA, but also of serotonin (Gray et al. 1999).

As seen in the treatment of diabetic neuropathy, the TCA imipramine has an NNT of 1.4 in a study with optimal doses. Other studies of tricyclics show an NNT of 2.4 in this pain disorder. Furthermore, SSRIs have an NNT of 6.7. The NNT is 3.3 for CBZ, 10.0 for mexiletine, 3.7 for GBP, 1.9 for dextromethorphan, 3.4 for both tramadol and levodopa, and 5.9 for capsaicin (Sindrup et al. 1999). In diabetic neuropathy, the NNT for anti-depressants was 3.4 and the NNT for anti-convulsants was 2.7 (Collins et al. 2000). Anti-depressants and anti-convulsants had the same efficacy and incidence of minor adverse effects in for diabetic neuropathy and PHN (Collins et al. 2000) In PHN, TCAs have an NNT of 2.3. The NNT for PHN is 3.2 for GBP, 2.5 for oxycodone and 5.3 for capsaicin. Dextromethorphan was inactive in PHN (Sindrup et al. 1999). In PHN, the NNT for anti-depressants was 2.1 and the NNT for anti-convulsants was 3.2 (Collins et al. 2000). The NNT was 2.5 for tricyclics and 3.5 for capsaicin in peripheral nerve injury (Sindrup et al. 1999).

In the treatment of pain in polyneuropathy, TCAs and anti-convulsants have become the conventional pharmacotherapy. According to the study by Sindrup and Jensen (2000) TCAs are the drugs of choice in the pharmacological treatment of pain in polyneuropathy. GBP, CBZ, and tramadol are good alternatives to TCAs if contraindications or tolerability problems are encountered with this class of drugs. Sindrup et al. (1999) found no obvious relationship between the mechanism of action of these drugs and their effect in distinct pain conditions or for specific drug classes and various pain conditions (Sindrup et al. 1999). McQuay et al. (1996) reviewed 21 placebo-controlled treatments including data on 10 different anti-depressants in 17 randomized controlled trials. An NNT of 3 for anti-depressants when compared with placebo shows significant pain relief in the 6 of 13 studies of diabetic neuropathy. PHN studies have an NNT of 2.3. The odds ratio for anti-depressants from two atypical facial pain studies is 4.1 and the NNT is 2.8. From the only central pain study with analysable dichotomous data, the NNT for anti-depressants was estimated to be 1.7 (McQuay et al. 1996).

However, since the early anti-depressants have a number of potential pharmacological targets, there may be non-monoamine actions of these compounds, although it is unclear that they contribute to the clinical effects of these compounds. Skolnick et al. (1996) examined the effect of chronic anti-depressant treatment on NMDA receptors. Adaptive changes in radioligand binding to NMDA receptors resulted from chronic (14 days), but not acute (1 day), anti-depressant administration to mice. The TCA imipramine, the SSRI citalopram, and electroconvulsive shock slowly produce these adaptive changes that persist for some time after treatment has been stopped. However, the ability of SSRIs, weakly effective in patients, to produce these actions, seemingly limited to the cerebral cortex, argue against a contribution to the clinical actions of anti-depressants in pain.

Valverde et al. (1994) have shown that anti-nociception associated with TCAs acts partly via the endogenous opioid system and partly by additional activation of noradrenergic and serotonergic pathways, although this study did not address nerve injury. De Felipe et al. (1985) found that rats treated chronically for 21 consecutive days with the typical anti-depressants clomipramine, desipramine and amitriptyline, as well as with the atypical anti-depressants iprindole and nomifensine, had increased levels of [Met5]enkephalin in striatum and nucleus accumbens.

Hamon et al. (1987) examined the central mechanisms involved in anti-depressant potentiation of morphine-induced analgesia. Levels of Leu-enkephalin, the opioid peptide, are markedly increased in the spinal cord, hypothalamus and cerebral cortex after a 14-day chronic treatment of amoxapine or amitriptyline. Met-enkephalin levels were increased after amitriptyline treatment in the spinal cord and hypothalamus. Chronic treatment with amoxapine or amitriptyline caused an increase of δ- and μ-opioid binding sites in the spinal cord and decreased in the hypothalamus; opioid receptor levels remained unchanged in the cerebral cortex (Hamon et al. 1987). However, due to the close relations between monoamine systems and opioids in the brainstem and midbrain, these secondary effects on opioid function are not unexpected.

Indeed, the anti-nociceptive properties of clomipramine and amitriptyline, as well as their ability to potentiate morphine-induced analgesia, seem to be linked to the activation of a serotonin-mediated endogenous opioid system. Sacerdote et al. (1987) have shown that acute administration of clomipramine and amitriptyline (acting on NA and 5HT), induce analgesia. Nortriptyline, a TCA that acts predominantly via the noradrenergic system, does not induce analgesia when administered acutely. However, acute dosing of nortriptyline, amitriptyline and clomipramine all potentiate the anti-nociceptive effects of morphine, which further exemplifies a relationship between the serotoninergic and the endogenous opioid systems (Sacerdote et al. 1987). Here as in many studies, the relation of effects seen with acute doses to the clinical profile of drugs used for chronic treatments is unclear.

Using a rat model of neuropathic pain, caffeine blocks the thermal anti-hyperalgesic effect of acute amitriptyline in a rat model of neuropathic pain. Concurrent systemic administration of both caffeine and amitriptyline blocked amitriptyline thermal anti-hyperalgesic effect. No observable effects inherent to caffeine were found at this dose. Spinally, the mild anti-hyperalgesic effect of amitriptyline was unchanged by pretreatment with intrathecal caffeine. Using brief anaesthesia, peripherally administered amitriptyline into the neuropathic paw resulted in anti-hyperalgesia. Furthermore, anti-hyperalgesia due to both doses of amitriptyline were partially antagonized with co-administration of caffeine. Ultimately, this study suggests that acute amitriptyline's thermal anti-hyperalgesic effects in this model may involve increase of a peripheral endogenous adenosine tone (Esser and Sawynok 2000). In a randomized, double-blind, placebo-controlled study of 200 adult patients, topically administered 3.3% doxepin hydrochloride, 0.025% capsaicin and a combination of 3.3% doxepin/0.025% capsaicin were found to provide similar levels of anti-nociception in human chronic neuropathic pain. However, a more rapid onset of analgesia was produced by the combination of doxepin/capsaicin (McCleane 2000).

In line with peripheral actions under some conditions, Abdi et al. (1998) examined the acute effects of amitriptyline and GBP on behavioural signs of mechanical allodynia using the Chung rat model of neuropathic pain. In a second experiment, continuous discharges in fascicles of injured afferent fibres were recorded. Amitriptyline and GBP increased the mechanical allodynia threshold and amitriptyline depressed the rate of continuing discharges of injured afferent fibres, whereas GBP had no effect on these discharges. Neuropathic pain behaviour in rats is clearly modulated by both amitriptyline and GBP. The site of action of GBP is exclusively central; amitriptyline appears to act both peripherally and centrally (Abdi et al. 1998), but with regard to the former, little is known whether this potential action acts on evoked responses or contributes to the effects seen in patients after systemic doses.

It is known that amitriptyline, as well as other anti-depressants, has a high binding affinity for NMDA receptors in vitro. Intrathecal amitriptyline completely antagonized thermal hyperalgesia induced by NMDA. Some authors have suggested that TCAs intrathecally administered may provide greater pain relief than systemically administered TCAs, which are known to provide modest activity in the treatment of clinical neuropathic pain. Inflammation-induced thermal hyperalgesia was reversed by intrathecal amitriptyline. The anti-nociceptive effect of amitriptyline was unaffected, except at the lowest dose, by block of NA and 5HT receptors. Hyperalgesia is reversed by amitriptyline in rats by a mechanism not linked to monoamine reuptake inhibition, and possibly due to NMDA receptor antagonism (Eisenach and Gebhart 1995).

However, these animal studies, often using thermal tests and acute doses, need to be expanded to include studies on allodynias and ongoing pain after nerve injury to better replicate the clinical situation. They also fail to explain why, if the effects of the TCAs are peripheral and/or central and not mediated by monoamines, sedation and cardiovascular effects, hallmarks of noradrenergic activity, are so common in patients. A significantly higher rate of serious adverse cardiac events occurs during nortriptyline treatment than during treatment with paroxetine (Roose et al. 1998).

Venlafaxine, a serotonin and noradrenergic reuptake inhibitor (SnaRI), is effective in multiple pain disorders and has an improved side-effect profile when compared to TCAs (Mattia et al. 2002).

Schreiber et al. (1999) have shown that the κ- and δ-opioid receptor subtypes strongly influenced the anti-nociceptive effect of venlafaxine, with the α_2-adrenergic receptor also contributing to the anti-nociceptive effect of this drug (Schreiber et al. 1999). α_2- and a minor α_1-adrenergic mechanisms of anti-nociception are implicated by tests where adrenergic and serotoninergic antagonists were used; venlafaxine-induced anti-nociception was decreased by yohimbine but not phentolamine or metergoline. Furthermore, clonidine, an α_2-adrenergic agonist, significantly potentiated venlafaxine-mediated anti-nociception (Schreiber et al. 1999).

5
Conclusion

As has been pointed out in this account, there are multiple mechanisms of neuropathic and other pains, and in the case of the many peripheral neuropathies, changes can be charted from the periphery, through the spinal cord and into the brain. Thus, the fact that both anti-depressants and anti-convulsants, with very different mechanisms, can be effective is not surprising since they target key but parallel systems involved in this pain state. A better understanding of the multiple mechanisms of neuropathic pain should lead to a more effective use of existing drugs, possibly allowing a greater number of patients to benefit, and provide a basis for the development of potential new therapies.

References

Abdi S, Lee DH, Chung JM (1998) The anti-allodynic effects of amitriptyline, gabapentin, and lidocaine in a rat model of neuropathic pain. Anesth Analg 87:1360–1366

Abe M, Kurihara T, Han W, Shinomiya K, Tanabe T (2002) Changes in expression of voltage-dependent ion channel subunits in dorsal root ganglia of rats with radicular injury and pain. Spine 27:1517–1524; discussion 1525

Ahmad M, Goucke CR (2002) Management strategies for the treatment of neuropathic pain in the elderly. Drugs Aging 19:929–945

Ardid D, Jourdan D, Mestre C, Villanueva L, Le Bars D, Eschalier A (1995) Involvement of bulbospinal pathways in the antinociceptive effect of clomipramine in the rat. Brain Res 695:253–256

Backonja M, Glanzman RL (2003) Gabapentin dosing for neuropathic pain: evidence from randomized, placebo-controlled clinical trials. Clin Ther 25:81–104

Backonja MM (2000) Anticonvulsants (antineuropathics) for neuropathic pain syndromes. Clin J Pain 16:S67–S72

Basbaum AI, Fields HL (1978) Endogenous pain control mechanisms: review and hypothesis. Ann Neurol 4:451–462

Bischofs S, Zelenka M, Sommer C (2004) Evaluation of topiramate as an anti-hyperalgesic and neuroprotective agent in the peripheral nervous system. J Peripher Nerv Syst 9:70–78

Bennett MI, Simpson KH (2004) Gabapentin in the treatment of neuropathic pain. Palliat Med 18:5–11

Blackburn-Munro G, Fleetwood-Walker SM (1999) The sodium channel auxiliary subunits beta1 and beta2 are differentially expressed in the spinal cord of neuropathic rats. Neuroscience 90:153–164

Blackburn-Munro G, Dickinson T, Fleetwood-Walker SM (2001) Non-opioid actions of lamotrigine within the rat dorsal horn after inflammation and neuropathic nerve damage. Neurosci Res 39:385–390

Bomholt SF, Mikkelsen JD, Blackburn-Munro G (2005) Antinociceptive effects of the antidepressants amitriptyline, duloxetine, mirtazapine and citalopram in animal models of acute, persistent and neuropathic pain. Neuropharmacology 48:252–263

Campbell FG, Graham JG, Zilkha KJ (1966) Clinical trial of carbazepine (tegretol) in trigeminal neuralgia. J Neurol Neurosurg Psychiatry 29:265–267

Canavero S, Bonicalzi V (1996) Lamotrigine control of central pain. Pain 68:179–181

Caraceni A, Zecca E, Martini C, De Conno F (1999) Gabapentin as an adjuvant to opioid analgesia for neuropathic cancer pain. J Pain Symptom Manage 17:441–445

Carrazana E, Mikoshiba I (2003) Rationale and evidence for the use of oxcarbazepine in neuropathic pain. J Pain Symptom Manage 25:S31–35

Chadda VS, Mathur MS (1978) Double blind study of the effects of diphenylhydantoin sodium on diabetic neuropathy. J Assoc Physicians India 26:403–406

Cheung H, Kamp D, Harris E (1992) An in vitro investigation of the action of lamotrigine on neuronal voltage-activated sodium channels. Epilepsy Res 13:107–112

Cheunsuang O, Maxwell D, Morris R (2002) Spinal lamina I neurones that express neurokinin 1 receptors. II. Electrophysiological characteristics, responses to primary afferent stimulation and effects of a selective mu-opioid receptor agonist. Neuroscience 111:423–434

Chong MS, Libretto SE (2003) The rationale and use of topiramate for treating neuropathic pain. Clin J Pain 19:59–68

Christensen D, Gautron M, Guilbaud G, Kayser V (2001) Effect of gabapentin and lamotrigine on mechanical allodynia-like behaviour in a rat model of trigeminal neuropathic pain. Pain 93:147–153

Clifford DB (1985) Treatment of pain with antidepressants. Am Fam Physician 31:181–185

Collins SL, Moore RA, McQuay HJ, Wiffen P (2000) Antidepressants and anticonvulsants for diabetic neuropathy and postherpetic neuralgia: a quantitative systematic review. J Pain Symptom Manage 20:449–458

Courteix C, Bardin M, Chantelauze C, Lavarenne J, Eschalier A (1994) Study of the sensitivity of the diabetes-induced pain model in rats to a range of analgesics. Pain 57:153–160

David G, Selzer ME, Yaari Y (1985) Suppression by phenytoin of convulsant-induced after-discharges at presynaptic nerve terminals. Brain Res 339:57–65

De Felipe MC, De Ceballos ML, Gil C, Fuentes JA (1985) Chronic antidepressant treatment increases enkephalin levels in N. accumbens and striatum of the rat. Eur J Pharmacol 112:119–122

Dickenson AH, Matthews EA, Suzuki R (2002) Neurobiology of neuropathic pain: mode of action of anticonvulsants. Eur J Pain 6 Suppl A:51–60

Dogrul A, Gardell LR, Ossipov MH, Tulunay FC, Lai J, Porreca F (2003) Reversal of experimental neuropathic pain by T-type calcium channel blockers. Pain 105:159–168

Dooley DJ, Donovan CM, Pugsley TA (2000) Stimulus-dependent modulation of [(3)H]norepinephrine release from rat neocortical slices by gabapentin and pregabalin. J Pharmacol Exp Ther 295:1086–1093

Duckrow RB, Taub A (1977) The effect of diphenylhydantoin on self-mutilation in rats produced by unilateral multiple dorsal rhizotomy. Exp Neurol 54:33–41

Dworkin RH, Backonja M, Rowbotham MC, Allen RR, Argoff CR, Bennett GJ, Bushnell MC, Farrar JT, Galer BS, Haythornthwaite JA, Hewitt DJ, Loeser JD, Max MB, Saltarelli M, Schmader KE, Stein C, Thompson D, Turk DC, Wallace MS, Watkins LR, Weinstein SM (2003) Advances in neuropathic pain: diagnosis, mechanisms, and treatment recommendations. Arch Neurol 60:1524–1534

Eisenach JC, Gebhart GF (1995) Intrathecal amitriptyline acts as an N-methyl-D-aspartate receptor antagonist in the presence of inflammatory hyperalgesia in rats. Anesthesiology 83:1046–1054

Eisenberg E, Lurie Y, Braker C, Daoud D, Ishay A (2001) Lamotrigine reduces painful diabetic neuropathy: a randomized, controlled study. Neurology 57:505–509

Erichsen HK, Hao JX, Xu XJ, Blackburn-Munro G (2003) A comparison of the antinociceptive effects of voltage-activated Na+ channel blockers in two rat models of neuropathic pain. Eur J Pharmacol 458:275–282

Esser MJ, Sawynok J (2000) Caffeine blockade of the thermal antihyperalgesic effect of acute amitriptyline in a rat model of neuropathic pain. Eur J Pharmacol 399:131–139

Farago F (1987) Trigeminal neuralgia: its treatment with two new carbamazepine analogues. Eur Neurol 26:73–83

Field MJ, McCleary S, Hughes J, Singh L (1999) Gabapentin and pregabalin, but not morphine and amitriptyline, block both static and dynamic components of mechanical allodynia induced by streptozocin in the rat. Pain 80:391–398

Fields H (2004) State-dependent opioid control of pain. Nat Rev Neurosci 5:565–575

Finnerup NB, Sindrup SH, Bach FW, Johannesen IL, Jensen TS (2002) Lamotrigine in spinal cord injury pain: a randomized controlled trial. Pain 96:375–383

Fishbain DA, Cutler R, Rosomoff HL, Rosomoff RS (2000) Evidence-based data from animal and human experimental studies on pain relief with antidepressants: a structured review. Pain Med 1:310–316

Flatters SJ, Bennett GJ (2004) Ethosuximide reverses paclitaxel- and vincristine-induced painful peripheral neuropathy. Pain 109:150–161

Fox A, Gentry C, Patel S, Kesingland A, Bevan S (2003) Comparative activity of the anti-convulsants oxcarbazepine, carbamazepine, lamotrigine and gabapentin in a model of neuropathic pain in the rat and guinea-pig. Pain 105:355–362

Gauriau C, Bernard JF (2004) A comparative reappraisal of projections from the superficial laminae of the dorsal horn in the rat: the forebrain. J Comp Neurol 468:24–56

Gee NS, Brown JP, Dissanayake VU, Offord J, Thurlow R, Woodruff GN (1996) The novel anticonvulsant drug, gabapentin (Neurontin), binds to the alpha2delta subunit of a calcium channel. J Biol Chem 271:5768–5776

Glauser TA (1999) Topiramate. Epilepsia 40 Suppl 5:S71–80

Gordon DB, Love G (2004) Pharmacologic management of neuropathic pain. Pain Manag Nurs 5:19–33

Grant SM, Faulds D (1992) Oxcarbazepine. A review of its pharmacology and therapeutic potential in epilepsy, trigeminal neuralgia and affective disorders. Drugs 43:873–888

Gray AM, Pache DM, Sewell RD (1999) Do alpha2-adrenoceptors play an integral role in the antinociceptive mechanism of action of antidepressant compounds? Eur J Pharmacol 378:161–168

Hamon M, Gozlan H, Bourgoin S, Benoliel JJ, Mauborgne A, Taquet H, Cesselin F, Mico JA (1987) Opioid receptors and neuropeptides in the CNS in rats treated chronically with amoxapine or amitriptyline. Neuropharmacology 26:531–539

Hansson PT, Dickenson AH (2005) Pharmacological treatment of peripheral neuropathic pain conditions based on shared commonalities despite multiple etiologies. Pain 113: 251–254

Hardy JR, Rees EA, Gwilliam B, Ling J, Broadley K, A'Hern R (2001) A phase II study to establish the efficacy and toxicity of sodium valproate in patients with cancer-related neuropathic pain. J Pain Symptom Manage 21:204–209

Hunt SP (2000) Pain control: breaking the circuit. Trends Pharmacol Sci 21:284–287

Hunter JC, Gogas KR, Hedley LR, Jacobson LO, Kassotakis L, Thompson J, Fontana DJ (1997) The effect of novel anti-epileptic drugs in rat experimental models of acute and chronic pain. Eur J Pharmacol 324:153–160

Ikeda H, Heinke B, Ruscheweyh R, Sandkuhler J (2003) Synaptic plasticity in spinal lamina I projection neurons that mediate hyperalgesia. Science 299:1237–1240

Inghilleri M, Conte A, Frasca V, Curra A, Gilio F, Manfredi M, Berardelli A (2004) Antiepileptic drugs and cortical excitability: a study with repetitive transcranial stimulation. Exp Brain Res 154:488–493

Jensen TS (2001) Recent advances in pain research: implications for chronic headache. Cephalalgia 21:765–769

Jensen TS (2002) Anticonvulsants in neuropathic pain: rationale and clinical evidence. Eur J Pain 6 Suppl A:61–68

Jensen TS, Gottrup H, Sindrup SH, Bach FW (2001a) The clinical picture of neuropathic pain. Eur J Pharmacol 429:1–11

Jensen TS, Gottrup H, Kasch H, Nikolajsen L, Terkelsen AJ, Witting N (2001b) Has basic research contributed to chronic pain treatment? Acta Anaesthesiol Scand 45:1128–1135

Johannessen CU (2000) Mechanisms of action of valproate: a commentatory. Neurochem Int 37:103–110

Johannessen CU, Johannessen SI (2003) Valproate: past, present, and future. CNS Drug Rev 9:199–216

Jun JH, Yaksh TL (1998) The effect of intrathecal gabapentin and 3-isobutyl gamma-aminobutyric acid on the hyperalgesia observed after thermal injury in the rat. Anesth Analg 86:348–354

Killian JM, Fromm GH (1968) Carbamazepine in the treatment of neuralgia. Use of side effects. Arch Neurol 19:129–136

Klamt JG (1998) Effects of intrathecally administered lamotrigine, a glutamate release inhibitor, on short- and long-term models of hyperalgesia in rats. Anesthesiology 88: 487–494

La Spina I, Porazzi D, Maggiolo F, Bottura P, Suter F (2001) Gabapentin in painful HIV-related neuropathy: a report of 19 patients, preliminary observations. Eur J Neurol 8:71–75

Lee WS, Limmroth V, Ayata C, Cutrer FM, Waeber C, Yu X, Moskowitz MA (1995) Peripheral GABAA receptor-mediated effects of sodium valproate on dural plasma protein extravasation to substance P and trigeminal stimulation. Br J Pharmacol 116:1661–1667

Leijon G, Boivie J (1989) Central post-stroke pain—a controlled trial of amitriptyline and carbamazepine. Pain 36:27–36

Levendoglu F, Ogun CO, Ozerbil O, Ogun TC, Ugurlu H (2004) Gabapentin is a first line drug for the treatment of neuropathic pain in spinal cord injury. Spine 29:743–751

Loscher W (1999) Valproate: a reappraisal of its pharmacodynamic properties and mechanisms of action. Prog Neurobiol 58:31–59

Luo ZD, Chaplan SR, Higuera ES, Sorkin LS, Stauderman KA, Williams ME, Yaksh TL (2001) Upregulation of dorsal root ganglion (alpha)2(delta) calcium channel subunit and its correlation with allodynia in spinal nerve-injured rats. J Neurosci 21:1868–1875

Luo ZD, Calcutt NA, Higuera ES, Valder CR, Song YH, Svensson CI, Myers RR (2002) Injury type-specific calcium channel alpha 2 delta-1 subunit up-regulation in rat neuropathic pain models correlates with antiallodynic effects of gabapentin. J Pharmacol Exp Ther 303:1199–1205

Maneuf YP, Gonzalez MI, Sutton KS, Chung FZ, Pinnock RD, Lee K (2003) Cellular and molecular action of the putative GABA-mimetic, gabapentin. Cell Mol Life Sci 60: 742–750

Marais E, Klugbauer N, Hofmann F (2001) Calcium channel alpha(2)delta subunits-structure and Gabapentin binding. Mol Pharmacol 59:1243–1248

Martin ED, Pozo MA (2004) Valproate reduced excitatory postsynaptic currents in hippocampal CA1 pyramidal neurons. Neuropharmacology 46:555–561

Matthews EA, Dickenson AH (2001) Effects of spinally delivered N- and P-type voltage-dependent calcium channel antagonists on dorsal horn neuronal responses in a rat model of neuropathy. Pain 92:235–246

Mattia C, Coluzzi F (2003) Antidepressants in chronic neuropathic pain. Mini Rev Med Chem 3:773–784

Mattia C, Paoletti F, Coluzzi F, Boanelli A (2002) New antidepressants in the treatment of neuropathic pain. A review. Minerva Anestesiol 68:105–114

Max MB (1994) Treatment of post-herpetic neuralgia: antidepressants. Ann Neurol 35 Suppl:S50–53

Maxwell DJ, Kerr R, Rashid S, Anderson E (2003) Characterisation of axon terminals in the rat dorsal horn that are immunoreactive for serotonin 5-HT3A receptor subunits. Exp Brain Res 149:114–124

McCleane G (1999) 200 mg daily of lamotrigine has no analgesic effect in neuropathic pain: a randomised, double-blind, placebo-controlled trial. Pain 83:105–107

McCleane G (2000) Topical application of doxepin hydrochloride, capsaicin and a combination of both produces analgesia in chronic human neuropathic pain: a randomized, double-blind, placebo-controlled study. Br J Clin Pharmacol 49:574–579

McCleane GJ, Suzuki R, Dickenson AH (2003) Does a single intravenous injection of the 5HT3 receptor antagonist ondansetron have an analgesic effect in neuropathic pain? A double-blinded, placebo-controlled cross-over study. Anesth Analg 97:1474–1478

McQuay H, Carroll D, Jadad AR, Wiffen P, Moore A (1995) Anticonvulsant drugs for management of pain: a systematic review. BMJ 311:1047–1052

McQuay HJ, Tramer M, Nye BA, Carroll D, Wiffen PJ, Moore RA (1996) A systematic review of antidepressants in neuropathic pain. Pain 68:217–227

Mico JA, Gibert-Rahola J, Casas J, Rojas O, Serrano MI, Serrano JS (1997) Implication of beta 1- and beta 2-adrenergic receptors in the antinociceptive effect of tricyclic antidepressants. Eur Neuropsychopharmacol 7:139–145

Millan MJ (2002) Descending control of pain. Prog Neurobiol 66:355–474

Miquel MC, Emerit MB, Nosjean A, Simon A, Rumajogee P, Brisorgueil MJ, Doucet E, Hamon M, Verge D (2002) Differential subcellular localization of the 5-HT3-As receptor subunit in the rat central nervous system. Eur J Neurosci 15:449–457

Monconduit L, Desbois C, Villanueva L (2002) The integrative role of the rat medullary subnucleus reticularis dorsalis in nociception. Eur J Neurosci 16:937–944

Nichols ML, Allen BJ, Rogers SD, Ghilardi JR, Honore P, Luger NM, Finke MP, Li J, Lappi DA, Simone DA, Mantyh PW (1999) Transmission of chronic nociception by spinal neurons expressing the substance P receptor. Science 286:1558–1561

Nicol CF (1969) A four year double-blind study of tegretol in facial pain. Headache 9:54–57

Oatway MA, Chen Y, Weaver LC (2004) The 5-HT3 receptor facilitates at-level mechanical allodynia following spinal cord injury. Pain 110:259–268

Okamoto K, Imbe H, Tashiro A, Kimura A, Donishi T, Tamai Y, Senba E (2005) The role of peripheral 5HT2A and 5HT1A receptors on the orofacial formalin test in rats with persistent temporomandibular joint inflammation. Neuroscience 130:465–474

Otto M, Bach FW, Jensen TS, Sindrup SH (2004) Valproic acid has no effect on pain in polyneuropathy: a randomized, controlled trial. Neurology 62:285–288

Peiris JB, Perera GL, Devendra SV, Lionel ND (1980) Sodium valproate in trigeminal neuralgia. Med J Aust 2:278

Perkin GD (1999) Trigeminal neuralgia. Curr Treat Options Neurol 1:458–465

Petersen KL, Maloney A, Hoke F, Dahl JB, Rowbotham MC (2003) A randomized study of the effect of oral lamotrigine and hydromorphone on pain and hyperalgesia following heat/capsaicin sensitization. J Pain 4:400–406

Porreca F, Burgess SE, Gardell LR, Vanderah TW, Malan TP Jr, Ossipov MH, Lappi DA, Lai J (2001) Inhibition of neuropathic pain by selective ablation of brainstem medullary cells expressing the mu-opioid receptor. J Neurosci 21:5281–5288

Porreca F, Ossipov MH, Gebhart GF (2002) Chronic pain and medullary descending facilitation. Trends Neurosci 25:319–325

Ren K, Dubner R (2002) Descending modulation in persistent pain: an update. Pain 100:1–6

Roose SP, Laghrissi-Thode F, Kennedy JS, Nelson JC, Bigger JT Jr, Pollock BG, Gaffney A, Narayan M, Finkel MS, McCafferty J, Gergel I (1998) Comparison of paroxetine and nortriptyline in depressed patients with ischemic heart disease. JAMA 279:287–291

Rowbotham M, Harden N, Stacey B, Bernstein P, Magnus-Miller L (1998) Gabapentin for the treatment of postherpetic neuralgia: a randomized controlled trial. JAMA 280:1837–1842

Rush AM, Elliott JR (1997) Phenytoin and carbamazepine: differential inhibition of sodium currents in small cells from adult rat dorsal root ganglia. Neurosci Lett 226:95–98

Sabatowski R, Galvez R, Cherry DA, Jacquot F, Vincent E, Maisonobe P, Versavel M (2004) Pregabalin reduces pain and improves sleep and mood disturbances in patients with post-herpetic neuralgia: results of a randomised, placebo-controlled clinical trial. Pain 109:26–35

Sacerdote P, Brini A, Mantegazza P, Panerai AE (1987) A role for serotonin and beta-endorphin in the analgesia induced by some tricyclic antidepressant drugs. Pharmacol Biochem Behav 26:153–158

Saudek CD, Werns S, Reidenberg MM (1977) Phenytoin in the treatment of diabetic symmetrical polyneuropathy. Clin Pharmacol Ther 22:196–199

Schreiber S, Backer MM, Pick CG (1999) The antinociceptive effect of venlafaxine in mice is mediated through opioid and adrenergic mechanisms. Neurosci Lett 273:85–88

Sierralta F, Pinardi G, Miranda HF (1995) Effect of p-chlorophenylalanine and alpha-methyltyrosine on the antinociceptive effect of antidepressant drugs. Pharmacol Toxicol 77:276–280

Simpson DM, Olney R, McArthur JC, Khan A, Godbold J, Ebel-Frommer K (2000) A placebo-controlled trial of lamotrigine for painful HIV-associated neuropathy. Neurology 54:2115–2119

Simpson DM, McArthur JC, Olney R, Clifford D, So Y, Ross D, Baird BJ, Barrett P, Hammer AE (2003) Lamotrigine for HIV-associated painful sensory neuropathies: a placebo-controlled trial. Neurology 60:1508–1514

Sindrup SH, Jensen TS (1999) Efficacy of pharmacological treatments of neuropathic pain: an update and effect related to mechanism of drug action. Pain 83:389–400

Sindrup SH, Jensen TS (2000) Pharmacologic treatment of pain in polyneuropathy. Neurology 55:915–920

Sindrup SH, Andersen G, Madsen C, Smith T, Brosen K, Jensen TS (1999) Tramadol relieves pain and allodynia in polyneuropathy: a randomised, double-blind, controlled trial. Pain 83:85–90

Skolnick P, Layer RT, Popik P, Nowak G, Paul IA, Trullas R (1996) Adaptation of N-methyl-D-aspartate (NMDA) receptors following antidepressant treatment: implications for the pharmacotherapy of depression. Pharmacopsychiatry 29:23–26

Sutton KG, Martin DJ, Pinnock RD, Lee K, Scott RH (2002) Gabapentin inhibits high-threshold calcium channel currents in cultured rat dorsal root ganglion neurones. Br J Pharmacol 135:257–265

Suzuki R, Dickenson AH (2000) Neuropathic pain: nerves bursting with excitement. Neuroreport 11:R17–21

Suzuki R, Morcuende S, Webber M, Hunt SP, Dickenson AH (2002) Superficial NK1-expressing neurons control spinal excitability through activation of descending pathways. Nat Neurosci 5:1319–1326

Suzuki R, Rygh LJ, Dickenson AH (2004a) Bad news from the brain: descending 5-HT pathways that control spinal pain processing. Trends Pharmacol Sci 25:613–617

Suzuki R, Rahman W, Hunt SP, Dickenson AH (2004b) Descending facilitatory control of mechanically evoked responses is enhanced in deep dorsal horn neurones following peripheral nerve injury. Brain Res 1019:68–76

Suzuki R, Rahman W, Rygh LJ, Webber M, Hunt SP, Dickenson AH (2005) Spinal-supraspinal serotonergic circuits regulating neuropathic pain and its treatment with gabapentin. Pain 117:292–303

Tanelian DL, Brose WG (1991) Neuropathic pain can be relieved by drugs that are use-dependent sodium channel blockers: lidocaine, carbamazepine, and mexiletine. Anesthesiology 74:949–951

Taylor CP (1997) Mechanisms of action of gabapentin. Rev Neurol (Paris) 153 Suppl 1:S39–45

Thienel U, Neto W, Schwabe SK, Vijapurkar U (2004) Topiramate in painful diabetic polyneuropathy: findings from three double-blind placebo-controlled trials. Acta Neurol Scand 110:221–231

Todd AJ (2002) Anatomy of primary afferents and projection neurones in the rat spinal dorsal horn with particular emphasis on substance P and the neurokinin 1 receptor. Exp Physiol 87:245–249

Todd AJ, McGill MM, Shehab SA (2000) Neurokinin 1 receptor expression by neurons in laminae I, III and IV of the rat spinal dorsal horn that project to the brainstem. Eur J Neurosci 12:689–700

Todd AJ, Puskar Z, Spike RC, Hughes C, Watt C, Forrest L (2002) Projection neurons in lamina I of rat spinal cord with the neurokinin 1 receptor are selectively innervated by substance p-containing afferents and respond to noxious stimulation. J Neurosci 22:4103–4113

Tremont-Lukats IW, Megeff C, Backonja MM (2000) Anticonvulsants for neuropathic pain syndromes: mechanisms of action and place in therapy. Drugs 60:1029–1052

Urban MO, Gebhart GF (1999) Supraspinal contributions to hyperalgesia. Proc Natl Acad Sci U S A 96:7687–7692

Valverde O, Mico JA, Maldonado R, Mellado M, Gibert-Rahola J (1994) Participation of opioid and monoaminergic mechanisms on the antinociceptive effect induced by tricyclic antidepressants in two behavioural pain tests in mice. Prog Neuropsychopharmacol Biol Psychiatry 18:1073–1092

Wallace MS, Quessy S, Schulteis G (2004) Lack of effect of two oral sodium channel antagonists, lamotrigine and 4030W92, on intradermal capsaicin-induced hyperalgesia model. Pharmacol Biochem Behav 78:349–355

Waxman SG (1999) The molecular pathophysiology of pain: abnormal expression of sodium channel genes and its contributions to hyperexcitability of primary sensory neurons. Pain Suppl 6:S133–140

Wieczorkiewicz-Plaza A, Plaza P, Maciejewski R, Czuczwar M, Przesmycki K (2004) Effect of topiramate on mechanical allodynia in neuropathic pain model in rats. Pol J Pharmacol 56:275–278

Wiffen P, Collins S, McQuay H, Carroll D, Jadad A, Moore A (2000) Anticonvulsant drugs for acute and chronic pain. Cochrane Database Syst Rev: CD001133

Zakrzewska JM, Patsalos PN (2002) Long-term cohort study comparing medical (oxcarbazepine) and surgical management of intractable trigeminal neuralgia. Pain 95:259–266

Zakrzewska JM, Chaudhry Z, Nurmikko TJ, Patton DW, Mullens EL (1997) Lamotrigine (Lamictal) in refractory trigeminal neuralgia: results from a double-blind placebo controlled crossover trial. Pain 73:223–230

Zeitz KP, Guy N, Malmberg AB, Dirajlal S, Martin WJ, Sun L, Bonhaus DW, Stucky CL, Julius D, Basbaum AI (2002) The 5-HT3 subtype of serotonin receptor contributes to nociceptive processing via a novel subset of myelinated and unmyelinated nociceptors. J Neurosci 22:1010–1019

Part III
Compounds in Preclinical Development

HEP (2006) 177:181–216
© Springer-Verlag Berlin Heidelberg 2006

Neuropeptide and Kinin Antagonists

R. G. Hill (✉) · K. R. Oliver

Merck, Sharp and Dohme Research Laboratories,
Terlings Park, Harlow, Essex CM20 2QR, UK
hillr@merck.com

1	**Introduction**	182
2	**Substance P**	185
2.1	Preclinical Studies with NK_1 Receptor Antagonists and Transgenic Mice	185
2.2	Clinical Trials with NK_1 Receptor Antagonists	189
2.3	Prospects for Further Studies?	190
3	**CGRP**	192
3.1	Evidence for a Role in Pain and Headache	192
3.2	CGRP Receptors	195
3.3	Studies with CGRP Receptor Antagonists	196
4	**Bradykinin**	198
4.1	Kinins as Mediators of Pain and Inflammation	198
4.2	Kinin Receptors and Pathophysiology	199
4.3	Studies on Transgenic Animals	201
4.4	Kinin Receptor Antagonists	202
5	**Overall Conclusions**	203
	References	203

Abstract Neuropeptides and kinins are important messengers in the nervous system and—on the basis of their anatomical localisation and the effects produced when the substances themselves are administered, to animals or to human subjects—a significant number of them have been suggested to have a role in pain and inflammation. Experiments in gene deletion (knock-out or null mutant) mice and parallel experiments with pharmacological receptor antagonists in a variety of species have strengthened the evidence that a number of peptides, notably substance P and calcitonin gene-related peptide (CGRP), and the kinins have a pathophysiological role in nociception. Clinical studies with non-peptide pharmacological antagonists are now in progress to determine if blocking the action of these peptides might have utility in the treatment of pain.

Keywords Peptides · Substance P · CGRP · Kinins · Bradykinin · Des-Arg bradykinin

1
Introduction

Progress in neuroscience research over the last five decades has led to changes in our understanding of the neurochemical events that underlie the function of both central (CNS) and peripheral nervous systems. Neuropeptides, originally considered exclusively in terms of regulation of hypothalamic-pituitary function, were found to be distributed all over the CNS and, therefore, likely to be involved in wider aspects of brain function (see Oliver et al. 2000). Several characteristics distinguish neuropeptides from biogenic amines. First, neuropeptides demonstrate very high affinity interactions with their receptors. Second, in neuropeptidergic systems, no specific uptake or catabolic systems have been demonstrated. Third, synapses are not usually of a classical type and peptides may act at a distance from their site of release. Fourth, peptides are synthesized on polyribosomes by messenger RNA (mRNA) molecules, transcribed from the genome, whilst biogenic amines are produced non-ribosomally under the control of biosynthetic enzymes (derived from cellular gene transcripts). As a result of genome structure, and particularly the involvement of intron regulation of tissue-specific gene transcription, two different peptides can result from the same gene. Two examples of such alternative splicing are calcitonin/calcitonin gene-related peptide (Amara et al. 1982) and the tachykinin family (Nawa et al. 1984).

The observation that some peptides have a pro-nociceptive role has led to the suggestion that antagonising the action of such peptides may lead to analgesia. This is not a new idea and indeed, one of the first hypotheses for explaining the analgesic action of aspirin was that this drug opposed the algogenic effect of the peptide bradykinin (Guzman et al. 1964), and the idea that substance P might have a special role in pain perception was suggested by Lembeck in the 1950s (cited in Salt and Hill 1983). The literature on neuropeptides in pain signalling is therefore very extensive and can only be covered in a single chapter by being extremely selective. After reviewing the topic in a general way, a more detailed treatment will be given to the roles of substance P, calcitonin gene-related peptide (CGRP) and bradykinin (together with its des-[Arg] analogues). This focus is a consequence of these peptides being the ones which have received most study and in particular because medicinal chemists have succeeded in making specific receptor antagonist drugs that block their actions. Some of these receptor antagonist drugs have already been evaluated for efficacy as analgesics in a clinical setting. In the previous volume of this *Handbook* series devoted to the topic of *Pain and Analgesia* (vol. 130: Dickenson and Besson 1997), peptides did receive some attention, with a chapter devoted to substance P, but because of the lack of clinical data it was not possible at that time for the authors to come to any firm conclusion on the therapeutic utility of antagonists.

There has been a great increase in our understanding of the process of nociception in the last decade (e.g. see reviews by Hill 2001; Hunt and Mantyh 2001;

Julius and Basbaum 2001) and this has enabled a more complete assessment of the role of peptide messengers. One special feature of the small unmyelinated fibres which contain peptides is that they are able to release them from both peripheral and central arborisations and thus may impinge on sensory transmission both in the peripheral innervated tissues and in the dorsal horn of the spinal cord (see Salt and Hill 1983; Hunt and Mantyh 2001; Jang et al. 2004). A variety of chemical and other stimuli, including H^+ ions, heat, intense mechanical pressure and kinins both stimulate peripheral peptide release (see Julius and Basbaum 2001) and generate impulses which travel rostrally to excite the central terminals within the dorsal horn of the spinal cord. The details of the nociceptive transmission process are described at length in the chapter by J.N. Wood of this volume. One important feature of peptide release from primary afferent fibres is that it is likely to be a parallel event, with glutamate and other transmitters being released in concert with one or more peptides (Salt and Hill 1983; Leah, Cameron and Snow 1985; Hill 2001). It has been suggested that neurokinin A, substance P and CGRP might be released together as co-transmitters from primary afferent fibres in the caudal trigeminal nucleus (Samsam et al. 2000). Antibody microprobe studies have shown that some neuropeptides can be detected at sites relatively distant to their site of release (see Duggan and Furmidge 1994) and that interaction between peptides (as competing peptidase substrates) may influence the levels that individual peptides reach in the dorsal horn of the spinal cord (DHSC). Gene array studies have also shown that spinal cord injury can result in an up-regulation of peptidase genes (Tachibana et al. 2002). It is also apparent that peptides can regulate receptor expression and, for example, CGRP can regulate the expression of the NK_1 receptors at which substance P acts (Seybold et al. 2003). The number and diversity of neuropeptides (see Oliver et al. 2000) is another complication of trying to ascribe a physiological or pathological role to any individual peptide, and a significant number of peptides also have extra-neuronal functions (Hokfelt et al. 2000). At the present time there are over 65 known neuropeptides (excluding the chemokines), receptors for over 20 neuropeptides have been cloned and many neuropeptides activate more than one receptor subtype (Oliver et al. 2000). It is of particular interest that a noxious insult in a neonatal rat results in the up-regulation of genes in the DHSC coding (amongst other things) for the synthesis of neuropeptides that persists into adulthood (Ren et al. 2005). It has been suggested that peptides have a particular role when the nervous system is under stress (Hokfelt et al. 2000), and many studies have been made of the effects of nerve injury on peptide expression. The changes seen are not especially helpful although it has been shown, for example, that injury to sensory nerves down-regulates CGRP and substance P yet up-regulates expression of vasoactive intestinal polypeptide (VIP), neuropeptide Y (NPY) and galanin, with inflammation producing a different expression pattern (Garry et al. 2004). Galanin is a 29-amino-acid peptide that is found both in dorsal root ganglion cells and in

DHSC interneurons and whose expression increases markedly after peripheral nerve lesions (Liu and Hokfelt. 2002), leading to the suggestion that it
may have a role in the processes leading to neuropathic pain. It has recently
been shown that the small proteins collectively known as chemokines might
have an important role in neuropathic pain, but this area has been considered
to be outside the scope of the present chapter (see Kinloch and Cox 2005;
White et al. 2005). The drug discovery scientist is faced with the dilemma
of too many potential targets and no easy way to determine which might
be the most productive for discovering a new analgesic drug (Boyce et al.
2001). Historically, discovery of a neuropeptide receptor was consequent on
the discovery of the neuropeptide itself, but with the advent of modern tech-
nologies this no longer necessarily applies. The rate-limiting factor in drug
discovery today is not the lack of attractive targets; indeed, the advent and
rapid development of molecular- and bioinformatics-related techniques has
created the problem of how to select the best targets from a rich supply of
receptor clones. So-called "orphan" G protein-coupled receptors (oGPCRs)
are being identified at a prolific rate, albeit with little information available
yet as to their endogenous ligands, many of which are likely to be peptides
(Oliver et al. 2000). There are neuropeptides for which we have as yet no
identified receptor, and paradoxically—through novel receptor research—we
have orphan receptors with unidentified ligands but which are structurally
related to known peptide receptor families. The vast majority of receptors for
neuropeptides discovered thus far are G protein coupled (GPCRs), with the
common basic structure of seven transmembrane domains and an extracellular 20- to 100-amino-acid residue extracellular tail. This receptor superfamily
has been divided into three subfamilies based on receptor sequence analysis:
(1) rhodopsin or β-adrenoceptor-like, (2) secretin or glucagon-like and (3)
metabotropic or chemosensor-like receptors. Peptide GPCRs are not structurally homogeneous and belong to both class 1 and class 2. Peptides that
act through GPCRs can be small—such as enkephalins, bradykinin, calcitonin
gene-related peptide, substance P and vasoactive intestinal peptide—or large
peptides, glycoproteins and hormones, or even enzymes such as trypsin and
thrombin (see Oliver et al. 2000).

   Much emphasis is now being placed on transgenic animals for the preclinical
validation of novel drug targets, including neuropeptide receptors. Thus, the
phenotype of a mouse resulting from a specific gene deletion or silencing may
provide information regarding the functional role of a specific receptor for
which the deleted gene codes in the tissue of interest and thus may predict
the action of a specific receptor antagonist. Transgenic technology has now
been used by numerous groups to elucidate the role of neuropeptides in vivo,
although at times some knock-out mice appear phenotypically normal. This
may be related to compensatory mechanisms occurring during development
probably due to up-regulation of molecules functionally related to the deleted
gene (see later and Oliver et al. 2000).

2
Substance P

2.1
Preclinical Studies with NK₁ Receptor Antagonists and Transgenic Mice

Evidence supporting the role of substance P as a pain transmitter comes from anatomical and immunocytochemical studies showing substance P is expressed in small unmyelinated sensory fibres (Nagy et al. 1981; Hokfelt et al. 2004) and it is released into the dorsal horn of the spinal cord following intense noxious stimulation (Duggan et al. 1987). In addition, substance P when applied onto the dorsal horn neurons produces prolonged excitation which resembles the activation observed following noxious stimulation (Henry 1976) and when given intrathecally produces behavioural hyperalgesia (Cridland and Henry 1986). More recently, it has been shown that following peripheral noxious stimulation NK_1 receptors become internalised on dorsal horn neurons and that this effect can be blocked by NK_1 receptor antagonists (Mantyh et al. 1995). In addition to its effects on spinal nociceptive processing, substance P has also been implicated in migraine headache. Sensory afferents that innervate meningeal tissues contain substance P and other neuropeptides (e.g. calcitonin gene related peptide; CGRP see later) and it has been suggested that release of these neuropeptides causes a neurogenic inflammation which could lead to activation of nociceptive afferents projecting to the brain stem (Shepheard et al. 1995; Williamson and Hargreaves 2001). The expectation was that therefore centrally acting NK_1 receptor antagonists would be anti-nociceptive in animals and analgesic in man and constitute a novel class of analgesic drug.

Compounds which have been optimised for activity at NK_1 receptors expressed in humans typically have low affinity for rats or mice, species used for anti-nociceptive studies (see Boyce and Hill 2004). Consequently, early studies with the NK_1 receptor antagonists which were performed in rats and mice required high doses to observe anti-nociceptive effects, and so interpretation of the data was confounded by potential off-target activity such as blockade of ion channels (Rupniak et al. 1993). There is now considerable evidence generated from well-controlled studies using enantiomeric pairs of a number of antagonist structures (one enantiomer having high affinity for the NK_1 receptor and the other low affinity) to control for non-specific effects. Analgesic tests have also been developed in appropriate species (gerbils, guinea-pigs) with similar NK_1 receptor pharmacology to human such that it has been possible to demonstrate unequivocally that NK_1 receptor antagonists do possess anti-nociceptive effects in animals. Nociception tests which demonstrate reproducible analgesic effects only with opioids such as morphine (hot plate, tail or paw flick and paw pressure tests) do not reveal anti-nociceptive effects of NK_1 receptor antagonists in any species even when these agents are administered at high doses (Rupniak et al. 1993). Similarly, NK$_1$ antagonists have little effect on baseline spinal nociceptive reflexes in anaesthetised animals (Laird et al. 1993). However, NK$_1$ receptor antagonists such as CP-96,345 and LY303870, but not their less active enantiomers, CP-96,344 and LY396155, were shown to be potent inhibitors of the excitation of dorsal horn neurons elicited by prolonged noxious mechanical or thermal peripheral stimulation or by iontophoretic application of substance P in cats (Radhakrishnan and Henry 1991; Radhakrishnan et al. 1998), indicating that these effects are due to a specific blockade of NK$_1$ receptors. In addition, aprepitant (MK-0869) or CP-99,994, but not its less active enantiomer CP-100,263, inhibited the facilitation or wind up of a spinal flexion reflex produced by C-fibre conditioning stimulation in decerebrate/spinalised rabbits (Boyce et al. 1993; see Boyce and Hill 2000), and RP67580, but not its less active enantiomer RP68651, inhibited facilitation of the hind limb flexor reflex in anaesthetised/spinalised rats (Laird et al. 1993).

In conscious animals, the first demonstration of a clear enantioselective analgesic effect came from studies using L-733,060, a highly selective and brain penetrant NK$_1$ receptor antagonist with long duration of action. This compound, but not its less active enantiomer L-733061, was able to inhibit the late phase nociceptive responses to intraplantar injection of formalin in gerbils (Rupniak et al. 1996). The poorly brain penetrant compound L-743,310, a potent inhibitor of peripherally mediated NK$_1$ receptor agonist-induced chromodacryorrhoea, failed to inhibit the late phase response, indicating that the anti-nociceptive effect of L-733,060 was via blockade of central NK$_1$ receptors. Consistent with a central anti-nociceptive action, intrathecal injection of CP-96,345, but not its less active enantiomer CP-96,344, attenuated the late phase formalin test response in rats (Yamamoto and Yaksh 1991) as did LY303870 (Iyengar et al. 1997). Oral administration of CP-99,994, SDZ NKT 343 (Novartis) or LY303870 have also been shown to attenuate mechanical hyperalgesia induced by carrageenan in guinea-pigs (Patel et al. 1996; Urban et al. 1999). L-733,060, but not its inactive isomer L-733,061, also reversed carrageenan-induced mechanical hyperalgesia in guinea-pigs (Boyce and Hill 2000).

In addition to their effects in assays of inflammatory hyperalgesia, NK$_1$ receptor antagonists are effective in a number of putative neuropathic pain assays. Urban and colleagues (1999) using partial sciatic nerve ligation in guinea-pigs showed that SDZ NKT 343 and LY303870 reduced established mechanical hyperalgesia following either oral or intrathecal administration. In contrast, RPR 100,893 was only active following intrathecal administration (Urban et al. 1999) probably due to poor brain penetration (Rupniak et al. 1997a). Likewise, CI-1021 was effective in reversing mechanical hypersensitivity (reduction in weight bearing) in guinea-pigs following sciatic nerve chronic constriction injury (CCI; Gonzalez et al. 2000) and it reduced mechanical hypersensitivity in rats following induction of diabetes by streptozotocin treatment (Field et al. 1998). Intrathecal administration of RP67580, but not its less active enantiomer, also reduced mechanical hyperalgesia in streptozotocin diabetic rats (Coudore-Civiale et al. 2000). GR205171 which has nanomolar affinity at rat NK_1 receptors, reversed both mechanical hypersensitivity and the increase in receptive field size of dorsal horn neurons in rats following CCI, effects which were not observed with its inactive enantiomer L-796,325 (Cumberbatch et al. 1998). In contrast, using the spinal nerve ligation (Chung) model, it was not possible to demonstrate an anti-algesic effect of GR205171 at doses that were effective in rats with CCI (M Sablad, A Hama and M Urban, personal communication; Boyce and Hill 2004). In addition to the nerve damage associated with CCI, a marked neurogenic inflammation also develops (Daemen et al. 1998) which could contribute to the development of hyperalgesia and allodynia. The analgesic effects of NK_1 antagonists in CCI and partial nerve ligation models may therefore relate to anti-inflammatory actions and not specifically to effects on neuropathic pain.

NK_1 receptor antagonists are effective in models of visceral pain. CP-99994 inhibited the nociceptive reflex response (depressor effect) to jejunal distension in rats (McLean et al. 1998) and TAK-637, but not its less active enantiomer, and CP-99994 reduced the number of abdominal contractions induced by colorectal distension in rabbits following sensitisation to acetic acid (Okano et al. 2002). Intrathecal administration of TAK-637 and CP-99994 inhibited abdominal contractions. In contrast, Julia et al. (1994) demonstrated that the NK_2 receptor antagonist SR-48,968, but not the NK_1 receptor antagonists CP-96345 or RP-67,580, inhibited abdominal contractions to rectal distension in rats. However, the NK_1 antagonists did prevent distension-induced inhibition of colonic motility in this study.

NK_1 receptor antagonists have also been shown to be active in tests involving inflammation associated with arthritic changes. Similar to indomethacin, daily administration of the NK_1 receptor antagonist L-760,735 (3 mg /kg s.c.) for 21 days reduced paw oedema and the associated thermal and mechanical hyperalgesia in Freund's adjuvant arthritic guinea-pigs (see Boyce and Hill 2000). Consistent with these findings, Binder et al. (1999) showed that repeated administration of GR205171, but not its less active enantiomer, also reduced arthritic joint damage (joint swelling, synovitis and bone demineralisation) caused by complete Freund's adjuvant (CFA) in rats. These findings suggest that NK_1 receptor antagonists may possess anti-inflammatory as well as anti-nociceptive activity. Other data suggest that NK_1 receptor antagonists are extremely potent inhibitors of neurogenic inflammation. The NK_1 receptor antagonists RP-67,580, CP-99,994, LY30380 and aprepitant block neurogenic plasma extravasation in the dura following trigeminal ganglion stimulation in rats or guinea-pigs (Shepheard et al. 1993; Shepheard et al. 1995; Phebus et al. 1997; Boyce and Hill 2000; Williamson and Hargreaves 2001). In addition to its actions on neurogenic extravasation, CP-99,994 has also been shown to reduce c-fos messenger RNA (mRNA) expression in the trigeminal nucleus caudalis in rats after trigeminal ganglion stimulation (Shepheard et al. 1995).

NK$_1$ receptor knock-out ($-/-$) mice exhibit little or no changes in acute nociception tests such as the hot plate, thermal paw withdrawal or responses to von Frey filaments (De Felipe et al. 1998; Mansikka et al. 1999). Acute nociceptive responses to intraplantar injection of chemical stimuli such as formalin or capsaicin, as well as the resultant mechanical/heat hypersensitivity, are slightly attenuated in the NK$_1$($-/-$) mice (De Felipe et al. 1998; Laird et al. 2001; Mansikka et al. 1999). However, these mice do develop hyperalgesia after induction of hind paw inflammation with CFA (De Felipe et a 1998), which contrasts with findings observed with NK$_1$ receptor antagonists (see Binder et al. 1999; Boyce and Hill 2000). Martinez-Caro and Laird (2000) failed to demonstrate any difference between responses of wild-type (WT) and NK$_1$($-/-$) mice following partial sciatic nerve ligation, whereas NK$_1$ receptor antagonists were effective in the same model in guinea-pigs (see above). Using the L5 spinal ligation (modified Chung) model, Mansikka et al. (2000) found that NK$_1$($-/-$) mice did not develop mechanical hypersensitivity but hyperalgesic responses to thermal stimuli (radiant heat or cooling) were unaltered in NK$_1$($-/-$) compared to WT mice.

Data from NK$_1$($-/-$) mice support a role of NK$_1$ receptors in visceral pain, particularly associated with neurogenic inflammation. Thus, instillation of capsaicin, which evokes neurogenic inflammation, into the colon of the NK$_1$($-/-$) mice produced fewer abdominal contractions than were observed in WT mice and they failed to develop referred hyperalgesia (Laird et al. 2000). Similarly, behavioural responses to cyclophosphamide and the acute nociceptive (pressor) reflex response or primary hyperalgesia following intracolonic acetic acid were impaired in NK$_1$($-/-$) mice. In contrast, nociceptive responses to intracolonic mustard oil which was found to evoke direct tissue damage were unchanged in the NK$_1$($-/-$) mice (Laird et al. 2000). Electrophysiological studies have also shown that the characteristic amplification ('wind up') of spinal nociceptive reflexes to repetitive high-frequency electrical stimulation is absent in NK$_1$($-/-$) mice (De Felipe et al. 1998), which is in agreement with the findings from studies with NK$_1$ receptor antagonist drugs. The evidence obtained from studies with the NK$_1$($-/-$) mice supporting the role of substance P and NK$_1$ receptors in pain is less compelling than has been reported for non-peptide antagonists. It is not clear why there should be differences in anti-nociceptive profile seen with NK$_1$ receptor antagonists and in the NK$_1$($-/-$) mice. Non-specific actions of NK$_1$ receptor antagonists contributing to the anti-nociceptive effects can be ruled out, as the studies outlined above are well-controlled with many demonstrating marked enantioselective inhibition. These differences may relate to compensatory changes in the knock-out mice as a result of the life-long absence of NK$_1$ receptors.

In summary, there is abundant preclinical data supporting the analgesic potential of NK$_1$ antagonists, particularly in pain conditions associated with inflammation or nerve injury.

2.2
Clinical Trials with NK$_1$ Receptor Antagonists

Only a single clinical study, with CP-99,994 in post-operative dental pain, has demonstrated analgesic activity in man (Dionne et al. 1999). In this study, CP-99,994 was administered as an intravenous infusion over 5 h, starting 30 min prior to surgery (total dose 0.75 mg/kg). CP-99,994 had comparable clinical efficacy to ibuprofen (Dionne et al. 1998). In contrast, the long-acting orally active NK$_1$ receptor antagonist aprepitant (300 mg p.o. given 2 h prior to surgery) was ineffective in post-operative dental pain (Reinhardt et al. 1998). The dental pain model is unlikely to be ideal for testing the analgesic effects of NK$_1$ receptor antagonists, especially as these agents are not effective against acute noxious stimuli in rodents (Urban and Fox 2000). A recent study which has utilised NK$_1$ receptor internalisation to determine the extent of substance P release in the spinal cord following dental tooth extraction in rodents (Sabino et al. 2002) demonstrated NK$_1$ receptor internalisation in neurons in the trigeminal nucleus caudalis and cervical spinal cord (100% of neurons within lamina I and 65% in lamina II–V) within 5 min following incisor extraction. The effect was relatively short-lived with only few neurons showing internalised receptor at 60 min. This suggests that substance P may play only a minor role in mediating pain associated with tooth extraction, limited to the initial phase of pain, which is not typically assessed in the clinical studies. A more appropriate model to evaluate NK$_1$ receptor antagonists may be dental pain associated with pulpal inflammation where elevated levels of substance P are found in dental pulp (Awawdeh et al. 2002).

NK$_1$ receptor antagonists have also been evaluated in patients with neuropathic pain and aprepitant (300 mg p.o. for 2 weeks) was ineffective in patients with established post-herpetic neuralgia (PHN; duration of 6 months to 6 years; Block et al. 1998). Lanepitant (LY303870; 50, 100 or 200 mg p.o. b.i.d. for 8 weeks) had no significant effect on pain intensity (daytime or night time) when compared to placebo in patients with painful diabetic neuropathy (Goldstein et al. 1999). Lanepitant (10, 30, 100, or 300 mg p.o. for 3 weeks) was also without effect in patients with moderate to severe osteoarthritis (Goldstein et al. 1998). To date, lanepitant and aprepitant are the only NK$_1$ receptor antagonists which have been evaluated in chronic pain conditions. The negative data obtained with aprepitant in PHN is not due to insufficient dose, as the same dose was shown by positron emission tomography (PET) to block central NK$_1$ receptors in man (Hargreaves 2002). Destruction of peptidergic C-fibre function has been reported in patients with long-established disease, and this loss in substance P function could therefore account, at least in part, for the failure of aprepitant to produce analgesia in patients with PHN.

Finally, clinical trials with NK$_1$ receptor antagonists for acute migraine and migraine prophylaxis have also been disappointing. L-758,298, an intravenous pro-drug of aprepitant (20, 40 or 60 mg i.v) failed to abort migraine pain as measured either by the time to meaningful relief or the number of patients reporting pain relief within 4 h (Norman et al. 1998). Similarly, GR205171 (25 mg i.v.; Connor et al. 1998) and lanepitant (30, 80 or 240 mg p.o., Goldstein et al. 1997) were ineffective as abortive treatments for migraine headache. Furthermore, prophylactic administration of lanepitant (200 mg p.o. per day) for 1 month had no effect on migraine frequency and severity compared to placebo (Goldstein et al. 1999). The hypothesis that NK_1 receptor antagonists would be effective anti-migraine agents was based on their ability to inhibit dural plasma extravasation (Shepheard et al. 1993), an effect shared with known anti-migraine drugs such as the triptans (Williamson et al. 1997; Williamson and Hargreaves 2001) but not established as the reason for their efficacy in migraine treatment.

The lack of clinical efficacy of aprepitant or GR205171 in pain or migraine trials is not due to insufficient dose or lack of brain penetration. At the dose used in the analgesia trials, aprepitant was found to produce more than 90% NK_1 receptor occupancy using PET (Hargreaves 2002) and is anti-emetic in cancer patients following chemotherapy (Navari et al. 1999). Similarly, the dose of GR205171 employed in the migraine trial was based on NK_1 receptor adequate occupancy calculated from PET studies (Connor et al. 1998). In view of these largely negative findings it has been concluded that NK_1 receptor antagonists are not effective as analgesic agents in man.

2.3
Prospects for Further Studies?

NK_1 receptor antagonists appear to reduce arthritic joint damage and resultant hypersensitivity in animals with adjuvant arthritis. There is high expression of NK_1 receptor mRNA in synovia taken from patients with rheumatoid arthritis, and NK_1 mRNA is positively correlated with serum C-reactive protein levels and radiological grade of joint destruction (Sakai et al. 1998), suggesting that NK_1 receptor gene expression may reflect the disease progression in rheumatoid arthritis. Achilles tendinosis is associated with sprouting of substance P-positive nerve fibres (Schubert et al. 2005). NK_1 receptor antagonists may have potential for alleviating other bone-generated pain including bone cancer pain and fractures. A preclinical study using a murine model of cancer pain has shown substantial internalisation of NK_1 receptors on NK_1 receptor-expressing neurons in lamina I of the spinal cord following non-noxious palpation of the tumourous bone which was positively correlated with the extent of bone destruction (Schwei et al. 1999). In addition, substance P, acting via the NK_1 receptor, stimulates osteoclast (OCL) formation and activates OCL bone resorption (Goto et al. 2001). Since bisphosphonates and osteoprotegerin reduce tumour-induced bone pain by blocking bone resorption (Honore and Mantyh 2000), NK_1 receptor antagonists could be effective in reducing bone cancer pain by blocking substance P-mediated bone resorption, as well as the spinal effects of substance P. Other chronic pain conditions in which NK_1 receptor antagonists may be worth testing include fibromyalgia, a syndrome in which elevated levels of substance P are found in the cerebrospinal fluid (Russell et al. 1994). Recently, Littman et al. (1999) reported that the NK_1 receptor antagonist CJ-11,974 (50 mg p.o. b.i.d. for 4 weeks) was able to reduce dysaesthesias in patients with fibromyalgia, and in a subset of patients there was some improvement in pain severity, morning stiffness and sleep disturbances. These findings warrant further investigation.

The clinical trials published to date have focussed on somatic pains, and none has reported on the effects of NK_1 receptor antagonists in visceral pain. The anatomical distribution of substance P certainly favours a major role in visceral rather than somatic pain as a greater number of visceral primary afferents (>80%) express substance P compared with only 25% in cutaneous afferents (Laird et al. 2001), and laminae I and X of the spinal dorsal horn, which receive afferents from the viscera, show the highest density of NK_1 receptors in the spinal cord (Li et al. 1998). It has recently been shown that cardiac somatic nociception involves NK_1 receptor activation in the parabrachial complex (Boscan et al. 2005). The preclinical findings described above support a potential utility of NK_1 receptor antagonists in visceral pain conditions.

The anomaly between data obtained in preclinical and clinical studies might be explained by species differences in physiology of substance P or distribution of NK_1 receptors or difference between clinical pain and the responses to noxious stimuli measured in small animals. Whereas in rats substance P is co-expressed in 5-HT dorsal raphe descending fibres (Neckers et al. 1979), in man it is restricted to dorsal raphe ascending fibres (Sergeyev et al. 1999), suggesting that it may play a greater role in supraspinal functions in man. It must be remembered that substance P is only one of many neurotransmitters expressed in primary sensory afferent neurons and that only a small proportion of these fibres (<25% of cutaneous fibres) contain substance P. Blocking the actions of substance P or NK_1 receptors alone might not be sufficient to produce clinical analgesia. It is interesting to note that animals injected intrathecally with saporin toxin conjugated to substance P to kill NK_1 receptor-expressing cells within the dorsal horn, display a more pronounced anti-nociception than was achieved by blocking NK_1 receptors (Mantyh et al. 1997; see also Morris et al. 2004) presumably by blocking all inputs to these neurons and not just by inhibiting the actions of substance P. Other studies have shown that the most important action of substance P might be to modulate the action of other transmitters in the spinal cord, particularly glutamate (Juranek and Lembeck 1997). Combination of RP-67580 (but not its inactive enantiomer) with the N-methyl-D-aspartate (NMDA)/glycine receptor antagonist (+)-HA-966 enhanced the anti-nociception in the rat formalin paw test (Seguin and Millan 1994). Similarly, Field and colleagues (2002) demonstrated a marked synergy of the anti-nociceptive effects of gabapentin when administered with the NK_1 receptor antagonists CI-1021 or CP-99994 in neuropathic (CCI or streptozotocin) rats.

In conclusion, although substance P, acting at NK_1 receptors, appears to play an important role in pain transmission in animals, it is clear that NK_1 receptor antagonists are not likely to be useable as simple analgesic drugs in the clinic although further clinical studies may be worthwhile. Some aspects of the action of substance P are hard to interpret and the clinical context is therefore obscure. It is noteworthy that the substance P locus of the preprotachykinin precursor is needed for transport of δ-opioid receptors in primary afferents (Julius and Basbaum 2005) and that substance P inhibits the production of neuroactive progesterone metabolites in spinal circuits (Patte-Mensah et al. 2005). NK_1 receptor neurotransmission has been suggested to have a role in the hyperalgesia following chronic morphine administration as a consequence of up-regulation of both substance P and NK_1 receptor expression (King et al. 2005).

3
CGRP

3.1
Evidence for a Role in Pain and Headache

Since its discovery in 1981 by Rosenfeld et al. (for review see Rosenfeld et al. 1992), CGRP has been shown to be an important neuropeptide that is widely distributed in both peripheral and central nervous systems (Hokfelt et al. 1992; Van Rossum et al. 1997). It is now known to be one of a family of structurally related peptides comprising calcitonin, amylin, CGRPα and β plus adrenomedullin, which act at a characteristic group of GPCRs made up from multiple subunits (Poyner et al. 2002). For the purposes of this chapter most attention will be given to CGRP itself and the reader interested in a general review of the properties of this peptide family and their role outside nociception is referred to Van Rossum et al. (1997).

CGRP is of particular interest in the context of nociception as it is the most abundant peptide in primary afferent fibres and has the widest distribution across subtypes of primary afferents including myelinated fibres. It is present in virtually all substance P-containing fibres and in many others (up to 80% of all primary afferents in the monkey; Hokfelt et al. 1992). Most of the CGRP immunoreactive terminals in the DHSC of the mouse are from primary afferents, as rhizotomy produces a dramatic depletion although there is a small population of CGRP mRNA positive cells in lamina III (Tie-Jun et al. 2001). There is a dense innervation of the cat caudal trigeminal nucleus by CGRP-containing fibres which synapse with intrinsic neurons of the nucleus (Henry et al. 1993). CGRP-containing fibres also richly innervate the human trigeminal nucleus caudalis (Smith et al. 2002). Inflammation of the craniofacial muscle or of the temporomandibular joint increases CGRP expression in the trigeminal ganglion and caudal trigeminal nucleus (Ambalavanar et al. 2006; Hutchins et al. 2006). In the lumbar dorsal root ganglion (DRG) there is up-regulation of CGRP expression after inflammation of the rat ankle (Hanesch et al. 1993). In collagen-induced arthritis in the rat (Nohr et al. 1999) or in an iodoacetate model of osteoarthritis (Fernihough et al. 2005) there was also a marked increase in the DRG expression of CGRP. In streptozotocin diabetic rats, in contrast, both CGRP and substance P expression were reduced several weeks after the induction of diabetes although an increase in mRNA in the DRG suggests this may have been associated with increased turnover of the peptides (Troger et al. 1999). In a mouse fibrosarcoma model of cancer pain it was found that hyperalgesic mice had tumours that were more densely innervated with CGRP immunoreactive fibres and less vascularised than tumours from non-hyperalgesic mice (Wacnik et al. 2005). The transforming growth factor (TGF)-β-related factor activin is released after damage or inflammation of peripheral tissues and has been shown to increase CGRP expression in sensory neurons and to produce tactile allodynia, leading to the suggestion that it may be the chemical mediator for this response (Xu et al. 2005). Partial sciatic nerve lesions in the rat produced increased expression of CGRP in those myelinated DRG neurons projecting to the gracile nucleus, again leading to the suggestion that CGRP may be involved in the production of tactile allodynia (Ma et al. 1999). Tumour necrosis factor (TNF)-α has been found to increase CGRP expression in rat trigeminal ganglion neurons (Bowen et al. 2006) and in DRG neurons (Opree and Kress 2000). The nociceptive acid sensing channel ASIC3 is co-localised with CGRP in trigeminal ganglion neurons retrogradely labelled from tooth pulp and facial skin (Ichikawa and Sugimoto 2002). Lumbar DRG neurons in the mouse co-express CGRP and voltage-gated calcium channels of N- and L-types (Just et al. 2001).

CGRP is distributed widely but unevenly across the CNS (Van Rossum et al. 1997). It has been found to co-exist with many other peptides; in motoneurons it is found together with VIP and somatostatin in many species including human (Hokfelt et al. 1992).

Clinical association of CGRP signalling and somatic pain are limited, but it has recently been shown that mice with a heterozygous mutation of the *Nf1* gene (analogous to human neurofibromatosis type 1) exhibit increased sensitivity to noxious stimuli that correlates with increased CGRP release (Hingten et al. 2006), and human patients with this disorder have abnormal pain sensitivity. Studies in strains of mice selected on the basis of their differential sensitivity to noxious heat using both electrophysiological and behavioural assays indicate that the observed differences are linked to strain-dependent CGRP expression. Linkage mapping suggests that a chromosome 7 polymorphism upstream of the *Calca* gene (coding CGRPα) is the cause of a heritable difference in both CGRP expression and noxious heat sensitivity (Mogil et al. 2005). The behavioural phenotype of mice in which the α-CGRP gene has been knocked out indicates that CGRP is involved in neurogenic inflammation and chemical nociception, but the full phenotype of these mice is complex (Muff et al. 2004). There is elevated sympathetic nervous system activity (Oh-hashi et al. 2001) but overall there is normal cardiovascular regulation and neuromuscular development (Lu et al. 1999). The knock-out protocol to deplete α-CGRP, however, leaves detectable amounts of β-CGRP in DRG and spinal cord (Schutz et al. 2004). It is relevant to note that the related peptide amylin is also found in primary afferent neurons in the mouse and rat, and knock-out mice lacking the amylin gene show reduced nociceptive responses in the formalin test (Gebre-Medhin et al. 1998). It has been reported that amylin can be anti-nociceptive when injected into the cerebral ventricles, but this is almost certain to be due to an action at calcitonin receptors (Sibilia et al. 2000)

Perhaps the most persuasive clinical association is between CGRP and the pathogenesis of migraine headache (Edvinsson 2001; Brain et al. 2002). For example, intravenous injection of CGRP induces a migraine-like headache in migraineurs (Lassen et al. 2002), levels of CGRP are elevated in the external jugular vein during a migraine headache and following treatment with triptans the plasma levels of CGRP return to control levels with successful ameliora- tion of the headache (Edvinsson and Goadsby 1995; Gallai et al. 1995). Plasma CGRP levels are higher than control in migraineurs even between attacks of headache (Ashina et al. 2000) and a similar relationship has recently been ob- served in salivary CGRP, which is elevated in migraineurs, rises further during a headache and returns to control levels after effective treatment with a triptan (Bellamy et al. 2006). It is not completely clear as yet whether the importance of CGRP in migraine is because it is a neuronally released vasodilator (Limmroth et al. 2001), a nociceptive neurotransmitter or both. However, the vascular link is a persuasive one (see Edvinsson et al. 1995) and those areas of the brainstem that have been suggested to be the migraine generator have only sparse CGRP fibres in comparison with other neuropeptides (Tajti et al. 2001). Dural vasodilatation produced by i.v. CGRP in the rat produces a sensitisation of the responses of neurons in the spinal trigeminal nucleus receiving input from low-threshold mechanoreceptors on the face (Cumberbatch et al. 1999) although CGRP dural vessel dilation does not activate or sensitise meningeal nociceptors (Levy et al. 2005). It is clear that cortical spreading depression (which has been linked to migraine aura) does not produce CGRP release into the jugular vein blood in the way that trigeminal ganglion stimulation or the headache phase of migraine does (Piper et al. 1993; Edvinsson and Goadsby 1995). It is not possible to make a general association between CGRP and all headaches however and, for example, there is no correlation between the severe headache caused by pituitary tumours and CGRP (Levy et al. 2004).

Some limited data have been obtained using selective antibodies to sequester CGRP and neutralise its physiological effects. These have helped to confirm its importance in neurogenic vasodilatation (Tan et al. 1994, 1995) and in the hyperalgesia following experimental arthritis (Kuraishi et al. 1988).

3.2
CGRP Receptors

Study of the receptors at which CGRP acts is complicated by their multi-subunit complexity, and until comparatively recently attempts to isolate or clone the receptor were hampered by the fact that it was not a single protein gene product. Some information on the localisation of the CGRP receptor was obtained from experiments with an antibody mixture raised against purified CGRP binding sites isolated from pig cerebellum (e.g. Ye et al. 1999), but as we know now that the receptor is made up from three different proteins that can individually also have roles in other receptors of the family, this earlier work should be treated with caution (see Brain et al. 2002; Poyner et al. 2002). The CGRP receptor consists of a seven-transmembrane G protein-coupled calcitonin-like receptor (CRLR) unit linked to receptor activity modifying protein 1 (RAMP1) and to receptor component protein (RCP), which is important in the coupling of receptor activation to stimulation of adenylyl cyclase (Brain et al. 2002). RAMPs and RCP are widely distributed in the body, suggesting that they interact with other receptors also (e.g see Oliver et al. 2001: Hay et al. 2006). It is important to note that CRLR can have different selectivity according to which RAMP it is associated with; with RAMP2, for example, it forms a receptor more selective for adrenomedullin and with RAMP3 a receptor sensitive to both CGRP and adrenomedullin (Hay et al. 2006). This makes it very difficult to use mapping of the localisation of an individual protein of the triad to identify where CGRP receptors are functionally located, although it has been claimed that RCP maps well with the location of CGRP immunoreactivity (Ma et al. 2003) and RCP expression is up-regulated in DRG and DHSC following peripheral inflammation. In addition to a widespread distribution in the CNS, the components of the CGRP receptor are also expressed in the human cerebral vasculature (Oliver et al. 2002). The receptor localisation issue is further complicated by the observation that some structures such as the cerebellum will bind CGRP, yet there is a relative lack of RAMP1 (Oliver et al. 2001).

Those receptors containing CRLR and RAMPs appear to signal through cyclic AMP (cAMP) and intracellular calcium with coupling by way of G_q or G_α (Hay et al. 2006). Intrathecal injection of CGRP in rats produced hyperalgesia that could be reduced with a protein kinase (PKA) or PKC blocker, suggesting the involvement of both these second messenger systems (Sun et al. 2004). In neonatal or adult rat DRG neurons, CGRP increased cAMP and produced phosphorylation of cAMP-response element binding protein (CREB), suggesting that CGRP can modulate gene expression (Anderson and Seybold 2004).

The complicated nature of the CGRP receptor has so far made it impossible to produce a genetically modified mouse lacking functional CGRP receptors. Thus, further elucidation of the function of CGRP in nociception has been crucially dependent on the availability of selective pharmacological antagonists.

3.3
Studies with CGRP Receptor Antagonists

The first useful antagonists of the effects of peptides of the CGRP family were truncated analogues of the peptides themselves such as CGRP 8–37 or amylin 22–52 (see Brain and Grant 2004; Hay et al. 2004; Van Rossum et al. 1997). In vascular and other smooth muscle tissues, especially in vitro, these peptide antagonists have proved generally useful in spite of some issues around lack of biological stability (see Brain and Grant 2004). In the CNS results have not been as consistent and CGRP 8–37 sometimes shows agonist properties (e.g. Riediger et al. 1999).

Low-intensity rat spinal cord electrical stimulation induces cutaneous vasodilatation that is blocked by CGRP 8–37 but not by hexamethonium (Tanaka et al. 2001) as is vasodilatation in the dental pulp and lip following stimulation of the rat inferior alveolar nerve (Kerezoudis et al. 1994) and the cerebro-dilator response following nasociliary nerve stimulation in the cat (Goadsby 1993). Using intravital microscopy in anaesthetised rats to visualise dural vessel dilatation, Williamson and colleagues (1997a, b) showed that the dilatation produced either by CGRP given systemically or neurogenic dilatation produced by perivascular electrical nerve stimulation were blocked by i.v. CGRP 8–37. This is suggestive of an anti-migraine profile for CGRP receptor antagonists which is also supported by the observation that triptans reduce the neurogenic dilatation of dural vessels (Williamson et al. 1997b) and that the terminals which release CGRP express the 5-HT$_{1B/D}$ receptors at which the triptans act to relieve migraine headache (Ma et al. 2001). The excitation of neurons within the dorsal horn of the rat spinal cord by noxious stimulation of the limbs in the presence or absence of inflammation and by ionophoretic application of exogenous CGRP was blocked by ionophoretic CGRP 8–37 (Ebersberger et al. 2000; Neugebauer et al. 1996). Excitatory responses evoked by ionophoretic application of substance P, neurokinin A or AMPA (S-α-amino-3-hydroxy-5-methyl-4-isoxazolepropionic acid) were unaffected by CGRP 8–37 co-application (Neugebauer et al. 1996). Deep tissue inflammation up-regulated CGRP expression within the trigeminal ganglion and lowered the somatic withdrawal thresholds to noxious stimulation, and this was prevented by infusing CGRP 8–37 prior to the inflammatory stimulus (Ambalavanar et al. 2006). Thermal injury to one hind paw of a rat produced swelling, inflammation and a lowered threshold for paw withdrawal which was reversed by intrathecal CGRP 8–37 (Lofgren et al. 1997) as was the thermal and mechanical allodynia in a chronic central pain model (Bennett et al. 2000). A colonic pain model where thresholds to distention were reduced by either CGRP instillation or by nerve growth factor (NGF) or brain-derived neurotrophic factor (BDNF) administration was also found to be sensitive to blockade by CGRP 8–37 (Delafoy et al. 2006). In contrast, exogenous CGRP microinjected into the periaqueductal grey matter can raise the nociceptive threshold in rats, but this effect too can be blocked by co-administration of CGRP 8–37 (Yu et al. 2003).

Non-peptide antagonists of the CGRP receptor have been sought for many years, but it is only recently that highly potent and selective agents that are active in vivo have been discovered. The discovery that SK-N-MC (neuroblastoma–neuroepithelioma) cells were a facile source of membranes expressing human CGRP receptors enabled a high-throughput screening campaign leading to quinuclidine compounds with micromolar affinity and antagonist properties as shown by blockade of the ability of CGRP to raise cAMP levels in SK-N-MC cells (Daines et al. 1997). SB-273779 is a more potent non-peptide antagonist (IC_{50} 310 nM) that showed some in vivo activity against CGRP-induced falls in systemic blood pressure but its low potency, short half-life and poor in vivo tolerability at higher doses limit its utility (Aiyar et al. 2001). Rudolph and colleagues (2005) were the first to report highly potent antagonists of the action of CGRP suitable for clinical evaluation. A high-throughput screening effort led them to a series of (R)-Tyr-(S)-Lys dipeptide-like compounds, and lead optimisation produced BIBN4096, the first picomolar antagonist that is active both in vitro and in vivo (Rudolph et al. 2005). The major drawback of this compound is low oral bioavailability (<1%) such that clinical proof of concept studies had to be performed with i.v. administration.

BIBN4096 was found to reduce both spontaneous and evoked activity of single neurons in the spinal trigeminal nucleus with receptive fields in the dura mater (Fischer et al. 2005). Supraspinal neurons within the central nucleus of the amygdala of anaesthetised rats showed an increase in plasticity after peripheral inflammation that was reversed after intra-amygdala injection of BIBN4096 or CGRP 8–37 (Han et al. 2005). Species selectivity has to be considered when using BIBN4096 as a tool in rodents, and doses tenfold higher than those effective at human or primate receptors may be needed (see Hershey et al. 2005). Dilation of human cerebral arteries in vitro by CGRP was potently reversed by BIBN4096 (Moreno et al. 2002). In the first reported randomised, double-blind, phase II clinical trial in migraine patients (Olesen et al. 2004) BIBN4096 at a dose of 2.5 mg i.v. was effective in relieving the headache and clearly differentiated from placebo. In a volunteer study (Petersen et al. 2005) BIBN4096 2.5 mg i.v. prevented the headache produced by an infusion of CGRP (1.5 µg/min for 20 min).

Indirect evidence on the putative role of CGRP in pain is provided from studies on the experimental analgesic drug cizolirtine as it has been shown to inhibit the spinal release of both substance P and CGRP in rats (Ballet et al. 2001) and is effective in rat models of neuropathic pain (Aubel et al. 2004; Kayser et al. 2003). Block of the effects of substance P does not produce analgesia in humans (see previous section of this chapter), thus any efficacy in cizolirtine is likely to be due to an effect on CGRP signalling. In a double-blind cross-over study in neuropathic pain patients, cizolirtine 200 mg p.o. b.i.d did not reduce overall pain experience but did reduce primary allodynia in the subgroup with this symptom (Shembalkar et al. 2001). At doses up to 150 mg it was ineffective against the pain following third molar extraction (Matthew et al. 2000); against the pain of renal colic, 350 mg of cizolirtine was also ineffective (Pavlik et al. 2004).

There is thus convincing preclinical and clinical evidence to show that blockade of CGRP receptors is likely to be an effective treatment for migraine headache. Some preclinical evidence suggests that blockade of CGRP receptors might have a more general utility in the treatment of painful conditions, but clinical studies with the release inhibitor cizolirtine (which must be treated cautiously given that a mechanism involving CGRP has not been confirmed in humans) only support a use against allodynia in patients with neuropathic pain.

4
Bradykinin

4.1
Kinins as Mediators of Pain and Inflammation

The topic of kinins as mediators of pain and inflammation has recently been reviewed in detail (Rupniak et al. 2000; Calixto et al. 2000; 2001; Couture et al. 2001) so it will only be dealt with briefly here. When kinins are produced by tissue damage the nonapeptide bradykinin appears rapidly followed by its metabolite des-[Arg^9] bradykinin and by des-[Arg^{10}] kallidin. All three peptides are pharmacologically active but with differing receptor selectivity (Rupniak et al. 2000). The production of bradykinin and kallidin from largely inactive precursors depends on cleavage by serine proteases known as kallikreins (although tissue and plasma kallikreins belong to different enzyme families). Bradykinin and its decapeptide analogue kallidin are then further cleaved by carboxypeptidase to produce the des-[Arg] analogues (Couture et al. 2001; Rupniak et al. 2000).

The kinins are directly algogenic and also release other mediators such as prostaglandins and cytokines which amplify the local inflammatory and nociceptive response. They also release transmitters from the terminals of primary afferents, including substance P and CGRP and may exert a pro-inflammatory effect by way of sympathetic fibres. Bradykinin (as a partially purified biological extract) was first shown to produce pain in humans by Armstrong and his colleagues in 1951 when they applied it to an exposed blister base in volunteers (cited by Rupniak et al. 2000). Bradykinin is released from muscles during contraction as part of normal physiology but when injected into a muscle it can evoke pain (Boix et al. 2005). Exercise studies show an association between perceived pain and levels of bradykinin and kallidin produced in the muscle (Boix et al. 2004). Bradykinin is able to increase the gain of peripheral nociceptive mechanisms by disinhibiting the TRPV1 receptor (Chuang et al. 2001) on primary afferents and also potentiates glutamate operated synaptic transmission in the spinal dorsal horn (Wang et al. 2005). It appears that roughly half of all primary afferent nociceptor fibres are sensitive to kinins under baseline conditions but that this proportion rises to 80% in the presence of inflammation (Rupniak et al. 2000).

The traditional idea of the kinin system being exclusively peripheral has now passed and it is accepted that kinins are found within the CNS, for example in the spinal cord (Lopes and Couture 1997). The increased sensitivity to opioids that has been reported in animals following the induction of peripheral inflammation may be due to a central action of kinins to increase opioid receptor trafficking (Patwardhan et al. 2005).

It is important to remember that kinins also have a role in smooth muscle contraction and relaxation, control of blood pressure, vasodilation and vascular permeability such that this may constrain the way in which their effects can be modulated to produced pain relief (Calixto et al. 2001).

4.2
Kinin Receptors and Pathophysiology

Kinins exert their effects through two receptors called the bradykinin 1 (B_1) and bradykinin 2 (B_2) receptors on the basis of a distinct pharmacological classification on isolated tissues obtained by a study of the agonist peptides themselves and of a number of peptide analogues with a variety of agonist, partial agonist and antagonist properties (Couture et al. 2001). The existence of the two distinct receptors has been confirmed by molecular cloning performed by Hess and his colleagues (cited in Rupniak et al. 2000). Both receptors are members of the GPCR family (see Oliver et al. 2000) and there is only some 38% structural homology between them (Couture et al. 2001). It has recently been shown that a proteolytic B_1 and B_2 receptor complex with enhanced signalling capacity can form and become inserted in the plasma membrane (Kang et al. 2004). Early pharmacological studies suggested clear species differences in the selectivity of kinin receptors for agonist and antagonist ligands, and this has now been confirmed by studies on cloned receptors from a number of species. For the B_1 receptor in particular, there are striking cross species differences, with des-[Arg^{10}] kallidin having much higher affinity for the human receptor than does des-[Arg^9] bradykinin whereas on rat and mouse B_1 receptors the situation is reversed (Jones et al. 1999; Rupniak et al. 2000). In most species, the preferred agonist for the B_2 receptor is bradykinin itself, whereas the des-[Arg] peptides are the preferred ligands for the B_1 receptor (Rupniak et al. 2000). Under most circumstances the B_2 receptor is constitutive, although it can be up-regulated by inflammatory mediators (Seabrook et al. 1997; Calixto et al. 2001) whereas the B_1 receptor is inducible and normally only expressed by peripheral tissues when they are exposed to an inflammatory or damaging stimulus (Couture et al. 2001; Marceau et al. 1998; Rupniak et al. 2000). Constitutive B_1 receptors may be found in the CNS, B_1 and B_2 receptors were found in the human brain by Raidoo and Bhoola (1997) and B_1 receptors have been found in spinal cord of rat, mouse, monkey and human (see Calixto et al. 2004). It appears that under some circumstances the expression of B_2 receptors can be down-regulated (Baptista et al. 2002; Kang et al. 2004). It is noteworthy that the human B_1 receptor has ligand-independent constitutive activity as it lacks critical epitopes that regulate activity (Leeb-Lundberg et al. 2001) although the physiological significance of this is unclear and homo-oligomerisation of this receptor may be needed for cell surface expression (Kang et al. 2005).

The role of B_1 receptors in pain and inflammation has recently been reviewed in depth (Calixto et al. 2004) and there is an extensive literature on the B_2 receptor (reviewed in Rupniak et al. 2000). Evidence from human studies, however, is limited at the present time. Tissue kallikrein, B_1 and B_2 receptors are expressed in mast and giant cells infiltrating oesophageal squamous cell carcinomas (Dlamini and Bhoola 2005) and receptors have been found in numerous other tumours (Calixto et al. 2004). It is likely that kinins act as mitogens to promote cell proliferation in addition to exacerbating any inflammatory response in the tumour. Studies in human volunteers have shown that UV-B irradiation of skin enhanced pain signalling through both B_1 and B_2 receptors activated by skin microdialysis of des-[Arg] kallidin or bradykinin respectively (Eisenbarth et al. 2004). Arthritic rats showed an enhanced B_1-mediated extravasation after 5 days of joint inflammation (Cruwys et al. 1994) and lipopolysaccharide (LPS)-induced paw oedema was potentiated by the B_1 agonist des-[Arg] bradykinin (Ferreira et al. 2000). Interleukin-1β seems to be an especially potent inducer of B_1 receptor expression and activation of nuclear factor (NF)-κB via B_2 receptors also stimulates B_1 expression (Couture et al. 2001). Platelet-activating factor (PAF) also activates NF-κB and up-regulates B_1 receptors and this is believed to be via TNF-α and subsequent interleukin (IL)-1β release (Fernandes et al. 2005). In adrenalectomised rats, B_1 receptor expression was increased and this could be reversed by administering dexamethasone or by inhibiting NF-κB with PDTC (pyrrolidine dithiocarbamate) (Cabrini et al. 2001). In sciatic nerve injured mice there was a switch from B_2 to B_1 receptor signalling with increased time after lesioning (Rashid et al. 2004). Functional B_1 receptors are expressed by nociceptive sensory neurons and expression is up-regulated by glia-derived neurotrophic factor (GDNF ;Vellani et al. 2004). There is also evidence for the involvement of p38 in the development of inflammation in the rat and the consequent increase in B_1 receptor expression (Ganju et al. 2001). Acute chronic cystitis in rat bladder induces expression of B_1 receptors whereas only B_2 receptors are seen in the non-inflamed state (Chopra et al. 2005). Intrathecal administration of a B_2 agonist to mice produces thermal hyperalgesia that peaks 10 min after injection whereas intrathecal injection of a B_1 agonist produces persistent thermal hyperalgesia lasting up to 1 h (Calixto et al. 2001), suggesting the receptors localised within the spinal cord are functional. In the cardiovascular system B_1 receptors are involved in inflammatory pathologies such as endotoxic shock, atheromatous disease and myocardial ischaemia, although it is not yet clear whether activation of B_1 receptors is pathological or protective (McLean et al. 2000). In rats with kindled epilepsy, induction of B_1 receptors resulted in potentiation of glutamate release in cortex and hippocampus (Bregola et al. 1994; Mazzuferi et al. 2005).

Both B_1 and B_2 receptors appear to be involved in nociception and inflammatory processes, and experiments with transgenic animals and/or selective receptor antagonists were needed to elucidate the respective role of each receptor (Calixto et al. 2004).

4.3
Studies on Transgenic Animals

The background presence of B_2 receptors and the inducible nature of B_1 receptors combine to make it difficult to assess the individual role of each receptor in pain and inflammation and hence which would make the best analgesic drug discovery target. The emergence of transgenic technology has thus been of crucial help in this research area.

The first knock-out produced (Borkowki et al. 1995) had a deletion of the entire coding region of the B_2 receptor gene. These mice are fertile and visually indistinguishable from WT littermates. Bradykinin fails to produce responses in ileum, uterus and superior cervical ganglia (SCG) in these mice, all tissues which express functional B_2 receptors in WT mice (Borkowki et al. 1995). The nociceptive response to intraplantar injection of bradykinin was absent in the −/− mice and there was no hyperalgesia following paw injection of carrageenan; however, the nociceptive response to formalin was preserved, as was the induction of thermal hyperalgesia following intraplantar Freund's adjuvant (Rupniak et al. 1997b).

Electrophysiological studies in isolated SCG showed that expression of functional B_1 receptors was stimulated by IL-1β in ganglia taken from the $B_2(-/-)$ mice (Seabrook et al. 1997), suggesting that the remaining nociceptive responses were operated through B_1 receptors. This was confirmed in studies on a mouse in which the B_1 receptor gene had been inactivated (Pesquero et al. 2000). These mice are healthy, fertile and normotensive yet have a reduced response to inflammation with LPS. Surprisingly, in the absence of any inflammatory stimulus these mice are analgesic in tests of thermal and chemical nociception in a similar manner to mice treated with an opioid analgesic. In an isolated spinal cord preparation there was a reduction in wind up of a nociceptive spinal reflex (Pesquero et al. 2000).

In contrast to the $B_2(-/-)$ mouse, in the $B_1(-/-)$ mouse thermal hyperalgesia following intraplantar CFA is absent both ipsilateral and, to a lesser extent, contralateral to the injected paw, reinforcing the idea that it is the spinal B_1 receptors which are crucial to spinal cord sensitisation in the nociceptive process (Calixto et al. 2001; Ferreira et al. 2001). Intrathecal injection of selective B_1 or B_2 receptor agonists failed to produce thermal hyperalgesia in the respective $-/-$ mice, confirming a functional role at the spinal level for both receptors (Ferreira et al. 2002). Partial lesion of the sciatic nerve in $B_1(-/-)$ mice produced much less mechanical allodynia and thermal hyperalgesia than was seen in WT animals subjected to the same procedure (Ferreira et al. 2005). In response to the pronounced species-to-species differences in the pharmacology of the B_1 receptor, both rats (Hess et al. 2004) and mice (Fox et al. 2005) have been engineered to express the human B_1 receptor so as to facilitate the evaluation of antagonists at the human B_1 receptor as putative analgesics (see the following section).

4.4
Kinin Receptor Antagonists

The elucidation of the role of the kinins has been dependent on the use of antagonists that were initially themselves analogues of the peptide agonists. Although this was a valuable step forward for work on isolated tissue pharmacology, the instability of most of these analogues limited their utility for in vivo studies. In some cases it appears that carboxypeptidases were able to convert peptide B_2 antagonists into B_1 receptor blockers; thus, on the basis of these tools the role of B_1 receptors in nociception may have been underestimated (Regoli et al. 1986 cited by Rupniak et al. 1997b). For this reason the more recently developed non-peptide antagonists will be emphasised here. This topic has been reviewed recently (Bock and Longmore 2000; Marceau and Regoli 2004). The first step towards improved molecules that had antagonist properties was to incorporate stable residues into a basic peptide structure, but many of these stable peptides were low-efficacy partial agonists rather than full antagonists. The most useful agent arising from work on peptide structures is probably the B_2 antagonist HOE 140 or icatibant (see Bock and Longmore 2000). The development of high-throughput functional assays using cloned and expressed human B_1 and B_2 receptors in mammalian cells (see Simpson et al. 2000) greatly facilitated the search for potent, bioavailable non-peptide antagonists. A number of companies had success in this area (see Bock and Longmore 2000; Marceau and Regoli 2004) and agents selective for rat (Burgess et al. 2000) and human (Dziadulewicz et al. 2002) that are orally bioavailable have now been produced. Icatibant was found to reduce the hyperalgesia following CCI in the rat sciatic nerve (Levy et al. 2000). Bradyzide, an orally active rodent selective B_2 receptor antagonist, was found to block Freund's adjuvant-induced hyperalgesia in the rat knee at a dose equipotent to morphine in the same assay (Burgess et al. 2000) and was superior to earlier agents of this type such as WIN64338 and FR173657 (see Calixto et al. 2000). The emphasis has switched to the B_1 receptor since the elucidation of the phenotype of the $B_1(-/-)$ mouse and because of concerns that blockade of the B_2

receptor may have cardiovascular liabilities. Several academic and pharmaceutical company groups have been successful in producing potent B_1 antagonists from a variety of different chemical scaffolds (see Fox et al. 2005; Gougat et al. 2004; Morissette et al. 2004; Ransom et al. 2004; Ritchie et al. 2004; Wood et al. 2003). In a rabbit spinal nerve reflex assay developed to evaluate B_1 antagonists for anti-nociceptive properties (see Mason et al. 2002), a novel non-peptide antagonist has been shown to be anti-nociceptive when given either intravenously of intrathecally (Conley et al. 2005). SSR240612, another novel B_1 receptor antagonist that is orally bioavailable (Gougat et al. 2004), inhibited capsaicin-induced ear oedema in the mouse, blocked thermal hyperalgesia following UV irradiation and reduced the late phase formalin response in the rat. It was also effective against thermal hyperalgesia after CCI in the rat sciatic nerve. NVP-SAA164, a B_1 receptor antagonist optimised for activity at the human receptor (Fox et al. 2005), produced a dose-related reversal of Freund's adjuvant-induced hyperalgesia in transgenic mice expressing a human B_1 receptor. Recent studies have shown that hyperalgesia in non-obese diabetic (NOD) mice and in streptozotocin diabetic rats is reduced by the B_1 antagonist R-954 (Gabra and Sirois 2005; Gabra et al. 2005).

Taken together with the phenotype of the receptor $-/-$ animals, the properties of the selective antagonist compounds suggest an analgesic potential in humans, especially for the B_1 receptor blocking agents.

5
Overall Conclusions

There is little doubt that neuropeptides, in particular substance P, CGRP and the kinins have a pivotal role in nociceptive processing. The failure of the substance P/NK_1 receptor antagonists to display analgesic properties in clinical trials either points to important species-specific differences in physiology or indicates that blocking a single channel of the multi-channel nociceptive pathway is not sufficient to produce analgesia. The clinical efficacy of the CGRP receptor antagonist BIBN4096 in migraine headache is very encouraging and leads us to the conclusion that if the correct peptide channel is blocked than clinical analgesia may well result. The bradykinin receptor antagonists that are moving forward to clinical evaluation will be the next big test of clinical relevance for this field of research.

References

Aiyar N, Daines RA, Disa J, et al (2001) Pharmacology of SB-273779, a non-peptide calcitonin gene related peptide 1 receptor antagonist. J Pharmacol Exp Ther 296:768–775

Amara SG, Jonas V, Rosenfeld MG, et al (1982) Alternative RNA processing in calcitonin gene expression generates mRNAs encoding different polypeptide products. Nature 298:240–244

Ambalavanar R, Moritani M, Moutanni A, et al (2006) Deep tissue inflammation upregulates neuropeptides and evokes nociceptive behaviours which are modulated by a neuropeptide antagonist. Pain 120:53–68

Anderson LE, Seybold VS (2004) Calcitonin gene related peptide regulates gene transcription in primary afferent neurons. J Neurochem 91:1417–1429

Ashina M, Bendtsen L, Jensen R, et al (2000) Evidence for increased plasma levels of calcitonin gene related peptide in migraine outside of attacks. Pain 86:133–138

Aubel B, Kayser V, Mauborgne A, et al (2004) Antihyperalgesic effects of cizolirtine in diabetic rats: behavioural and biochemical studies. Pain 110:22–32

Awawdeh L, Lundy FT, Shaw C, et al (2002) Quantitative analysis of substance P, neurokinin A and calcitonin gene-related peptide in pulp tissue from painful and healthy human teeth. Int Endod J 35:30–36

Ballet S, Aubel B, Mauborgne A, et al (2001) The novel analgesic cizolirtine inhibits the spinal release of substance P and CGRP in rats. Neuropharmacology 40:578–589

Baptista HA, Avellar MCW, Araujo RC, et al (2002) Transcriptional regulation of the rat bradykinin B2 receptor gene: identification of a silencer element. Mol Pharmacol 62:1344–1355

Bellamy JL, Cady RK, Durham PL (2006) Salivary levels of CGRP and VIP in rhinosinusitis and migraine patients. Headache 46:24–33

Bennett AD, Chastain KM, Hulseboch CE (2000) Alleviation of mechanical and thermal allodynia by CGRP 8–37 in a rodent model of chronic central pain. Pain 86:163–175

Beresford IJ, Birch PJ, Hagan RM, et al (1991) Investigation into species variants in tachykinin NK1 receptors by use of the non-peptide antagonist, CP-96,345. Br J Pharmacol 104: 292–293

Binder W, Scott C, Walker JS (1999) Involvement of substance P in the anti-inflammatory effects of the peripherally selective kappa-opioid asimadoline and the NK1 antagonist GR 205171. Eur J Neurosci 11:2065–2072

Block GA, Rue D, Panebianco D, et al (1998) The substance P receptor antagonist L-754,030 (MK-0869) is ineffective in he treatment of postherpetic neuralgia. Neurology 4:A225

Bock MG, Longmore J (2000) Bradykinin antagonists: new opportunities. Curr Opin Chem Biol 4:401–406

Boix F, Roe C, Rosenborg L, Knardahl S (2005) Kinin peptides in human trapezius muscle during sustained isometric contraction and their relation to pain. J Appl Physiol 98: 534–540

Borkowki JA, Ransom RW, Seabrook GR, et al (1995) Targeted disruption of a B2 bradykinin receptor gene in mice eliminates bradykinin action in smooth muscle and neurons. J Biol Chem 270:13706–13710

Boscan P, Dutschmann M, Herbert H, Paton JFR (2005) Neurokininergic mechanism within the lateral crescent nucleus of the parabrachial complex participates in the heart rate response to nociception. J Neurosci 25:1412–1420

Bowen EJ, Schmidt TW, Firm CS, et al (2006) Tumour necrosis factor α stimulation of calcitonin gene related peptide expression and secretion from rat trigeminal ganglion neurons. J Neurochem 96:65–77

Boyce S, Hill RG (2000) Discrepant results from preclinical and clinical studies on the potential of substance P-receptor antagonists compounds as analgesics. In: Devor M, Rowbotham MC, Wiesenfeld-Hallin Z (eds) Proceedings of the 9th World Congress on Pain. IASP press, Seattle, pp 313–324

Boyce S, Hill RG (2004) Substance P (NK1) receptor antagonists—analgesics or not? In: Holzer P (ed) Tachykinins. (Handbook of experimental pharmacology, vol 164) Springer, Berlin Heidelberg New York, pp 441–457

Boyce S, Laird JMA, Tattersall FD, et al (1993) Antinociceptive effects of NK1 receptor antagonists: comparison of behavioural and electrophysiological tests. 7th World Congress on Pain. Abstr 641

Boyce S, Ali Z, Hill RG (2001) New developments in analgesia. Drug Discov World 4:31–35

Brain SD, Grant AD (2004) Vascular actions of calcitonin gene related peptide and adrenomedullin. Physiol Rev 84:903–934

Brain SD, Poyner DR, Hill RG (2002) CGRP receptors: a headache to study, but will antagonists prove therapeutic in migraine? Trends Pharmacol Sci 23:51–53

Bregola G, Varani K, Gessi S, et al (1999) Changes in hippocampal and cortical B1 bradykinin receptor biological activity in two experimental models of epilepsy. Neuroscience 92: 1043–1049

Burgess GM, Perkins MN, Rang HP, et al (2000) Bradyzide, a potent non-peptide B2 bradykinin receptor antagonist with long-lasting oral activity in animal models of inflammatory hyperalgesia. Br J Pharmacol 129:77–86

Cabrini DA, Campos MM, Tratsk KS, et al (2001) Molecular and pharmacological evidence for modulation of kinin B1 receptor expression by endogenous glucocorticoid hormones in rats. Br J Pharmacol 132:567–577

Calixto JB, Cabrini DA, Ferreira J, et al (2000) Kinins in pain and inflammation. Pain 87:1–5

Calixto JB, Cabrini DA, Ferreira J, et al (2001) Inflammatory pain: kinins and antagonists. Curr Opin Anaesthesiol 14:519–526

Calixto JB, Medeiros R, Fernandes ES, et al (2004) Kinin B1 receptors: key G-protein-coupled receptors and their role in inflammatory and painful processes. Br J Pharmacol 143:803–818

Cascieri MA, Ber E, Fong TM, et al (1992) Characterization of the binding of a potent, selective, radioiodinated antagonist to the human neurokinin-1 receptor. Mol Pharmacol 42:458–463

Chopra B, Barrick SR, Meyers S, et al (2005) Expression and function of bradykinin B1 and B2 receptors in normal and inflamed rat urinary bladder urothelium. J Physiol 562:859–871

Chuang HH, Prescott ED, Kong H, et al (2001) Bradykinin and nerve growth factor release the capsaicin receptor from PtdIns (4,5)P2-mediated inhibition. Nature 411:957–962

Conley RK, Wheeldon A, Webb JK, et al (2005) Inhibition of acute nociceptive responses in rat spinal cord by a bradykinin B1 receptor antagonist. Eur J Pharmacol 527:44–51

Connor HE, Bertin L, Gillies S, et al (1998) Clinical evaluation of a novel, potent, CNS penetrating NK1 receptor antagonist in the acute treatment of migraine. Cephalalgia 18:392

Coudore-Civiale M, Courteix C, Boucher M, et al (2000) Evidence for an involvement of tachykinins in allodynia in streptozocin-induced diabetic rats. Eur J Pharmacol 40: 47–53

Couture R, Harrisson M, Vianna RM, et al (2001) Kinin receptors in pain and inflammation. Eur J Pharmacol 429:161–176

Cridland RA, Henry JL (1986) Comparison of the effects of substance P, neurokinin A, physalaemin and eledoisin in facilitating a nociceptive reflex in the rat. Brain Res 381: 93–99

Cruwys SC, Garrett NE, Perkins MN, et al (1994) The role of bradykinin B1 receptors in the maintenance of intra-articular plasma extravasation in chronic antigen-induced arthritis. Br J Pharmacol 113:940–944

Cumberbatch MJ, Carlson E, Wyatt A, et al (1998) Reversal of behavioural and electrophysiological correlates of experimental peripheral neuropathy by the NK1 receptor antagonist GR205171 in rats. Neuropharmacology 37:1535–1543

Cumberbatch MJ, Williamson DJ, Mason GS, et al (1999) Dural vasodilation causes a sensitization of rat caudal trigeminal nucleus neurons in vivo that is blocked by a 5-HT 1B/1D agonist. Br J Pharmacol 126:1478–1486

Daemen MA, Kurvers HA, Kitslaar PJ, et al (1998) Neurogenic inflammation in an animal model of neuropathic pain. Neurol Res 20:41–45

Daines RA, Sham KKC, Taggart JJ, et al (1997) Quinine analogues as non-peptide calcitonin gene related peptide (CGRP) receptor antagonists. Bioorg Med Chem Lett 7:2673–2676

De Felipe C, Herrero JF, O'Brien A, et al (1998) Altered nociception, analgesia and aggression in mice lacking the receptor for substance P. Nature 392:394–397

Delafoy L, Gelot A, Ardid D, et al (2006) Interactive involvement of BDNF, NGF and CGRP in colonic hypersensitivity in the rat. Gut. Published online 9 Jan 2006. http://gut.bmjjournals.com/cgi/content/abstract/gut.2005.064063v1. Cited 16 May 2006

Dickenson A, Besson JM (eds) (1997) The pharmacology of pain. (Handbook of experimental pharmacology, vol 130) Springer, Berlin Heidelberg New York

Dionne RA (1999) Clinical analgesic trials of NK1 antagonists. Curr Opin Investig Drugs 1:82–85

Dionne RA, Max MB, Gordon SM, et al (1998) The substance P receptor antagonist CP-99,994 reduces acute postoperative pain. Clin Pharmacol Ther 64:562–568

Dlamini Z, Bhoola KD (2005) Upregulation of tissue kallikrein, kinin B1 receptor, and kinin B2 receptor in mast and giant cells infiltrating oesophageal squamous cell carcinoma. J Clin Pathol 58:915–922

Duggan AW, Furmidge LJ (1994) Probing the brain and spinal cord with neuropeptides in pathways related to pain and other functions. Front Neuroendocrinol 15:275–300

Duggan AW, Morton CR, Zhao ZQ, et al (1987) Noxious heating of the skin releases immunoreactive substance P in the substantia gelatinosa of the cat: a study with antibody microprobes. Brain Res 403:345–349

Dziadulewicz EK, Ritchie TJ, Hallett A, et al (2002) Nonpeptide bradykinin B2 receptor antagonists: conversion of rodent-selective bradyzide analogues into potent, orally-active human bradykinin B2 receptor antagonists. J Med Chem 45:2160–2172

Ebersberger A, Charbel Issa P, Vanegas H, Schaible HG (2000) Differential effects of calcitonin gene related peptide and calcitonin gene related peptide 8–37 upon responses to NMDA or AMPA in spinal nociceptive neurons with knee joint input in the rat. Neuroscience 99:171–178

Edvinsson L (2001) Calcitonin gene-related peptide (CGRP) and the pathophysiology of headache: therapeutic implications. CNS Drugs 15:745–753

Edvinsson L, Goadsby PJ (1995) Neuropeptides in the cerebral circulation: relevance to headache. Cephalalgia 15:272–276

Edvinsson L, Olesen IJ, Kingman TA, et al (1995) Modification of vasoconstrictor responses in cerebral blood vessels by lesioning of the trigeminal nerve: possible involvement of CGRP. Cephalalgia 15:373–383

Eisenbarth H, Rukwied R, Petersen M, et al (2004) Sensitization to bradykinin B1 and B2 receptor activation in UV-B irradiated human skin. Pain 110:197–204

Fang LN, Wang ZZ, Wang YL, et al (2004) Expression of calcitonin gene related peptide type 1 receptor mRNA and the activity modifying proteins in the rat nucleus accumbens. Neurosci Lett 362:146–149

Fernandes ES, Passos GF, Campos MM, et al (2005) Cytokines and neutrophils as important mediators of platelet-activating factor-induced kinin B1 receptor expression. Br J Pharmacol 146:209–216

Fernihough J, Gentry C, Bevan S, Winter J (2005) Regulation of calcitonin gene related peptide and TRPV1 in a rat model of osteoarthritis. Neurosci Lett 388:75–80

Ferreira J, Campos MM, Pesquero JB, et al (2001) Evidence for the participation of kinins in Freund's adjuvant-induced inflammatory and nociceptive responses in kinin B1 and B2 receptor knockout mice. Neuropharmacology 41:1006–1012

Ferreira J, Campos MM, Araújo R, et al (2002) The use of kinin B1 and B2 receptor knockout mice and selective antagonists to characterise the nociceptive responses caused by kinins at the spinal level. Neuropharmacology 43:1188–1197

Ferreira J, Beirith A, Mori MAS, et al (2005) Reduced nerve injury-induced neuropathic pain in kinin B1 receptor knock-out mice. J Neurosci 25:2405–2412

Ferreira PK, Campos MM, Calixto JB (2000) The role of sensorial neuropeptides in the edematogenic responses mediated by B1 agonist des-Arg^9-BK in rats pre-treated with LPS. Regul Pept 89:29–35

Field MJ, McCleary S, Boden P, et al (1998) Involvement of the central tachykinin NK1 receptor during maintenance of mechanical hypersensitivity induced by diabetes in the rat. J Pharmacol Exp Ther 285:1226–1232

Field MJ, Gonzalez MI, Tallarida RJ, et al (2002) Gabapentin and the neurokinin(1) receptor antagonist CI-1021 act synergistically in two rat models of neuropathic pain. J Pharmacol Exp Ther 303:730–735

Fischer MJM, Koulchitsky S, Messlinger K (2005) The nonpeptide calcitonin gene related peptide receptor antagonist BIBN4096BS lowers the activity of neurons with meningeal input in the rat spinal trigeminal nucleus. J Neurosci 25:5877–5883

Fox A, Kaur S, Li B, et al (2005) Antihyperalgesic activity of a novel nonpeptide bradykinin B1 receptor antagonist in transgenic mice expressing the human B1 receptor. Br J Pharmacol 144:889–899

Gabra BH, Sirois P (2005) Hyperalgesia in non-obese diabetic (NOD) mice: a role for the inducible bradykinin B1 receptor. Eur J Pharmacol 514:61–67

Gabra BH, Benrezzak O, Pheng LH, et al (2005) Inhibition of type 1 diabetic hyperalgesia in streptozotocin-induced Wistar versus spontaneous gene-prone BB/Worcester rats: efficacy of a selective bradykinin B1 receptor antagonist. J Neuropathol Exp Neurol 64:782–789

Gallai V, Sarchielli P, Floridi A, et al (1995) Vasoactive peptide levels in the plasma of young migraine patients with and without aura assessed both interictally and ictally. Cephalalgia 15:384–390

Ganju P, Davis A, Patel S, et al (2001) p38 stress-activated protein kinase inhibitor reverses bradykinin B1 receptor-mediated component of inflammatory hyperalgesia. Eur J Pharmacol 421:191–199

Garret C, Carruette A, Fardin V, et al (1992) RP 67580, a potent and selective substance P non-peptide antagonist. C R Acad Sci III 314:199–204

Garry EM, Jones E, Fleetwood-Walker SM (2004) Nociception in vertebrates: key receptors participating in spinal mechanisms of chronic pain in animals. Brain Res Rev 46:216–224

Gebre-Medhin S, Mulder H, Zhang Y, et al (1998) Reduced nociceptive behaviour in islet amyloid polypeptide (amylin) knockout mice. Mol Brain Res 63:180–183

Goadsby PJ (1993) Inhibition of calcitonin gene related peptide by h-CGRP (8–37) antagonises the cerebral dilator response from nasociliary nerve stimulation in the cat. Neurosci Lett 151:13–16

Goldstein DJ, Wang O (1999) Lanepitant, an NK1 antagonist, in painful diabetic neuropathy. Clin Pharmacol Therap 65 (Abstr)

Goldstein DJ, Wang O, Saper JR, et al (1997) Ineffectiveness of neurokinin-1 antagonist in acute migraine: a crossover study. Cephalalgia 17:785–790

Goldstein DJ, Wang O, Todd TE (1998) Lanepitant in osteoarthritis pain. Clin Pharmacol Ther 63:168

Goldstein DJ, Offen WW, Klein EG (1999) Lanepitant, an NK1 antagonist, in migraine prophylaxis. Clin Pharmacol Ther 65:Abstr

Gonzalez MI, Field MJ, Hughes J, Singh L (2000) Evaluation of selective NK(1) receptor antagonist CI-1021 in animal models of inflammatory and neuropathic pain. J Pharmacol Exp Ther 294:444–450

Goto T, Tanaka T (2002) Tachykinins and tachykinin receptors in bone. Microsc Res Tech 58:91–97

Gougat J, Ferrari B, Sarran L, et al (2004) SSR240612 [(2R)-2-[((3R)-3-(1,3-benzodioxol-5-yl)-3-[(6-methoxy-2-naphthyl)sulfonyl]aminopropanoyl)amino]-3-(4-[2R,6S)-2,6-di methylpiperidinyl]methylphenyl)-N-isopropyl –N-methylpropanamide hydrochloride], a new nonpeptide antagonist of the bradykinin B1 receptor: biochemical and pharmacological characterization. J Pharmacol Exp Ther 309:661–669

Guzman F, Braun C, Lim RKS, et al (1964) Narcotic and non-narcotic analgesics which block visceral pain evoked by intra-arterial injection of bradykinin and other algesic agents. Arch Int Pharmacodyn Ther 149:571–588

Han JS, Li W, Neugebauer V (2005) Critical role of calcitonin gene related peptide 1 receptors in the amygdala in synaptic plasticity and pain behaviour. J Neurosci 25:10717–10728

Hanesch U, Pfrommer U, Grubb BD, Schaible HG (1993) Acute and chronic phases of unilateral inflammation in rat's ankle are associated with an increase in the proportion of calcitonin gene related peptide-immunoreactive dorsal root ganglion cells. Eur J Neurosci 5:154–161

Hargreaves R (2002) Imaging substance P receptors (NK1) in the living human brain using positron emission tomography. J Clin Psychiatry 63 Suppl:18–24

Hay DL, Conner AC, Howitt SG, et al (2004) The pharmacology of adrenomedullin receptors and their relationship to CGRP receptors. J Mol Neurosci 22:105–113

Hay DL, Poyner DR, Sexton PM (2006) GPCR modulation by RAMPs. Pharmacol Ther 109:173–197

Henry JL (1976) Effects of substance P on functionally identified units in cat spinal cord. Brain Res 114:439–451

Henry MA, Nouser-Goebl NA, Westrum LE (1993) Light and electron microscopic localization of calcitonin gene related peptide immunoreactivity in lamina II of the feline trigeminal pars caudalis/medullary dorsal horn. Synapse 13:99–107

Hershey JC, Corcoran HA, Baskin EP, et al (2005) Investigation of the species selectivity of a non-peptide CGRP receptor antagonist using a novel pharmacodynamic assay. Regul Pept 127:71–77

Hess JF, Ransom RW, Zeng Z, et al (2004) Generation and characterization of a human bradykinin receptor B1 transgenic rat as a pharmacodynamic model. J Pharmacol Exp Ther 10:488–497

Hill RG (2001) Molecular basis for the perception of pain. Neuroscientist 7:282–292

Hill RG, Rupniak NMJ (1999) Tachykinin receptors and the potential of tachykinin antagonists as clinically effective analgesics and anti-inflammatory agents. In: Brain SB, Moore PK (eds) Pain and neurogenic inflammation. Birkhauser, Basel, pp 313–333

Hingten CM, Roy SL, Clapp DW (2006) Stimulus-evoked release of neuropeptides is enhanced in sensory neurons from mice with a heterozygous mutation of the Nf1 gene. Neuroscience 137:637–645

Hokfelt T, Arvidsson U, Ceccatelli S, et al (1992) Calcitonin-gene related peptide in the brain, spinal cord and some peripheral systems. Ann NY Acad Sci 657:119–134

Hokfelt T, Broberger C, Xu ZQ, Sergeyev V, Ubink R, Diez M (2000) Neuropeptides—an overview. Neuropharmacology 39:1337–1356

Hokfelt T, Kuteeva E, Stanic D, Ljungdahl A (2004) The histochemistry of tachykinin systems in the brain. In: Holzer P (ed) Tachykinins (Handbook of experimental pharmacology, vol 164). Springer, Berlin, Heidelberg, New York, pp 64–120

Honore P, Mantyh P (2000) Bone cancer pain: from mechanism to model to therapy. Pain Med 1:303–309

Hunt SP, Mantyh PW (2001) The molecular dynamics of pain control. Nat Rev Neurosci 2:83–91

Hutchins B, Spears R, Hinton RJ, Harper RP (2000) Calcitonin gene related peptide and substance P immunoreactivity in rat trigeminal ganglia and brainstem following adjuvant-induced inflammation of the temporomandibular joint. Arch Oral Biol 45:335–345

Ichikawa H, Sugimoto T (2002) The co-expression of ASIC3 with calcitonin gene related peptide and parvalbumin in the rat trigeminal ganglion. Brain Res 943:287–291

Iyengar S, Hipskind PA, Gehlert DR, et al (1997) LY303870, a centrally active neurokinin-1 antagonist with a long duration of action. J Pharmacol Exp Ther 280:774–785

Jang JH, Nam TS, Paik KS, Leem JW (2004) Involvement of peripherally released substance P and calcitonin gene related peptide in mediating mechanical hyperalgesia in a traumatic neuropathy model of the rat. Neurosci Lett 360:129–132

Jones C, Phillips E, Davis C, et al (1999) Molecular characterisation of cloned bradykinin B1 receptors from rat and human. Eur J Pharmacol 374:423–433

Julius D, Basbaum A (2005) A neuropeptide courier for δ-opioid receptors? Cell 122:496–498

Julius D, Basbaum AI (2001) Molecular mechanisms of nociception. Nature 413:203–210

Juranek I, Lembeck F (1997) Afferent C-fibres release substance P and glutamate. Can J Physiol Pharmacol 75:661–664

Just S, Leipold-Buttner C, Heppelmann B (2001) Histological demonstration of voltage dependent calcium channels on calcitonin gene related peptide immunoreactive nerve fibres in the mouse knee joint. Neurosci Lett 312:133–136

Kang DS, Ryberg K, Morgelin M, Leeb-Lundberg LM (2004) Spontaneous formation of a proteolytic B1 and B2 bradykinin receptor complex with enhanced. signaling capacity. J Biol Chem 279:22102–22107

Kang DS, Gustafsson C, Mörgelin M, et al (2005) B1 bradykinin receptor homo-oligomers in receptor cell surface expression and signaling: effects of receptor fragments. Mol Pharmacol 67:309–318

Kayser V, Farre A, Hamon M, Bourgoin S (2003) Effects of the novel analgesic cizolirtine in a rat model of neuropathic pain. Pain 104:169–177

Kerezoudis NP, Olgart L, Edwall L (1994) CGRP(8–37) reduces the duration but not the maximal increase of antidromic vasodilation in dental pulp and lip of the rat. Acta Physiol Scand 151:73–81

King T, Gardell LR, Wang R, et al (2005) Role of NK-1 transmission in opioid-induced hyperalgesia. Pain 116:276–288

Kinloch RA, Cox PJ (2005) New targets for neuropathic pain therapeutics. Expert Opin Ther Targets 9:685–698

Kuraishi Y, Nanayama T, Ohno H, et al (1988) Antinociception induced in rats by intrathecal administration of antiserum against calcitonin gene related peptide. Neurosci Lett 92:325–329

Laird JM, Hargreaves RJ, Hill RG (1993) Effect of RP 67580, a non-peptide neurokinin1 receptor antagonist, on facilitation of a nociceptive spinal flexion reflex in the rat. Br J Pharmacol 109:713–718

Laird JM, Olivar T, Roza C, et al (2000) Deficits in visceral pain and hyperalgesia of mice with a disruption of the tachykinin NK1 receptor gene. Neuroscience 98:345–352

Laird JM, Roza C, De Felipe C, et al (2001) Role of central and peripheral tachykinin NK1 receptors in capsaicin-induced pain and hyperalgesia in mice. Pain 90:97–103

Lassen LH, Haderslev PA, Jacobsen VB, et al (2002) CGRP may play a causative role in migraine. Cephalalgia 22:54–61

Leah JD, Cameron AA, Snow PJ (1985) Neuropeptides in physiologically identified mammalian sensory neurons. Neurosci Lett 23:257–263

Leeb-Lundberg LM, Kang DS, Lamb ME, et al (2001) The human B1 bradykinin receptor exhibits high ligand-independent, constitutive activity. J Biol Chem 276:8785–8792

Levy D, Zochodne DW (2000) Increased mRNA expression of the B1 and B2 bradykinin receptors and antinociceptive effects of their antagonists in an animal model of neuropathic pain. Pain 86:265–271

Levy D, Burstein R, Strassman AM (2005) Calcitonin gene related peptide does not excite or sensitise meningeal nociceptors: implications for the pathophysiology of migraine. Ann Neurol 58:698–705

Levy MJ, Classey JD, Manreesri S, et al (2004) The association between calcitonin gene related peptide (CGRP), substance P and headache in pituitary tumours. Pituitary 7:67–71

Li JL, Ding YQ, Xiong KH, Li JS, et al (1998) Substance P receptor (NK1)-immunoreactive neurons projecting to the periaqueductal gray: distribution in the spinal trigeminal nucleus and the spinal cord of the rat. Neurosci Res 30:219–225

Limmroth V, Katsarava Z, Liedert B, et al (2001) An in vivo model to study calcitonin gene related peptide release following activation of the trigeminal vascular system. Pain 92:101–106

Littman B, Newton FA, Russell IJ (1999) Substance P antagonism in fibromyalgia: a trial with CJ-11,974. 9th World Congress of Pain, abstr 218, p 67

Liu HX, Hokfelt T (2002) The participation of galanin in pain processing at the spinal level. Trends Pharmacol Sci 23:468–474

Lofgren O, Yu LC, Theodorsson E, et al (1997) Intrathecal CGRP (8–37) results in a bilateral increase in the hindpaw withdrawal latency in rats with a unilateral thermal injury. Neuropeptides 31:601–607

Lopes P, Couture R (1997) Localization of bradykinin-like immunoreactivity in the rat spinal cord: effects of capsaicin, melittin, dorsal rhizotomy and peripheral axotomy. Neuroscience 78:481–497

Lu JT, Son YJ, Lee J, et al (1999) Mice lacking α-calcitonin gene related peptide exhibit normal cardiovascular regulation and neuromuscular development. Mol Cell Neurosci 14:99–120

Ma QP, Hill R, Sirinathsinghji D (2001) Colocalization of CGRP with 5-HT 1B/1D receptors and substance P in trigeminal ganglion neurons in rats. Eur J Neurosci 13:2099–2104

Ma W, Ramer MS, Bisby MA (1999) Increased calcitonin related peptide immunoreactivity in gracile nucleus after partial sciatic nerve injury: age dependent and originating from spared sensory neurons. Exp Neurol 159:459–473

Ma W, Chabot JG, Powell KJ, et al (2003) Localization and modulation of calcitonin gene related peptide receptor component protein immunoreactive cells in the rat central and peripheral nervous systems. Neuroscience 120:677–694

Mansikka H, Shiotani M, Winchurch R, et al (1999) Neurokinin-1 receptors are involved in behavioral responses to high-intensity heat stimuli and capsaicin-induced hyperalgesia in mice. Anesthesiology 90:1643–1649

Mansikka H, Sheth RN, DeVries C, Lee H, Winchurch R, Raja SN (2000) Nerve injury-induced mechanical but not thermal hyperalgesia is attenuated in neurokinin-1 receptor knockout mice. Exp Neurol 162:343–349

Mantyh PW, Hunt SP (1985) The autoradiographic localization of substance P receptors in the rat and bovine spinal cord and the rat and cat spinal trigeminal nucleus pars caudalis and the effects of neonatal capsaicin. Brain Res 332:315–324

Mantyh PW, DeMaster E, Malhotra A, et al (1995) Receptor endocytosis and dendrite reshaping in spinal neurons after somatosensory stimulation. Science 268:1629–1632

Mantyh PW, Rogers SD, Honore P, et al (1997) Inhibition of hyperalgesia by ablation of lamina I spinal neurons expressing the substance P receptor. Science 278:275–279

Marceau F, Regoli D (2004) Bradykinin receptor ligands: therapeutic perspectives. Nat Rev Drug Discov 3:845–852

Marceau F, Hess JF, Bachvarov DR (1998) The B1 receptor for kinins. Pharmacol Rev 50:358–382

Martinez-Caro L, Laird JM (2000) Allodynia and hyperalgesia evoked by sciatic mononeuropathy in NK1 receptor knockout mice. Neuroreport 11:1213–1217

Mason GS, Cumberbatch MJ, Hill RG, et al (2002) The bradykinin B1 receptor antagonist B9858 inhibits a nociceptive spinal reflex in rabbits. Can J Physiol Pharmacol 80:264–268

Matthew IR, Ogden GR, Frame JW, Wight AJ (2000) Dose response and safety of cizolirtine citrate (E-4018) in patients with pain following extraction of third molars. Curr Med Res Opin 16:107–114

Max MB, Schafer SC, Culnane M, et al (1988) Association of pain relief with drug side-effects in postherpetic neuralgia: a single-dose study clonidine, codeine, ibuprofen and placebo. Clin Pharmacol Ther 43:363–371

Mazzuferi M, Binaschi A, Rodi D, et al (2005) Induction of B1 bradykinin receptors in the kindled hippocampus increases extracellular glutamate levels: a microdialysis study. Neuroscience 135:979–986

McLean PG, Perretti M, Ahluwalia A (2000) Kinin B1 receptors and the cardiovascular system: regulation of expression and function. Cardiovasc Res 48:194–210

McLean S, Ganong AH, Seeger TF, et al (1991) Activity and distribution of binding sites in brain of a nonpeptide substance P (NK1) receptor antagonist. Science 251:437–439

Mogil JS, Miermeister F, Seifert F, et al (2005) Variable sensitivity to noxious heat is mediated by differential expression of the CGRP gene. Proc Natl Acad Sci U S A 102:12938–12943

Molander C, Ygge J, Dalsgaard CJ (1987) Substance P-, somatostatin- and calcitonin gene-related peptide-like immunoreactivity and fluoride resistant acid phosphatase-activity in relation to retrogradely labeled cutaneous, muscular and visceral primary sensory neurons in the rat. Neurosci Lett 74:37–42

Moreno MJ, Abounader R, Hebert E, et al (2002) Efficacy of the non-peptide CGRP receptor antagonist BIBN4096BS in blocking CGRP-induced dilations in human and bovine cerebral arteries: potential implications in acute migraine treatment. Neuropharmacology 42:568–576

Morissette G, Fortin JP, Otis S, et al (2004) A novel nonpeptide antagonist of the kinin B1 receptor: effects on the rabbit receptor. J Pharmacol Exp Ther 311:1121–1130

Morris R, Cheunsuang O, Stewart A, Maxwell D (2004) Spinal dorsal horn neurone targets for nociceptive primary afferents: do single neurone morphological characteristics suggest how nociceptive information is processed at the spinal level. Brain Res Brain Res Rev 46:173–190

Muff R, Born W, Lutz TA, Fischer JA (2004) Biological importance of the peptides of the calcitonin family as revealed by disruption and transfer of corresponding genes. Peptides 25:2027–2038

Nagy JI, Hunt SP, Iversen LL, et al (1981) Biochemical and anatomical observations on the degeneration of peptide-containing primary afferent neurons after neonatal capsaicin. Neuroscience 6:1923–1934

Natsugari H, Ikeura Y, Kiyota Y, et al (1995) Novel, potent, and orally active substance P antagonists: synthesis and antagonist activity of N-benzylcarboxamide derivatives of pyrido[3,4-b]pyridine. J Med Chem 38:3106–3120

Navari RM, Reinhardt RR, Gralla RJ, et al (1999) Reduction of cisplatin-induced emesis by a selective neurokinin-1-receptor antagonist. L-754,030 Antiemetic Trials Group. N Engl J Med 340:190–195

Nawa H, Kotani H, Nakanishi S (1984) Tissue-specific generation of two preprotachykinin mRNAs from one gene by alternative RNA splicing. Nature 312:729–734

Neckers LM, Schwartz JP, Wyatt RJ, et al (1979) Substance P afferents from the habenula innervate the dorsal raphe nucleus. Exp Brain Res 37:619–623

Neugebauer V, Rumenapp P, Schaible HG (1996) Calcitonin gene related peptide is involved in the spinal processing of mechanosensory input from the rat's knee joint and in the generation and maintenance of hyperexcitability of dorsal horn neurons during development of acute inflammation. Neuroscience 71:1095–1109

Nohr D, Schafer MKH, Persson S, et al (1999) Calcitonin gene related peptide gene expression in collagen-induced arthritis is differentially regulated in primary afferents and motoneurons: influence of glucocorticoids. Neuroscience 93:759–773

Norman B, Panebianco D, Block GA (1998) A controlled, in clinic study to explore the preliminary safety and efficacy of intravenous L-758,298 (a prodrug of the NK1 receptor antagonist L-754,030) in the acute treatment of migraine [abstract]. Cephalalgia 18:407

Oh-hashi Y, Shindo T, Kurihara Y, et al (2001) Elevated sympathetic nervous activity in mice deficient in α-CGRP. Circ Res 89:983–990

Okano S, Ikeura Y, Inatomi N (2002) Effects of tachykinin NK1 receptor antagonists on the viscerosensory response caused by colorectal distention in rabbits. J Pharmacol Exp Ther 300:925–931

Okayama Y, Ono Y, Nakazawa T, et al (1998) Human skin mast cells produce TNF-alpha by substance P. Int Arch Allergy Immunol 117 Suppl 1:48

Olesen J, Diener HC, Husstedt IW, et al (2004) Calcitonin gene related peptide receptor antagonist BIBN4096BS for the acute treatment of migraine. N Engl J Med 350:1104–1110

Oliver KR, Sirinathsinghji DJ, Hill RG (2000) From basic research on neuropeptide receptors to clinical benefit. Drug News Perspect 13:530–542

Oliver KR, Kane SA, Salvatore CA, et al (2001) Cloning, characterization and central nervous system distribution of rat receptor activity modifying proteins. Eur J Neurosci 14:618–628

Oliver KR, Wainright A, Edvinsson L, Pickard JD, Hill RG (2002) Immunochemical localization of calcitonin-like receptor and receptor activity-modifying proteins in the human cerebral vasculature. J Cereb Blood Flow Metab 22:620–629

Opree A, Kress M (2000) Involvement of the proinflammatory cytokines tumor necrosis factor α, IL-1β and IL-6 but not IL-8 in the development of heat hyperalgesia: effects on heat-evoked calcitonin gene-related peptide release from rat skin. J Neurosci 20:6289–6293

Patel S, Gentry CT, Campbell EA (1996) A model for in vivo evaluation of tachykinin NK1 receptor antagonists using carrageenan-induced hyperalgesia in the guinea pig paw. Br J Pharmacol 117:248P

Patte-Mensah C, Kibaly C, Mensah-Nyagan AG (2005) Substance P inhibits progesterone conversion to neuroactive metabolites in spinal sensory circuit: a potential component of nociception. Proc Natl Acad Sci U S A 102:9044–9049

Patwardhan AM, Berg KA, Akopain AN, et al (2005) Bradykinin-induced functional competence and trafficking of the δ-opioid receptor in trigeminal nociceptors. J Neurosci 25:8825–8832

Pavlik I, Suchy J, Pac D, et al (2004) Comparison of cizolirtine citrate and metamizol sodium in the treatment of adult acute renal colic: a randomized double blind clinical pilot study. Clin Ther 26:1061–1072

Pesquero JB, Araujo RC, Heppenstall PA, et al (2000) Hypoalgesia and altered inflammatory responses in mice lacking kinin B1 receptors. Proc Natl Acad Sci U S A 97:8140–8145

Petersen KA, Lassen LH, Birk S, et al (2005) BIBN4096BS antagonizes human α-calcitonin gene related peptide-induced headache and extracerebral artery dilatation. Clin Pharmacol Ther 77:202–213

Phebus LA, Johnson KW, Stengel PW, et al (1997) The non-peptide NK-1 receptor antagonist LY303870 inhibits neurogenic dural inflammation in guinea pigs. Life Sci 60:1553–1561

Piper RD, Edvinsson L, Ekman R, Lambert GA (1993) Cortical spreading depression does not result in the release of calcitonin gene related peptide into the external jugular vein of the cat: relevance to human migraine. Cephalalgia 13:180–183

Poyner DR, Sexton PM, Marshall I, et al (2002) International Union of Pharmacology. XXXII. The mammalian calcitonin gene related peptide, adrenomedullin, amylin and calcitonin receptors. Pharmacol Rev 54:233–246

Radhakrishnan V, Henry JL (1991) Novel substance P antagonist, CP-96,345, blocks responses of cat spinal dorsal horn neurons to noxious cutaneous stimulation and to substance P. Neurosci Lett 132:39–43

Radhakrishnan V, Iyengar S, Henry JL (1998) The nonpeptide NK-1 receptor antagonists LY303870 and LY306740 block the responses of spinal dorsal horn neurons to substance P and to peripheral noxious stimuli. Neuroscience 83:1251–1260

Raidoo DM, Bhoola KD (1997) Kinin receptors on human neurons. J Neuroimmunol 77:39–44

Ransom RW, Harrell CM, Reiss D, et al (2004) Pharmacological characterization and radioligand binding properties of a high-affinity, nonpeptide, bradykinin B1 receptor antagonist. Eur J Pharmacol 499:77–84

Rashid MH, Inoue M, Matsumoto M, et al (2004) Switching of bradykinin-mediated nociception following partial sciatic nerve injury in mice. J Pharmacol Exp Ther 308:1158–1164

Reinhardt RR, Laub JB, Fricke JR, et al (1998) Comparison of the neurokinin-1 antagonist, L-754,030, to placebo, acetaminophen and ibuprofen in the dental pain model. Clin Pharmacol Ther 63:168

Ren K, Novikova SI, He F, et al (2005) Neonatal local noxious insult affects gene expression in the spinal dorsal horn of adult rats. Mol Pain 1:27

Richie TJ, Dziadulewicz EK, Culshaw AJ, et al (2004) Potent and orally bioavailable nonpeptide antagonists at the human bradykinin B1 receptor based on a 2-alkylamino-5-sulfamoylbenzamide core. J Med Chem 47:4642–4644

Riediger T, Schmid HA, Young AA, Simon E (1999) Pharmacological characterization of amylin-related peptides activating subfornical organ neurons. Brain Res 837:161–168

Rosenfeld MG, Emeson RB, Yeakley JM, et al (1992) Calcitonin gene related peptide: a peptide generated as a consequence of tissue-specific developmentally regulated alternative RNA processing events. Ann N Y Acad Sci 657:1–17

Rudolf K, Eberlein W, Engel W, et al (2005) Development of human calcitonin gene related peptide (CGRP) receptor antagonists .1. potent and selective small molecule CGRP antagonists. 1-[N2[3,5 dibromo-N-[[4-(3,4-dihydro-2)1H)-oxoquinazolin-3yl)-1-piperidinyl]carbonyl]-D-tyrosyl]-L-lysyl]-4-(4-pyridinyl)piperazine: the first CGRP antagonist for clinical trials in acute migraine. J Med Chem 48:5921–5931

Rupniak NM, Boyce S, Williams AR, et al (1993) Antinociceptive activity of NK1 receptor antagonists: non-specific effects of racemic RP67580. Br J Pharmacol 110:1607–1613

Rupniak NM, Carlson E, Boyce S, et al (1996) Enantioselective inhibition of the formalin paw late phase by the NK1 receptor antagonist L-733,060 in gerbils. Pain 67:189–195

Rupniak NM, Tattersall FD, Williams AR, et al (1997a) In vitro and in vivo predictors of the anti-emetic activity of tachykinin NK1 receptor antagonists. Eur J Pharmacol 326:201–209

Rupniak NMJ, Boyce S, Webb JK, et al (1997b) Effects of the bradykinin B1 receptor antagonist des-Arg^9[Leu^8] bradykinin and genetic disruption of the B2 receptor on nociception in rats and mice. Pain 7:89–97

Rupniak NMJ, Longmore J, Hill RG (2000) Role of bradykinin B1 and B2 receptors in nociception and inflammation. In: Wood JN (ed) Molecular basis of pain induction. Wiley-Liss, Toronto, pp 149–173

Russell IJ, Orr MD, Littman B, et al (1994) Elevated cerebrospinal fluid levels of substance P in patients with the fibromyalgia syndrome. Arthritis Rheum 37:1593–1601

Sabino MA, Honore P, Rogers SD, et al (2002) Tooth extraction-induced internalization of the substance P receptor in trigeminal nucleus and spinal cord neurons: imaging the neurochemistry of dental pain. Pain 95:175–186

Sakai K, Matsuno H, Tsuji H, et al (1998) Substance P receptor (NK1) gene expression in synovial tissue in rheumatoid arthritis and osteoarthritis. Scand J Rheumatol 27:135–141

Salt TE, Hill RG (1983) Neurotransmitter candidates of somatosensory primary afferent fibres. Neuroscience 4:1083–1103

Samsam M, Covenas R, Ahangari R, et al (2000) Simultaneous depletion on neurokinin A, substance P and calcitonin gene related peptide from the caudal trigeminal nucleus of the rat during electrical stimulation of the trigeminal ganglion. Pain 84:389–395

Schubert TEO, Weidler C, Lerch K, et al (2005) Achilles tendinosis is associated with sprouting of substance P positive nerve fibres. Ann Rheum Dis 64:1083–1086

Schutz B, Mauer D, Salmon AM, et al (2004) Analysis of the cellular expression pattern of β-CGRP in α-CGRP deficient mice. J Comp Neurol 476:32–43

Schwei MJ, Honore P, Rodgers SD, et al (1999) Neurochemical and cellular reorganization of the spinal cord in a murine model of bone cancer pain. J Neurosci 19:10886–10897

Seabrook GR, Bowery BJ, Heavens R, et al (1997) Expression of B1 and B2 bradykinin receptor mRNA and their functional roles in sympathetic ganglia and sensory dorsal root ganglia neurons from wild-type and B2 receptor knockout mice. Neuropharmacology 36:1009–1017

Seguin L, Millan MJ (1994) The glycine B receptor partial agonist (+)-HA966, enhances induction of antinociception by RP 67580 and CP-99,994. Eur J Pharmacol 253:R1–3

Sergeyev V, Hokfelt T, Hurd Y (1999) Serotonin and substance P co-exist in dorsal raphe neurons of the human brain. Neuroreport 10:3967–3970

Seybold VS, McCarson KE, Mermelstein PG, et al (2003) Calcitonin gene related peptide regulates expression of neurokinin 1 receptors by rat spinal neurons. J Neurosci 23: 1816–1824

Shembalkar P, Taubel J, Abadias M, et al (2001) Cizolirtine citrate (E-4018) in the treatment of chronic neuropathic pain. Curr Med Res Opin 17:262–266

Shepheard SL, Williamson DJ, Hill RG, et al (1993) The non-peptide neurokinin1 receptor antagonist, RP 67580, blocks neurogenic plasma extravasation in the dura mater of rats. Br J Pharmacol 108:11–12

Shepheard SL, Williamson DJ, Williams J, et al (1995) Comparison of the effects of suma-triptan and the NK1 antagonist CP-99,994 on plasma extravasation in Dura mater and c-fos mRNA expression in trigeminal nucleus caudalis of rats. Neuropharmacology 34:255–261

Sibilia V, Pagani F, Lattuada N, et al (2000) Amylin compared with calcitonin: competitive binding studies in rat brain and antinociceptive activity. Brain Res 854:79–84

Simpson PB, Woollacott AJ, Hill RG, et al (2000) Functional characterization of bradykinin analogues on recombinant human bradykinin B1 and B2 receptors. Eur J Pharmacol 392:1–9

Smith D, Hill RG, Edvinsson L, Longmore J (2002) An immunohistochemical investigation of human trigeminal nucleus caudalis: CGRP, substance P and 5-HT1D receptor immunoreactivities are expressed by trigeminal sensory fibres. Cephalalgia 22:424–431

Su DS, Markowitz MK, DiPardo RM, et al (2003) Discovery of a potent, non-peptide bradykinin B1 receptor antagonist. J Am Chem Soc 125:7516–7517

Sun RQ, Tu YJ, Lawand NB, et al (2004) Calcitonin gene related peptide receptor activation produces PKA- and PKC-dependent mechanical hyperalgesia and central sensitization. J Neurophysiol 92:2859–2866

Tachibana T, Noguchi K, Ruda MA (2002) Analysis of gene expression following spinal cord injury in rat using complementary DNA microarray. Neurosci Lett 327:133–137

Tajti J, Uddman R, Edvinsson L (2001) Neuropeptide localization in the 'migraine generator' region of the human brainstem. Cephalalgia 21:96–101

Tan KK, Brown MJ, Hargreaves RJ, et al (1995) Calcitonin gene related peptide as an endogenous vasodilator: immunoblockade studies in vivo with an anti-calcitonin gene related peptide monoclonal antibody and its Fab' fragment. Clin Sci 89:565–573

Tan KKC, Brown MJ, Longmore J, et al (1994) Demonstration of the neurotransmitter role of calcitonin gene related peptide (CGRP) by immuno-blockade with anti-CGRP monoclonal antibodies. Br J Pharmacol 111:703–710

Tanaka S, Barron KW, Chandler MJ, et al (2001) Low intensity spinal cord stimulation may induce cutaneous vasodilation via CGRP release. Brain Res 896:183–187

Troger J, Humpel C, Kremser B, et al (1999) The effects of streptozotocin-induced diabetes mellitus on substance P and calcitonin gene related peptide expression in the rat trigeminal ganglion. Brain Res 842:84–91

Urban L, Gentry C, Patel S, et al (1999) Selective NK1 receptor antagonists block neuropathic and inflammatory pain in the guinea pig. 9th World Congress on Pain (abstr 125), p 40

Urban LA, Fox AJ (2000) NK1 receptor antagonists—are they really without effect in the pain clinic? Trends Pharmacol Sci 21:462–464

Van Rossum D, Hanisch UK, Quirion R (1997) Neuroanatomical localization, pharmacological characterization and functions of CGRP, related peptides and their receptors. Neurosci Biobehav Rev 21:649–678

Vellani V, Zachrisson O, McNaughton PA (2004) Functional bradykinin B1 receptors are expressed in nociceptive neurones and are upregulated by the neurotrophin GDNF. J Physiol 560:391–401

Wacnik PW, Baker CM, Herron MJ, et al (2005) Tumor-induced mechanical hyperalgesia involves CGRP receptors and altered innervation and vascularization of DsRed2 fluorescent hindpaw tumors. Pain 115:95–106

Wang H, Kohno T, Amaya F, et al (2005) Bradykinin produces pain hypersensitivity by potentiating spinal cord glutamatergic synaptic transmission. J Neurosci 25:7986–7992

White FA, Bhangoo SK, Miller RJ (2005) Chemokines: integrators of pain and inflammation. Nat Rev Drug Discov 4:834–844

Williamson DJ, Hargreaves RJ (2001) Neurogenic inflammation in the context of migraine. Microsc Res Tech 53:167–178

Williamson DJ, Shepheard SL, Hill RG, et al (1997) The novel anti-migraine agent rizatriptan inhibits neurogenic dural vasodilation and extravasation. Eur J Pharmacol 328:61–64

Williamson DJ, Hargreaves RJ, Hill RG, Shepheard SL (1997a) Intravital microscope studies on the effects of neurokinin agonists and calcitonin gene related peptide on dural vessel diameter in the anesthetized rat. Cephalalgia 17:518–524

Williamson DJ, Hargreaves RJ, Hill RG, Shepheard SL (1997b) Sumatriptan inhibits neurogenic vasodilation of dural blood vessels in the anaesthetized rat—intravital microscope studies. Cephalalgia 17:525–531

Wood MR, Kim JJ, Han W, et al (2003) Benzodiazepines as potent and selective bradykinin B1 antagonists. J Med Chem 46:1803–1806

Xu P, Van Slambrouck C, Berti-Mattera L, Hall AK (2005) Activin induces tactile allodynia and increases calcitonin gene related peptide after peripheral inflammation. J Neurosci 25:9227–9235

Yamamoto T, Yaksh TL (1991) Stereospecific effects of a nonpeptidic NK1 selective antagonist, CP-96,345: antinociception in the absence of motor dysfunction. Life Sci 49: 1955–1963

Yasuda T, Iwamoto T, Ohara M, et al (1999) The novel analgesic compound OT-7100 (5-n-butyl-7-(3,4,5-trimethoxybenzoylamino)pyrazolo[1,5-a]pyrimidine) attenuates mechanical nociceptive responses in animal models of acute and peripheral neuropathic hyperalgesia. Jpn J Pharmacol 79:65–73

Ye Z, Wimalaswansa SJ, Westlund KN (1999) Receptor for calcitonin gene related peptide: localization in the dorsal and ventral spinal cord. Neuroscience 92:1389–1397

Yu LC, Weng XH, Wang JW, Lundeberg T (2003) Involvement of calcitonin gene related peptide and its receptor in anti-nociception in the periaqueductal grey of rats. Neurosci Lett 349:1–4

HEP (2006) 177:217–249

Glutamate Receptor Ligands

V. Neugebauer

Department of Neuroscience and Cell Biology, The University of Texas Medical Branch,
301 University Blvd., Galveston TX, 77555-1069, USA
voneugeb@utmb.edu

1	**Glutamate Receptors**	218
1.1	Ionotropic Glutamate Receptors	218
1.1.1	NMDA Receptors	219
1.1.2	Non-NMDA Receptors	221
1.2	Metabotropic Glutamate Receptors	222
2	**Glutamatergic Nociceptive Transmission in the Peripheral and Central Nervous System**	224
2.1	Ionotropic Glutamate Receptors	224
2.1.1	Periphery	224
2.1.2	Spinal Cord	225
2.1.3	Brain	226
2.2	Metabotropic Glutamate Receptors	227
2.2.1	Periphery	227
2.2.2	Spinal Cord	228
2.2.3	Brain	229
3	**Preclinical Studies**	230
3.1	Ionotropic Glutamate Receptors	231
3.1.1	Periphery	231
3.1.2	Spinal Cord	231
3.1.3	Brain	232
3.2	Metabotropic Glutamate Receptors	234
3.2.1	Periphery	234
3.2.2	Spinal Cord	235
3.2.3	Brain	236
4	**Clinical Studies**	237
4.1	NMDA Receptor Antagonists	237
4.1.1	Ketamine	238
4.1.2	Memantine	238
4.1.3	Dextromethorphan	239
4.1.4	NR2B-Selective Antagonists	240
4.1.5	GlycineB Site Antagonists	240
4.1.6	Side Effects	240
4.2	Non-NMDA Receptor Antagonists	241
4.2.1	LY293558	241
4.2.2	Side Effects	242
5	**Conclusions**	242
	References	243

Abstract Glutamate acts through a variety of receptors to modulate neurotransmission and neuronal excitability. Glutamate plays a critical role in neuroplasticity as well as in nervous system dysfunctions and disorders. Hyperfunction or dysfunction of glutamatergic neuro-transmission also represents a key mechanism of pain-related plastic changes in the central and peripheral nervous system. This chapter will review the classification of glutamate receptors and their role in peripheral and central nociceptive processing. Evidence from preclinical pain models and clinical studies for the therapeutic value of certain glutamate receptor ligands will be discussed.

Keywords Ionotropic glutamate receptors · NMDA and non-NMDA receptor antagonists · Metabotropic glutamate receptors · Neurotransmission · Nociception · Plasticity · Analgesia · Preclinical · Clinical

1
Glutamate Receptors

Glutamate is the major excitatory amino acid in the mammalian nervous system. A highly flexible molecule, glutamate binds to a number of diverse families of receptors and transporters. These include the ionotropic glutamate receptors (iGluRs), which are ligand-gated ion channels, and the metabotropic glutamate receptors (mGluRs), which couple through different G proteins to a variety of signal transduction pathways. Vesicular transporters (vGluT1 and 2) package glutamate into vesicles for synaptic exocytosis whereas plasma membrane glutamate transporters (excitatory amino acid transporters EAAT1–5) remove glutamate from the synaptic space. Glutamate receptor classification, structure, and function have been reviewed. This chapter will focus on the role of iGluRs and mGluRs in nociception and pain (for reviews of glutamate receptor classification, structure, and function see Michaelis 1998; Anwyl 1999; Dingledine et al. 1999; Schoepp et al. 1999; Lerma et al. 2001; Wollmuth and Sobolevsky 2004; Mayer and Armstrong 2004; Swanson et al. 2005; Mayer 2005).

1.1
Ionotropic Glutamate Receptors

The iGluRs allow the flow of cations through the channel in the center of the receptor complex upon binding of an extracellular ligand (glutamate). Typically, this results in the depolarization of the plasma membrane and the generation of an electrical signal, the action potential, that propagates along the axon and triggers the release of transmitter(s) from the synaptic terminal. The iGluRs are tetrameric complexes of subunits transcribed from separate genes (Michaelis 1998; Dingledine et al. 1999; Wollmuth and Sobolevsky 2004; Mayer and Armstrong 2004; Mayer 2005). Each subunit has four hydrophobic domains but only three transmembrane segments because the second domain forms a pore loop at the inner opening of the ion channel and does not go through the membrane. Thus, different from other ionotropic receptors, iGluRs have an extracellular N-terminal and an intracellular C-terminal domain. The C-terminus contains sites for phosphorylation and protein–protein interaction and is subject to posttranscriptional processes such as RNA editing and alternative splicing. Phosphorylation of iGluRs by various kinases (including PKA, PKC, CaM kinase II, tyrosine kinase) can increase the ion channel function. Interaction with intracellular scaffolding and cytoskeletal proteins may be important for receptor trafficking, anchoring, and signaling.

The iGluRs are subdivided into three major groups based on their pharmacology, structural similarities, and sequence homology (Table 1; Michaelis 1998; Dingledine et al. 1999; Lerma et al. 2001; Wollmuth and Sobolevsky 2004; Mayer and Armstrong 2004; Mayer 2005). Each group includes different subunits that are encoded by different genes: N-methyl-D-aspartate (NMDA) receptors (NR1, NR2A-D, NR3A, and NR3B subunits); α-amino-3-hydroxy-5-methyl-4-isoxazolepropionic acid (AMPA) receptors (GluR1–4); and kainate receptors (GluR5–7, KA1 and KA2). Two orphan receptor subtypes (δ1 and δ2) also have been cloned, which share sequence homology with other iGluRs, but their ligand-binding and functional properties remain to be determined. AMPA and kainate receptors are also referred to as non-NMDA receptors.

1.1.1
NMDA Receptors

Functional NMDA receptors are obligate heteromeric assemblies of NR1 subunits with NR2A-D or, less commonly, with NR3A,B subunits (Michaelis 1998; Dingledine et al. 1999; Wollmuth and Sobolevsky 2004; Mayer and Armstrong 2004; Mayer 2005). NMDA receptors have binding sites for glutamate (formed by the NR2 subunits) and the co-agonist glycine (strychnine-insensitive glycineB site formed by NR1) as well as binding sites for polyamines (NR2B) and phencyclidine (PCP site inside the ion channel), which can modulate NMDA receptor function. Ion currents through NR2B-containing NMDA receptor heteromers have a much slower decay time (i.e., longer duration) compared to NR2A-containing receptors. NMDA receptors are unique in that occupation of the glycine binding site and removal of the Mg^{2+} blockade of the ion channel are required for full activation. Furthermore, NMDA receptors are tonically inhibited by protons, and Zn^{2+} (NR2A>NR2B) enhances whereas polyamines (NR2B) relieve proton inhibition. Compared to non-NMDA receptors, NMDA receptors respond more slowly to glutamate due to the tonic and voltage-dependent inhibition by Mg^{2+}; they participate in slow synaptic transmission, desensitize only weakly, and have a high permeability to Ca^{2+} (tenfold greater than to Na^+).

NMDA is the diagnostic ligand for these receptors. D-AP5 (D-2-amino-5-phosphonopentanoic acid) is the most commonly used competitive antagonist at the glutamate binding site. Noncompetitive antagonists that bind to the PCP site in the NMDA receptor channel include the high-affinity compound MK-801 (dizocilpine; 10,11-dihydro-5-methyldibenzocyclohepten-5,10-imine) and

Table 1 Glutamate receptor classification

Group	Ionotropic			Metabotropic		
	NMDA	AMPA	Kainate	Group I	Group II	Group III
Subtype	NR1 NR2A, B,C,D NR3A,B	GluR1–4	GluR5–7 KA1, KA2	mGluR1,5	mGluR2,3	mGluR4,6–8
Agonist	NMDA	AMPA	Kainate	DHPG (1,5) CHPG (5)	LY354740* LY379268 APDC	LAP4 LSOP
Antagonist	AP5 DXM* Ketamine* Memantine* Ifenprodil (2B) *+ CP-101606 (2B) * Ro 25–6981 (2B)	GYKI53655	UBP302 LY382884 (5) NBQX LY293558*	CPCCOEt (1) LY367385 (1) MPEP (5)	EGLU LY341495	UBP1112
Effector	Ion-channel Na$^+$ K$^+$ Ca^{2+}	Ion-channel Na$^+$ K$^+$ (Ca^{2+})	Ion-channel Na$^+$ K$^+$ (Ca^{2+})	G$_q$-protein PLC ↑ ERK ↑ (AC ↑)	G$_{i/o}$-protein AC ↓ GIRK ↑ VGCC ↓	G$_{i/o}$-protein AC ↓ GIRK ↑ VGCC ↓

AC, adenylyl cyclase; AMPA, α-amino-3-hydroxy-5-methyl-4-isoxazolepropionic acid; AP5, D-2-amino-5-phosphonopentanoic acid; APDC, (2R,4R)-4-aminopyrrolidine-2,4-dicarboxylate; CHPG, (RS)-2-chloro-5-hydroxyphenylglycine; CNQX, cyano-7-nitroquinoxaline-2,3-dione; CP-101606 (traxoprodil; (1S,2S)-1-(4-hydroxyphenyl)-2-(4-hydroxy-4-phenylpiperidino)-1-propanol); CPCCOEt, 7-(hydroxy-imino) cyclopropa[b]chromen-1a-carboxylate ethyl ester; DHPG, (S)-3,5-dihydroxyphenylglycine; DXM, dextromethorphan; EGLU, (2S)-alpha-ethylglutamic acid; GIRK, G protein-activated inwardly rectifying potassium channels; LAP4, L-(+)-2-amino-4-phosphonobutyric acid; LSOP, L-serine-O-phosphate; LY293558, (3S,4aR,6R, 8aR)-6-[2-(1(2)H-tetrazole-5-yl)ethyl] decahydroisoquinoline-3-carboxylic acid; LY341495, 2S-2-amino-2-(1S,2S-2-carboxycyclopropyl-1-yl)-3-(xanth-9-yl)propanoic acid; LY354740, [1S, 2S,5R,6S]-2-aminobicyclo[3.1.0] hexane-2,6-dicarboxylic acid; LY367385, (S)-(+)-α-amino-4-carboxy-2-methylbenzeneacetic acid; LY379268, (−)-2-oxa-4-aminobicylco hexane-4,6-dicarboxylic acid; LY382884, (3S, 4aR, 6S, 8aR)-6-(4-carboxyphenyl)methyl-1,2,3,4,4a,5,6,7,8,8a-decahydroisoquinoline-3-carboxylic acid; MPEP, 2-methyl-6-(phenylethynyl)pyridine; NBQX, 2,3-dioxo-6-nitro-1,2,3,4-tetrahydrobenzo[f]quinoxaline-7-sulphonamide; NMDA, N-methyl-D-aspartic acid; Ro 25–6981, (R-R*,S*)-alpha-(4-hydroxyphenyl)-β-methyl-4-(phenylmethyl)-1-piperidine propanol; UBP1112, α-methyl-3-methyl-4-phosphonophenylglycine; UBP302, (S)-1-(2-amino-2-carboxyethyl)-3-(2-carboxybenzyl)pyrimidine-2,4-dione; VGCC, voltage-gated calcium channel
Numbers in parentheses refer to receptor subtype/subunit selectivity *Denotes drugs tested/used clinically +Also binds to other classes of receptors (α1, 5HT1α, and σ)

clinically used agents such as ketamine, memantine, and dextromethorphan with its main metabolite dextrorphan. Noncompetitive antagonists selective for NR2B subunit-containing NMDA receptors include CP-101606 [traxoprodil; (1S,2S)-1-(4-hydroxyphenyl)-2-(4-hydroxy-4-phenylpiperidino)-1-propanol) and Ro 25–6981 (R-R*,S*)-α-(4-hydroxyphenyl)-β-methyl-4-(phenylmethyl)-1-piperidine propanol] and their parent compound ifenprodil, which also binds to other receptors besides glutamate receptors (Table 1; Michaelis 1998; Dingledine et al. 1999; Parsons 2001; Wollmuth and Sobolevsky 2004; Mayer 2005).

1.1.2
Non-NMDA Receptors

AMPA and kainate receptors can be homo- or heteromeric tetramers. AMPA receptors (Michaelis 1998; Dingledine et al. 1999; Wollmuth and Sobolevsky 2004; Mayer 2005) are composed of subunits GluR1–4, which are encoded by separate genes. All AMPA receptor subunits exist as two splice variants, *flip* and *flop*, which yield altered kinetics such that the flop forms show more rapid desensitization. Each subunit has a ligand binding site made up from the N-terminal region; the C-terminus plays a role in receptor trafficking. Different from NMDA receptors, native AMPA receptors mediate fast synaptic transmission, have fast gating kinetics, desensitize rapidly, and show a lower permeability to Ca^{2+}. Ca^{2+} permeability of AMPA receptors is determined by the GluR2 subunit, which in its native form is impermeable to Ca^{2+} due to posttranscriptional RNA editing that changes a single amino acid in the pore-forming second membrane domain from glutamine (Q) to arginine (R). Most neurons express GluR2 in combination with one or more of the GluR1, 3, and 4 subunits, yielding AMPA receptors with low Ca^{2+} permeability.

Kainate receptors (Michaelis 1998; Dingledine et al. 1999; Chittajallu et al. 1999; Lerma 2003; Wollmuth and Sobolevsky 2004; Mayer 2005) are tetrameric assemblies of low-affinity GluR5–7 subunits and high-affinity KA1 and 2 subunits. Homomeric expression of KA1 and KA2 does not form functional ion channels, but KA1 and KA2 contribute to heteromeric receptor complexes when expressed with the other subunits. GluR5–7 can form homomeric and heteromeric kainate receptors. Like the other iGluRs, kainate receptor subunits undergo alternate splicing and RNA editing, yielding a number of pharmacologically and functionally distinct receptors. Similar to AMPA receptors, kainate receptors with Q to R editing in the GluR5 or GluR6 subunits are impermeable to Ca^{2+}; receptors with unedited subunits are calcium permeable. Interestingly, some actions of kainate may involve the interaction of ionotropic kainate receptors with a G protein. Kainate receptors contribute to postsynaptic excitatory responses and plasticity; presynaptic kainate receptors can increase or decrease the release of glutamate and inhibit the release of the inhibitory transmitter γ-aminobutyric acid (GABA) (resulting in disinhibition).

The pharmacological differentiation of AMPA and kainate receptors has been difficult (see Table 1; Michaelis 1998; Dingledine et al. 1999; Chittajallu et al. 1999; Wollmuth and Sobolevsky 2004). Naturally, AMPA and kainate show some selectivity for AMPA- and kainate-preferring receptors, respectively. ATPA [(RS)-2-amino-3-(3-hydroxy-5-tert-butyl-4-isoxazolyl) propionic acid] is a more selective kainate receptor agonist, particularly for GluR5. The most commonly used non-NMDA receptor antagonists are CNQX (cyano-7-nitroquinoxaline-2,3-dione) and NBQX (2,3-dioxo-6-nitro-1,2,3,4-tetrahydro-benzo[f]quinoxaline-7-sulfonamide), which have limited selectivity for AMPA over kainate receptor subunits. GYKI53655, a 2,3-benzodiazepine, is currently the most selective AMPA receptor antagonist (non-competitive allosteric modulator). The competitive antagonist LY293558 [(3S,4aR,6R, 8aR)-6-[2-(1(2)H-tetrazole-5-yl)ethyl] decahydroisoquinoline-3-carboxylic acid], which has been tested in phase II clinical trials, shows higher selectivity for AMPA receptors over GluR6 and GluR7 kainate receptors, but it is also active at the GluR5 subunit (Sang et al. 2004). Antagonists that distinguish kainate from AMPA receptors have only recently become available. LY382884 [(3S, 4aR, 6S, 8aR)-6-(4-carboxyphenyl)methyl-1,2,3,4,4a,5,6,7,8,8a-decahydroisoquinoline-3-carboxylic acid] and UBP302 [(S)-1-(2-Amino-2-carboxyethyl)-3-(2-carboxybenzyl)pyrimidine-2,4-dione] are GluR5-selective antagonists at concentrations that do not affect AMPA receptors (Bortolotto et al. 2003; More et al. 2004).

1.2
Metabotropic Glutamate Receptors

mGluRs belong to family 3 of G protein-coupled receptors, which can trigger long-lasting intracellular processes and plastic changes. They are characterized by a seven-transmembrane domain topology and a large N-terminal extracellular domain, which contains important residues for ligand binding and forms two lobes that close like a Venus' flytrap upon ligand binding (Bockaert and Pin 1999). The second intracellular loop determines G protein specificity and the intracellular C-terminal interacts directly with intracellular proteins such as Homer, which are involved in receptor trafficking, synaptic anchoring, cell signaling, and constitutive (basal) receptor activity (Bockaert and Pin 1999; De Blasi et al. 2001; Gasparini et al. 2002; Bhave et al. 2003). Eight mGluR subtypes have been cloned and are classified into groups I (mGluRs 1 and 5), II (mGluRs 2 and 3), and III (mGluRs 4, 6, 7, and 8) based on their sequence homology, signal transduction mechanisms, and pharmacological profile (Schoepp et al. 1999; De Blasi et al. 2001; Neugebauer 2001; Gasparini et al. 2002; Varney and Gereau 2002; Lesage 2004; Swanson et al. 2005; see Table 1). Several splice variants have been identified that may differ with regard to their pharmacology and G protein coupling.

Group I mGluRs couple through G_q proteins to the activation of phospholipase C (PLC), which leads to the formation of inositol-1,4,5-trisphosphate (IP3) and diacylglycerol (DAG), resulting in calcium release from intracellular stores and activation of protein kinase C (PKC), respectively (Anwyl 1999; Schoepp et al. 1999; Neugebauer 2001; Gasparini et al. 2002). Tyrosine kinase activation is another signaling pathway of group I mGluRs. Both PKC- and tyrosine kinase-dependent pathways can involve mitogen-activated protein (MAP) kinases such as the extracellular signal-regulated kinases 1/2 (ERK1/2) (Varney and Gereau 2002). Stimulation of adenylyl cyclase (AC) by group I mGluRs has been reported but the underlying mechanism is not yet known. Group II and group III mGluRs are negatively coupled to AC through G_i/G_o proteins, thereby inhibiting cyclic AMP (cAMP) formation and cAMP-dependent protein kinase (PKA) activation (Anwyl 1999; Schoepp et al. 1999; Neugebauer 2001; Gasparini et al. 2002).

Individual mGluR subtypes show distinct synaptic localization and function (Schoepp et al. 1999; Neugebauer 2001; Gasparini et al. 2002; Varney and Gereau 2002; Lesage 2004; Swanson et al. 2005). Group I mGluR1 and 5 are most often localized postsynaptically whereas group II mGluR2 and group III mGluR8 are largely presynaptic. Group II mGluR3 and group III mGluR4 and 7 can be found both pre- and postsynaptically. In general, the predominant effect of group I mGluR activation is enhanced neuronal excitability and synaptic transmission whereas groups II and III typically mediate inhibitory effects, although exceptions exist. The mGluRs can regulate neuronal excitability through direct or indirect effects on a variety of voltage-sensitive ion channels, including high voltage-activated Ca^{2+} channels, K^+ channels, and nonselective cationic channels (Anwyl 1999; Schoepp et al. 1999; Neugebauer 2001). The modulation of ligand-gated ion channels by mGluRs includes the group I mGluR-mediated enhancement of ionotropic glutamate receptor function, which likely involves receptor phosphorylation (Anwyl 1999; Fundytus 2001; Neugebauer 2001). Group I mGluRs also potentiate the function of the capsaicin/vanilloid receptor, TRPV1 (Hu et al. 2002). Convincing evidence suggests that mGluRs interact with the opioid system and play a role in the development of opioid tolerance and dependence (Fundytus 2001). mGluRs can also modulate the release of transmitters by acting as autoreceptors (glutamate) or heteroreceptors (GABA, substance P, serotonin, dopamine, and acetylcholine) (Cartmell and Schoepp 2000).

Several potent and mGluR subgroup/subtype-selective compounds have been developed (Schoepp et al. 1999; Neugebauer 2001; Gasparini et al. 2002; Varney and Gereau 2002; Lesage 2004; Swanson et al. 2005; see Table 1). Currently available agonists are selective for subgroups I (DHPG, (S)-3,5-dihydroxyphenylglycine), II (LY354740, [1S, 2S,5R,6S]-2-aminobicyclo[3.1.0] hexane-2,6-dicarboxylic acid; LY379268, (−)-2-oxa-4-aminobicylco hexane-4,6-dicarboxylic acid), and III (LAP4, L-(+)-2-amino-4-phosphonobutyric-acid). LY354740 has been tested in phase II clinical trials. Several subtype-selective agonists have become available. (RS)-2-chloro-5-hydroxyphenylglyine (CHPG) is selective for mGluR5. (S)-3,4-dicarboxyphenylglycine [(S)-3,4-

DCPG] activates mGluR8 with nanomolar potency and has greater than 280-fold selectivity over other mGluR subtypes (Thomas et al. 2001). Positive allosteric activators have been identified for mGluR4 (N-phenyl-7-(hydroxylimino)cyclopropa[b]chromen-1a-carboxamide [PHCCC]; Maj et al. 2003; Shipe et al. 2005) and mGluR7 (N,N'-dibenzhydrylethane-1,2-diamine dihydrochloride [AMN082]; Conn and Niswender 2006; Mitsukawa et al. 2005). Antagonists for group I mGluRs include the competitive mGluR1 subtype-selective antagonist LY367385 [(S)-(+)-α-amino-4-carboxy-2-methylbenzeneacetic acid] and noncompetitive (allosteric) antagonists for mGluR1 [CPCCOEt, 7-(hydroxyimino-breakno) cyclopropa[b]chromen-1a-carboxylate ethyl ester] and mGluR5-(MPEP, 2-methyl-6-(phenylethynyl)pyridine). Competitive group II and group III mGluR antagonists are available; they are subgroup- but not subtype-selective (Table 1). The activity of mGluRs can be regulated not only by receptor agonists and antagonists but also through receptor phosphorylation, including PKC-mediated desensitization of group I mGluRs and uncoupling of groups II and III mGluRs from G proteins by PKC and PKA (Karim et al. 2001; Neugebauer 2001; Varney and Gereau 2002).

2
Glutamatergic Nociceptive Transmission in the Peripheral and Central Nervous System

The role of iGluRs and mGluRs in nociceptive transmission has been reviewed in detail in a number of recent articles (Fisher et al. 2000; Carlton 2001; Willis 2001; Neugebauer and Carlton 2002; Neugebauer 2002; Varney and Gereau 2002; Ruscheweyh and Sandkuhler 2002; Hewitt 2003; Garry et al. 2004; Lesage 2004). The following is a summary of glutamate receptor function in nociceptive processing in naïve animals; the involvement of iGluRs and mGluRs in pain-related plasticity will be discussed in the context of preclinical pain models (Sect. 3).

2.1
Ionotropic Glutamate Receptors

Functional NMDA, AMPA, and kainate receptors are present along the pain neuraxis from the peripheral nervous system to the brain.

2.1.1
Periphery

It is firmly established now that iGluRs (particularly NR2B, GluR1, and GluR5) are localized in the periphery on nociceptive primary afferent terminals and on their cell bodies (Carlton 2001). Injections of NMDA, AMPA, or kainate into peripheral tissues excite and sensitize nociceptors in electrophysiological studies and produce pronociceptive behavioral effects including thermal and mechanical hyperalgesia as well as spontaneous lifting and licking behaviors (Lawand et al. 1997; Carlton 2001). These effects can be blocked by the appropriate antagonists. Although the details of iGluR-mediated signal transduction at the peripheral nerve terminals need to be determined, it is clear that neuronal as well as nonneuronal elements serve as the sources for glutamate (Carlton 2001). Importantly, glutamate levels are increased in the joints of patients with arthritis, which may suggest a role of peripheral iGluRs in clinical pain associated with tissue damage (McNearney et al. 2000).

2.1.2
Spinal Cord

In the spinal dorsal horn, NMDA, AMPA, and kainate receptors have now been shown to be localized pre- and postsynaptically, particularly in the superficial laminae I and II (Tolle et al. 1993; Willis and Coggeshall 2004; Lu et al. 2005). NMDA receptors (NR1) are present on the terminals of primary afferents and of GABAergic interneurons as well as on nearly all dorsal horn neurons. The distribution of the different NR2 subunits appears to be more complex, but NR2B is found predominantly in small-diameter primary afferents and in the superficial dorsal horn whereas NR2A is highly concentrated in the deep dorsal horn (Nagy et al. 2004). AMPA receptors are expressed on the terminals of unmyelinated (GluR1) and myelinated (GluR2) afferents and of GABAergic interneurons (GluR4) as well as on neurons in the superficial (GluR1 and 2) and deep (GluR3 and 4) dorsal horn. Although the AMPA receptor subunit distribution is controversial, it has been suggested that unmyelinated C-fibers are positioned to activate calcium-permeable AMPA receptors (lacking GluR2) on inhibitory (and some excitatory) interneurons in the superficial dorsal horn whereas (small) myelinated fibers make contact with GluR2-containing AMPA receptors on excitatory interneurons (Willis and Coggeshall 2004). Such an arrangement would limit the nociceptive transmission from C-fibers under normal conditions. Kainate receptor subunits KA1 and KA2 are found presynaptically on primary afferents and GABAergic interneurons as well as postsynaptically on dorsal horn neurons (Willis and Coggeshall 2004; Lu et al. 2005). Importantly, essentially all of the kainate receptor-expressing primary afferents appear to be nociceptors, and GluR5 is the predominant kainate receptor subunit expressed in primary afferents (Carlton 2001).

Presynaptic NMDA, AMPA, and kainate receptors have been shown to act as autoreceptors on primary afferents to decrease the release of glutamate through a mechanism that involves primary afferent depolarization, thus preventing the propagation of action potentials into the central terminals or, more likely, reducing their size (Lee et al. 2002; Bardoni et al. 2004). The consequence of such inhibitory action for spinal nociceptive processing remains to be determined, but inhibitory effects of kainate receptor activation on spinal excitatory neurotransmission have been described (Ruscheweyh and Sandkuhler 2002; Youn and Randic 2004). The predominant effect, however, of spinal NMDA, AMPA, or kainate receptor activation is the excitation of spinal dorsal horn neurons and the increases of their responses to innocuous and noxious stimuli (Fundytus 2001; Ruscheweyh and Sandkuhler 2002; Youn and Randic 2004). Accordingly, intrathecal administration of NMDA, AMPA, and kainate receptor agonists produces spontaneous nociceptive behavior and thermal and mechanical hyperalgesia (Fundytus 2001). Conversely, there is good evidence that spinal administration of NMDA, AMPA, and kainate receptor antagonists can inhibit nociceptive transmission in dorsal horn neurons and pain behavior (Stanfa and Dickenson 1999; Moore et al. 2000; Fundytus 2001; Willis 2001; Schaible et al. 2002; Ruscheweyh and Sandkuhler 2002; Garry et al. 2004). It should be noted, however, that AMPA receptor activation is also involved in the transmission of non-nociceptive information whereas blockade of NMDA and kainate receptors does not affect all forms of nociceptive transmission. NMDA receptors may be involved predominantly in tonic pain responses and persistent pain states (see Sect. 3). The role of kainate receptors is only beginning to emerge.

2.1.3
Brain

Activation of NMDA and AMPA receptors in the brainstem, including peri-aqueductal gray (PAG) and rostral ventromedial medulla (RVM), produces antinociceptive effects, which is consistent with the key role of these brainstem areas in the descending inhibition of nociception and pain (Berrino et al. 2001; Ren and Dubner 2002; Gebhart 2004; Vanegas and Schaible 2004). More recently, however, it has been shown that glutamate or NMDA, but not AMPA, micro-injected into the RVM facilitates spinal nociceptive processing (Ren and Dubner 2002; Gebhart 2004). The dual facilitatory and inhibitory role of iGluRs in the brainstem reflects the bidirectional modulation of pain by the descending control system. These differential effects appear to be activity and time-dependent as is evident in pain models (see Sect. 3). Antagonists for non-NMDA, but not NMDA, receptors in the RVM produce facilitation of nociceptive responses in naïve animals, suggesting that a glutamatergic descending inhibitory system is tonically active (Urban et al. 1999). The role of kainate receptors in descending pain modulation is not yet known.

The contribution of iGluRs to nociceptive processing in higher brain areas has been determined in the thalamus (Salt 2002) and amygdala (Neugebauer et al. 2004). Sensory thalamic relay nuclei such as the ventrobasal thalamus (VB) play an important role in gating and processing sensory information transmitted to the cerebral cortex. Sensory transmission to the VB complex involves both NMDA and non-NMDA receptors. NMDA receptors contribute strongly to nociceptive responses of VB neurons and prolonged or repetitive synaptic input. Non-NMDA receptors mediate non-nociceptive responses and the fast component of sensory-evoked synaptic responses but contribute little to nociceptive transmission. Kainate receptors do not appear to contribute to the responses of thalamic relay cells to sensory inputs, but studies using LY382884 (kainate GluR5 antagonist) suggest there is activation of kainate receptors on GABAergic axons from the thalamic reticular nucleus, which results in disinhibition through decreased recurrent inhibition. This has been proposed to play an important novel role in extracting sensory information from background noise (Salt 2002).

The latero-capsular part of the central nucleus of the amygdala (CeLC) represents the nociceptive amygdala, which is believed to be concerned with the emotional-affective component and modulation of pain (Neugebauer et al. 2004). Nociceptive responses of CeLC neurons in naïve animals are mediated by a combination of NMDA and non-NMDA receptors whereas non-nociceptive inputs and basal synaptic transmission activate only non-NMDA receptors (Li and Neugebauer 2004b; Bird et al. 2005). The relative contribution of AMPA and kainate receptors is not yet known. Enhanced NMDA receptor function appears to be an important mechanism in pain-related plasticity in the CeLC (see Sect. 3).

2.2
Metabotropic Glutamate Receptors

The important role of group I mGluRs in peripheral and central nociceptive processing and pain behavior is now well established whereas the functions of groups II and III mGluRs are less well known (Fundytus 2001; Neugebauer 2001; Neugebauer 2002; Varney and Gereau 2002; Lesage 2004).

2.2.1
Periphery

Group I mGluR1 and mGluR5 have been demonstrated on a subset (~20%–30%) of unmyelinated and myelinated peripheral axons (Neugebauer and Carlton 2002; Lesage 2004). There is evidence for a colocalization of mGluR5 with the capsaicin/vanilloid receptor (TRPV1), while mGluR1 may also be present on sympathetic efferent fibers. Group II mGluR2 and mGluR3 and group III mGluR7 and mGluR8 are also present in a subpopulation of small-diameter primary afferent neurons, and there is some colocalization of group I and group II mGluRs (Neugebauer and Carlton 2002; Varney and Gereau 2002). Exogenous activation of peripheral group I mGluRs (Neugebauer and Carlton 2002; Varney and Gereau 2002; Lesage 2004) produced long-lasting thermal hyperalgesia in mice (but not rats), which was significantly reduced by peripheral injections of mGluR1 antagonists (CPCCOEt and LY367385) and completely blocked by an mGluR5 antagonist (MPEP). Peripheral injections of a selective mGluR5 agonist (CHPG) and the mGluR1/5 agonist (DHPG) were equally potent in producing mechanical allodynia in rats. The mechanical allodynia was blocked by a selective mGluR5 antagonist (MPEP) but not by a selective mGluR1 antagonist (4CPG, (S)-4-carboxy-phenylglycine). These data may suggest a role of peripheral mGluR5 in mechanical allodynia whereas both mGluR1 and mGluR5 are involved in thermal hyperalgesia.

There is good evidence to suggest the involvement and endogenous activation of peripheral group I mGluRs in persistent pain states (see Sect. 3) but not in normal nociception. Subcutaneous injection of a group II mGluR agonist (APDC; 2R,4R-4-aminopyrrolidine-2,4-dicarboxylate) into the mouse hindpaw did not alter mechanical and thermal sensitivity in behavioral studies (Yang and Gereau 2002; Yang and Gereau 2003), but very low concentrations of APDC inhibited the extracellularly recorded responses of nociceptive fibers to heat stimuli in an in vitro skin-nerve preparation (Neugebauer and Carlton 2002). Peripheral group II mGluRs may be particularly useful targets in pain states (see Sect. 3). The role of peripheral group III mGluRs remains to be determined.

2.2.2
Spinal Cord

Group I mGluR1 and mGluR5 are functionally expressed in the spinal dorsal horn: mGluR5 expression is particularly strong in the superficial laminae whereas high levels of mGluR1 are found in the deep dorsal horn. Anatomical and electrophysiological data further suggest that mGluR1 and mGluR5 are mainly postsynaptic but can also act presynaptically to facilitate spinal neurotransmission (Neugebauer 2001, 2002; Varney and Gereau 2002; Lesage 2004). Importantly, mGluR5 was identified on GABA and non-GABAergic dorsal horn neurons. Activation of spinal group I mGluRs generally produces pronociceptive effects in behavioral and electrophysiological assays, although mixed excitatory and inhibitory effects have been reported (Fundytus 2001; Neugebauer 2001; Varney and Gereau 2002; Lesage 2004). Intrathecal administration of group I agonists such as DHPG evokes spontaneous nociceptive behavior, thermal and mechanical hyperalgesia, and mechanical allodynia, which can be blocked with antagonists or antibodies for mGluR1 or mGluR5, where tested (Fundytus 2001; Neugebauer 2001; Varney and Gereau 2002; Lesage 2004). Activation of spinal group I mGluRs can produce facilitation or inhibition of synaptic transmission and of dorsal horn neuron responses to innocuous and noxious stimuli (Gerber et al. 2000a; Neugebauer 2001; Lesage 2004). Antagonists selective for mGluR1 (CPCCOEt) or mGluR5 (MPEP) can block these facilitatory effects but do not appear to affect nociceptive behavior under normal conditions (Fundytus 2001; Neugebauer 2001; Varney and Gereau 2002; Lesage 2004; Soliman et al. 2005). Spinal mGluR5 may mediate the inhibitory effects of group I mGluR activation.

The roles of group II and group III mGluRs in spinal nociceptive processing are less clear (Neugebauer 2001; Neugebauer 2002; Varney and Gereau 2002). Both group II mGluR2/3 and group III mGluR4 and 7, but not mGluR6 and 8, are present in the spinal cord. Group III mGluRs are localized predominantly on presynaptic terminals in the dorsal and ventral horns whereas group II mGluRs have been detected on presynaptic terminals in the superficial dorsal horn as well as on postsynaptic elements in deeper laminae. Agonists of group II (LCCG, (2S,1′S,2′S)-2-(carboxycyclopropyl)glycine) and III (LAP4) mGluRs can inhibit synaptic transmission in the dorsal horn in spinal cord slices in vitro (Gerber et al. 2000b), but behavioral studies found little evidence for antinociceptive effects of group II or group III mGluR activation (Neugebauer 2001; Neugebauer 2002; Varney and Gereau 2002). Intrathecal administration of selective group II (APDC) and group III (LAP4) agonists had no effect on mechanical withdrawal response thresholds in the absence of tissue damage (Soliman et al. 2005). Similarly, systemic administration of a selective group II agonist (LY379268) had no significant effects on the tail flick or paw withdrawal tests of acute thermal nociceptive function (Simmons et al. 2002). Intraspinal administration of LY379268 had no effect on the responses of nociceptive dorsal horn neurons (spinothalamic tract cells) recorded under normal conditions whereas LAP4 inhibited the responses to brief noxious and innocuous mechanical cutaneous stimuli (Neugebauer et al. 2000).

2.2.3
Brain

In the brainstem, activation of group I mGluR1/5 (DHPG) or mGluR5 (CHPG) in the PAG had antinociceptive effects in the hotplate test in naïve animals (Maione et al. 1998; Lesage 2004). Intra-PAG administration of an mGluR1 antagonist (CPCCOEt) attenuated the effect of DHPG whereas an mGluR5 antagonist (MPEP) blocked the effect of CHPG, indicating the involvement of both mGluR1 and mGluR5 subtypes. When administered without exogenous agonists, MPEP, but not CPCCOEt, had pronociceptive effects, suggesting the presence of tonic descending inhibition mediated by mGluR5 in the PAG. Activation of mGluR5 (CHPG) in the RVM, however, produced cold hypersensitivity that was prevented by MPEP (Lesage 2004). The possibly differential roles of mGluR1 and mGluR5 in descending inhibitory and facilitatory systems await a detailed analysis. Different from group I mGluRs, activation of groups II and III mGluRs in the PAG appears to decrease the descending inhibition of pain behavior (Maione et al. 1998). Agonists of group II (LCCG) and III (LSOP, L-serine-O-phosphate) receptors administered into the PAG decreased the latency of the nociceptive reaction in the hot plate test. Antagonists of group II [EGLU, (2S)-α-ethylglutamic acid] and III [MSOP, (RS)-α-methylserine-O-phosphate] receptors antagonized these pronociceptive effects of LCCG and LSOP. Interestingly, MSOP, but not EGLU, alone increased the latency in the hot plate test, perhaps suggesting the tonic activation of group III mGluRs in the PAG.

In the VB, mGluR1 and mGluR5 are involved in the processing of nociceptive, but not non-nociceptive, information (Salt and Binns 2000; Lesage 2004). Intrathalamic administration of antagonists selective for mGluR1 (LY367385) and mGluR5 (MPEP) inhibited the responses of VB neurons to brief noxious heat but not innocuous stimuli. Intrathalamic MPEP had no effect on noxious mechanical stimuli; the role of thalamic mGluR1 in mechanonociception remains to be determined. Group II and III mGluRs mediate the presynaptic reduction of GABAergic inhibition in the VB, producing disinhibition of sensory (including nociceptive) processing (Salt et al. 1996; Salt 2002). Agonists of group II (LY354740 and APDC) and III (LAP4) decreased the inhibitory transmission from the thalamic reticular nucleus and the respective antagonists [MCCG (α-methyl-CCG-I) and MAP4 (α-methyl-L-AP4)] blocked these disinhibitory effects. Accordingly, administration of a group II antagonist (EGLU) in the thalamic reticular nucleus produced antinociceptive effects presumably by blocking the activation of group II mGluRs by the noxious input, thus disinhibiting the GABAergic neurons that inhibit thalamic relay neurons (Neto and Castro-Lopes 2000). When evaluating the therapeutic potential of these drug targets, it is important to consider possible facilitatory effects of otherwise inhibitory groups II and III mGluRs in brain areas such as the PAG and thalamus.

In the amygdala (Neugebauer et al. 2004), activation of group I mGluR1/5 (DHPG) or mGluR5 (CHPG) enhanced the responses of CeLC neurons to innocuous and noxious stimuli in naïve animals (Li and Neugebauer 2004a). Likewise, DHPG and CHPG potentiated normal synaptic transmission of presumed nociceptive input from the pontine parabrachial area to the CeLC in brain slices (Neugebauer et al. 2003). An mGluR5 antagonist (MPEP) inhibited brief nociceptive responses of CeLC neurons under normal conditions whereas an mGluR1 antagonist (CPCCOEt) had no effect. Similarly, MPEP, but not CPC-COEt, inhibited basal synaptic transmission in CeLC neurons in slices from naïve animals. The role of group II and III mGluRs in nociceptive processing in the amygdala is not yet known.

3
Preclinical Studies

The analysis of pain mechanisms in preclinical animal models of inflammatory and neuropathic pain has shown that iGluRs and mGluRs play important roles in peripheral sensitization, central sensitization, and descending pain modulation (Fisher et al. 2000; Fundytus 2001; Carlton 2001; Willis 2001; Parsons 2001; Neugebauer and Carlton 2002; Neugebauer 2002; Varney and Gereau 2002; Ruscheweyh and Sandkuhler 2002; Lesage 2004; Woolf 2004).

3.1
Ionotropic Glutamate Receptors

3.1.1
Periphery

Peripheral administration of NMDA or non-NMDA receptor antagonists inhibits nociceptive behavior in the second phase of the formalin test and thermal and mechanical hyperalgesia associated with inflammation of the hindpaw (complete Freund's adjuvant CFA- or carrageenan-induced) and knee joint (kaolin/carrageenan-induced) (Carlton 2001; Parsons 2001; Du et al. 2003). NMDA receptor antagonists tested in these studies include the clinically used compounds dextrorphan (a metabolite of dextromethorphan), ketamine, and memantine. Peripheral NMDA receptors might also be involved in visceral pain, as memantine was shown to inhibit the responses of single fibers in the decentralized pelvic nerves to colorectal distention (McRoberts et al. 2001). In a model of neuropathic pain, block of peripheral NMDA receptors (by MK-801), but not non-NMDA receptors (by NBQX), attenuated and delayed the onset of mechanical hyperalgesia (Jang et al. 2004). The potential therapeutic value of peripheral NMDA, AMPA, and kainate receptor antagonists still awaits a systematic analysis in models of inflammatory and, particularly, neuropathic pain.

3.1.2
Spinal Cord

Spinal administration of NMDA or non-NMDA antagonists is well known to inhibit central sensitization in various models of inflammatory and neuropathic pain (Fisher et al. 2000; Fundytus 2001; Willis 2001; Parsons 2001). NMDA or non-NMDA receptor antagonists in the spinal cord reversed the enhanced responses of dorsal horn neurons, including spinothalamic tract cells, in inflammatory pain states induced by intradermal capsaicin, intraplantar carrageenan, or intraarticular kaolin and carrageenan (Stanfa and Dickenson 1999; Fisher et al. 2000; Fundytus 2001; Willis 2001; Parsons 2001; Schaible et al. 2002). Compounds tested in these studies include the clinically used NMDA receptor antagonists ketamine and memantine, a somewhat AMPA receptor-preferring antagonist (NBQX), and a GluR5 kainate receptor-selective antagonist (LY382884). Central sensitization of dorsal horn neurons, including spinothalamic tract cells, in models of neuropathic pain has also been shown to be inhibited by spinal administration of NMDA (memantine, dextrorphan, and MK-801) and non-NMDA (CNQX and LY382884) receptor antagonists (Carlton et al. 1997; Carlton et al. 1998; Parsons 2001; Palecek et al. 2004; Willis and Coggeshall 2004).

Behavioral data also show that NMDA and non-NMDA receptor antagonists are antinociceptive in inflammatory and neuropathic pain models (Fisher et al.

2000; Fundytus 2001; Willis 2001; Parsons 2001; Soliman et al. 2005). Spinally or systemically administered NMDA receptor antagonists, including memantine and dextromethorphan, inhibit nociceptive behavior, thermal hyperalgesia, and mechanical allodynia associated with peripheral inflammation as well as visceral hypersensitivity. NMDA receptor antagonists also reduce heat hyperalgesia and, less consistently, mechanical allodynia associated with peripheral nerve injury. Interestingly, intrathecal administration of an NR2B subunit-selective antagonist (CP-101606) inhibited mechanical allodynia in a model of postoperative pain (Nishimura et al. 2004) but had no effect on mechanical allodynia in a neuropathic pain model whereas memantine was antinociceptive in that model (Nakazato et al. 2005), suggesting differential roles of spinal NR2B in different forms of pain. Systemic administration of another agent with NR2B-selective antagonistic properties (ifenprodil) had antinociceptive effects in inflammatory and neuropathic pain models but, unlike MK-801 and memantine, did not inhibit NMDA-evoked responses of dorsal horn neurons (Nakazato et al. 2005). Thus the role of spinal NR2B subunit-containing NMDA receptors in nociceptive processing remains unclear.

Intrathecally or systemically administered non-NMDA receptor antagonists, including NBQX, have antinociceptive effects in animal models of inflammatory and neuropathic pain, but they also produce side effects such as ataxia. A selective AMPA receptor antagonist (GYKI53655), however, did not produce antinociception in the formalin pain test at doses that did not cause ataxia (Simmons et al. 1998), suggesting that kainate rather than AMPA receptors may be useful targets. Indeed, more recent studies focused on kainate receptors and showed that systemic administration of a GluR5/6-selective antagonist (SYM 2081; 2S,4R-4-methylglutamic acid; Sutton et al. 1999) and GluR5-selective antagonists such as LY382884 (Simmons et al. 1998) and orally active compounds LY467711 and LY525327 (Dominguez et al. 2005) inhibited nociceptive behavior in the formalin test, thermal hyperalgesia, and mechanical allodynia induced by carrageenan or capsaicin, and thermal hyperalgesia and mechanical allodynia in a model of peripheral nerve injury. The site or sites of action of these systemically administered drugs remain to be determined.

3.1.3
Brain

In the brainstem (RVM), NMDA receptor activation is involved in descending facilitation whereas inhibition involves activation of non-NMDA receptors (Ren and Dubner 2002; Gebhart 2004; Vanegas and Schaible 2004). NMDA-dependent descending facilitation appears to be particularly important for the development of secondary thermal hyperalgesia and mechanical allodynia in the early stages of inflammatory pain; it may be important for maintenance rather than initiation of neuropathic pain states as well (Ren and Dubner 2002; Porreca et al. 2002; Heinricher et al. 2003; Gebhart 2004; Vanegas and

Schaible 2004). Microinjection of NMDA receptor antagonists such as AP5 into the RVM inhibited hyperalgesic behavior produced by injection of formalin into the hindpaw, carrageenan-induced hindpaw inflammation, application of mustard oil to the hindlimb skin (topical), and colon inflammation. In contrast, block of non-NMDA receptors in the RVM further enhanced the hyperalgesic response, suggesting the presence of descending inhibition. Differential effects of NMDA and non-NMDA receptor antagonists on antinociceptive "off-cells" and pronociceptive "on-cells" in the RVM also suggest that distinct pharmacological profiles of inhibitory and facilitatory circuits may be a neural mechanism of bidirectional descending control (Heinricher et al. 2003). Descending modulation may undergo time-dependent functional changes such that facilitation decreases or inhibition increases (or both) at the later stages of inflammatory pain. These changes and their role in primary versus secondary hyperalgesia await a detailed analysis.

The role of iGluRs in the PAG in prolonged or chronic pain states is less well understood. Block of NMDA receptors in the PAG inhibited pain in the formalin test, but not the hotplate test, suggesting that NMDA receptors are involved in tonic, but not phasic, pain (Vaccarino et al. 1997). In another study, however, NMDA receptor antagonists in the PAG were ineffective in the formalin test but activation of NMDA receptors produced antinociception (Berrino et al. 2001). The role of non-NMDA receptors in the PAG remains to be determined.

In higher brain areas, intrathalamic injection of an NMDA receptor antagonist (AP5) reduced thermal and mechanical hyperalgesia in the acute and subacute phases of the carrageenan-induced hindpaw inflammation model. The effects were confined to the withdrawal responses evoked from the injected paw. Pretreatment with intrathalamic injections of antisense oligodeoxynucleotides directed against the NR1 subunit prevented the development of thermal hyperalgesia and attenuated the development of mechanical hyperalgesia (Kolhekar et al. 1997). The pharmacology of thalamic pain mechanisms has yet to be analyzed at the single cell level in preclinical pain models.

In the amygdala both NMDA (AP5) and non-NMDA (NBQX) receptor antagonists inhibited the nociceptive responses of CeLC neurons in the kaolin/carrageenan-induced arthritis pain model (Li and Neugebauer 2004b). However, increased function of NMDA receptors rather than non-NMDA receptors appears to be a key mechanism of pain-related synaptic plasticity recorded in brain slices from arthritic animals compared to naïve controls (Bird et al. 2005).

In the anterior cingulate cortex (ACC), bilateral microinjections of an NMDA receptor antagonist (AP5) significantly inhibited bilateral mechanical allodynia in the CFA-induced inflammatory pain model (posttreatment on day 1; Wei et al. 2002). Conversely, overexpression of NR2B in the forebrain, including the ACC and insular cortex, increased formalin-induced pain behavior and mechanical allodynia associated with CFA-induced hindpaw inflammation (Wei et al. 2001). However, pretreatment with bilateral injections of NMDA (AP5) or non-NMDA (DNQX) receptor antagonists into the ACC had no effect on acute nociceptive behaviors in the formalin test whereas affect-related behavior (formalin-induced conditioned place avoidance) was effectively eliminated by intra-ACC microinjection of AP5 but not DNQX (Lei et al. 2004).

3.2
Metabotropic Glutamate Receptors

3.2.1
Periphery

There is good evidence to suggest the involvement and endogenous activation of peripheral group I mGluRs in models of inflammatory and neuropathic pain but not in normal nociception (Carlton 2001; Neugebauer 2001, 2002; Neugebauer and Carlton 2002; Varney and Gereau 2002; Lesage 2004). Peripheral injections of antagonists for mGluR1 (including CPCCOEt) or mGluR5 (MPEP) inhibited nociceptive behavior in the second, but not the first, phase of the formalin test. Similarly, peripheral administration of MPEP reversed mechanical allodynia in carrageenan- and CFA-induced inflammatory pain models. The antagonists did not inhibit normal nociception and had no effect when injected into the contralateral non-inflamed paw. Peripheral group I mGluRs may also play a role in neuropathic pain. In the spinal nerve ligation model, peripheral injections of an mGluR5 antagonist (SIB-1757, 6-methyl-2-(phenylazo)-3-pyridinol) into the injured hindlimb, but not the contralateral paw, reversed thermal hyperalgesia, but not mechanical allodynia, and had no effect in sham-operated animals.

Peripheral injection of a group II mGluR agonist (APDC) inhibited nociceptive behavior in the first and the second phase of formalin-induced pain (Neugebauer and Carlton 2002). APDC also blocked prostaglandin E2 (PGE2)-induced thermal hyperalgesia and PGE2- and carrageenan-induced mechanical allodynia (Yang and Gereau 2002; Yang and Gereau 2003). However, APDC had no effect on basal thermal and mechanical thresholds in naïve animals. The antinociceptive effects of APDC were antagonized by a selective group II antagonist (LY341495) when tested. Importantly, blockade of peripheral group II mGluRs (LY341495) prolonged PGE2- and carrageenan-induced mechanical allodynia, suggesting that peripheral group II mGluRs mediate endogenous anti-allodynic effects (Yang and Gereau 2003). Similarly, peripheral injection of a group II/III antagonist (MSOPPE, (RS)-α-methylserine-O-phosphate monophenyl ester) enhanced glutamate-induced mechanical allodynia (Neugebauer and Carlton 2002). In the spinal nerve lesion model of neuropathic pain, pre-treatment with APDC delayed the onset of mechanical allodynia but post-treatment with APDC had no effect (Jang et al. 2004). The contribution of peripheral mGluRs to nociceptive processes associated with inflammatory and neuropathic pain would suggest that peripherally acting group I antagonists and group II agonists may have a therapeutic value in the treatment of pain states arising from peripheral tissue injury. The role of group III mGluRs remains to be determined.

3.2.2
Spinal Cord

The endogenous activation and involvement of spinal group I mGluRs, particularly mGluR1, in prolonged nociception and persistent pain states is well documented in behavioral and electrophysiological studies using antagonists, antibodies, and antisense oligonucleotides in models of inflammatory pain (induced by formalin, intradermal capsaicin, intraplantar carrageenan or CFA, and intraarticular kaolin/carrageenan) and neuropathic pain (Neugebauer et al. 1999; Fundytus 2001; Karim et al. 2001; Neugebauer 2001; Neugebauer 2002; Varney and Gereau 2002; Lesage 2004; Soliman et al. 2005). Electrophysiological studies of spinal dorsal horn neurons, including spinothalamic tract cells, showed antinociceptive effects of spinally administered group I antagonists, including mGluR1-selective compounds (CPCCOEt), or antisense oligodeoxynucleotides directed against mGluR1, in pain-related central sensitization following intradermal capsaicin, topical application of mustard oil to the skin, or intraarticular kaolin/carrageenan injections (Neugebauer et al. 1999; Fundytus 2001; Neugebauer 2001; Varney and Gereau 2002). The involvement and intrinsic activation of mGluR5 in spinal neurons in pain models is not entirely clear yet.

Intrathecal administration of group I antagonists, including CPCCOEt-(mGluR1) and MPEP (mGluR5), inhibited nociceptive behavior in the formalin test, thermal hyperalgesia and mechanical allodynia following intraplantar carrageenan, and capsaicin-induced mechanical, but not thermal, hypersensitivity (Fundytus 2001; Neugebauer 2001; Neugebauer 2002; Varney and Gereau 2002; Lesage 2004; Soliman et al. 2005). Group I antagonists had also antinociceptive effects in models of neuropathic pain. Whereas mGluR1-selective antagonists inhibited thermal hyperalgesia and mechanical allodynia, the role of mGluR5 in neuropathic pain is controversial, but a number of studies have shown antinociceptive effects of systemically or intrathecally applied blockers of mGluR5 (Varney and Gereau 2002; Lesage 2004). When directly compared, systemic administration of an mGluR1 antagonist [LY456236, (4-methoxy-phenyl)-(6-methoxy-quinazolin-4-yl)-amine HCl] reversed mechanical allodynia in a neuropathic pain model whereas mGluR5 antagonists (including MPEP) only attenuated it; however, both strongly inhibited formalin-induced nociceptive behavior (Varty et al. 2005). It is possible that mGluR5 receptors play a more prominent role in inflammatory than neuropathic pain states, but mGluR1 appears to be important for both.

The roles of group II and group III mGluRs in spinal pain mechanisms are less clear. Intrathecal administration of a group III agonist (LAP4) produced antinociceptive effects in the second phase of the formalin test whereas intrathecally administered group II agonists such as LY379268 were ineffective in this pain model (Neugebauer and Carlton 2002; Varney and Gereau 2002; Jones et al. 2005). Intrathecal administration of group II (APDC) and III (LAP4) agonists inhibited mechanical allodynia following intradermal capsaicin but had little effect on thermal hyperalgesia (Soliman et al. 2005). Electrophysiological studies showed that activation of spinal group II mGluRs inhibited electrically evoked nociceptive responses of dorsal horn neurons in carrageenan-induced hindpaw inflammation whereas mixed effects (inhibition and facilitation) were observed in control rats. A selective group II agonist (LY379268) inhibited capsaicin-induced central sensitization of spinothalamic tract cells but had no effect on the responses of non-sensitized neurons (Neugebauer et al. 2000). In contrast, a group III agonist (LAP4) inhibited the responses of spinothalamic tract cells to brief innocuous and noxious stimuli under normal condition as well as capsaicin-induced central sensitization (Neugebauer et al. 2000). These data suggest a dramatic change in the functional role of spinal group II, rather than group III, mGluRs in inflammatory pain.

3.2.3
Brain

In the brainstem, administration of group I (DHPG) and II (LCCG) agonists into the PAG decreased the nociceptive response in the second phase of the formalin test. These antinociceptive effects were antagonized by the respective antagonists (CPCCOEt, group I mGluR1; EGLU, group II) (Maione et al. 2000). A group III agonist (LSOP) increased the formalin-evoked nociceptive response. This facilitatory effect was antagonized by a group III antagonist (MSOP). Interestingly, an antagonist for mGluR5 (MPEP) potentiated per se the early nociceptive phase of the formalin test, suggesting mGluR5 in the PAG is endogenously activated to produce descending inhibition (Berrino et al. 2001). EGLU and MSOP had no effects on their own. It has been suggested that group I and group II mGluRs in the PAG positively modulate descending pain inhibition whereas group III mGluRs inhibit this antinociceptive pathway (Maione et al. 2000; Berrino et al. 2001).

In higher brain areas, the function of mGluRs in prolonged or chronic pain states is still largely unknown. Recent electrophysiological and behavioral studies in the amygdala suggested an important role for group I mGluRs, particularly mGluR1, in nociceptive plasticity and pain behavior (Neugebauer et al. 2004). In the kaolin/carrageenan arthritis pain model, administration of antagonists selective for mGluR1 (CPCCOEt) or mGluR5 (MPEP) into the amygdala inhibited the increased responses of sensitized CeLC neurons whereas the responses of these neurons under normal conditions before arthritis were inhibited by MPEP but not by CPCCOEt (Li and Neugebauer 2004a). Accordingly, CPCCOEt had no effect on basal synaptic transmission in CeLC neurons recorded in slices from normal animals but inhibited pain-related synaptic plasticity in slices from arthritic rats. MPEP inhibited basal synaptic transmission as well as synaptic plasticity (Neugebauer et al. 2003). Thus, enhanced receptor activation of mGluR1 appears to be a key mechanism of pain-related synaptic plasticity in the CeLC. Importantly, behavioral studies that addressed the significance of mGluR1 and mGluR5 function in the amygdala showed that CPCCOEt administration into the CeLC inhibited higher integrated behavior organized in the amygdala (vocalization afterdischarges) and in the brainstem (vocalizations during stimulation) as well as spinal nociceptive withdrawal reflexes. MPEP inhibited only vocalizations organized in the amygdala. It appears that activation of mGluR1 in the amygdala contributes to pain production through descending facilitation whereas mGluR5 is involved in intrinsic amygdala processes (Han and Neugebauer 2005). The roles of group II and III mGluRs in nociception and plasticity in the amygdala remain to be determined.

4
Clinical Studies

A number of glutamate receptor ligands have been tested in humans and are in clinical trials as analgesics. A main focus has been on their therapeutic potential for neuropathic pain, a condition that continues to be notoriously difficult to treat. Clinically tested compounds include antagonists for NMDA receptors and AMPA/kainate receptors. None of the mGluR compounds appear to have been studied clinically as potential analgesics. However, a group II agonist (LY354740) has been successfully tested in clinical trials for generalized anxiety disorders, and mGluR5 antagonists such as MPEP are on their way to clinical trials as well (Swanson et al. 2005).

4.1
NMDA Receptor Antagonists

Commercially available NMDA receptor antagonists, including ketamine, memantine, dextromethorphan, and its main metabolite dextrorphan, showed antinociceptive effects in preclinical studies (Sect. 3) and are analgesic in humans (Parsons et al. 1999; Fisher et al. 2000; Weinbroum et al. 2000; Fundytus 2001; Parsons 2001; Kilpatrick and Tilbrook 2002; Henriksson and Sorensen 2002; Hewitt 2003; Carlsson et al. 2004). Evidence from preclinical and earlier clinical studies further suggested that NMDA receptor antagonists enhanced opioid analgesia and prevented the development of tolerance (Fundytus 2001; Parsons 2001), but a recent report of three controlled clinical trials failed to demonstrate such effects of a combination of morphine and dextromethorphan (Galer et al. 2005).

4.1.1
Ketamine

The noncompetitive NMDA receptor antagonist ketamine has long been used to induce and maintain anesthesia. Ketamine, which has analgesic properties at subanesthetic doses, is one of the most extensively studied NMDA receptor antagonists. The antinociceptive effects of ketamine in preclinical models of inflammatory and neuropathic pain have been well documented (Sect. 3; Fundytus 2001; Parsons 2001; Hewitt 2003). Ketamine is also analgesic in experimental pain induced in healthy human subjects by intradermal capsaicin, ischemia, or burn (Fundytus 2001; Hewitt 2003). Interestingly, burn-induced pain was also inhibited by peripherally injected ketamine (Carlton 2001). In case reports and controlled studies, systemic (intravenous) ketamine produced relief of various forms of peripheral and central neuropathic pain (including postherpetic and posttraumatic neuralgias, phantom limb pain, and spinal cord injury), cancer pain, and pain in fibromyalgia patients (Fisher et al. 2000; Fundytus 2001; Parsons 2001; Henriksson and Sorensen 2002; Hewitt 2003). Oral and epidural administrations of ketamine have also been reported to be effective. There is little evidence to support long-term treatment of chronic pain with ketamine. The usefulness of perioperative ketamine for the treatment of postoperative pain is controversial. Some studies reported benefits of preemptive ketamine analgesia such as reduced postoperative pain and/or decreased analgesic consumption, but others found little or no evidence (Fundytus 2001; McCartney et al. 2004; Ong et al. 2005). Likewise, postoperative treatment has produced mixed results. Interestingly, intravenous administration of ketamine may be used as a diagnostic test to predict the analgesic response of neuropathic pain patients to dextromethorphan, which has a better side effect profile (Cohen et al. 2004). Undesirable side effects of ketamine include dizziness, sedation, perceptual changes, and dissociative symptoms, which typically disappear fairly quickly (Fisher et al. 2000; Fundytus 2001; Parsons 2001; Henriksson and Sorensen 2002). In summary, ketamine is effective in the treatment of neuropathic pain and perhaps fibromyalgia but its usefulness is limited by the well-documented albeit temporary side effects, abuse potential, and lack of evidence for long-term treatment benefits.

4.1.2
Memantine

A noncompetitive NMDA receptor antagonist memantine has been used for many years in the treatment of Parkinson's disease and, more recently, dementia (Parsons et al. 1999; Kilpatrick and Tilbrook 2002). Memantine is clinically well tolerated and shows little of the side effects typically seen with NMDA receptor antagonists, possibly because of the strong voltage dependence and rapid kinetics of its NMDA channel-blocking effects. Psychotomimetic effects, agitation/excitation, increased motor activity, and insomnia have been reported but appear to be sporadic and at doses outside the recommend range (Parsons et al. 1999; Kilpatrick and Tilbrook 2002). Preclinical studies showed antinociceptive effects in animal models of inflammatory and neuropathic pain (see Sect. 3) although relatively high doses were used (Parsons et al. 1999). However, clinical trials have yielded less conclusive data on its usefulness in the treatment of neuropathic pain (Parsons 2001; Kilpatrick and Tilbrook 2002). Memantine reduced nocturnal pain in patients with diabetic neuropathy but was not effective on spontaneous or evoked pain in patients with nerve injury from amputation or surgery (Kilpatrick and Tilbrook 2002). In summary, memantine may still have a place in the treatment of neuropathic pain because it is well tolerated and neuropathic pain represents one of the therapeutically most challenging pain conditions.

4.1.3
Dextromethorphan

An orally available non-competitive NMDA receptor antagonist, dextromethorphan, has a long history as a safe cough suppressant with few side effects (Fisher et al. 2000; Weinbroum et al. 2000; Fundytus 2001; Carlsson et al. 2004). Dextromethorphan showed antinociceptive effects in preclinical models of inflammatory and neuropathic pain (Sect. 3). In clinical studies, pretreatment with dextromethorphan provided preemptive analgesia for acute postoperative pain, although others observed no such effect (Weinbroum et al. 2000; Fundytus 2001; McCartney et al. 2004; Ong et al. 2005). There is, however, little evidence for analgesic effects of dextromethorphan in experimental pain in healthy human volunteers and in neuropathic pain, although a relatively high dose was analgesic in patients with diabetic or posttraumatic neuropathy (Weinbroum et al. 2000; Fundytus 2001; Henriksson and Sorensen 2002; Hewitt 2003; Carlsson et al. 2004). Intravenous ketamine has been proposed to have predictive value for the effectiveness of dextromethorphan in neuropathic pain (Cohen et al. 2004). Dextromethorphan appeared to be effective in a subgroup of patients with fibromyalgia and again, intravenous ketamine may help to select these patients (Henriksson and Sorensen 2002). It has also been suggested that dextromethorphan may enhance the analgesic effects of opioids and prevent opioid tolerance, but a recent study failed to show any clinical benefit of MorphiDex (Endo Pharmaceuticals, Chadds Ford, PA), a combination of morphine and dextromethorphan (Galer et al. 2005).

4.1.4
NR2B-Selective Antagonists

Commercially available NR2B receptors antagonists such as CP-101606 (traxo-prodil) and ifenprodil were antinociceptive in preclinical models of inflammatory and neuropathic pain (Sect. 3; Parsons 2001; Chizh et al. 2001; Nakazato et al. 2005). CP-101606 showed analgesic effects in pain patients with peripheral neuropathy and spinal cord injury (Nakazato et al. 2005). CP-101606 and ifen-prodil have also been tested in clinical trials for the treatment of ischemic brain injury or stroke. They were well tolerated and did not cause ataxia, sedation, or impaired learning and memory at therapeutic concentrations, suggesting a better therapeutic index than other NMDA receptor antagonists (Chizh et al. 2001; Wang and Shuaib 2005). Unfortunately, some NR2B-selective antagonists produced electrocardiographic abnormalities such as a prolonged Q-T interval through blockade of potassium channels (Parsons 2001). There is not enough clinical evidence yet to suggest any therapeutic advantages of NR2B antagonists in the treatment of pain.

4.1.5
GlycineB Site Antagonists

The presence of glycine at the strychnine-insensitive recognition site (glycineB) of the NMDA receptor is required for channel activation by glutamate or NMDA (Michaelis 1998; Dingledine et al. 1999; Wollmuth and Sobolevsky 2004; Mayer and Armstrong 2004; Mayer 2005). GlycineB site antagonists have been reported to lack the typical side effects of NMDA receptor antagonists (Parsons 2001; Wallace et al. 2002). A glycineB antagonist (GV196771) showed antinociceptive effects in preclinical models of inflammatory (formalin and carrageenan evoked) and neuropathic pain (Parsons 2001; Wallace et al. 2002). However, a clinical study found no significant effects of GV196771 on spontaneous and mechanically or thermally evoked pain in patients with neuropathic pain associated with diabetic neuropathy, postherpetic neuralgia, complex regional pain syndrome, or peripheral nerve injury (Wallace et al. 2002). A significant decrease of the size of the allodynic area was observed but did not translate into a reduction of pain (Wallace et al. 2002). The therapeutic value of glycineB antagonists for pain relief remains to be determined.

4.1.6
Side Effects

Side effects typically associated with NMDA receptor antagonists include memory impairment, psychomimetic effects, ataxia, and motor incoordination as well as neurotoxicity (Parsons 2001; Haberny et al. 2002; Low and Roland 2004). Noncompetitive NMDA receptor antagonists such as memantine and dextromethorphan are better tolerated and have fewer side effects, which has been explained by their relatively low affinity, fast kinetics, and strong voltage dependence (Parsons et al. 1999; Parsons 2001). GlycineB- and NR2B-selective antagonists show a much better profile in animal models of chronic pain than high-affinity channel blockers and competitive NMDA receptor antagonists (Parsons 2001; Chizh et al. 2001), but their clinical value as analgesics is not yet clear. Neurotoxic effects of NMDA receptor antagonists such as vacuolizations were observed with competitive and some noncompetitive NMDA receptor antagonists whereas glycineB and NR2B antagonists did not show neurotoxicity (Low and Roland 2004). They appear to be dose and time dependent. Most studies, however, were done in animals (rats) and it is not clear if NMDA receptor antagonists induce neurotoxic effects in humans. Furthermore, several compounds have been shown to prevent NMDA antagonist induced neurotoxicity; these include GABAergic, α2-adrenergic, anticholinergic, serotonergic, antipsychotic, and antiepileptic drugs (Haberny et al. 2002; Low and Roland 2004).

4.2
Non-NMDA Receptor Antagonists

Non-NMDA receptor antagonists produce antinociceptive effects in preclinical pain models but also inhibit normal nociceptive and non-nociceptive processing, which would suggest a narrow therapeutic window and make them unlikely drug targets for pain relief. Still, a systemically active non-NMDA receptor antagonist (LY293558, see the following section) has been tested in phase II clinical trials for pain. A selective AMPA receptor antagonist (YM872, zonampanel) is being studied in phase II clinical trials for potentially neuroprotective effects in stroke. In preclinical studies, YM872 inhibited normal nociceptive responses and formalin-induced pain behavior (Nishiyama et al. 2004).

4.2.1
LY293558

LY293558 is a competitive AMPA(GluR2)/kainate(GluR5) antagonist that showed antinociceptive effects in a preclinical study of formalin-induced pain behavior (Simmons et al. 1998; Gilron 2001) but also inhibited nociceptive baseline responses (Von Bergen et al. 2002). In healthy human volunteers, systemic LY293558 significantly reduced capsaicin-evoked pain and mechanical hyperalgesia and allodynia but had no effect on mechanical or heat pain evoked from normal skin (Sang et al. 1998). In clinical studies, LY293558 reduced spontaneous and movement-evoked postoperative pain following oral surgery (Gilron et al. 2000) and inhibited headache pain in patients with acute moderate or severe migraine attacks (Sang et al. 2004). It has been hypothesized that the analgesic effects of LY293558 involve its GluR5 antagonist action whereas GluR2 antagonism accounts for the side effects (see the following section).

4.2.2
Side Effects

In preclinical tests, LY293558 produced ataxia and motor deficits, but no serious side effects were observed in clinical studies involving humans. Side effects included a mild transient visual impairment (hazy vision), dizziness, and sedation (Gilron 2001). Although LY293558 was reported to be well tolerated, the therapeutic range, duration of drug action, and effect of repeated dosing remain to be determined.

5
Conclusions

Ionotropic and metabotropic glutamate receptors (iGluRs and mGluRs) regulate and fine-tune neurotransmission and neuronal excitability throughout the nervous system and along the pain neuraxis through a variety of mechanisms. They are involved in a number of physiological and pathological processes and are emerging as promising therapeutic targets for the treatment of certain pain conditions in preclinical and some clinical studies. Despite the diversity of iGluR and mGluR mediated effects, it appears that antagonists for iGluRs and group I mGluRs and agonists for group II and III mGluRs can inhibit nociceptive processing in various parts of the nervous system. Among the iGluRs, NMDA and kainate receptors are more useful targets than AMPA receptors. It has also been suggested that group I mGluR1 antagonists may be better candidates for pain relief than mGluR5 antagonists particularly for the treatment of neuropathic pain. Group II agonists appear to hold more promise than group III agonists, but the latter have been not been studied extensively and subtype-selective agonists are still largely missing.

Although some evidence suggests distinct antinociceptive effects of subtype-selective agents on mechanical versus thermal and inflammatory versus neuropathic pain and in different parts of the nervous system, a consistent pattern has yet to emerge. The continued development of subtype-selective agents and analysis of their antinociceptive effects in different parts of the nervous system and in different pain models will provide answers in the near future. Of particular importance may be the fact that in the brainstem (PAG) some iGluRs and mGluRs produce effects opposite to those observed in the periphery and spinal cord. The role of glutamate receptors in higher brain centers in preclinical pain models is still understudied and awaits a systematic and comparative analysis. The increasing availability of orally active compounds that can be tested and used clinically is extremely promising and suggests that certain iGluR and mGluR ligands can become novel pharmacological therapeutics for pain relief. Glutamate receptor ligands may provide new alternatives or supplements to currently available analgesics.

Acknowledgements Work in the author's laboratory is supported by National Institutes of Health (NIH) grants NS38261 and NS11255.

References

Anwyl R (1999) Metabotropic glutamate receptors: electrophysiological properties and role in plasticity. Brain Res Brain Res Rev 29:83–120

Bardoni R, Torsney C, Tong CK, Prandini M, MacDermott AB (2004) Presynaptic NMDA receptors modulate glutamate release from primary sensory neurons in rat spinal cord dorsal horn. J Neurosci 24:2774–2781

Berrino L, Oliva P, Rossi F, Palazzo E, Nobili B, Maione S (2001) Interaction between metabotropic and NMDA glutamate receptors in the periaqueductal grey pain modulatory system. Naunyn Schmiedebergs Arch Pharmacol 364:437–443

Bhave G, Nadin BM, Brasier DJ, Glauner KS, Shah RD, Heinemann SF, Karim F, Gereau RW IV (2003) Membrane topology of a metabotropic glutamate receptor. J Biol Chem 278:30294–30301

Bird GC, Lash LL, Han JS, Zou X, Willis WDNeugebauer V (2005) PKA-dependent enhanced NMDA receptor function in pain-related synaptic plasticity in amygdala neurons. J Physiol Online 564.3:907–921

Bockaert J, Pin JP (1999) Molecular tinkering of G protein-coupled receptors: an evolutionary success. EMBO J 18:1723–1729

Bortolotto ZA, Lauri S, Isaac JT, Collingridge GL (2003) Kainate receptors and the induction of mossy fibre long-term potentiation. Philos Trans R Soc Lond B Biol Sci 358:657–666

Carlsson KC, Hoem NO, Moberg ER, Mathisen LC (2004) Analgesic effect of dextromethorphan in neuropathic pain. Acta Anaesthesiol Scand 48:328–336

Carlton SM (2001) Peripheral excitatory amino acids. Curr Opin Pharmacol 1:52–56

Carlton SM, Rees H, Gondesen KWillis WD (1997) Dextrorphan attenuates responses of spinothalamic tract cells in normal and nerve-injured monkeys. Neurosci Lett 229:169–172

Carlton SM, Rees H, Tsuruoka MWillis WD (1998) Memantine attenuates responses of spinothalamic tract cells to cutaneous stimulation in neuropathic monkeys. Eur J Pain 2:229–238

Cartmell J, Schoepp DD (2000) Regulation of neurotransmitter release by metabotropic glutamate receptors. J Neurochem 75:889–907

Chittajallu R, Braithwaite SP, Clarke VR, Henley JM (1999) Kainate receptors: subunits, synaptic localization and function. Trends Pharmacol Sci 20:26–35

Chizh BA, Headley PM, Tzschentke TM (2001) NMDA receptor antagonists as analgesics: focus on the NR2B subtype. Trends Pharmacol Sci 22:636–642

Cohen SP, Chang AS, Larkin T, Mao J (2004) The intravenous ketamine test: a predictive response tool for oral dextromethorphan treatment in neuropathic pain. Anesth Analg 99:1753–1759

Conn PJ, Niswender CM (2006) mGluR7's lucky number. Proc Natl Acad Sci U S A 103:251–252

De Blasi A, Conn PJ, Pin J, Nicoletti F (2001) Molecular determinants of metabotropic glutamate receptor signaling. Trends Pharmacol Sci 22:114–120

Dingledine R, Borges K, Bowie D, Traynelis SF (1999) The glutamate receptor ion channels. Pharmacol Rev 51:7–61

Dominguez E, Iyengar S, Shannon HE, Bleakman D, Alt A, Arnold BM, Bell MG, Bleisch TJ, Buckmaster JL, Castano AM, Del Prado M, Escribano A, Filla SA, Ho KH, Hudziak KJ, Jones CK, Martinez-Perez JA, Mateo A, Mathes BM, Mattiuz EL, Ogden AM, Simmons RM, Stack DR, Stratford RE, Winter MA, Wu Z, Ornstein PL (2005) Two prodrugs of potent and selective GluR5 kainate receptor antagonists actives in three animal models of pain. J Med Chem 48:4200–4203

Du J, Zhou S, Coggeshall RE, Carlton SM (2003) N-methyl-D-aspartate-induced excitation and sensitization of normal and inflamed nociceptors. Neuroscience 118:547–562

Fisher K, Coderre TJ, Hagen NA (2000) Targeting the N-methyl-D-aspartate receptor for chronic pain management. Preclinical animal studies, recent clinical experience and future research directions. J Pain Symptom Manage 20:358–373

Fundytus ME (2001) Glutamate receptors and nociception. Implications for the drug treatment of pain. CNS Drugs 15:29–58

Galer BS, Lee D, Ma T, Nagle B, Schlagheck TG (2005) MorphiDex[trademark] (morphine sulfate/dextromethorphan hydrobromide combination) in the treatment of chronic pain: three multicenter, randomized, double-blind, controlled clinical trials fail to demonstrate enhanced opioid analgesia or reduction in tolerance. Pain 115:284–295

Garry EM, Jones E, Fleetwood-Walker SM (2004) Nociception in vertebrates: key receptors participating in spinal mechanisms of chronic pain in animals. Brain Res Brain Res Rev 46:216–224

Gasparini F, Kuhn R, Pin JP (2002) Allosteric modulators of group I metabotropic glutamate receptors: novel subtype-selective ligands and therapeutic perspectives. Curr Opin Pharmacol 2:43–49

Gebhart GF (2004) Descending modulation of pain. Neurosci Biobehav Rev 27:729–737

Gerber G, Youn DH, Hsu CH, Isaev D, Randic M (2000a) Spinal dorsal horn synaptic plasticity: involvement of group I metabotropic glutamate receptors. Prog Brain Res 129:115–134

Gerber G, Zhong J, Youn D, Randic M (2000b) Group II and group III metabotropic glutamate receptor agonists depress synaptic transmission in the rat spinal cord dorsal horn. Neuroscience 100:393–406

Gilron I (2001) LY-293558. Eli Lilly and Co. Curr Opin Investig Drugs 2:1273–1278

Gilron I, Max MB, Lee G, Booher SL, Sang CN, Chappell AS, Dionne RA (2000) Effects of the 2-amino-3-hydroxy-5-methyl-4-isoxazole-proprionic acid/kainate antagonist LY293558 on spontaneous and evoked postoperative pain. Clin Pharmacol Ther 68:320–327

Haberny KA, Paule MG, Scallet AC, Sistare FD, Lester DS, Hanig JP, Slikker W Jr (2002) Ontogeny of the N-methyl-D-aspartate (NMDA) receptor system and susceptibility to neurotoxicity. Toxicol Sci 68:9–17

Han JSNeugebauer V (2005) mGluR1 and mGluR5 antagonists in the amygdala inhibit different components of audible and ultrasonic vocalizations in a model of arthritic pain. Pain 113:211–222

Heinricher MM, Pertovaara AOssipov MH (2003) Descending modulation after injury. Prog Pain Res Manag 24:251–260

Henriksson KG, Sorensen J (2002) The promise of N-methyl-D-aspartate receptor antagonists in fibromyalgia. Rheum Dis Clin North Am 28:343–351

Hewitt DJ (2003) N-methyl-D-aspartate-enhanced analgesia. Curr Pain Headache Rep 7: 43–47

Hu HJ, Bhave G, Gereau RW IV (2002) Prostaglandin and protein kinase A-dependent modulation of vanilloid receptor function by metabotropic glutamate receptor 5: potential mechanism for thermal hyperalgesia. J Neurosci 22:7444–7452

Jang JH, Kim DW, Sang Nam T, Se Paik K, Leem JW (2004) Peripheral glutamate receptors contribute to mechanical hyperalgesia in a neuropathic pain model of the rat. Neuroscience 128:169–176

Jones CK, Eberle EL, Peters SC, Monn JA, Shannon HE (2005) Analgesic effects of the selective group II (mGlu2/3) metabotropic glutamate receptor agonists LY379268 and LY389795 in persistent and inflammatory pain models after acute and repeated dosing. Neuropharmacology 49:206–218

Karim F, Wang CC, Gereau RW (2001) Metabotropic glutamate receptor subtypes 1 and 5 are activators of extracellular signal-regulated kinase signaling required for inflammatory pain in mice. J Neurosci 21:3771–3779

Kilpatrick GJ, Tilbrook GS (2002) Memantine. Merz. Curr Opin Investig Drugs 3:798–806

Kolhekar R, Murphy S, Gebhart GF (1997) Thalamic NMDA receptors modulate inflammation-produced hyperalgesia in the rat. Pain 71:31–40

Lawand NB, Willis WD, Westlund KN (1997) Excitatory amino acid receptor involvement in peripheral nociceptive transmission in rats. Eur J Pharmacol 324:169–177

Lee CJ, Bardoni R, Tong CK, Engelman HS, Joseph DJ, Magherini PC, MacDermott AB (2002) Functional expression of AMPA receptors on central terminals of rat dorsal root ganglion neurons and presynaptic inhibition of glutamate release. Neuron 35:135–146

Lei LG, Sun S, Gao YJ, Zhao ZQ, Zhang YQ (2004) NMDA receptors in the anterior cingulate cortex mediate pain-related aversion. Exp Neurol 189:413–421

Lerma J (2003) Roles and rules of kainate receptors in synaptic transmission. Nat Rev Neurosci 4:481–495

Lerma J, Paternain AV, Rodriguez-Moreno A, Lopez-Garcia JC (2001) Molecular physiology of kainate receptors. Physiol Rev 81:971–998

Lesage ASJ (2004) Role of group I metabotropic glutamate receptors mGlu1 and mGlu5 in nociceptive signalling. Curr Neuropharmacol 2:363–393

Li W, Neugebauer V (2004a) Differential roles of mGluR1 and mGluR5 in brief and prolonged nociceptive processing in central amygdala neurons. J Neurophysiol 91:13–24

Li W, Neugebauer V (2004b) Block of NMDA and non-NMDA receptor activation results in reduced background and evoked activity of central amygdala neurons in a model of arthritic pain. Pain 110:112–122

Low SJ, Roland CL (2004) Review of NMDA antagonist-induced neurotoxicity and implications for clinical development. Int J Clin Pharmacol Ther 42:1–14

Lu CR, Willcockson HH, Phend KD, Lucifora S, Darstein M, Valtschanoff JG, Rustioni A (2005) Ionotropic glutamate receptors are expressed in GABAergic terminals in the rat superficial dorsal horn. J Comp Neurol 486:169–178

Maj M, Bruno V, Dragic Z, Yamamoto R, Battaglia G, Inderbitzin W, Stoehr N, Stein T, Gasparini F, Vranesic I (2003) (−)-PHCCC, a positive allosteric modulator of mGluR4: characterization, mechanism of action, and neuroprotection. Neuropharmacology 45: 895–906

Maione S, Marabese I, Leyva J, Palazzo E, de Novellis V, Rossi F (1998) Characterisation of mGluRs which modulate nociception in the PAG of the mouse. Neuropharmacology 37:1475–1483

Maione S, Oliva P, Marabese I, Palazzo E, Rossi F, Berrino L, Rossi F, Filippelli A (2000) Periaqueductal gray matter metabotropic glutamate receptors modulate formalin-induced nociception. Pain 85:183–189

Mayer ML (2005) Glutamate receptor ion channels. Curr Opin Neurobiol 15:282–288

Mayer ML, Armstrong N (2004) Structure and function of glutamate receptor ion channels. Annu Rev Physiol 66:161–181

McCartney CJ, Sinha A, Katz J (2004) A qualitative systematic review of the role of N-methyl-D-aspartate receptor antagonists in preventive analgesia. Anesth Analg 98:1385–1400

McNearney T, Speegle D, Lawand N, Lisse J, Westlund KN (2000) Excitatory amino acid profiles of synovial fluid from patients with arthritis. J Rheumatol 27:739–745

McRoberts JA, Coutinho SV, Marvizon JC, Grady EF, Tognetto M, Sengupta JN, Ennes HS, Chaban VV, Amadesi S, Creminon C (2001) Role of peripheral N-methyl-D-aspartate (NMDA) receptors in visceral nociception in rats. Gastroenterology 120:1737–1748

Michaelis EK (1998) Molecular biology of glutamate receptors in the central nervous system and their role in excitotoxicity, oxidative stress and aging. Prog Neurobiol 54:369–415

Mitsukawa K, Yamamoto R, Ofner S, Nozulak J, Pescott O, Lukic S, Stoehr N, Mombereau C, Kuhn R, McAllister KH, van der Putten H, Cryan JF, Flor PJ (2005) A selective metabotropic glutamate receptor 7 agonist: activation of receptor signaling via an allosteric site modulates stress parameters in vivo. Proc Natl Acad Sci U S A 102:18712–18717

Moore KA, Baba H, Woolf CJ (2000) Synaptic transmission and plasticity in the superficial dorsal horn. Prog Brain Res 129:63–80

More JC, Nistico R, Dolman NP, Clarke VR, Alt AJ, Ogden AM, Buelens FP, Troop HM, Kelland EE, Pilato F, Bleakman D, Bortolotto ZA, Collingridge GL, Jane DE (2004) Characterisation of UBP296: a novel, potent and selective kainate receptor antagonist. Neuropharmacology 47:46–64

Nagy GG, Watanabe M, Fukaya M, Todd AJ (2004) Synaptic distribution of the NR1, NR2A and NR2B subunits of the N-methyl-D-aspartate receptor in the rat lumbar spinal cord revealed with an antigen-unmasking technique. Eur J Neurosci 20:3301–3312

Nakazato E, Kato A, Watanabe S (2005) Brain but not spinal NR2B receptor is responsible for the anti-allodynic effect of an NR2B subunit-selective antagonist CP-101,606 in a rat chronic constriction injury model. Pharmacology 73:8–14

Neto FL, Castro-Lopes JM (2000) Antinociceptive effect of a group II metabotropic glutamate receptor antagonist in the thalamus of monoarthritic rats. Neurosci Lett 296:25–28

Neugebauer V (2001) Metabotropic glutamate receptors: novel targets for pain relief. Expert Rev Neurother 1:207–224

Neugebauer V (2002) Metabotropic glutamate receptors—important modulators of nociception and pain behavior. Pain 98:1–8

Neugebauer V, Chen P-SWillis WD (2000) Groups II and III metabotropic glutamate receptors differentially modulate brief and prolonged nociception in primate STT cells. J Neurophysiol 84:2998–3009

Neugebauer V, Chen PS, Willis WD (1999) Role of metabotropic glutamate receptor subtype mGluR1 in brief nociception and central sensitization of primate STT cells. J Neurophysiol 82:272–282

Neugebauer V, Li W, Bird GC, Bhave GGereau RW (2003) Synaptic plasticity in the amygdala in a model of arthritic pain: differential roles of metabotropic glutamate receptors 1 and 5. J Neurosci 23:52–63

Neugebauer V, Li W, Bird GCHan JS (2004) The amygdala and persistent pain. Neuroscientist 10:221–234

Neugebauer VCarlton SM (2002) Peripheral metabotropic glutamate receptors as drug targets for pain relief. Expert Opin Ther Targets 6:349–361

Nishimura W, Muratani T, Tatsumi S, Sakimura K, Mishina M, Minami T, Ito S (2004) Characterization of N-methyl-D-aspartate receptor subunits responsible for postoperative pain. Eur J Pharmacol 503:71–75

Nishiyama T, Kawasaki-Yatsugi S, Yamaguchi T, Hanaoka K (2004) Spinal neurotoxicity and tolerance after repeated intrathecal administration of YM 872, an AMPA receptor antagonist, in rats. J Anesth 18:113–117

Ong CK, Lirk P, Seymour RA, Jenkins BJ (2005) The efficacy of preemptive analgesia for acute postoperative pain management: a meta-analysis. Anesth Analg 100:757–773

Palecek J, Neugebauer V, Carlton SM, Iyengar S, Willis WD (2004) The effect of a kainate GluR5 receptor antagonist on responses of spinothalamic tract neurons in a model of peripheral neuropathy in primates. Pain 111:151–161

Parsons CG (2001) NMDA receptors as targets for drug action in neuropathic pain. Eur J Pharmacol 429:71–78

Parsons CG, Danysz W, Quack G (1999) Memantine is a clinically well tolerated N-methyl-D-aspartate (NMDA) receptor antagonist—a review of preclinical data. Neuropharmacology 38:735–767

Porreca F, Ossipov MH, Gebhart GF (2002) Chronic pain and medullary descending facilitation. Trends Neurosci 25:319–325

Ren K, Dubner R (2002) Descending modulation in persistent pain: an update. Pain 100:1–6

Ruscheweyh R, Sandkuhler J (2002) Role of kainate receptors in nociception. Brain Res Brain Res Rev 40:215–222

Salt TE (2002) Glutamate receptor functions in sensory relay in the thalamus. Philos Trans R Soc Lond B Biol Sci 357:1759–1766

Salt TE, Binns KE (2000) Contributions of mGlu1 and mGlu5 receptors to interactions with N-methyl-D-aspartate receptor-mediated responses and nociceptive sensory responses of rat thalamic neurons. Neuroscience 100:375–380

Salt TE, Eaton SA, Turner JP (1996) Characterization of the metabotropic glutamate receptors (mGluRs) which modulate GABA-mediated inhibition in the ventrobasal thalamus. Neurochem Int 29:317–322

Sang CN, Hostetter MP, Gracely RH, Chappell AS, Schoepp DD, Lee G, Whitcup S, Caruso R, Max MB (1998) AMPA/kainate antagonist LY293558 reduces capsaicin-evoked hyperalgesia but not pain in normal skin in humans. Anesthesiology 89:1060–1067

Sang CN, Ramadan NM, Wallihan RG, Chappell AS, Freitag FG, Smith TR, Silberstein SD, Johnson KW, Phebus LA, Bleakman D, Ornstein PL, Arnold B, Tepper SJ, Vandenhende F (2004) LY293558, a novel AMPA/GluR5 antagonist, is efficacious and well-tolerated in acute migraine. Cephalalgia 24:596–602

Schaible HG, Ebersberger A, von Banchet GS (2002) Mechanisms of pain in arthritis. Ann N Y Acad Sci 966:343–354

Schoepp DD, Jane DE, Monn JA (1999) Pharmacological agents acting at subtypes of metabotropic glutamate receptors. Neuropharmacology 38:1431–1476

Shipe WD, Wolkenberg SE, Williams DL Jr, Lindsley CW (2005) Recent advances in positive allosteric modulators of metabotropic glutamate receptors. Curr Opin Drug Discov Devel 8:449–457

Simmons RM, Li DL, Hoo KH, Deverill M, Ornstein PL, Iyengar S (1998) Kainate GluR5 receptor subtype mediates the nociceptive response to formalin in the rat. Neuropharmacology 37:25–36

Simmons RM, Webster AA, Kalra AB, Iyengar S (2002) Group II mGluR receptor agonists are effective in persistent and neuropathic pain models in rats. Pharmacol Biochem Behav 73:419–427

Soliman AC, Yu JSC, Coderre TJ (2005) mGlu and NMDA receptor contributions to capsaicin-induced thermal and mechanical hypersensitivity. Neuropharmacology 48:325–332

Stanfa LC, Dickenson AH (1999) The role of non-N-methyl-D-aspartate ionotropic gluta-mate receptors in the spinal transmission of nociception in normal animals and animals with carrageenan inflammation. Neuroscience 93:1391–1398

Sutton JL, Maccecchini ML, Kajander KC (1999) The kainate receptor antagonist 2S,4R-4-methylglutamate attenuates mechanical allodynia and thermal hyperalgesia in a rat model of nerve injury. Neuroscience 91:283–292

Swanson CJ, Bures M, Johnson MP, Linden AM, Monn JA, Schoepp DD (2005) Metabotropic glutamate receptors as novel targets for anxiety and stress disorders. Nat Rev Drug Discov 4:131–144

Thomas NK, Wright RA, Howson PA, Kingston AE, Schoepp DD, Jane DE (2001) (S)-3,4-DCPG, a potent and selective mGlu8a receptor agonist, activates metabotropic glutamate receptors on primary afferent terminals in the neonatal rat spinal cord. Neuropharma-cology 40:311–318

Tolle TR, Berthele A, Zieglgansberger W, Seeburg PH, Wisden W (1993) The differential expression of 16 NMDA and non-NMDA receptor subunits in the rat spinal cord and in periaqueductal gray. J Neurosci 13:5009–5028

Urban MO, Coutinho SV, Gebhart GF (1999) Involvement of excitatory amino acid re-ceptors and nitric oxide in the rostral ventromedial medulla in modulating secondary hyperalgesia produced by mustard oil. Pain 81:45–55

Vaccarino AL, Clemmons HR, Mader J, Magnusson JE (1997) A role of periaqueductal grey NMDA receptors in mediating formalin-induced pain in the rat. Neurosci Lett 236:117–119

Vanegas H, Schaible HG (2004) Descending control of persistent pain: inhibitory or facili-tatory? Brain Res Brain Res Rev 46:295–309

Varney MAGereau RW (2002) Metabotropic glutamate receptor involvement in models of acute and persistent pain: prospects for the development of novel analgesics. Curr Drug Targets 1:215–225

Varty GB, Grilli M, Forlani A, Fredduzzi S, Grzelak ME, Guthrie DH, Hodgson RA, Lu SX, Nicolussi E, Pond AJ, Parker EM, Hunter JC, Higgins GA, Reggiani A, Bertorelli R (2005) The antinociceptive and anxiolytic-like effects of the metabotropic glutamate receptor 5 (mGluR5) antagonists, MPEP and MTEP, and the mGluR1 antagonist, LY456236, in rodents: a comparison of efficacy and side-effect profiles. Psychopharmacology (Berl) 179:207–217

Von Bergen NH, Subieta A, Brennan TJ (2002) Effect of intrathecal non-NMDA EAA receptor antagonist LY293558 in rats: a new class of drugs for spinal anesthesia. Anesthesiology 97:177–182

Wallace MS, Rowbotham MC, Katz NP, Dworkin RH, Dotson RM, Galer BS, Rauck RL, Backonja MM, Quessy SN, Meisner PD (2002) A randomized, double-blind, placebo-controlled trial of a glycine antagonist in neuropathic pain. Neurology 59:1694–1700

Wang CX, Shuaib A (2005) NMDA/NR2B selective antagonists in the treatment of ischemic brain injury. Curr Drug Targets CNS Neurol Disord 4:143–151

Wei F, Wang GD, Kerchner GA, Kim SJ, Xu HM, Chen ZF, Zhuo M (2001) Genetic enhance-ment of inflammatory pain by forebrain NR2B overexpression. Nat Neurosci 4:164–169

Wei F, Qiu CS, Kim SJ, Muglia L, Maas J, Pineda VV, Xu HM, Chen ZF, Storm DR (2002) Genetic elimination of behavioral sensitization in mice lacking calmodulin-stimulated adenylyl cyclases. Neuron 36:713–726

Weinbroum AA, Rudick V, Paret G, Ben-Abraham R (2000) The role of dextromethorphan in pain control. Can J Anaesth 47:585–596

Willis WD (2001) Role of neurotransmitters in sensitization of pain responses. Ann N Y Acad Sci 933:142–156

Willis WD, Coggeshall RE (2004) Sensory mechanisms of the spinal cord. Kluwer Academic/Plenum, New York

Wollmuth LP, Sobolevsky AI (2004) Structure and gating of the glutamate receptor ion channel. Trends Neurosci 27:321–328

Woolf CJ (2004) Pain: moving from symptom control toward mechanism-specific pharmacologic management. Ann Intern Med 140:441–451

Yang D, Gereau RW (2002) Peripheral group II metabotropic glutamate receptors (mGluR2/3) regulate prostaglandin E2-mediated sensitization of capsaicin responses and thermal nociception. J Neurosci 22:6388–6393

Yang D, Gereau RW (2003) Peripheral group II metabotropic glutamate receptors mediate endogenous anti-allodynia in inflammation. Pain 106:411–417

Youn DH, Randic M (2004) Modulation of excitatory synaptic transmission in the spinal substantia gelatinosa of mice deficient in the kainate receptor GluR5 and/or GluR6 subunit. J Physiol 555:683–698

HEP (2006) 177:251–264

Adrenergic and Cholinergic Compounds

R. D. Sanders · M. Maze (✉)

Academic Anaesthetics, Imperial College, Chelsea and Westminster Hospital, 369 Fulham Road, London SW10 9NH, UK
m.maze@ic.ac.uk

1   Introduction   252

2   Adrenergic Compounds   252
2.1   α₂ Adrenergic Receptors and Substrates   253
2.1.1 Pharmacogenetic Studies   253
2.1.2 Site of Action   253
2.2   Supraspinal Effects   254
2.3   Spinal Effects   254
2.3.1 Clinical Application: Acute Pain   255
2.3.2 Clinical Application: Chronic Pain   256

3   Conclusion: α₂ Adrenergic Agonists   256

4   Cholinergic Agents   256
4.1   Cholinergic Receptors and Substrates   257
4.2   Pharmacogenetic Studies   257
4.3   Anti-cholinesterase Inhibitors   258
4.4   Nicotinic Agonists   258
4.5   Muscarinic Agonists   259

5   Conclusion: Cholinergic Agents   260

References   260

Abstract Adrenergic and cholinergic signalling contributes significantly to the endogenous antinociceptive system. Exogenous α₂ adrenergic agonists have a well-established analgesic profile; however, recent investigations suggest that this class of agents is underused, and herein we highlight the potential for both current application and future development of these agents. Nicotinic and muscarinic cholinergic ligands represent a novel class of agents with much promise for the management of problematic pain. In this chapter we review advances in both preclinical and clinical arenas and highlight potential avenues for further research.

Keywords Pain · Antinociception · Adrenergic · Clonidine · Dexmedetomidine · Cholinergic · Nicotinic · Muscarinic

1
Introduction

Pain management remains a real and current problem in clinical medicine; in the United States 70%–80% of surgical patients experience moderate to severe post-operative pain (Owen et al. 1990; Svensson et al. 2000; Thomas et al. 1998). This does not merely reflect inadequate pain management strategies at a local level but also poor efficacy and poor tolerability of the analgesic agents. For example, opioid administration is commonly limited by side-effects from respiratory and gastrointestinal symptoms. To enable more effective therapy multi-modal strategies are now employed; however, new agents with improved efficacy are required to help combat problematic pain management. In addition, chronic and neuropathic pain syndromes remain resistant to current approaches, with only a minority of patients responding mostly at the expense of significant side-effects (Arner and Meyerson 1988).

With administration via systemic or regional approaches for acute, chronic and neuropathic pain, α_2 adrenergic agonists remain a potent but relatively underused class of analgesic agents. Below we review supporting evidence for an expanding role of this class of agents and explore their mechanisms of action.

At present, cholinergic compounds, both nicotinic and muscarinic, are being developed as novel analgesics and herein we review their progress. Furthermore, there is substantial overlap in the mechanisms of action of both of these classes of agents; further scientific exploration is required to inform us about their potential adjuvant administration.

2
Adrenergic Compounds

Adrenergic signalling is one of the primary components of the endogenous antinociceptive system that modulates pain responses. Acting at spinal and supraspinal sites, norepinephrine release is involved in the control of a wide range of pain responses via activation of α_2 and α_1 adrenoceptors. Descending inhibitory neurons (DINs) are an important component of the antinociceptive system. Activated from supraspinal sites such as the periaqueductal grey and dorsal raphe nucleus (Jones and Gebhart 1984; Tjolsen et al. 1990) as well as other brainstem nuclei such as the A5 and A7, they inhibit the nociceptive responses in the dorsal horn of the spinal cord via release of norepinephrine, serotonin and acetylcholine (Li and Zhuo 2001). In the dorsal horn, norepinephrine depresses wide-dynamic-range neuron responses after Aδ and C nociceptive fibre activation by stimulation of α_2 adrenoceptors (Jones and Gebhart 1984). This effect of norepinephrine is mimicked by exogenous α_2 adrenoceptor agonists (Millar et al. 1993) and is thought to be dependent on stimulation of spontaneously active neurons in the deep layer of the spinal cord which release acetylcholine and enkephalins. Further indirect evidence is provided by the observation that acute pain increases norepinephrine and acetylcholine levels in the cerebrospinal fluid (CSF), and the α_2 adrenoceptor agonist clonidine increases acetylcholine in the CSF (Eisenach et al. 1996; Detweiler et al. 1993). This also indicates an interdependent antinociceptive effect exerted between the cholinergic and adrenergic systems.

2.1
α_2 Adrenergic Receptors and Substrates

When stimulated, α_2 adrenoceptors inhibit adenyl cyclase via pertussis-sensitive G proteins. These receptors are coupled, via the subunits of the G protein, to ligand-gated ion channels including the N-type calcium channel (inhibition; Adamson et al. 1989), the P/Q-type calcium channel (inhibition; Ishibashi et al. 1995), the I_A potassium channel (activation; North et al. 1987), the calcium activated potassium channel (activation; Ryan et al. 1998), the ATP-sensitive potassium channel (activation; Galeotti et al. 1999), the voltage-dependent potassium channels (activation; Galeotti et al. 1999) and the Na+/H+ antiporter (activation; Ryan et al. 1998). Furthermore, recent work has highlighted the association of α_2 adrenoceptors with G protein-coupled inwardly rectifying potassium (GIRK) channels (Blednov et al. 2003; Mitrovic et al. 2003).

2.1.1
Pharmacogenetic Studies

Using D79N mice which express dysfunctional α_{2A} adrenoceptors, Lakhlani and colleagues showed that adrenoceptor agonist antinociception (assessed by the hot plate test) and sedation were dependent on this receptor subtype (Lakhlani et al. 1997). In the absence of functional α_{2A} adrenoceptors, the agents could not suppress voltage-gated calcium or activate potassium currents. This mutation did not affect morphine analgesia. It is noteworthy, though, that pharmacogenetic analysis of different inbred mouse strains showed significant correlation between strain dependence of morphine and clonidine analgesia (in hot plate and formalin tests; Wilson et al. 2003). Furthermore, as the interaction between clonidine and morphine is synergistic (Wilcox et al. 1987) and there are overlapping pharmacogenomic substrates, investigation of downstream effectors beyond the receptor may lead to the development of novel agents which separate analgesic and sedative effects of α_2 adrenoceptor agonists.

2.1.2
Site of Action

Supraspinal and spinal targets contribute to the potent antinociceptive efficacy of α_2 adrenoceptor agonists. This is of importance because drugs which rely on DINs such as nitrous oxide are ineffective in the young, as DINs are immature in early development (Ohashi et al. 2002). The α_{2A} adrenoceptor agonist dexmedetomidine (Dex) is effective in the immature phenotype as it targets both supraspinal and spinal sites, circumventing DINs (Sanders et al. 2005).

2.2
Supraspinal Effects

The locus coeruleus (LC) is an adrenergic centre in the brainstem that tonically inhibits the A5 and A7, which are then coupled to DINs. Activation of α_2 adrenoceptors in the LC inhibits neuronal firing in this region (Guo et al. 1996). Inhibition of the LC by discrete administration of α_2 adrenoceptor agonists leads to 'disinhibition' (i.e. activation) of the A5 and A7 and therefore DINs.

2.3
Spinal Effects

Comparison between the analgesic effectiveness of clonidine after systemic or neuraxial (spinal or epidural) administration revealed that the spinal cord was an important site of action for α_2 adrenoceptor agonist-induced analgesia (Bernard et al. 1995; Eisenach et al. 1998). Furthermore, in human volunteers intrathecal (IT) clonidine was superior to intravenous clonidine against capsaicin and thermal pain (Eisenach et al. 1998).

In the dorsal horn of the spinal cord, activation of pre-synaptic α_2 adrenoceptors reduces glutamate (Li and Eisenach 2001), substance P and calcitonin gene-related peptide (CGRP) release (Takano and Yaksh 1993). Post-synaptic effects are related to activation of voltage-dependent potassium channels (Galeotti et al. 1999) and GIRK channels (Blednov et al. 2003; Mitrovic et al. 2003). In two separate studies the action of clonidine was examined in GIRK-2-null mutant mice using the hot plate test and tail flick latency (Blednov et al. 2003; Mitrovic et al. 2003); the mutation reduced clonidine antinociception almost to baseline, indicating primarily a post-synaptic action of clonidine. We have previously found electrophysiological evidence to support this genetic evidence of a post-synaptic action for α_2 adrenoceptor agonists as Dex reduces ventral root potentials (induced by substance P) in an ex vivo isolated neonatal rat spinal cord preparation. In addition, α_2 adrenoceptor agonists inhibit adenyl cyclase, which is a pivotal enzymatic step in the development of hyperalgesia at post-synaptic sites (Hoeger-Bement and Sluka 2003; Sanders et al. 2005).

Systemic administration of α_2 adrenoceptor agonists induces antinociception in several animal models with effects both at supraspinal and spinal sites. Both clonidine and dexmedetomidine increase latency of tail flick during the hot plate test in a dose-related manner (Sabbe et al. 1994). Formalin and capsaicin induce inflammatory pain with a typical biphasic pain response (acute pain and secondary hyperalgesia). α_2 Adrenoceptor agonists inhibit this pain response (Wilson et al. 2003; Sanders et al. 2005) likely via both pre-synaptic (reduction of glutamate, substance P and CGRP release) and post-synaptic (activation of GIRK channels and inhibition of adenyl cyclase) mechanisms. This underlies the known efficacy of α_2 adrenoceptor agonists in hyperalgesia and neuropathic pain-associated allodynia; α_2 adrenoceptor agonists may even show increased efficacy against neuropathic pain (Puke and Wiesenfeld-Hallin 1993). Furthermore, α_2 adrenoceptor agonists reduce allodynia after nerve lesioning models of neuropathic pain (Poree et al. 1998), which may be related to peripheral adrenoceptor activation. This potent anti-neuropathic pain effect is also reduced by acetylcholine depletion in the spinal cord (Paqueron et al. 2001) and muscarinic cholinergic antagonists (Pan et al. 1999) likely via M4 receptors (Kang and Eisenach 2003). The α_2 adrenoceptor agonists also show efficacy against visceral pain (Harada et al. 1995; Iwasaki et al. 1991) and at peripheral—such as intra-articular injection—sites (potentially mediated by local enkephalin release; Nakamura and Ferreira 1988).

Likewise, α_2 adrenoceptor agonists have long been administered for regional anaesthesia; after spinal administration in sheep they interact synergistically with opioid and cholinergic agonists and cholinesterase inhibitors such as neostigmine (Detweiler et al. 1993). This synergistic interaction has yet to be observed in humans, but opioid analgesia is enhanced in the presence of clonidine (at doses of up to 75 µg IT; Grace et al. 1994). Similarly, combination of spinal neostigmine and clonidine prolongs post-operative analgesia (Pan et al. 1998). Therefore, whether administered systemically or neuraxially, α_2 adrenoceptor agonists exert their primary analgesic effect at the level of the spinal cord.

2.3.1
Clinical Application: Acute Pain

IT administration of clonidine with local anaesthetic (LA) improves the quality and duration of the LA block but may cause greater hypotension (Bonnet et al. 1989). Similarly, epidural clonidine ($1–4\ \mu g\,kg^{-1}$) with LA improves the quality and duration of the block but does not increase hypotension. Caudal administration ($0.75–3\ \mu g\,kg^{-1}$) with LA increases anaesthesia duration two-to threefold (Lee and Rubin 1994). This may be of especial utility in paediatric anaesthesia, as children appear less susceptible to adverse haemodynamic changes (as blood pressure is less dependent on sympathetic tone at this age). Clonidine is also efficacious for labour analgesia (epidural doses of $1\ \mu g kg^{-1}$) with the epidural combination of 75 µg clonidine and 50 µg fentanyl more than doubling the duration of analgesia produced by bupivacaine alone (Celleno et al. 1995). Furthermore, clonidine is a commonly employed adjuvant for brachial plexus blocks as it significantly prolongs the duration of anaesthesia provided (Bernard and Macaire 1997).

2.3.2
Clinical Application: Chronic Pain

Epidural administration of clonidine has been associated with significant analgesia for deafferentation pain post spinal cord injury (Glynn et al. 1986), spasticity (Rémy-Néris et al. 1999), chronic arachnoiditis (Glynn et al. 1988) and for chronic sharp and shooting pains (Byas-Smith et al. 1995). Furthermore, in the treatment of intractable cancer pain, epidural clonidine (100–900 µg) produces a dose-dependent analgesia lasting up to 8 h (Eisenach et al. 1989). Two weeks of analgesia is also produced by continuous epidural infusion of 30 µg h^{-1} during which time the initial sedative effect disappears (Eisenach et al. 1995). Clonidine is now regarded a second line pharmacotherapy for the treatment of cancer pain as an adjunct or an alternative to opioids.

3
Conclusion: α_2 Adrenergic Agonists

In both the acute and chronic pain settings, α_2 adrenergic agonists remain relatively underused. With the expanding role of dexmedetomidine in the intensive care setting (Coursin et al. 2001) further information about the analgesic action of this class of agents will become available. A recent study of the systemic administration of dexmedetomidine in human volunteers found significant analgesia against thermal-induced pain (Cortinez et al. 2004), although the modality of experimental pain influences the estimation of analgesic efficacy in this type of study (Maze and Angst 2004). In addition, a recent randomised controlled trial of 34 post-operative patients showed that Dex provided more efficacious analgesia than morphine (Arain et al. 2004). However, as described above (Sect. 2.3), regional rather than systemic approaches appear more efficacious, although further clinical studies are required to quantify the systemic analgesia afforded by α_2 adrenoceptor agonists. Preclinical investigation into the downstream effectors beyond surface receptor signalling may facilitate the development of a new class of drugs to allow more effective pain relief.

4
Cholinergic Agents

As discussed in Sect. 2, the intrinsic antinociceptive system involves cholinergic signalling to modulate pain responses. Acetylcholine release induced by DINs or exogenous sources such as α_2 adrenoceptor and opiate agonists induces an antinociceptive effect (Chen and Pan 2001). Recent interest in this class of agents has been sparked by a series of interesting discoveries using genetic and pharmacological approaches.

Cholinesterase inhibitors have been used in anaesthesia for many years and their analgesic potential was highlighted over 70 years ago; recently their IT administration for analgesia has gained deserved interest (Hood et al. 1997). In human volunteers, neostigmine was shown to have an analgesic effect when given intrathecally and to potentiate systemic alfentanil analgesia. This effect was correlated with increased CSF acetylcholine.

Nicotinic acetylcholine receptor (nAChR) and muscarinic acetylcholine receptor (mAChR) agonists are antinociceptive (Traynor 1998; Eisenach 1999). Cholinergic agonists have similar efficacy to morphine; they lack the long-term addiction and withdrawal side-effects (Bannon et al. 1998; Swedberg et al. 1997) and thus may have utility in both acute and chronic pain settings. Furthermore, intranasal nicotine has recently shown potency as a post-operative analgesic (Flood and Daniel 2004).

4.1
Cholinergic Receptors and Substrates

Nicotinic cholinergic receptors are ligand-gated ion channels formed from pentamers of α subunits (containing the ACh binding site) with β, γ, δ or ϵ subunits. Neuronal nAChR are considered more diverse than their muscle equivalents, with $\alpha2$–10 and $\beta2$–4 subunits cloned in neurons. $\alpha2$–4 and 6 can form heteromeric channels with $\beta2$–4 subunits; $\alpha7$–9 form homomeric channels. In the rat brain, messenger RNA (mRNA) for $\alpha4$, $\alpha7$ and $\beta2$ subunits are widely expressed, though the $\beta2$ subunit is less abundant in the brain of primates (Tassonyi et al. 2002; Gotti et al. 2004). nAChR are excitatory in nature and likely influence learning, memory, arousal and analgesia.

mAChR are G protein-coupled channels which are either excitatory (M2 and 4) or inhibitory (M1, M3, M5) in nature. Even-numbered channels inhibit adenylyl cyclase via G_i/G_o while odd-numbered channels, coupled to G_q/G_{11}, activate phospholipase C (Caulfield and Birdsall 1998). Similar to α_2 adrenoceptors, M2 receptor activation also activates GIRK channels (Fernandez-Fernandez et al. 1999).

4.2
Pharmacogenetic Studies

Investigation of the receptor subtypes involved has been furthered greatly by the use of genetic manipulation. Knock-out mice lacking the α_4 or β_2 nAChR subunit showed reduced nicotine-elicited antinociception in the hot plate test (Marubio et al. 1999). In addition, morphine antinociception is reduced in M_4 and M_4/M_2 knock-out mice (Duttaroy et al. 2000). Similar to α_2 adrenoceptor agonists, M_2 and M_4 receptors are coupled to G_i proteins and are inhibitory in nature, and dual knock-out of both receptors abolished the antinociception induced by oxotremorine, a muscarinic agonist (Duttaroy et al. 2002). Sole knock-out of the M_2 receptor reduced antinociception (but to a lesser extent than dual knock-out) and also reduced the inhibitory action of muscarine on CGRP release from peripheral nerve endings (Bernardini et al. 2002). The antinociceptive action of oxotremorine, the muscarinic agonist, is reduced in mice with a GIRK-2-null mutation, indicating primarily a post-synaptic action of this drug via GIRK channels. As M2 channels are known to activate GIRK channels and knock-out of either reduced muscarinic receptor antinociception, it is likely that M2 and GIRK channels mediate muscarinic antinociception, at least in mice. Therefore the likely cholinergic receptor subtypes modulating pain are the nAChR α_4 or β_2, and mAChR M_2 and M_4.

4.3
Anti-cholinesterase Inhibitors

Potentiation of endogenous acetylcholine by the IT use of anti-cholinesterase inhibitors has recently gained renewed interest after recent clinical trials. Acting via both muscarinic and nicotinic receptors, acetylcholine is known to play a role in both endogenous and exogenous analgesia. Neostigmine (IT) potentiates opioid and α_2 adrenoceptor agonist-induced analgesia (Detweiler et al. 1993; Hood et al. 1997). Clinically the combination of neostigmine IT and opioid analgesia has been used successfully in gynaecological and obstetric anaesthesia; particular utility for mobile epidurals has been noted (Lauretti et al. 1998; Roelants and Lavand'homme 2004). However, nausea remains a limitation of this novel strategy and further investigation is required to fully describe the extent of this side-effect.

4.4
Nicotinic Agonists

Recent interest in nAChR agonists as analgesics was prompted by epibatidine, a compound isolated from the Ecuadorian tree frog, *Epipedobates tricolor*. Epibatidine is 200 times more potent than morphine but has a narrow therapeutic window with significant toxicity problems, including cardiovascular and motor effects (Decker and Meyer 1999). Newer compounds such as ABT-594 (Bannon et al. 1998) have an improved safety profile but similar efficacy. Importantly, ABT-594 also lacks the withdrawal side-effects and physical dependence of opioid analgesics, at least in rats. In a series of studies, Bannon and colleagues investigated the systemic efficacy of ABT-594 in models of thermal, inflammatory and neuropathic pain; the compound proved superior to morphine. The neuroanatomical locus for this effect is still under discussion but activation of the LC and serotonergic neurons in the nucleus raphe magnus which in turn activates DINs is likely to mediate the systemic analgesia of nAChR agonists (Bannon et al. 1998; Bitner et al. 1998). Consistent with this concept, intracerebroventricular pre-treatment with an α_4 antisense oligonucleotide attenuated systemic nAChR agonist analgesia. At the level of the spinal cord, serotonin release contributes to nAChR agonist analgesia likely via activation of non-$\alpha_4\beta_2$ nAChR. Activation of these receptors likely acts via 'volume transmission' whereby pre-synaptic nAChR increase serotonin release rather than directly stimulate neuronal firing (Cordero-Erausquin and Changeux 2001). nAChR agonists also activate noradrenergic and muscarinic DINs (Rogers and Iwamoto 1993) when administered systemically. Significant controversy still plagues the analgesic effects of nAChR agonists administered intrathecally with both pro- and antinociceptive actions reported (Rueter et al. 2000); therefore, further study is required before use of these compounds for regional analgesia. Systemic administration of nAChR agonists likely induces analgesia predominantly through supraspinal mechanisms with subsequent activation of DINs.

4.5
Muscarinic Agonists

Activation of muscarinic receptors induces antinociception in various pain paradigms including thermal, inflammatory and neuropathic pain (Wess et al. 2003; Kang and Eisenach 2003; Shannon et al. 2001). Both central and peripheral mechanisms of mAChR agonist analgesia exist. Central effects are likely targeted to the dorsal horn of spinal cord where M2 receptors predominate. Peripheral activation of M2 receptors likely contributes to analgesia via reduced CGRP release. However, peripheral mechanisms lead to some concern about autonomic effects of these ligands which will require careful evaluation; mAChR agonists may lend themselves to regional techniques rather than systemic approaches (potentially in contrast to nAChR agonists). Furthermore, as there is little evidence for supraspinal effects of muscarinic agonists there may be little need to employ systemic administration.

As vedaclidine exhibits the typical antinociceptive profile of a muscarinic agonist and activates M2 and M4 receptor subtypes but inhibits the odd numbered receptors (Shannon et al. 2001), it is likely that the inhibitory action of the even-numbered channels is the predominant antinociceptive mediator. Furthermore, consistent with pharmacogenomic data, muscarinic antinociception is pertussis toxin sensitive, which indicates the role of inhibitory G protein signalling, likely via M2 and M4 receptors. Further evidence that even numbered channels mediate muscarinic agonist antinociception is that M2 receptors are known to couple to GIRK receptors and GIRK-null mutants exhibit reduced muscarinic antinociception. This also indicates a post-synaptic mechanism of action; however, muscarinic antinociception is also reduced in the presence of the γ-aminobutyric acid (GABA)$_B$ receptor antagonist CGP55845, which is thought to represent a pre-synaptic effect of augmented endogenous GABA release inhibiting neurotransmitter release (Li et al. 2002). Antagonists of the M2, M3 and M4 receptor subtypes inhibit this GABA release (Zhang et al. 2005). In addition, as M4 receptors play a crucial role in the potency of α_2 adrenoceptor agonists against neuropathic pain (Kang and Eisenach 2003), targeting this receptor subtype may prove useful for problematic pain management.

5
Conclusion: Cholinergic Agents

Cholinergic agents represent a novel and potent class of new analgesics. We await the results of clinical trials to investigate their role in clinical medicine, but we hope they will enjoy clinical utility as independent and adjunctive analgesic therapy. Further investigation into the neural substrates and the receptor subtypes involved will allow further development of cholinergic strategies to combat pain.

References

Adamson P, Xiang JZ, Mantzourides T, Brammer MJ, Campbell IC (1989) Presynaptic alpha 2-adrenoceptor and kappa-opiate receptor occupancy promotes closure of neuronal (N-type) calcium channels. Eur J Pharmacol 174:63–70

Arain SR, Ruehlow RM, Uhrich TD, Ebert TJ, Arain SR, Ruehlow RM, Uhrich TD, Ebert TJ (2004) The efficacy of dexmedetomidine versus morphine for postoperative analgesia after major inpatient surgery. Anesth Analg 98:153–158

Arner S, Meyerson BA (1988) Lack of analgesic effect of opioids on neuropathic and idiopathic forms of pain. Pain 33:11–23

Bannon AW, Decker MW, Holladay MW, Curzon P, Donnelly-Roberts D, Puttfarcken PS, Bitner RS, Diaz A, Dickenson AH, Porsolt RD, Williams M, Arneric SP (1998) Broad-spectrum, non-opioid analgesic activity by selective modulation of neuronal nicotinic acetylcholine receptors. Science 279:77–81

Bernard JM, Macaire P (1997) Dose-range effects of clonidine added to lidocaine for brachial plexus block. Anesthesiology 87:277–284

Bernard JM, Kick O, Bonnet F (1995) Comparison of intravenous and epidural clonidine for postoperative patient-controlled analgesia. Anesth Analg 81:706–712

Bernardini N, Roza C, Sauer SK, Gomeza J, Wess J, Reeh PW (2002) Muscarinic M2 receptors on peripheral nerve endings: a molecular target of antinociception. J Neurosci 22:RC229

Bitner RS, Nikkel AL, Curzon P, Arneric SP, Bannon AW, Decker MW (1998) Role of the nucleus raphe magnus in antinociception produced by ABT-594: immediate early gene responses possibly linked to neuronal nicotinic acetylcholine receptors on serotonergic neurons. J Neurosci 18:5426–5432

Blednov YA, Stoffel M, Alva H, Harris RA (2003) A pervasive mechanism for analgesia: activation of GIRK2 channels. Proc Natl Acad Sci U S A 100:277–282

Bonnet F, Diallo A, Saada M, Belon M, Guilbaud M, Boico O (1989) Prevention of tourniquet pain by spinal isobaric bupivacaine with clonidine. Br J Anaesth 63:93–96

Byas-Smith MG, Max MB, Muir J, Kingman A (1995) Transdermal clonidine compared to placebo in painful diabetic neuropathy using a two-stage "enriched enrollment" design. Pain 60:267–274

Caulfield MP, Birdsall NJ (1998) International Union of Pharmacology. XVII. Classification of muscarinic acetylcholine receptors. Pharmacol Rev 50:279–290

Celleno P, Capogna G, Costantino P (1995) Comparison of fentanyl with clonidine as adjuvants for epidural analgesia with 0.125% bupivacaine in the first stage of labor. Int J Obstet Anesth 4:26–29

Chen SR, Pan HL (2001) Spinal endogenous acetylcholine contributes to the analgesic effect of systemic morphine in rats. Anesthesiology 95:525–530

Chen SR, Wess J, Pan HL (2005) Functional activity of the m2 and m4 receptor subtypes in the spinal cord studied with muscarinic acetylcholine receptor knockout mice. J Pharmacol Exp Ther 313:765–770

Cordero-Erausquin M, Changeux JP (2001) Tonic nicotinic modulation of serotoninergic transmission in the spinal cord. Proc Natl Acad Sci U S A 98:2803–2807

Cortinez LI, Hsu YW, Sum-Ping ST, Young C, Keifer JC, Macleod D, Robertson KM, Wright DR, Moretti EW, Somma J (2004) Dexmedetomidine pharmacodynamics. Part II. Crossover comparison of the analgesic effect of dexmedetomidine and remifentanil in healthy volunteers. Anesthesiology 101:1077–1083

Coursin DB, Coursin DB, Maccioli GA (2001) Dexmedetomidine. Curr Opin Crit Care 7:221–226

Decker MW, Meyer MD (1999) Therapeutic potential of neuronal nicotinic acetylcholine receptor agonists as novel analgesics. Biochem Pharmacol 58:917–923

Detweiler DJ, Eisenach JC, Tong C, Jackson C (1993) A cholinergic interaction in alpha2 adrenoreceptor-mediated antinociception in sheep. J Pharmacol Exp Ther 265:536–542

Duttaroy A, Gomeza J, Gan JW, Basile AS, Harman WD, Smith PL, Felder CC, Wess J (2000) Analysis of muscarinic agonist-induced analgesia by the use of receptor knockout mice (abstract). Neurosci Abstr 26:616–618

Duttaroy A, Gomeza J, Gan JW, Siddiqui N, Basile AS, Harman WD, Smith PL, Felder CC, Levey AI, Wess J (2002) Evaluation of muscarinic agonist-induced analgesia in muscarinic acetylcholine receptor knockout mice. Mol Pharmacol 62:1084–1093

Eisenach J, Rauck RLR, Buzzanell C, Lysak SZ (1989) Epidural clonidine analgesia for intractable cancer pain: phase I. Anesthesiology 71:647–652

Eisenach JC (1999) Muscarinic-mediated analgesia. Life Sci 64:549–554

Eisenach JC, DuPen S, Dubois M, Miguel R, Allin D (1995) Epidural clonidine analgesia for intractable cancer pain. The Epidural Clonidine Study Group. Pain 61:391–399

Eisenach JC, Detweiler DJ, Tong C, D'Angelo R, Hood DD (1996) Cerebrospinal fluid norepinephrine and acetylcholine concentrations during acute pain. Anesth Analg 82:621–626

Eisenach JC, Hood DD, Curry R (1998) Intrathecal, but not intravenous, clonidine reduces experimental thermal or capsaicin-induced pain and hyperalgesia in normal volunteers. Anesth Analg 87:591–596

Fernandez-Fernandez JM, Wanaverbecq N, Halley P, Caulfield MP, Brown DA (1999) Selective activation of heterologously expressed G protein-gated K+ channels by M2 muscarinic receptors in rat sympathetic neurones. J Physiol 515:631–637

Flood P, Daniel D (2004) Intranasal nicotine for postoperative pain treatment. Anesthesiology 101:1417–1421

Galeotti N, Ghelardini C, Vinci MC, Bartolini A (1999) Role of potassium channels in the antinociception induced by agonists of alpha2-adrenoceptors. Br J Pharmacol 126:1214–1220

Glynn C, Dawson D, Sanders R (1988) A double-blind comparison between epidural morphine and epidural clonidine, in patients with chronic non-cancer pain. Pain 34:123–128

Glynn CJ, Jamous MA, Teddy PJ, Moore RA, Lloyd JW (1986) Role of spinal noradrenergic system in transmission of pain in patients with spinal cord injury. Lancet 2:1249–1250

Gotti C, Clementi F (2004) Neuronal nicotinic receptors: from structure to pathology. Prog Neurobiol 74:363–396

Grace D, Bunting H, Milligan KR, Fee JP (1995) Postoperative analgesia after co-administration of clonidine and morphine by the intrathecal route in patients undergoing hip replacement. Anesth Analg 80:86–91

Guo TZ, Jiang JY, Buttermann AE, Maze M (1996) Dexmedetomidine injection into the locus ceruleus produces antinociception. Anesthesiology 84:873–881

Harada Y, Nishioka K, Kitahata LM, Kishikawa K, Collins JG (1995) Visceral antinociceptive effects of spinal clonidine combined with morphine, [D-Pen2, D-Pen5] enkephalin, or U50,488H. Anesthesiology 83:344–352

Hoeger-Bement MK, Sluka KA (2003) Phosphorylation of CREB and mechanical hyperalgesia is reversed by blockade of the cAMP pathway in a time-dependent manner after repeated intramuscular acid injections. J Neurosci 23:5437–5445

Hood DD, Mallak KA, James RL, Tuttle R, Eisenach JC (1997) Enhancement of analgesia from systemic opioid in humans by spinal cholinesterase inhibition. J Pharmacol Exp Ther 282:86–92

Ishibashi H, Akaike N (1995) Norepinephrine modulates high voltage-activated calcium channels in freshly dissociated rat nucleus tractus solitarii neurons. Neuroscience 68:1139–1146

Iwasaki H, Collins JG, Saito Y, Uchida H, Kerman-Hinds A (1991) Low dose clonidine enhances pregnancy-induced analgesia to visceral but not somatic stimuli in rats. Anesth Analg 72:325–329

Jones SL, Gebhart GF (1986) Characterization of coerulospinal inhibition of the nociceptive tail-flick reflex in the rat: mediation by spinal a2-adrenoreceptors. Brain Res 364:315–330

Kang YJ, Eisenach JC (2003) Intrathecal clonidine reduces hypersensitivity after nerve injury by a mechanism involving spinal m4 muscarinic receptors. Anesth Analg 96:1403–1408

Lakhlani PP, MacMillan LB, Guo TZ, McCool BA, Lovinger DM, Maze M, Limbird LE (1997) Substitution of a mutant alpha2a-adrenergic receptor via "hit and run" gene targeting reveals the role of this subtype in sedative, analgesic, and anesthetic-sparing responses in vivo. Proc Natl Acad Sci U S A 94:9950–9955

Lauretti GR, Hood DD, Eisenach JC, Pfeifer BL (1998) A multi-center study of intrathecal neostigmine for analgesia following vaginal hysterectomy. Anesthesiology 89:913–918

Lee JJ, Rubin AP (1994) Comparison of a bupivacaine-clonidine mixture with plain bupivacaine for caudal analgesia in children. Br J Anaesth 72:258–262

Li DP, Chen SR, Pan YZ, Levey AI, Pan HL (2002) Role of presynaptic muscarinic and GABA(B) receptors in spinal glutamate release and cholinergic analgesia in rats. J Physiol 543:807–818

Li P, Zhuo M (2001) Cholinergic, noradrenergic, and serotonergic inhibition of fast synaptic transmission in spinal lumbar dorsal horn of rat. Brain Res Bull 54:639–647

Li X, Eisenach JC (2001) alpha2A-adrenoceptor stimulation reduces capsaicin-induced glutamate release from spinal cord synaptosomes. J Pharmacol Exp Ther 299:939–944

Marubio LM, del Mar Arroyo-Jimenez M, Cordero-Erausquin M, Lena C, Le Novere N, de Kerchove d'Exaerde A, Huchet M, Damaj MI, Changeux JP (1999) Reduced antinociception in mice lacking neuronal nicotinic receptor subunits. Nature 398:805–810

Maze M, Angst MS (2004) Dexmedetomidine and opioid interactions: defining the role of dexmedetomidine for intensive care unit sedation. Anesthesiology 101:1059–1061

Millar J, O'Brien FE, Williams GV, Wood J (1993) The effect of iontophoretic clonidine on neurones in the rat superficial dorsal horn. Pain 53:137–145

Mitrovic I, Margeta-Mitrovic M, Bader S, Stoffel M, Jan LY, Basbaum AI (2003) Contribution of GIRK2-mediated postsynaptic signaling to opiate and alpha 2-adrenergic analgesia and analgesic sex differences. Proc Natl Acad Sci U S A 100:271–276

Nakamura M, Ferreira SH (1998) Peripheral analgesic action of clonidine: mediation by enkephalin-like substances. Eur J Pharmacol 146:223–228

North RA, Williams JT, Surprenant A, Christie MJ (1997) Mu and delta opioid receptors belong to a family of receptors that are coupled to potassium channels. Proc Natl Acad Sci U S A 84:5487–5491

Ohashi Y, Stowell JM, Nelson LE, Hashimoto T, Maze M, Fujinaga M (2002) Nitrous oxide exerts age-dependent antinociceptive effects in Fischer rats. Pain 100:7–18

Owen H, McMillan V, Rogowski D (1990) Postoperative pain therapy: a survey of patients' expectations and their experiences. Pain 41:303–307

Pan HL, Chen SR, Eisenach JC (1999) Intrathecal clonidine alleviates allodynia in neuropathic rats: interaction with spinal muscarinic and nicotinic receptors. Anesthesiology 90:509–514

Pan PM, Huang CT, Wei TT, Mok MS (1998) Enhancement of analgesic effect of intrathecal neostigmine, clonidine on bupivacaine spinal anesthesia. Reg Anesth Pain Med 23:49–56

Paqueron X, Li X, Bantel C, Tobin JR, Voytko ML, Eisenach JC (2001) An obligatory role for spinal cholinergic neurons in the antiallodynic effects of clonidine after peripheral nerve injury. Anesthesiology 94:1074–1081

Poree LR, Guo TZ, Kingery WS, Maze M (1998) The analgesic potency of dexmedetomidine is enhanced after nerve injury: a possible role for peripheral a2-adrenoreceptors. Anesth Analg 87:941–948

Puke MJ, Wiesenfeld-Hallin Z (1993) The differential effects of morphine and the [alpha]2-adrenoceptor agonists clonidine and dexmedetomidine on the prevention and treatment of experimental neuropathic pain. Anesth Analg 77:104–109

Rémy-Néris O, Barbeau H, Daniel O, Boiteau F, Bussel B (1999) Effects of intrathecal clonidine injection on spinal reflexes and human locomotion in incomplete paraplegic subjects. Exp Brain Res 129:433–440

Roelants F, Lavand'homme PM (2004) Epidural neostigmine combined with sufentanil provides balanced and selective analgesia in early labor. Anesthesiology 101:439–444

Rogers DT, Iwamoto ET (1993) Multiple spinal mediators in parenteral nicotine-induced antinociception. J Pharmacol Exp Ther 267:341–349

Rueter LE, Meyer MD, Decker MW (2000) Spinal mechanisms underlying A-85380-induced effects on acute thermal pain. Brain Res 872:93–101

Ryan JS, Tao QP, Kelly ME (1998) Adrenergic regulation of calcium-activated potassium current in cultured rabbit pigmented ciliary epithelial cells. J Physiol 511:145–157

Sabbe MB, Penning JP, Ozaki GT, Yaksh TL (1994) Spinal and systemic action of the alpha 2 receptor agonist dexmedetomidine in dogs. Anesthesiology 80:1057–1072

Sanders RD, Giombini M, Ma D, Ohashi Y, Hossain M, Fujinaga M, Maze M (2005) Dexmedetomidine exerts dose-dependent age-independent antinociception but age-dependent hypnosis in Fischer rats. Anesth Analg 100:1295–1302

Shannon HE, Sheardown MJ, Bymaster FP, Calligaro DO, Delapp NW, Gidda J, Mitch CH, Sawyer BD, Stengel PW, Ward JS, Wong DT, Olesen PH, Suzdak PD, Sauerberg P, Swedberg MD (1997) Pharmacology of butylthio[2. 2 2] (LY297802/NNC11-1053): a novel analgesic with mixed muscarinic receptor agonist and antagonist activity. J Pharmacol Exp Ther 281:884–894

Shannon HE, Jones CK, Li DL, Peters SC, Simmons RM, Iyengar S (2001) Antihyperalgesic effects of the muscarinic receptor ligand vedaclidine in models involving central sensitization in rats. Pain 93:221–227

Sheardown MJ, Shannon HE, Swedberg MD, Suzdak PD, Bymaster FP, Olesen PH, Mitch CH, Ward JS, Sauerberg P (1997) M1 receptor agonist activity is not a requirement for muscarinic antinociception. J Pharmacol Exp Ther 281:868–875

Svensson I, Sjostrom B, Haljamae H (2000) Assessment of pain experiences after elective surgery. J Pain Symptom Manage 20:193–201

Swedberg MD, Sheardown MJ, Sauerberg P, Olesen PH, Suzdak PD, Hansen KT, Bymaster FP, Ward JS, Mitch CH, Calligaro DO, Delapp NW, Shannon HE (1997) Butylthio[2. 2 2] (NNC 11-1053/LY297802): an orally active muscarinic agonist analgesic. J Pharmacol Exp Ther 281:876–883

Takano Y, Yaksh TL (1998) Release of calcitonin gene-related peptide (CGRP), substance P (SP), and vasoactive intestinal polypeptide (VIP) from rat spinal cord: modulation by alpha 2 agonists. Peptides 14:371–378

Tassonyi E, Charpantier E, Muller D, Dumont L, Bertrand D (2002) The role of nicotinic acetylcholine receptors in the mechanisms of anesthesia. Brain Res Bull 57:133–150

Thomas T, Robinson C, Champion D, McKell M, Pell M (1998) Prediction and assessment of the severity of postoperative pain and of satisfaction with management. Pain 75:177–185

Tjolsen A, Lund A, Hole K (1990) The role of descending noradrenergic systems in regulation of nociception: the effects of intrathecally administered alpha-adrenoreceptor antagonists and clonidine. Pain 43:113–120

Traynor JR (1998) Epibatidine and pain. Br J Anaesth 81:69–76

Wess J, Duttaroy A, Gomeza J, Zhang W, Yamada M, Felder CC, Bernardini N, Reeh PW (2003) Muscarinic receptor subtypes mediating central and peripheral antinociception studied with muscarinic receptor knockout mice: a review. Life Sci 72:2047–2054

Wilcox GL, Carlsson KH, Jochim A, Jurna I (1987) Mutual potentiation of antinociceptive effects of morphine and clonidine on motor and sensory responses in rat spinal cord. Brain Res 405:84–93

Wilson SG, Smith SB, Chesler EJ, Melton KA, Haas JJ, Mitton B, Strasburg K, Hubert L, Rodriguez-Zas SL, Mogil JS (2003) The heritability of antinociception: common pharmacogenetic mediation of five neurochemically distinct analgesics. J Pharmacol Exp Ther 304:547–559

Zhang HM, Li DP, Chen SR, Pan HL (2005) M2, m3, and m4 receptor subtypes contribute to muscarinic potentiation of GABAergic inputs to spinal dorsal horn neurons. J Pharmacol Exp Ther 313:697–704

HEP (2006) 177:265–306
© Springer-Verlag Berlin Heidelberg 2006

Cannabinoids and Pain

I. J. Lever · A. S. C. Rice (✉)

Pain Research Group, Department of Anaesthetics, Intensive Care and Pain Medicine,
Imperial College London, Chelsea and Westminster Hospital Campus, 369 Fulham Road,
London SW10 9NH, UK
a.rice@imperial.ac.uk

1	**The CB Signalling System**	266
1.1	CB Receptors	266
1.2	Molecular and Cellular Consequences of CB Receptor Activation	268
1.3	Tissue Expression of CB Receptors in Nociceptive Pathways	269
1.3.1	CB Receptors in Brain	269
1.3.2	CB Receptors in Spinal Cord	269
1.3.3	Peripheral CB Receptors	271
1.4	CB Receptor Ligands	273
1.4.1	Endocannabinoids	273
2	**Analgesic Actions of CBs in Animal Models**	275
2.1	Inflammatory Pain	275
2.2	Neuropathic Pain	278
3	**Mechanisms of CB-Mediated Analgesia**	279
3.1	Central Mechanisms	280
3.1.1	CB Receptors in Brain	280
3.1.2	CB Receptors in Spinal Cord	282
3.2	Peripheral Mechanisms	285
4	**Analgesic Actions of CBs in Humans**	288
4.1	Evidence from Volunteer Studies	288
4.2	Evidence from Randomised Controlled Clinical Trials	289
4.3	Side-Effects	290
5	**Concluding Remarks**	290
	References	291

Abstract Convincing evidence from preclinical studies demonstrates that cannabinoids can reduce pain responses in a range of inflammatory and neuropathic pain models. The anatomical and functional data reveal cannabinoid receptor-mediated analgesic actions operating at sites concerned with the transmission and processing of nociceptive signals in brain, spinal cord and the periphery. The precise signalling mechanisms by which cannabinoids produce analgesic effects at these sites remain unclear; however, significant clues point to cannabinoid modulation of the functions of neurone and immune cells that mediate nociceptive and inflammatory responses. Intracellular signalling mechanisms engaged by cannabinoid receptors—like the inhibition of calcium transients and adenylate cyclase, and pre-synaptic modulation of transmitter release—have been demonstrated in some of these cell types and are predicted to play a role in the analgesic effects of cannabinoids. In contrast, the clinical effectiveness of cannabinoids as analgesics is less clear. Progress in this area requires the development of cannabinoids with a more favourable therapeutic index than those currently available for human use, and the testing of their efficacy and side-effects in high-quality clinical trials.

Keywords CB_1 · CB_2 · Endocannabinoid · Spinal cord · Sensory neurone · G protein-coupled receptor

1
The CB Signalling System

Although the psychotropic and therapeutic properties of the marijuana plant (*Cannabis sativa*) have been documented for thousands of years, it was not until 1964 that Gaoni and Mechoulam first identified Δ^9 tetrahydrocannabinol (Δ^9THC) as a major psychoactive constituent of *C. sativa* and elucidated its structure. Since then, more than 60 bioactive components have been identified (Howlett et al. 2002; Mechoulam 2000). These, including synthetic molecules and endogenous compounds derived from animal tissues, are collectively known as the cannabinoids (CBs). Two membrane receptors for CBs have been identified and cloned, events which preceded the discovery of several endogenous CB ligands that bind to these receptors. CB pharmacology is still in the process of identifying all the signalling pathways that mediate the cellular actions of CBs and the processes governing production and degradation of endogenous CB ligands, which together make up the endocannabinoid system.

This chapter will outline our current knowledge of the endocannabinoid signalling system. It will then focus on evidence for the analgesic properties of CBs; initially from the perspective of animal models and the insights that such research has provided into possible analgesic mechanisms for CBs operating at different sites along the pain signalling pathway, from the peripheral nervous system to the brain. It will then discuss evidence from the clinical use of CBs, which leads to perspectives on the likely therapeutic usefulness of CBs as analgesics.

1.1
CB Receptors

The first evidence for the existence of CB-responsive receptors came from radioligand binding studies that reported the presence of saturable, stereoselective, high-affinity CB binding sites in mammalian brain (Devane et al. 1988). Subsequently, the first CB receptor subtype, CB_1, was cloned from a rat complementary DNA (cDNA) library (Matsuda et al. 1990). It is 473 amino acids in length and has a molecular weight of 53 kDa, although variants of 59 and 64 kDa also exist. Cloning of human CB_1 (hCB_1) (Gerard et al. 1991) and mouse (Chakrabarti et al. 1995) homologues that share close sequence homology (>97%) with rat CB_1 followed. Two splice variants of human CB_1 (CB_{1a} and CB_{1b}) have been identified. Both have truncated amino terminals, conferring altered ligand binding and activation properties, but have relatively low tissue abundance compared to full-length CB_1 (Shire et al. 1995; Ryberg et al. 2005). The second CB receptor, CB_2, was first identified in a human promyelocytic leukaemia cell line (Munro et al. 1993). Subsequently, the murine and rat homologues of CB_2 have been cloned, revealing 82% (Shire et al. 1996) and 81% (Brown et al. 2002; Griffin et al. 2000) sequence homology with hCB_2 respectively and 90% homology between them. CB_1 and CB_2 receptors are both seven trans-membrane domain, G protein-coupled receptors (GPCRs) with C and N terminals. The distinction between them is firstly based on their predicted amino acid sequences: hCB_2 is shorter than hCB_1 (360 amino acids, 40 kDa) with only 44% sequence homology (rising to 68% in the transmembrane regions) (Munro et al. 1993). The two receptor subtypes are also distinguished by their signalling mechanisms (Sect. 1.2) and tissue distribution (Sect. 1.3). CB_1 (Ledent et al. 1999; Zimmer et al. 1999), CB_2 (Buckley et al. 2000) and CB_1/CB_2 (Járai et al. 1999) knock-out mice have been created and phenotyped.

Residual pharmacological activity of CBs in CB receptor knock-out mice or following the administration of receptor antagonists in rodents, has suggested the existence of additional CB receptors (Begg et al. 2005; Howlett et al. 2002). Bioassays from mesenteric artery preparations (Járai et al. 1999) and binding studies in CNS tissue (Breivogel et al. 2001) have uncovered residual effects of both endogenous and synthetic CBs. These are thought to be mediated by several pharmacologically distinct non-CB_1/CB_2 GPCR systems. One is known to be expressed on blood vessel endothelium and is responsive to the endocannabinoid anandamide (AEA) (Sect. 1.4.1.1) and abnormal cannabidiol (Abn-CBD), a synthetic form of the phytocannabinoid cannabidiol (Járai et al. 1999; Offertaler et al. 2003). Another is distinctively responsive to the vanilloid capsaicin, as well as to the synthetic CBs WIN55,212-2 and CP55,940 (Sect. 1.4; Breivogel et al. 2001; Hájos and Freund 2002). In addition, the anti-inflammatory effects of the endogenous cannabimimetic compound palmitoylethanolamide (PEA) are not likely to be explained by its binding to either CB_1 or CB_2 receptors (Griffin et al. 2000). Instead, research in mice suggests these effects may be mediated by activation of the nuclear receptor peroxisome proliferator-activated receptor-α (PPARα) (Lo et al. 2005). CBs are also reported to have agonist activity at two of the transient receptor potential (TRP) type of ligand-gated cation channels that are expressed by sensory neurones. The capsaicin receptor TRPV1 and the TRPA1 receptor are respectively implicated in the transduction of noxious heat and noxious cold sensory stimuli by primary afferents (Bandell et al. 2004). Several studies have demonstrated the ability of anandamide to induce membrane currents and increase intracellular calcium in both rat and human cells expressing TRPV1 receptors (Zygmunt et al. 1999; Smart et al. 2000; Ross et al. 2001; Roberts et al. 2002; Dinis et al. 2004; Ross; 2004). More recently, Jordt et al. (2004) described the ability of THC and cannabidiol to activate TRPA1-expressing transfected cells and rat sensory neurones in culture, providing an explanation for the non-CB_1/CB_2 mediated excitatory effects of AEA on perivascular sensory nerves from TRPV1 knock-out mice (Zygmunt et al. 1999).

1.2
Molecular and Cellular Consequences of CB Receptor Activation

CB_1 receptors are coupled to pertussis toxin (PTX)-sensitive G (α_i) and G (α_o) ($G_i/_o$) signalling proteins that function to recruit signal transduction pathways and engage various effector mechanisms within cells (Pertwee 1997; Howlett et al. 2002; McAllister and Glass 2002). The intracellular C-terminal domain of the receptor mediates signalling functions (Nie and Lewis 2001a), controls receptor internalisation/recycling in the membrane after ligand binding (Coutts et al. 2001) and regulates desensitisation after prolonged (>2 h) agonist exposure (Kouznetsova et al. 2002). The proximal part of this domain is critical for G protein binding (Nie and Lewis 2001b). CB_1 receptor signalling via G_i/G_o inhibits cyclic adenosine monophosphate (cAMP) production by adenylate cyclase (Howlett et al. 1988) and modulates ion channel function; including inhibition of voltage gated calcium channels (VGCC) (Mackie and Hille 1992; Twitchell et al. 1997; Chemin et al. 2001). Forskolin-induced production of cAMP [measured in cultured dorsal root ganglion (DRG) cells] can be reduced by CBs (Ross et al. 2001; Oshita et al. 2005), and CB_1-mediated inhibition of the N-type VGCC is implicated in the reduction of stimulus-evoked Ca^{2+} influx and rises in $[Ca^{2+}]_i$ produced by CB agonists applied to cultured sensory neurones (Ross et al. 2001; Khasabova et al. 2004). CB_1 activity also modulates K^+ channel conductances, enhancing the activity of both A-type and inwardly rectifying potassium channels (K_{ir} current) (Deadwyler et al. 1995; Mackie et al. 1995; Shen et al. 1996). Where CB_1 receptors exist on pre-synaptic nerve terminals, the effect of these actions is to reduce the probability of activity-regulated transmitter release. Exogenous CBs act pre-synaptically to inhibit glutamatergic (Shen et al. 1996) and γ-aminobutyric acid (GABA)ergic (Katona et al. 1999) transmission in various brain regions including hippocampus, cerebellum, striatum and nucleus accumbens. CB_2 receptors also couple to inhibitory G proteins to modulate adenylate cyclase activity but not ion channel function. This difference may be explained by the receptor's low affinity for the G_o protein subtype compared to CB_1 (McAllister and Glass 2002). CB receptors also couple to signalling pathways related to cell proliferation, which in turn can recruit mitogen activated protein (MAP) kinase and protein kinase (PK)B signalling systems (Derkinderen et al. 2001; Bouaboula et al. 1999 see Howlett et al. 2002). For example, PKB activation has been implicated in the CB receptor-mediated survival of oligodendrocytes after trophic factor withdrawal (Molina-Holgado et al. 2002).

1.3
Tissue Expression of CB Receptors in Nociceptive Pathways

CB_1 receptors are found primarily in CNS neurones (Egertova et al. 2000; Herkenham et al. 1991; Matsuda et al. 1993; Tsou et al. 1998; Mailleux and Vanderhaeghen 1992), and the majority of CB_2 receptors are expressed by cells with inflammatory and immune response functions, including glia (Pertwee 1997; Howlett et al. 2002; Walter and Stella 2004). However, there are reports of CB_1 receptor expression on peripheral neurones (Bridges et al. 2003) as well as on glial (Salio et al. 2002b; Molina-Holgado et al. 2002) and immune cell types (Galiègue et al. 1995), although in non-neuronal tissues such as spleen, levels of CB_1 messenger RNA (mRNA) are lower than CB_2 receptor mRNA (Galiègue et al. 1995; Carlisle et al. 2002; Walter and Stella 2004). CB_2 mRNA has also been detected in CNS (spinal cord) tissue from injured but not naïve rats (Zhang et al. 2003). CB receptors have been identified at tissue sites associated with the transmission and processing of nociceptive information. These are the putative cellular targets responsible for mediating the analgesic effects of CB treatment.

1.3.1
CB Receptors in Brain

CB_1 receptors are expressed at their highest levels in brain and are particularly enriched in cerebral cortex, hippocampus, basal ganglia and cerebellum (Herkenham et al. 1991; Mailleux and Vanderhaeghen 1992; Masuda et al. 1993; Glass et al. 1997). The receptors have also been located in pain-modulating regions like periaqueductal grey (PAG), rostro-ventromedial medulla (RVM) and thalamus (Herkenham et al. 1991; Tsou et al. 1998). In the lateral and basal nuclei of the amygdala, CB_1 receptors have been localised to a population of cholecystokinin (CCK)-containing interneurones which are activated to inhibit pre-synaptic release of GABA (Katona et al. 2001). There are relatively low levels of CB_1 mRNA in thalamus (Mailleux and Vanderhaeghen 1992; Masuda et al. 1993); however, one study reports an up-regulation of CB_1 receptors in this area following injury to peripheral nerve (Siegling et al. 2001).

1.3.2
CB Receptors in Spinal Cord

CB_1 receptors have been localised in spinal cord tissue (Farquhar-Smith et al. 2000; Hohmann et al. 1999a; Ong et al. 1999; Sanudo-Pena et al. 1999) where they are distributed in areas that are important for nociceptive processing. Microarray experiments reveal a 2.9-fold greater abundance of the CB_1-encoding gene in the dorsal compared with the ventral spinal horn (Sun et al. 2002). Detailed analysis of CB_1 immunoreactivity (CB_1-ir) in the spinal cord (Farquhar-Smith et al. 2000) revealed a concentration in superficial dorsal horn (laminae I and II), the termination area for nociceptive primary afferent fibres, as well as the dorso-lateral funiculus and lamina X (Farquhar-Smith et al. 2000; Tsou et al. 1998). In lamina II, CB_1-ir has been localised to the inner part of lamina II (IIi) – the termination zone of non-peptidergic C-fibre afferents – using antibodies to the C-terminal of the receptor (Farquhar-Smith et al. 2000). Alternatively, using antibodies raised to N-terminal regions of the receptor, CB_1-ir is described in the outer part (IIo) of lamina II, which is the termination zone of peptidergic C-fibres (Tsou et al. 1998; Salio et al. 2002a, b). CB_1-ir in the superficial dorsal horn is likely to be located at both pre- and post-synaptic sites, with the major population being expressed by intrinsic spinal neurones (Hohmann et al. 1999a; Hohmann and Herkenham 1999b; Salio et al. 2001; Salio et al. 2002a).

Ultrastructural analysis identified CB_1 receptors on unmyelinated afferent fibre terminals (as well as on astrocytic cells) within superficial spinal cord laminae (Salio et al. 2002a, b). This report of pre-synaptic CB_1 receptors would appear to correlate well with the 50% reduction to CB binding sites in the cord reported after an extensive unilateral dorsal rhizotomy (Hohmann and Herkenham 1999a). However, more restricted lumbar rhizotomy experiments report only a less than 5% reduction to the levels of CB_1-ir in the superficial dorsal horn (Farquhar-Smith et al. 2000). In accordance with this study, a modest 16% reduction in CB receptor binding was attributed to TRPV1-responsive afferents ablated by neonatal capsaicin treatment (Hohmann and Herkenham 1998).

The expression of CB_1 in the dorso-lateral funiculus (Farquhar-Smith et al. 2000) is consistent with observations that endocannabinoids are involved in descending modulation of nociceptive processing (Meng et al. 1998; Meng and Johansen 2004). Using immunohistochemistry, a progressive ipsilateral up-regulation of CB_1 receptors in the spinal cord has been reported following a chronic constriction injury to rat sciatic nerve, in a mechanism that putatively involves the MAP kinase and PKC signalling pathways (Lim et al. 2003). The induction of CB_2 receptor mRNA expression in the ipsilateral spinal cord also occurs in this neuropathy model, where the location and timing of expression correlate with the appearance of activated microglial markers (Zhang et al. 2003).

De-afferentation studies suggest that the contribution of central primary afferent terminals to the total CB_1-ir in the spinal cord is likely to be small, making it likely that the receptor is expressed on intrinsic neurones, in the spinal cord. Co-staining with markers for intrinsic dorsal horn neurones shows that CB_1 receptors are indeed expressed on both excitatory interneurones containing PKCγ (Farquhar-Smith et al. 2000) as well as inhibitory ones containing GABA (Hohmann et al. 1999a; Salio et al. 2002a). Another population co-expresses CB_1 and type 1 μ-opioid receptors and is likely to exist separately from GABAergic interneurones (Salio et al. 2001; Kemp et al. 1996). Enkephalinergic interneurones also contain CB_1 mRNA, and it is possible that a proportion of the CB_1-ir in the spinal cord exists on the efferent terminals of supraspinal neurones, including CB_1-expressing neurones from the RVM and PAG that send descending inputs to the spinal cord (Hohmann et al. 1999a; Tsou et al. 1998; Farquhar-Smith et al. 2000). In summary, the anatomical evidence suggests that CBs could potentially operate at both pre- and post-synaptic loci in order to modulate neurotransmission at nociceptor synapses in the dorsal horn.

1.3.3
Peripheral CB Receptors

Anatomical and functional evidence supports the presence of CB receptors in peripheral nervous tissue. CB_1 mRNA has been detected in superior cervical ganglia (Ishac et al. 1996) as well the cell bodies of primary afferent sensory nerves contained within DRG (Hohmann and Herkenham 1999b; Salio et al. 2002a; Bridges et al. 2003; Sanudo-Pena et al. 1999) trigeminal ganglia (TG) (Price et al. 2003) and nodose ganglia (Burdyga et al. 2004). CB binding sites have also been shown to undergo peripherally directed axonal transport in the sciatic and vagus nerves (Hohmann and Herkenham 1999a; Burdyga et al. 2004). Twenty-three percent of lumbar 4/5 DRG soma and 30% of TG soma expressed CB_1 receptor mRNA. CB_1 mRNA has been found in DRG neurones of all sizes, including 13% of those containing substance P (SP) mRNA (Hohmann and Herkenham 1999b). The distribution of CB_1-positive cells among the small, TRPV1-positive soma that are typical of nociceptive nerve fibres, was found to be limited in favour of intermediate to large-sized cells immunopositive for 200-kDa neurofilament protein (75% in TG, 69%–82% in DRG) (Bridges et al. 2003; Price et al. 2003). CB_1 receptors have been immuno-labelled on primary cultures of both neonatal (Ross et al. 2001) and adult DRG sensory neurones (Ahluwalia et al. 2000, 2002; Khasabova et al. 2002, 2004). In some studies, 47%–57% of cultured DRG were CB_1 positive, of which a large majority were small and co-labelled by TRPV1 antibodies (Ahluwalia et al. 2000, 2002).

The activity of cultured DRG neurones (measured by calcium imaging and whole patch-clamp electrophysiological techniques) has provided functional evidence for the existence of CB receptors on cutaneous sensory neurones. Taking the various studies into account, CBs have been shown to modulate the activity of neurones from a range of cultured DRG sub-populations, including large-sized, non-capsaicin-responsive cells (Khasabova et al. 2002, 2004) small, capsaicin-sensitive cells (Millns et al. 2001; Ross et al. 2001) and cells from both large and small size classes (Evans et al. 2004). In another functional assay, CB_1 receptor activation has been demonstrated to modulate neurosecretion of the vasodilatatory peptide calcitonin gene-related peptide (CGRP) from peripheral terminals of capsaicin-sensitive sensory neurones in isolated rat paw skin (Richardson et al. 1998b; Ellington et al. 2002). A recent immunohistochemistry study identified CB_1 and CB_2 receptors on both myelinated and unmyelinated CGRP immunoreactive nerve fibres in human skin, as well as on non-neuronal cells such as keratinocytes (Ständer et al. 2005). CB_2 has also been localised on epidermal keratinocytes from glabrous skin of the rat hind paw (Ibrahim et al. 2005).

Functional evidence for the existence of skin CB_2 receptors was provided by in vitro release studies. These experiments demonstrated that superfusion of the selective agonist for the CB_2 receptor, AM1251, evoked the release of β-endorphin from excised sections of rat skin (Ibrahim et al. 2005). Further evidence for CB receptors in skin is derived from studies where topical application of CBs to human skin has been reported to reduce histamine-evoked itch (Dvorak et al. 2003) and capsaicin-evoked pain responses (Rukwied et al. 2003) produced by excitation of unmyelinated nerve fibre terminals in skin. In these experiments, the efferent functions of sensory neurones in skin were shown to be modulated by CBs. Activation of cutaneous sensory nerve terminals by histamine or capsaicin causes an antidromic activation of collateral fibres, depolarising their terminals to release vasoactive neuropeptides, including CGRP. Measurements used to gauge the extent of this neurogenic inflammation—laser Doppler imaging of cutaneous blood flow, measurement of protein extravasation and the area of skin flare—were all reportedly reduced by topical CB application.

In contrast to CB_1, CB_2 receptor mRNA has not yet been detected in adult rat DRG or TG neurones by in situ hybridisation (Hohmann and Herkenham 1999b; Price et al. 2003). If expression levels of CB_2 are low in sensory ganglia, however, its expression might be detectable using the more sensitive technique of reversed transcription coupled to the polymerase chain reaction (RT-PCR). This has previously been used to reveal the presence of both CB_1 and CB_2 mRNA in immune cells (Galiègue et al. 1995; Pertwee 1997). In contrast to reports of an up-regulation of CB receptors in the spinal cord following chronic constriction injury (CCI) to the sciatic nerve, a microarray study of gene expression in DRG 3 days after sciatic axotomy indicates that CB_1 expression is down-regulated. This study showed a 1.5-fold down-regulation of CB_1 gene expression in the DRG as verified by Northern blotting (1.2-fold decrease), which is just at the threshold for biological significance (Costigan et al. 2002). A preliminary immunohistochemistry study in DRG supports these data, as sciatic axotomy is reported to produce a 70% reduction in the number of neuronal soma that immunostain for CB_1 lateral to the injury (Bridges et al. 2002).

Non-neuronal cells in peripheral tissues also express CB receptors. CB_2 is present on cells that are functionally involved in immune responses to tissue injury, including B and T cells, natural killer cells, neutrophils, macrophages and mast cells (see Pertwee 1997; Howlett et al. 2002; Samson et al. 2003; Walter and Stella 2004). Furthermore, mitogen activation of some immune cells, such as human lymphocytes, has been shown to stimulate an up-regulation of CB receptors and also to trigger the production of endocannabinoids (Pertwee 1997; Howlett et al. 2002; Walter and Stella 2004).

1.4
CB Receptor Ligands

Compounds that bind to CB receptors have been classified into four groups according to their chemical structure (see reviews by Howlett et al. 2002 and Pertwee 1997). The classical CB group includes plant-derived CBs like Δ^9THC and their synthetic analogues (e.g. HU210). The non-classical group contains the next series of synthetic CB compounds to be developed. These lack the dihydropyran ring of THC-based molecules. CP55,940 is an example of a potent CB receptor agonist from this group (Melvin et al. 1993; Pertwee 1997). The third group of aminoalkylindole compounds were the first discovered to have cannabimimetic properties without being structurally related to THC (Bell et al. 1991). The Sterling Winthrop compound WIN55,212-2 is an important example. This has a high affinity for both CB receptors, with moderate selectivity for CB_2 (Bouaboula et al. 1997), and is chemically related to cyclo-oxygenase (COX) inhibitors. The final class of CBs are the eicosanoid group containing the five endocannabinoid molecules discovered so far (De Petrocellis et al. 2004).

1.4.1
Endocannabinoids

Endocannabinoids are endogenous compounds isolated from animal tissue and identified as ligands at CB receptors. The prototypical endocannabinoid compound is the fatty acid amide N-arachidonoyl-ethanolamine, also known as anandamide (Devane et al. 1992). Subsequently, a number of other endocannabinoids have been proposed, including the monoacylglycerol ester 2-arachidonoylglycerol (2-AG) (Mechoulam et al. 1995), noladin ether, virodhamine and N-arachidonoyl-dopamine (reviewed in Petrocellis et al. 2004). They are all derivatives of long chain polyunsaturated fatty acids, specifically arachidonic acid (Di Marzo et al. 2004). There is also a growing list of endogenous lipid mediators with related structures. Many of these have cannabimimetic effects but do not necessarily bind to known CB receptors (Bradshaw and Walker 2005).

1.4.1.1
Anandamide

Anandamide binds to both CB receptors but has a higher affinity for CB_1 (K_i ~89 nM) than CB_2. Although it is a relatively weak agonist of CB_1, compared with other classes of CBs, it does evoke the classical 'tetrad' of antinociception, catalepsy, hypothermia and hypolocomotion (Di Marzo et al. 1998; Felder et al. 1993; Martin et al. 1991) of CB effects (Jaggar et al. 1998; Calignano et al. 1998). AEA activates the G protein-coupled signalling systems of CB receptors (Breivogel et al. 1998; Kearn et al. 1999) to activate effector mechanisms including modulation of voltage-gated ion channels (Felder et al. 1993; Gebremedhin et al. 1999; Mackie et al. 1993; Mackie et al. 1995) and inhibition of adenylate cyclase (Bayewitch et al. 1995; Felder et al. 1993). Due to its high lipophilicity, AEA production and inactivation processes are likely to differ from those of conventional transmitter molecules. Indeed, evidence shows that instead of vesicular storage of pre-formed transmitter, AEA is rapidly synthesised on demand by activity-dependent cleavage from membrane phospholipid precursors (Piomelli et al. 1998). Activity-linked synthesis, demonstrated initially in cultured neurones and by microdialysis of freely moving rats (Di Marzo et al. 1994; Giuffrida et al. 1999; Walker et al. 1999; Stella and Piomelli 2001), is thought to be due to rises in $[Ca^{2+}]_i$ increasing the activity of enzymes that catalyse phospholipid conversion (Di Marzo et al. 1994; Okamoto et al. 2004). AEA synthesis and release has been demonstrated in several different cell types including capsaicin-sensitive sensory neurones (Ahluwalia et al. 2003b), vascular endothelium (Randall et al. 1997), immune cells (Pestojamasp and Burstein 1998) and glia (Walter and Stella 2004).

Once formed, the bioactivity of AEA is thought to be terminated by three mechanisms: desensitisation and internalisation of CB receptors transducing the AEA signal, facilitated diffusion of AEA from the extracellular space and external CB receptor binding sites into post-synaptic cells, followed by degradation by hydrolysis or oxidation. Rapid AEA uptake into neurones is a temperature-sensitive, saturable and selective process (Beltramo et al. 1997; Di Marzo et al. 1994), suggesting the existence of a membrane transport which has yet to be characterised and is the subject of some controversy (see Fowler and Jacobsson 2002 for reviews). The membrane-bound serine hydrolase enzyme fatty acid amide hydrolase (FAAH) catalyses the hydrolysis of AEA into arachidonic acid and ethanolamine (Deutsch et al. 1993; Cravatt et al. 1996; Bracey et al. 2002). FAAH mRNA and protein has been mapped to intracellular membranes in the soma and dendrites of principle neurones in various parts of the CNS (Romero et al. 2002; Thomas et al. 1997; Guylas et al. 2004) where its distribution is frequently but not exclusively complimentary to CB_1 on pre-synaptic axons (Egertova et al. 1998; Egertova et al. 2003). There is also evidence for oxidative metabolism of AEA by lipoxygenase and COX enzymes involved in arachidonic acid metabolism (Yu et al. 1997).

1.4.1.2
2-Arachidonoylglycerol

The monoacylglycerol ester 2-AG usually has higher measurable tissue concentrations than AEA and binds to both CB receptors to produce cannabimimetic effects (Mechoulam et al. 1995; Stella et al. 1997; Mechoulam et al. 1998). 2-AG is a full agonist at the CB_1 receptor (K_i 14 nM), and it has been suggested that it is the optimal known candidate for the natural ligand at CB_2 receptors (K_i 58 nM) (Hillard 2000; McAllister and Glass 2002; Sugiura et al. 2000). Various stimuli lead to the formation of 2-AG in cells (Sugiura et al. 2002) including membrane depolarisation in neurones (Stella et al. 1997). Several biosynthetic pathways for the formation of 2-AG are likely to exist. Of these, the phospholipase C-dependent pathway, involving hydrolysis of diacylglycerol membrane phosphoproteins by diacylglycerol lipase, has been most studied (Sugiura et al. 2002; reviewed by De Petrocellis et al. 2004). Although there are less data for 2-AG than for AEA, it is also likely to be inactivated by cellular uptake (Bisogno et al. 2001) and enzymatic hydrolysis involving monoacyl-glycerol lipases (MAGLs) (Bisogno et al. 1997; Di Marzo et al. 1999) rather than FAAH (Lichtman et al. 2002). Like FAAH, MAGL is also expressed in brain regions containing a high density of CB_1 receptors, but it is not restricted to cell membranes and occurs in pre-synaptic neurones where it is likely to co-exist with CB_1 receptors (Dinh et al. 2002; Guylas et al. 2004). As for AEA, alternative mechanisms of 2-AG inactivation have also been proposed (see De Petrocellis et al. 2004).

2
Analgesic Actions of CBs in Animal Models

There are a substantial number of animal studies reporting both anti-nociceptive and anti-hyperalgesic effects of CB compounds in acute nociceptive, inflammatory and neuropathic pain models (see Rice 2005). CBs applied systemically (Fox et al. 2001)—as well as intrathecally (Hohmann et al. 1998; Scott et al. 2004), intracerebroventricularly (Raffa et al. 1999) or to the skin area receiving the stimulus (Calignano et al. 1998; Yesilyurt et al. 2003; Malan et al. 2001)—have been shown to increase the time taken for withdrawal from a noxious stimulus (reviewed in Pertwee et al. 2001).

2.1
Inflammatory Pain

The injection of inflammatory agents such as carrageenan, complete Freund's adjuvant (CFA), formalin, yeast, nerve growth factor (NGF) or capsaicin (usually into rodent hind paw skin), produces a localised inflammatory hyperalgesia. CB compounds from all four chemical subtypes–applied through various routes–have been reported to reduce hyperalgesic responses in these models. For example, Δ^9THC, CP55,940, WIN55,212-2 and AEA are all systemically active against behavioural measures of inflammatory hyperalgesia in the formalin test (Jaggar et al. 1998; Moss and Johnson 1980; Tsou et al. 1996; Hohmann et al. 1999b; Calignano et al. 1998). WIN55,212-2, HU210 and PEA are also effective if injected locally with formalin into the hind paw skin (Calignano et al. 1998). Injection of carrageenan into the rodent hind paw shortens limb withdrawal times measured in response to a noxious thermal stimulus. These response times can be increased by either intrathecal administration of AEA (Richardson et al. 1998a) or oral administration of cannabidiol (Costa et al. 2004a, b). Behavioural responses to mechanical (Clayton et al. 2002; Nackley et al. 2003a) as well as thermal stimuli (Malan et al. 2001; Quartilho et al. 2003; Nackley et al. 2003b) can be reduced by administration of CBs to carrageenan-inflamed rodents. As an alternative measure of allodynia and hyperalgesia in this model, the application of mechanical and thermal stimuli to the inflamed paw increases the activity of neurones in the spinal cord that receive sensory input from the inflamed limb. This change can be monitored either by electrophysiological recording from dorsal horn neurones or the induction of an activity-regulated protein, Fos, visualised by immunohistochemistry in spinal cord tissue. In rat electrophysiological experiments, the enhanced responses of dorsal horn neurones (as evoked by innocuous and noxious mechanical stimulation) were reduced by CBs when these were applied locally to the site of inflammation (Sokal et al. 2003). CB agonists selective for either CB_1 (Kelly et al. 2003) or CB_2 (Elmes et al. 2004; Nackley et al. 2004) receptors were also peripherally effective using this outcome measure. Capsaicin injected into rat paw skin has similarly been used to sensitise the responses of dorsal horn neurones to mechanical stimuli. The enhanced responses of these cells were attenuated by intrathecal injections of CP55,940 (Johanek and Simone 2005). As might be expected, behavioural hyperalgesic responses induced by topical capsaicin are reduced by CBs (Ko et al. 1999; Johanek et al. 2001; Li et al. 1999; Quartilho et al. 2003; Hohmann et al. 2004).

In immunohistochemical studies, local application of either WIN55,212-2 or the selective CB_2 receptor agonist, AM1241, can reduce the levels of carrageenan-evoked Fos protein in the superficial dorsal horn of the spinal cord (Nackley et al. 2003a, b). Intrathecal administration of WIN55,212-2, which reversed mechanical allodynia following subcutaneous injection of CFA into the hind paw, also prevented the associated appearance of Fos-like immunoreactivity in spinal cord neurones (Martin et al. 1999c). In a rodent model of persistent visceral inflammatory pain produced by inflaming the bladder wall with turpentine or NGF, the induction of spinal Fos protein can also be reduced by AEA and PEA. Behavioural correlates of hyperalgesia are also reduced by CBs in this model (Jaggar et al. 1998; Farquhar-Smith and Rice 2001; Farquhar-Smith et al. 2002).

CBs have reported anti-hyperalgesic efficacy in other related models; such as chemical irritation of the peritoneum (Burstein et al. 1998; Calignano et al. 2001). Additionally, in a model of deep tissue pain produced by carrageenan inflammation of the triceps muscle, WIN55,212-2 is demonstrated to produce a complete reversal of inflammatory hyperalgesia (measured by reduction to limb grip force) (Kehl et al. 2003). Chronic inflammatory pain of the kind associated with arthritis in humans, has been studied in rats by intradermal injection of CFA to the tail. Inflammation proceeds to a generalised polyarthritis within 19 days. THC and AEA have anti-nociceptive effects in tests of mechanical nociception as reported in both arthritic and non-arthritic rats (Cox and Welch 2004; Smith et al. 1998).

In addition to effects on pain responses, CB treatment also has potent anti-inflammatory actions that have been observed in several of these animal models. For example, after acute inflammation of rodent skin, both plasma extravasation and tissue oedema can be measurably reduced by CB treatment (Mazzari et al. 1996; Richardson et al. 1998b; Hanus et al. 1999; Clayton et al. 2002; Lodzki et al. 2003; Costa et al. 2004a). The anti-inflammatory actions of CBs are thought to be mediated in part by their suppression of pro-inflammatory mediators such as cytokines, prostanoids and neuropeptides (Sect. 3.2). CBs reduce capsaicin-evoked release of the vasodilatory peptide CGRP from carrageenan-inflamed rat paw skin (Richardson et al. 1998b; Ellington et al. 2002). The resulting localised increase in cutaneous blood flow (producing a skin flare) is also measurably reduced by topical HU210 in human iontophoresis studies (Dvorak et al. 2003). Cannabidiol, administered to mice with collagen-induced arthritis, was associated with the reduced production of tumour necrosis factor-α (TNF-α) and interferon gamma (IFN-γ) cytokines by synovial cells and a concomitant reduction of inflammatory joint damage (Malfait et al. 2000). Increases in plasma levels of prostaglandin E_2 (measured after carrageenan inflammation of hind paw skin) were also attenuated by cannabidiol treatment. COX activity and the levels endothelial nitric oxide synthase (eNOS) and NO production assayed in inflamed paw tissue were also reduced by cannabidiol in this study (Costa et al. 2004a). Production of NO and neutrophil-derived oxygen radicals are implicated in the cytotoxic effects of the inflammatory process. Systemic administration of PEA, but not AEA, was demonstrated to reduce neutrophil accumulation in rat hind paw skin inflamed by intradermal injections of NGF. Both of these endogenous compounds were effective at reducing thermal hyperalgesic responses in this model (Farquhar-Smith and Rice 2003). However, in the rat model of persistent visceral inflammation, the extent of plasma extravasation of Evan's blue dye was not affected by systemic treatment with either PEA or AEA (Jaggar et al. 1998).

Elevated concentrations of PEA and AEA have been measured in formalin-inflamed rat hind paw skin (Calignano et al. 1998) and 2-AG levels are increased in inflamed mouse ear tissue (Oka et al. 2005), suggesting that the levels of the endogenous activators of CB_1 and CB_2 receptors are likely to be increased by inflammation. Co-administration of CB_1 receptor antagonists prior to tissue inflammation, indicates that endogenous activity at these receptors acts to tonically suppress hyperalgesic responses (Calignano et al. 1998). The work of Cravatt and co-workers (Cravatt et al. 1996, 2001, 2004; Lichtman et al. 2004a, b) has demonstrated that disrupting the activity of AEA's degradation enzyme, FAAH, can artificially enhance tissue levels of AEA. Pharmacological inhibition of this enzyme—or its genetic deletion to produce FAAH knock-out mice ($FAAH^{-/-}$)—has the effect of prolonging withdrawal latencies to acute noxious stimuli (Lichtman et al. 2004a, b; Cravatt et al. 2001). $FAAH^{-/-}$ mice also have reduced paw oedema and thermal hyperalgesic responses in both the formalin and carrageenan models of cutaneous inflammation, which are postulated to arise as a consequence of higher tissue levels of endocannabinoids (Lichtman et al. 2004a; Cravatt et al. 2004).

2.2
Neuropathic Pain

In animal experiments, some of the sensory abnormalities associated with neuropathic pain—allodynia and hyperalgesia—have been reproduced by injury to peripheral nerves (Bridges et al. 2001b). CB treatment has been demonstrated to reduce some of these behavioural effects of neuropathic pain in animal models. After a unilateral CCI to the rat sciatic nerve, behavioural hypersensitivity to cold, mechanical and thermal stimuli can be measured by timing hind paw withdrawal latencies. At doses (2.14 mg/kg) that did not affect withdrawal latencies of hind paws contralateral to the injury, systemic application of WIN55,212-2 was effective at reducing heat and mechanical hyperalgesia and mechanical and cold allodynia following the induction of neuropathy (Herzberg et al. 1997). The same rodent neuropathy model was used to show that intrathecal injections of Δ^9THC were also effective at lengthening withdrawal latencies to thermal stimuli (Mao et al. 2000). In contrast, the dose-response curve produced for the thermal anti-nociceptive effects of intrathecally injected morphine, underwent a rightward shift after CCI. In an alternative neuropathic pain model, partial ligation of the rat sciatic nerve produces similar changes to hind limb sensory stimulus thresholds, that manifest as allodynia and hyperalgesia (Seltzer et al. 1990). Systemic treatment with WIN55,212-2, CP55,940 or HU210, 12–15 days after nerve injury, produced a dose-related reversal of mechanical hyperalgesia measured from 1 h to 6 h after drug administration (Fox et al. 2001). With higher doses of these CBs, anti-nociceptive effects on contralateral withdrawal thresholds and side-effects of catalepsy and sedation were also observed. Of these three CBs, WIN55,2212-2 had the best side-effect profile and was also reported to reverse mechanical allodynia (0.3–3 mg/kg) and reduce thermal hyperalgesia (3 mg/kg). In addition, intrathecal injections of WIN55,212-2 (as well as local injections into hind paw tissue) were effective at reducing mechanical hyperalgesia. AM404, an inhibitor of anandamide uptake, has been shown to enhance the anti-nociceptive and hypotensive effects of anandamide in vivo (Beltramo et al. 1997; Calignano et al. 1997). This drug also decreases spinal cord Fos immunoreactivity produced in the CCI model (Rodella et al. 2005). In support of these studies, 7 days after a ligation injury to the L5 spinal nerve in rat, systemic administration of WIN55,212-2 (0.5–2.5 mg/kg) dose-dependently reduced cold allodynia and thermal hyperalgesia, with higher doses reducing hypersensitivity to mechanical stimuli (Bridges et al. 2001a). In a subsequent study, tactile and thermal hypersensitivity produced by the ligation of both L6 and L5 spinal nerves was dose-dependently inhibited by systemic administration of the CB_2 receptor agonist AM1251. This effect could be reproduced in $CB_1{}^{-/-}$ and $CB_1{}^{+/+}$ mice with the same nerve injury, thus claiming the advantage of circumventing side-effects mediated by CBs active at CB_1 receptors in the CNS (Ibrahim et al. 2003; Malan et al. 2001). The analgesic action of AM1241 injected directly into the hind paw skin, has been demonstrated in both acute and inflammatory pain models (Malan et al. 2001, 2003; Nackley et al. 2003a; Quartilho et al. 2003) but not so far in neuropathic animals. In an electrophysiological study, however, local injection of the CB_2-selective agonist JWH-133 into the hind paw is reported to directly reduce the mechanically evoked responses of spinal cord neurones in the same L5/L6 spinal nerve ligation (SNL) neuropathy model (Elmes et al. 2004). Intrathecal injection of CP55,940 was also effective at inhibiting tactile allodynia in this model, although treatment was associated with significant behavioural toxicity that could be alleviated by treatment with CB_1 but not CB_2 receptor antagonists (Scott et al. 2004).

In an interesting study on CCI-induced neuropathy (Costa et al. 2004c), rats were given daily systemic injections of a low, sub-effective (0.1 mg/kg) dose of WIN55,212-2 from day 1 to days 7 or 14 after injury. This dose does not produce CNS side-effects or have any effect on sensory thresholds in the contralateral paw, nor does it affect ipsilateral sensory thresholds when injected after the development of neuropathic pain (Costa et al. 2004c; Bridges et al. 2001a). Repeated administration of WIN55,212-2 during the development of neuropathy, effectively normalised mechanical hypersensitivity and reduced thermal hyperalgesia compared to vehicle-treated nerve-injured controls. Indicators of inflammatory injury, like plasma elevations of PGE_2 and increased levels of neuronal NOS and NO production in sciatic nerve tissue, were also attenuated by WIN55,212-2 treatment (Costa et al. 2004c). Furthermore, CBs have been shown to have analgesic properties in a model of peripheral nerve demyelination-associated pain (Wallace et al. 2003). Intrathecal administration of WIN55,212-2 reverses, in a CB_1-mediated manner, the thermal hyperalgesia and mechanical allodynia in mice that had been rendered neuropathic following injection topical application of lysolecithin into peripheral nerves of the hind limb. This CB is also reported to be effective against behavioural signs of neuropathic pain in a model of diabetic neuropathy induced in mice. Both systemic and local hind paw skin injections of WIN55,212-2 were effective at reducing mechanical sensitivity in this model (Dogrul et al. 2003; Ulugol al. 2004).

3
Mechanisms of CB-Mediated Analgesia

Targeted application of CB receptor agonists and antagonists to supraspinal (Martin et al. 1998), spinal (Richardson et al. 1998a) and peripheral sites

(Malan et al. 2001) in the pain pathway has provided evidence for CB-mediated analgesic signalling mechanisms operating at these loci. Interestingly, other intrinsic pain control signalling systems like the GABAergic (Naderi et al. 2005), nor-adrenergic (Gutierrez et al. 2003) and opioidergic systems (Manzanares et al. 1999) are also known to operate at these sites. The cellular mechanisms by which CBs mediate their analgesic effects have yet to be fully elucidated, as has the degree to which the operations of parallel analgesic signalling systems in these regions might be integrated. In addition, a recent study has suggested that endogenous CBs mediate the non-opioid component of stress-induced analgesia (Hohmann et al. 2005)

3.1
Central Mechanisms

The central pain modulatory systems operating in mammals are thought to consist of neural circuits in the forebrain, brain stem regions like PAG and RVM and the spinal cord. Major evidence for the involvement of these regions in pain processing was derived from experiments that demonstrated their role in the anti-nociceptive effects of systemically administered analgesics such as morphine. Repetitions of these experiments have recently shown that some of these same neural circuits are also involved in the anti-nociceptive effects of systemically applied CBs.

3.1.1
CB Receptors in Brain

The anti-nociceptive effects of CBs, as measured using the tail flick assay, can be reproduced by brain area-specific microinjection into the RVM, PAG and central and basolateral nuclei of the amygdala (Martin et al. 1998, 1999b; Monhemius et al. 2001; Meng et al. 1998). The amygdala region of the limbic forebrain is implicated in the processing of emotional information. Its functional repertoire also includes modulation of pain sensations such as the induction of stress-induced anti-nociception. Targeted inactivation of the central nucleus region of the amygdala (CeA) in rhesus monkeys and rodents was shown to attenuate the anti-nociceptive effects of systemically administered morphine (Manning et al. 2001, 2003). In rats, this was assessed by two outcome measures: an increase to tail flick latencies and a decrease in the level of Fos protein in the spinal cord evoked by the injection of formalin into the hind paw. Chemical activation of nociceptors in hind paw skin by formalin produces a bi-phasic nociceptive behaviour that is strongly correlated to the level of Fos protein induced in the lumbar spinal cord (Presley et al. 1990). The activity of spinal cord neurones receiving nociceptive input from the hind paw is modulated by descending inputs. Inactivation of the CeA region results in dysfunction of these inputs, as indicated by a decrease in the extent to which morphine is able to reduce Fos levels. Repetition of these experiments with systemic administration of WIN55212-2 similarly demonstrated that inactivation of the CeA region was also effective at reducing the full anti-nociceptive effects of this CB. WIN55,212-2 reduction of formalin-induced Fos was similarly affected, implicating the role of descending inputs in the systemic anti-nociceptive effects of CBs, as well as opioids, in the spinal cord (Manning et al. 2003). CB_1 receptors are enriched in the limbic system and are the likely targets for CB-mediated effects on both the anxiolytic and analgesic functions of this region (Herkenham et al. 1990; Glass et al. 1997).

As further evidence for the involvement of descending nociceptive pathways, the selective depletion of noradrenaline in the terminals of descending projections to the rat lumbar spinal cord was effective at suppressing the anti-nociceptive efficacy of both opioids and WIN55,212-2 in both acute and tonic nociception assays (Martin et al. 1999a; Gutierrez et al. 2003). Consistent with these results, CB-mediated anti-nociception can be attenuated by antagonising α2-noradrenaline receptors (Martin et al. 1991). The microinjection of WIN55,212-2 directly to the A5 noradrenergic nucleus in the brain stem also produces anti-nociceptive effects in the tail flick test (Martin et al. 1999b). This microinjection study also implicated the superior colliculus and lateral posterior and submedius regions of the thalamus in CB-mediated analgesia. The presence of injury-regulated CB_1 receptor expression in the thalamus lends support to this evidence (Siegling et al. 2001).

Neural circuits located in the RVM and PAG regions of the brain stem also contribute to opioid and CB-mediated analgesia. Microinjections of CBs into the RVM suppress pain-related behaviour (Martin et al. 1998; Monhemius et al. 2001) and targeted inactivation of the RVM (by pharmacological activation of $GABA_A$ receptors) prevents the analgesic action of systemic CBs (Meng et al. 1998; Meng and Johansen; 2004). In vitro recordings from brain stem slices have demonstrated a CB_1-mediated pre-synaptic inhibition of GABAergic neurotransmission in the RVM (Vaughan et al. 1999). Extracellular single unit recordings, conducted during local microinfusion of WIN55,212-2 to the RVM, has determined its effect on the activity of individual neurones involved in withdrawal reflexes (Meng and Johansen 2004). Before a withdrawal reflex, the activity of RVM 'on-cells' increases whilst 'off-cell' activity decreases. CB-mediated activation of CB_1 receptors prolongs tail withdrawal latencies by inhibiting the activity of on-cells and disinhibiting off-cell firing. Endogenous opioids released in the RVM operate via μ-opioid receptors to inhibit limb withdrawals by the same mechanism. However, pretreatment with μ-opioid receptor antagonists have demonstrated that the analgesic effects of WIN55,212-2 in the RVM occur independently (Meng et al. 1998). Pre-treatment with the selective CB_1 receptor antagonist SR141716a also provided evidence that RVM CB_1 receptors are tonically activated to suppress nociceptive behaviours. In a separate study, microinfusions of WIN55,212-2 or SR141716a into the nucleus reticularis gigantocellularis pars α (GiA) region of the RVM also demonstrated

CB_1-mediated inhibition of nociceptive behaviours in the tail flick and formalin tests (Monhemius et al. 2001). The results suggested that sustained input from ascending nociceptive pathways (provided by peripheral formalin injection or nerve injury) is required to stimulate endocannabinoid production in the RVM and drive descending inhibition.

Further evidence that endocannabinoid production in the brain stem modulates pain responses, is provided by a microdialysis study in rats (Walker et al. 1999). Release of AEA in the periaqueductal grey was measured after formalin injection into the hind paw or local electrical stimulation of the dorsal and lateral PAG. Enhancement of AEA levels in the PAG, by direct electrical stimulation, produced an analgesic effect that was mediated by CB_1 receptors. In support of this mechanism, formalin-evoked Fos protein, induced in the PAG, was attenuated by a local microinjection of HU210 (Finn et al. 2003). In vitro electrophysiological studies have revealed a CB_1-dependant modulation of excitatory and inhibitory post-synaptic currents in the PAG. The pre-synaptic inhibitory mechanisms mediating this action were also exhibited by μ-opioids (Vaughan et al. 2000).

3.1.2
CB Receptors in Spinal Cord

The importance of supraspinal mechanisms to the anti-nociceptive action of systemically administered CBs, is highlighted by the finding that spinal transection reduces the anti-nociceptive effect of systemically administered Δ^9THC and CP55,940, as measured by tail flick latency (Lichtman and Martin 1991) and noxious heat-evoked activity in spinal wide dynamic range neurones (Hohmann et al. 1999b). Yet there is evidence that CBs can also operate via local analgesic mechanisms sited in the spinal cord. CBs applied directly to the spinal cord suppress the responses of dorsal horn neurones to nociceptive input from C-fibres (Tsou et al. 1996; Hohmann et al. 1995, 1998; Drew et al. 2000; Harris et al. 2000) and have the ability to raise nociceptive thresholds in normal animals (Richardson et al. 1997; Pertwee et al. 2001). Analgesic effects can persist even after spinal transection (Smith and Martin 1992), suggesting that at least some of the anti-nociceptive actions of CBs are intrinsic to CB signalling mechanisms in the spinal cord (Lichtman and Martin 1991). Intrathecal delivery of CBs also reduces pain behaviours associated with tissue injury: inflammatory thermal hyperalgesia was decreased by intrathecal AEA in a manner that was reversed by intrathecal administration of the selective CB_1 antagonist SR141716a (Richardson et al. 1997). Intrathecal WIN55,212-2 attenuated pain behaviour following formalin injection via a CB_1—but not a CB_2—receptor-dependent mechanism (Rice et al. 2002). Intrathecally administered HU210 was found to be more effective than morphine in attenuating formalin-evoked pain behaviour (Guhring et al. 2001).

Spinal CBs also suppress mechanical hypersensitivity after inflammatory (Martin et al. 1999c) and neuropathic (Fox et al. 2001) injury. Furthermore, hyperalgesia (evoked by injections of capsaicin into the hind paw) can be suppressed by spinal CP55,940 (Johanek et al. 2001). Electrophysiological recordings have shown that the sustained noxious input generated by capsaicin in this model potentiates the activity of spinal nociceptive neurones, allowing them to be activated by sub-threshold sensory stimuli. In this study, the sensitised responses of dorsal horn cells to mechanical stimuli could be attenuated by activation of spinal CB_1 receptors with CP55,940. This suggests that the hyperexcitability of dorsal horn neurones (an underlying mechanism for hypersensitivity after tissue injury) can be inhibited by CBs applied directly to the spinal cord. In support of this claim, short-term potentiation or 'wind-up' responses in these neurones and the induction of Fos protein are both suppressed by WIN55,212-2 applied directly to the spinal cord (Strangman and Walker 1999; Martin et al. 1999c).

The mechanism of action to explain the inhibitory effect of CBs at the central synapses of nociceptive C-fibres has not yet been fully elucidated. The location of CB_1 receptors in this area indicates that there could be several sites of action for exogenous CBs applied to the cord surface (Sect. 1.3.2). Functional evidence from patch clamp studies—recording from second order neurones in adult rat trigeminal caudal nucleus (Liang et al. 2004) and spinal cord slices (Morisset et al. 2001)—provides evidence for CB inhibition of glutamate transmission from pre-synaptic C-fibre terminals. WIN55,212-2 is proposed to operate at CB_1 receptors located pre-synaptically on the central terminals of sensory afferents by inhibiting calcium influx via N-type voltage-gated calcium channels (Liang et al. 2004). This mechanism is further supported by peptide release studies from spinal cord tissue, which also serve to strengthen the evidence for a spinal site of CB analgesia. Using ex vivo spinal cord tissue mounted in a superfusion chamber, the excitation-mediated release of peptides found in the central terminals of C-fibres can be measured in the superfusate fluid in response to C-fibre stimulation. CB application to the tissue reduces the release of CGRP and SP peptides after electrical or capsaicin stimulation of C-fibres, an effect that can be attenuated by CB_1 receptor antagonists (Richardson et al. 1998b; Tognetto et al. 2001; Lever et al. 2002; Brooks et al. 2004). Likewise, in cultured sensory neurones, voltage-activated Ca^{2+} currents can be attenuated by CB_1-mediated inhibition of N-type VGCC (Ross et al. 2001; Khasabova et al. 2004), and capsaicin-evoked increases in $[Ca^{2+}]_i$ are also suppressed by CBs (Millns et al. 2001; Oshita et al. 2005).

Collectively, the evidence suggests that CB_1 receptor activity can reduce the increases in $[Ca^{2+}]_i$ that drive transmitter exocytosis in sensory neurones. It is plausible that this mechanism also operates at the central terminals of cutaneous sensory neurones in the spinal cord; however, there is a paucity of anatomical evidence for CB_1 receptors in this location (Sect. 1.3.3).

Several studies also suggest that there maybe tonic inhibitory control over dorsal horn neurones receiving nociceptive input exerted by endogenous CBs acting at pre-synaptic CB_1 receptors. Spinal administration of SR141716a has been shown to facilitate responses of dorsal horn neurones to noxious C-fibre input (Chapman et al. 1999) and reduce the threshold for thermal nociceptive responses in rats (Richardson et al. 1997). This effect is possibly due to the increased release of excitatory transmitters from stimulated C-fibre terminals, as evidence for this was provided by the ability of SR141716a to increase capsaicin-evoked peptide release from both spinal cord tissue and cultured DRGs (Lever et al. 2002; Ahluwalia et al. 2003a). However, the application of SR141716a to spinal cord slices had no effect on the excitability of dorsal horn neurones (Morisset et al. 2001). The production of endocannabinoids from C-fibre-responsive dorsal horn neurones has been proposed to explain the ability of AMPA (S-alpha-amino-3-hydroxy-5-methyl-4-isoxazolepropionic acid) superfusion to reduce electrically evoked CGRP release from spinal cord slices, as this inhibitory effect can be reversed by SR141716a (Brooks et al. 2004). In this setting, endocannabinoids produced by excitation of post-synaptic neurones may signal retrogradely back onto pre-synaptic CB_1 receptors in order to reduce excitatory transmission from these fibres. In support of this effect, the increased production of endogenous CBs by systemic treatment with the AEA uptake inhibitor AM404, reduces Fos protein induction (Rodella et al. 2005). Endocannabinoid signalling at CB_1 receptors in the dorsal horn is also cited to explain the analgesic effects of some nonsteroidal anti-inflammatory drug (NSAIDs) (Ates et al. 2003).

As a substantial proportion of dorsal horn CB_1 receptors are expressed by interneurone populations, including GABAergic neurones and those expressing opioid receptors (Sect. 1.3.2), the spinal analgesic action of CBs may operate via other intrinsic inhibitory systems. Interaction between CB and opioid signalling is consistent with reports of synergism and cross-tolerance between their analgesic effects in the spinal cord (Manzanares et al. 1999). Delivery of intrathecal CBs has been used to enhance endogenous opioid levels measured in the spinal cord (see Welch and Eads 1999). In addition, opioid receptor antagonists can be used to reverse the anti-hyperalgesic effects of intrathecal CBs (Thorat and Bhargava 1994; Welch and Eads 1999). This is except in models of neuropathic pain (Fox et al. 2001; Bridges et al. 2001a; Mao et al. 2000), where the reduction of spinal opioid binding sites is more extensive compared to CB_1 (Hohmann et al. 1999a) and may explain why, in contrast to opioids, the anti-nociceptive potency of CBs remains unchanged after a nerve injury (Mao et al. 2000; Dogrul et al. 2003). A recent study by Naderi et al. (2005) has demonstrated that spinal $GABA_B$ receptors do not mediate the analgesic effects of intrathecal CP55490 measured in the formalin test. Conversely, the analgesic effect of intrathecal baclofen (a $GABA_B$ receptor agonist) is prevented by pretreatment with SR141716a. Interestingly, this suggests that endocannabinoid signalling at CB_1 receptors is required for baclofen-mediated analgesia in this model.

It has recently become clear that not only spinal neurones but also microglia play a role in the CNS responses to inflammation and peripheral nerve injury that underlie persistent pain (DeLeo et al. 2001; Watkins et al. 2001; Watkins et al. 2003; Tsuda et al. 2005). Evidence suggests that microglia express functional CB_2 receptors and synthesise endocannabinoids and that CBs can influence microglial migration (Walter et al. 2003). Furthermore, CBs block cytokine mRNA expression in cultured microglial cells (Puffenbarger et al. 2000) and are implicated in anti-inflammatory and neuroprotective effects mediated by CB receptors on glial and neuronal cells (Molina-Holgado et al. 2003; see Walter and Stella 2004). The appearance of CB_2 mRNA in the spinal cord after nerve injury coincident with microglial activation (Zhang et al. 2003), together with the analgesic efficacy of selective CB_2 agonists in inflammatory and neuropathic pain (Malan et al. 2001; Ibrahim et al. 2003), may implicate the function of spinal CB_2 receptors in CB-mediated analgesia. Most of the experimental evidence so far indicates that the analgesic effects of spinally administered CBs are predominately mediated via CB_1 receptors.

3.2
Peripheral Mechanisms

A number of recent studies have demonstrated that pain responses can be reduced by CBs applied locally to peripheral tissues at systemically inactive doses. These effects are locally reversed by CB receptor antagonists, implying that the analgesic mechanisms involve peripheral CB receptors and are distinct from the actions of CBs at receptors in the brain and spinal cord.

After inflammatory injury, both the effects of paw oedema and thermal hyperalgesia can be attenuated by a local injection of a low dose of AEA into the paw skin, but not when the same dose of AEA was applied systemically. Co-administration of the CB_1 receptor antagonist SR141716a reversed the effect of AEA on thermal hypersensitivity. It also attenuated the CB-mediated reduction of plasma extravasation after capsaicin inflammation, thus demonstrating both an anti-hyperalgesic and anti-inflammatory action for CBs operating via peripheral CB_1 receptors (Richardson et al. 1998b). The peripheral anti-hyperalgesic actions of CBs, after capsaicin-induced inflammation, were also attenuated by CB_1 receptor antagonists (Johanek et al. 2001; Ko et al. 1999). Local injection of WIN55,212-2, HU210, AEA or methanandamide in the formalin model of the rat hind paw skin inflammation confirmed a reduction in pain behaviour via the activation of peripheral CB_1 receptors, excluding effects via CB_2 or opioid receptors (Calignano et al. 1998). However, hind paw injection of PEA, reduced pain behaviour via a CB_2-dependent mechanism, and co-injection of AEA and PEA produced a synergistic analgesic effect. This suggested the existence of two separate analgesic mechanisms operating via peripheral CB_1 and CB_2 receptors. In support of this hypothesis, the peripheral analgesic effects of WIN55,212-2-mediating the reduction of hyperalgesia or spinal Fos induction after carrageenan inflammation-can be blocked separately by CB_1 and CB_2 receptor antagonists (Nackley et al. . 2003a; Kehl et al. 2003). A peripheral analgesic action of CBs mediated by CB_2 receptors has been confirmed in several inflammatory pain models by the use of CB_2-selective agonists and antagonists (Hanus et al. 1999; Malan et al. 2001; Quartilho et al. 2003; Malan et al. 2003; Hohmann et al. 2004; Elmes et al. 2004).

Systemic CB_2 receptor-selective agonists are also effective against paw tissue oedema (Clayton et al. 2002; Malan et al. 2003). In electrophysiological studies, local injection of CB_2 agonists could inhibit both the normal and potentiated responses of dorsal horn neurones (after inflammation of the hind paw, CB_2 agonists suppressed both the receptive field expansion and wind-up responses in spinal cord neurones) (Sokal et al. 2003; Nackley et al. 2004; Elmes et al. 2004). Local injection of a CB_1-selective agonist also suppresses responses to mechanical stimuli in carrageenan inflamed and non-inflamed rats (Kelly et al. 2003). Interestingly, however, the peripheral effects of AEA on these responses were attenuated by a CB_2 antagonist (Sokal et al. 2003).

Peripheral CB_1 and CB_2 receptors have both been implicated in the anti-hyperalgesic effects of locally injected CBs after nerve injury (Fox et al. 2001; Ibrahim et al. 2003; Elmes et al. 2004; Ulugol et al. 2004; see Sect. 2.2). Thus, CBs have anti-inflammatory, anti-hyperalgesic and anti-nociceptive actions that can be mediated by peripheral CB_1 and CB_2 receptors.

Endogenous CBs have been measured in skin (the site of the peripheral analgesic action of CBs) and their levels here are increased by tissue injury (Calignano et al. 1998; Oka et al. 2005). Therefore, CBs in the skin may interact directly with receptors on the peripheral endings of cutaneous nociceptive sensory neurones to modulate the transmission of nociceptive signals to the spinal cord. As evidence of this direct mechanism, functional CB_1 receptors have been demonstrated on cultured sensory neurones (Ross et al. 2001; Khasabova et al. 2004; Millns et al. 2001; Oshita et al. 2005) where inhibition of excitatory calcium transients reduces the exocytosis of neuropeptides both from sensory neurone cell bodies (Ahluwalia et al. 2003a; Oshita et al. 2005) and the peripheral terminals of these cells stimulated in skin (Richardson et al. 1998b; Ellington et al. 2002). The suppressive effects of topical CBs on efferent C-fibre functions in vivo (Sect. 1.3.3) are also thought to be mediated by the inhibition of excitatory neuropeptide release. The release of AEA—stimulated by $[Ca^{2+}]_i$ increases in these neurones in culture (Ahluwalia et al. 2003b)—may provide the means for a negative feedback on excitatory transmitter release from sensory neurones. Nerve injury, involving transection of the nerve trunk and disruption of distal axonal transport, is likely to reduce peripheral CB receptor levels (Bridges et al. 2002). This may explain why the anti-nociceptive phenotype exhibited by $FAAH^{-/-}$ mice is retained by inflammatory injury but lost after nerve injury (Lichtman et al. 2004a). So far the anatomical evidence does not fully support the hypothesis that direct activation of CB_1 receptors on peripheral nociceptive sensory neurones mediates the local anti-nociceptive and anti-hyperalgesic actions of CBs (see Sect. 1.3.3). Anatomical and functional evidence for CB_2 receptors on these fibres is also limited. Instead, stimulation of β-endorphin release by AM1241 acting on CB_2 receptors in skin keratinocytes has been proposed as a mechanism to explain the peripheral analgesic actions of this compound, as these effects are critically dependent on μ-opioid receptor activity (Ibrahim et al. 2005). In support of this mechanism, topical application of WIN55,212-2 and morphine were demonstrated to have synergistic effects in the mouse tail flick test (Yesilyurt et al. 2003).

An alternative mechanism to explain the peripheral anti-hyperalgesic action of CBs is linked to anti-inflammatory effects of these compounds in peripheral tissues. CB agonists may indirectly inhibit transmission in nociceptive afferents by reducing the release of by-products of inflammatory and excitotoxic processes, which serve to sensitise peripheral nociceptive fibres to mechanical and thermal stimuli. CB_1 and CB_2 receptor-mediated inhibition of cAMP formation could act to reduce the potentiating effects of PKA on TRPV1 receptor-mediated responses in these neurones (see Ross et al. 2004; Oshita et al. 2005). CBs are reported to reduce the production and release of pro-inflammatory signalling molecules, including TNF, NO and interleukin (IL)-1, and to enhance the release of anti-inflammatory cytokines like the IL-1 receptor antagonist, IL-4 and IL-10 (Molina-Holgado et al. 2003; Howlett et al. 2002; Walter and Stella 2004).

Mast cells synthesise and release inflammatory mediators that increase local vascular permeability, and others, like serotonin and NGF, can directly sensitise receptors involved in transducing noxious stimuli on sensory neurones. The ability of CB_1 and CB_2 receptor signalling to reduce inflammatory responses has been linked to their regulation of mast cell function (Samson et al. 2003; Mazzari et al. 1996). CB_1 receptor activation on mast cell lines is linked to the suppression of serotonin secretory responses, whereas co-expressed CB_2 receptors regulate the activation of signalling pathways that regulate gene expression. CBs are also reported to suppress immune cell proliferation and chemotactic processes that contribute to the establishment of inflammatory sites in tissues (Howlett et al. 2002; Walter and Stella 2004). Specifically, PEA has been shown to reduce neutrophil accumulation in hind paw skin inflamed by NGF injections (Farquhar-Smith and Rice 2003). This is speculated to involve peripheral CB_2-like receptor signalling pathways that act to reduce the production and/or release of mast cell-derived neutrophil chemotactic factors, such as leukotriene B4 or even NGF itself. Components of the inhibitory action of CBs on oedema and plasma extravasation are also likely to be mediated by suppression of the pro-inflammatory functions of glial and immune cells (see Walter and Stella 2004). The reduced paw oedema observed in inflamed $FAAH^{-/-}$ mice (Lichtman et al. 2004a) was maintained in conditional (non-neuronal cell) FAAH knock-outs, but was not sensitive to CB_1 or CB_2 receptor antagonists (Cravatt et al. 2004), thus implicating the involvement of other CB-sensitive receptors (Sect. 1.1).

The peripheral anti-inflammatory, anti-nociceptive and anti-hyperalgesic actions of CB_1 and CB_2 receptor agonists are of potential therapeutic importance because they may present a way of delivering the analgesic benefit of CB compounds without their centrally mediated psychoactive side-effects. The CB_2 receptor agonist AM1251 maybe useful in this context, as systemic administration produces no CNS side-effect in animal models (Malan et al. 2001).

4
Analgesic Actions of CBs in Humans

Reports from animal studies provide strong evidence to support the analgesic effects of CBs; however, studies in human volunteers and patients are at a much earlier stage and the evidence is, at present, weak. Nevertheless, patient surveys report the use of cannabis for pain relief: in a recent survey of 2,969 UK patients, medicinal use of cannabis is reported by those with chronic pain (25%) multiple sclerosis (22%), arthritis (21%) and neuropathy (19%) (Ware et al. 2005). Of a sample of 209 Canadian chronic non-cancer pain sufferers, 15% reported having used cannabis at least once for the control of their pain, with approximately 38% using cannabis at least daily (Ware et al. 2003). There is also evidence that a significant proportion of people living with human immunodeficiency virus (HIV) in London use cannabis for symptom control (Woolridge et al. 2005).

4.1
Evidence from Volunteer Studies

There is a relatively small literature on the effects of CBs in human volunteer models of pain. Application of HU210 to human skin has been reported to have inhibitory effects on histamine-evoked itch (Dvorak et al. 2003) and capsaicin-evoked pain responses (Rukwied et al. 2003). In the latter study, the rate of increase in pain intensity following capsaicin application was lower in the HU210-treated compared to the placebo (ethanol)-treated group, and a similar temporary slowing in the development phase of capsaicin-associated mechanical allodynia was reported. However, there was no overall difference in pain intensity. Anti-nociceptive properties of smoked marijuana have also been reported in a noxious thermal stimulus withdrawal test (Greenwald and Stitzer 2000). In contrast, a study on 12 volunteers reported that a single does of oral THC (20 mg) did not have significant anti-nociceptive effects on responses to thermal, mechanical or electrical stimuli. Interestingly, 30 mg of morphine was effective in most of the tests, and some analgesic effects were reported when THC was administered with 30 mg of morphine before electrical stimulation (Naef et al. 2003).

4.2
Evidence from Randomised Controlled Clinical Trials

The data from clinical trials to date indicate that the efficacy of currently available CBs in humans is modest and that their effectiveness is hampered by an unfavourable therapeutic index.

A qualitative systematic review of trials published up to 1999 identified nine clinical trials of CBs of sufficient quality for inclusion in the analysis (Campbell et al. 2001). Five of these trials used cancer pain as a model, two used chronic non-malignant pain and two acute pain. Most of the trials examined the effects of either Δ^9THC or levonantradol. The analgesic effect of these CBs was estimated to be approximately equi-analgesic to codeine 50–120 mg, but adverse effects were common, being reported in all studies. One study showed the adverse effects to be dose-related and it is possible that these obfuscated a greater analgesic effect at the higher dose of Δ^9THC which was examined (Noyes et al. 1975).

Since 1999, several clinical trials have been published in which the analgesic effects of CBs in chronic, especially neuropathic, pain conditions were investigated. One trial examined the efficacy of CBs in alleviating neuropathic symptoms in multiple sclerosis (Wade et al. 2003). In this study, a self-titration regimen was used in which either plant-derived Δ^9THC, cannabidiol, a 1:1 mixture of Δ^9THC and cannabidiol, or placebo were administered by sublingual spray. Data on a range of symptoms were collected and modest analgesic effects were evident. Whilst the fixed ratio preparation (mean dose 22 mg/day) was not associated with a significant reduction in baseline pain intensity scores, Δ^9THC (23.5 mg/day) and cannabidiol (22 mg/day) were, when compared to the effect of placebo. Adverse effects were common; 30%–67% of subjects reporting more than one adverse event, and 17% of patients withdrew from the trial because of adverse effects. A cross-over trial of 24 multiple sclerosis patients with central pain investigated the effects of a 3-week course of daily treatment with oral dronabinol (maximum 10 mg dose) (Svendsen et al. 2004). The authors report a modest but significant analgesic effect of the active treatment on median spontaneous pain intensity scores, calculating a number needed to treat (NNT) value for 50% pain relief at 3.5. A study of 48 patients with central neuropathic pain resulting from brachial plexus avulsion injury reported that short-term treatment with oral cannabis extract (as an adjunct to existing medication) revealed no improvement in the primary pain efficacy measure (Berman et al. 2004). Furthermore, a complicated trial of 21 patients with chronic neuropathic pain, in which patients received two daily doses of ajulemic acid (the synthetically modified metabolite of THC) for a week, did reveal evidence of analgesic efficacy for this compound (Karst et al. 2003). No significant effects of the drug on mechanical hypersensitivity were reported in this trial; however, there was evidence of an analgesic effect. Pain relief from conventional CBs was also measured as a secondary outcome in a very large study in multiple sclerosis patients (Zajicek et al. 2003): although there was no effect of CBs on the primary efficacy measures, a modest analgesic effect was reported.

4.3
Side-Effects

In addition to efficacy, adverse effects are important in determining the clinical effectiveness of any novel therapy, and an acceptable therapeutic index for short-term adverse events will have to be proved for CBs. Furthermore, concerns relating to the long-term risk of developing mental illness in regular cannabis users have obvious relevance for the patients electing to undergo long-term, regular medication with CBs in conditions such as chronic pain. For example, a 27-year cohort study of 50,000 Swedish military conscripts found a dose-dependant increased risk of schizophrenia (once confounding factors such as cannabis use in prodromal schizophrenia and concomitant drug abuse had been excluded) in regular cannabis users (Zammit et al. 2002). Similar findings for depression and anxiety (Patton et al. 2002) and psychosis (Arseneault et al. 2002; D'Souza et al. 2004; Henquet et al. 2005) have also been reported in smaller cohort studies. There is also evidence that the risk of cannabis-induced psychosis is substantially greater in those individuals who have a predisposition to developing psychosis (Henquet et al. 2005) or genetic functional polymorphisms (Caspi et al. 2005). There are also data indicating cumulative, dose-dependent deficits in cognitive function in regular cannabis users (Solowij et al. 2002).

5
Concluding Remarks

There are compelling laboratory data supporting the analgesic effects of CBs; however, before CB-based drugs can be used therapeutically in humans, they must be shown to be both effective and safe in long-term regular use. Well-designed clinical trials are therefore required, but are perhaps premature until suitable CBs with a satisfactory therapeutic index for analgesia and proven bioavailability when administered by a practical route of administration are available for human study. Current strategies to circumvent side-effects but retain analgesic efficacy include the development of non-psychoactive or peripherally active CBs, such as cannabidiol, ajulemic acid and CB_2 receptor selective agonists (Fride et al. 2004; Salim et al. 2005; Ibrahim et al. 2005). Whilst new drugs are being trialled, the prospective clinical uses for CBs could lie with chronic pain patients in whom fear contributes to abnormal pain behaviour (Marsicano et al. 2002) or in situations where the adverse effects of CBs might confer additional benefit over existing therapies, for example by exploiting their anti-inflammatory or anti-emetic properties.

Acknowledgements   The authors receive support from the Wellcome Trust.

References

Ahluwalia J, Urban L, Capogna M, Bevan S, Nagy I (2000) Cannabinoid 1 receptors are expressed in nociceptive primary sensory neurones. Neuroscience 100:685–688

Ahluwalia J, Urban L, Bevan S, Capogna M, Nagy I (2002) Cannabinoid 1 receptors are expressed by nerve growth factor- and glial cell-derived neurotrophic factor-responsive primary sensory neurones. Neuroscience 110:747–753

Ahluwalia J, Urban L, Bevan S, Nagy I (2003a) Anandamide regulates neuropeptide release from capsaicin-sensitive primary sensory neurones by activating both the cannabinoid 1 receptor and the vanilloid receptor 1 in vitro. Eur J Neurosci 17:2611–2618

Ahluwalia J, Yacoob M, Urban L, Bevan S, Nagy I (2003b) Activation of capsaicin-sensitive primary sensory neurones induces anandamide production and release. J Neurochem 84:585–591

Arseneault L, Cannon M, Poulton R, Murray R, Caspi A, Moffitt TE (2002) Cannabis use in adolescence and risk for adult psychosis: longitudinal prospective study. Br Med J 325:1212–1213

Ates M, Hamza M, Seidel K, Kotalla CE, Ledent C, Guhring H (2003) Intrathecally applied flurbiprofen produces an endocannabinoid-dependent antinociception in the rat formalin test. Eur J Neurosci 17:597–604

Bandell M, Story GM, Hwang SW, Viswanath V, Eid SR, Petrus MJ, Earley TJ, Patapoutian A (2004) Noxious cold ion channel TRPA1 is activated by pungent compounds and bradykinin. Neuron 41:849–857

Bayewitch M, Avidor Reiss T, Levy R, Barg J, Mechoulam R, Vogel Z (1995) The peripheral cannabinoid receptor: adenylate cyclase inhibition and G protein coupling. FEBS Lett 375:143–147

Begg M, Pacher P, Batkai S, Osei-Hyiaman D, Offertaler L, Mo FM, Liu J, Kunos G (2005) Evidence of for novel cannabinoid receptors. Pharmacol Ther 106:133–145

Bell MR, D'Ambra TE, Kumar V, Eissenstat MA, Herrmann JL Jr, Wetzel JR, Rosi D, Philion RE, Daum SJ, Hlasta DJ (1991) Antinociceptive (aminoalkyl)indoles. J Med Chem 34:1099–1110

Beltramo M, Stella N, Calignano A, Lin SY, Makriyannis A, Piomelli D (1997) Functional role of high-affinity anandamide transport, as revealed by selective inhibition. Science 277:1094–1097

Berman JS, Symonds C, Birch R (2004) Efficacy of two cannabis based medicinal extracts for relief of central neuropathic pain from brachial plexus avulsion: results of a randomised controlled trial. Pain 112:299–306

Bisogno T, Maurelli S, Melck D, De Petrocellis L, Di Marzo V (1997) Biosynthesis, uptake, and degradation of anandamide and palmitoylethanolamide in leukocytes. J Biol Chem 272:3315–3323

Bisogno T, Hanus L, De Petrocellis L, Tchilibon S, Ponde DE, Brandi I, Schiano Moriello A, Davis JB, Mechoulam R, Di Marzo V (2001) Molecular targets for cannabidiol and its synthetic analogues: effect on vanilloid VR1 receptors and on the cellular uptake and enzymatic hydrolysis of anandamide. Br J Pharmacol 134:845–852

Bouaboula M, Perrachon S, Milligan L, Canat X, Rinaldi-Carmona M, Portier M, Barth F, Calandra B, Pecceu F, Lupker J, Maffrand JP, Le Fur G, Casellas P (1997) A selective inverse agonist for central cannabinoid receptor inhibits mitogen-activated protein kinase activation stimulated by insulin or insulin-like growth factor 1. Evidence for a new model of receptor/ligand interactions. J Biol Chem 272:22330–22339

Bouaboula M, Desnoyer N, Carayon P, Combes T, Casellas P (1999) Gi protein modulation induced by a selective inverse agonist for the peripheral cannabinoid receptor CB2: implication for intracellular signalization cross-regulation. Mol Pharmacol 55:473–480

Bracey MH, Hanson MA, Masuda KR, Stevens RC, Cravatt BF (2002) Structural adaptations in a membrane enzyme that terminates endocannabinoid signaling. Science 298: 1793–1796

Bradshaw HB, Walker JM (2005) The expanding field of cannabimimetic and related lipid mediators. Br J Pharmacol 144:459–465

Breivogel CS, Selley DE, Childers SR (1998) Cannabinoid receptor agonist efficacy for stimulating [35S]GTPgammaS binding to rat cerebellar membranes correlates with agonist-induced decreases in GDP affinity. J Biol Chem 273:16865–16873

Breivogel CS, Griffin G, Di Marzo V, Martin BR (2001) Evidence for a new G-protein coupled cannabinoid receptor in mouse brain. Mol Pharmacol 60:155–163

Bridges D, Ahmad KS, Rice ASC (2001a) The synthetic cannabinoid WIN55,212-2 attenuates hyperalgesia and allodynia in a rat model of neuropathic pain. Br J Pharmacol 133: 586–594

Bridges D, Thompson SWN, Rice ASC (2001b) Mechanisms of neuropathic pain. Br J Anaesth 87:12–26

Bridges D, Rice ASC, Egertova M, Elphick MR, Winter J (2002) The distribution of cannabinoid CB1 receptor within the dorsal root ganglion following peripheral nerve injury. 10th World Congress of Pain, Abstr 371-P5

Bridges D, Rice ASC, Egertova M, Elphick MR, Winter J, Michael GJ (2003) Localisation of cannabinoid receptor 1 in rat dorsal root ganglion using in situ hybridisation and immunohistochemistry. Neuroscience 119:803–812

Brooks JW, Thompson SW, Rice AS, Malcangio M (2004) (S)-AMPA inhibits electrically evoked calcitonin gene-related peptide (CGRP) release from the rat dorsal horn: reversal by cannabinoid receptor antagonist SR141716A. Neurosci Lett 372:85–88

Brown SM, Wager-Miller J, Mackie K (2002) Cloning and molecular characterization of the rat CB2 cannabinoid receptor. Biochim Biophys Acta 1576:255–264

Buckley NE, McCoy KL, Mezey E, Bonner T, Zimmer A, Felder CC, Glass M (2000) Immunomodulation by cannabinoids is absent in mice deficient for the cannabinoid CB(2) receptor. Eur J Pharmacol 396:141–149

Burdyga G, Lal S, Varro A, Dimaline R, Thompson DG, Dockray GJ (2004) Expression of CB1 receptors in vagal afferent neurons in inhibited by cholecystokinin. J Neurosci 24:2708–2715

Burstein SH, Friderichs E, Kogel B, Schneider J, Selve N (1998) Analgesic effects of 1′,1′ dimethylheptyl-delta8-THC-11-oic acid (CT3) in mice. Life Sci 63:161–168

Calignano A, La Rana G, Beltramo M, Makriyannis A, Piomelli D (1997) Potentiation of anandamide hypotension by the transport inhibitor, AM404. Eur J Pharmacol 337:R1–2

Calignano A, La Rana G, Giuffrida A, Piomelli D (1998) Control of pain initiation by endogenous cannabinoids. Nature 394:277–281

Calignano A, La Rana G, Piomelli D (2001) Antinociceptive activity of the endogenous fatty acid amide, palmitylethanolamide. Eur J Pharmacol 419:191–198

Campbell F, Tramer M, Carroll D, Reynolds DJM, Moore RA, McQuay HJ (2001) Are cannabinoids an effective and safe option in the management of pain? A qualitative systematic review. Br Med J 323:13–16

Carlisle SJ, Marciano-carbral F, Staab A, Ludwick C, Cabral GA (2002) Differential expression of the CB2 cannabinoid receptor by rodent macrophages and macrophage-like cells in relation to cell activation. Int Immunopharmacol 2:69–82

Caspi A, Moffitt TE, Cannon M, McClay J, Murray R, Harrington H, Taylor A, Arseneault L, Williams B, Braithwaite A (2005) Moderation of the effect of adolescent-onset cannabis use on adult psychosis by a functional polymorphism in the catechol-o-methyltransferase gene: longitudinal evidence of a gene X environment interaction. Biol Psychiatry 57:1117–1127

Chakrabarti A, Onaivi ES, Chaudhuri G (1995) Cloning and sequencing of a cDNA encoding the mouse brain-type cannabinoid receptor protein. DNA Seq 5:385–388

Chapman V (1999) The cannabinoid CB1 receptor antagonist, SR141716A, selectively facilitates nociceptive responses of dorsal horn neurones in the rat. Br J Pharmacol 127:1765–1767

Chemin J, Monteil A, Perez-Reyes E, Nargot J, Lory P (2001) Direct inhibition of T-type calcium channels by the endogenous cannabinoid anandamide. EMBO J 20:7033–7040

Clayton N, Marshall FH, Bountra C, O'Shaughnessy CT (2002) CB1 and CB2 cannabinoid receptors are implicated in inflammatory pain. Pain 96:253–260

Costa B, Colleoni M, Conti S, Parolaro D, Trovato AE, Franke CM, Giagnoni G (2004) Oral anti-inflammatory activity of cannabidiol, a non-psychoactive constituent of cannabis, in acute carrageenan-induced inflammation in the rat paw. Naunyn Schmiedebergs Arch Pharmacol 369:294–299

Costa B, Giagnoni G, Franke CM, Trovato AE, Colleoni M (2004b) Vanilloid TRPV1 receptor mediated the antihyperalgesic effect of the nonpsychoactive cannabinoid, cannabidiol, in a rat model of acute inflammation. Br J Pharmacol 143:247–250

Costa B, Colleoni M, Conti S, Trovato AE, Bianchi M, Sotgiu ML, Giagnoni G (2004c) Repeated treatment with the synthetic cannabinoid WIN55,212-2 reduces both hyperalgesia and production of pronociceptive mediators in a rat model of neuropathic pain. Br J Pharmacol 141:4–8

Costigan M, Befort K, Karchewski L, Griffin R, D'Urso D, Allchorne A, Sitarski J, Mannion J, Pratt R, Woolf C (2002) Replicate high-density rat genome oligonucleotide microarrays reveal hundreds of regulated genes in the dorsal root ganglion after peripheral nerve injury. BMC Neurosci 3:16

Coutts AA, Anavi-Goffer S, Ross RA, MacEwan DJ, Mackie K, Pertwee RG, Irving AJ (2001) Agonist-induced internalisation and trafficking of cannabinoid CB1 receptors in hippocampal neurons. J Neurosci 21:2425–2433

Cox ML, Welch SP (2004) The antinociceptive effect of Delta9-tetrahydrocannabinol in the arthritic rat. Eur J Pharmacol 493:65–74

Cravatt BF, Giang DK, Mayfield SP, Boger DL, Lerner RA, Gilula NB (1996) Molecular characterization of an enzyme that degrades neuromodulatory fatty-acid amides. Nature 384:83–87

Cravatt BF, Demarest K, Patricelli MP, Bracey MH, Giang DK, Martin BR, Lichtman AH (2001) Supersensitivity to anandamide and enhanced endogenous cannabinoid signaling in mice lacking fatty acid amide hydrolase. Proc Natl Acad Sci USA 98:9371–9376

Cravatt BF, Saghatelian A, Hawkins EG, Clement AB, Bracey MH, Lichtman AH (2004) Functional disassociation of the central and peripheral fatty acid amide signaling systems. Proc Natl Acad Sci USA 101:10821–10826

D'Souza DC, Perry E, MacDougall L, Yola Ammerman Y, Thomas Cooper T, Wu T, Braley G, Gueorguieva R, Krystal JH (2004) The psychotomimetic effects of intravenous delta-9-tetrahydrocannabinol in healthy individuals: implications for psychosis. Neuropsychopharmacology 29:1558–1572

De Petrocellis L, Cascio MG, Di Marzo V (2004) The endocannabinoid system: a general view and latest editions. Br J Pharmacol 141:765–774

Deadwyler SA, Hampson RE, Mu J, Whyte A, Childers S (1995) Cannabinoids modulate voltage sensitive potassium A-current in hippocampal neurons via a cAMP-dependent process. J Pharmacol Exp Ther 273:734–743

DeLeo JA, Yezierski RP (2001) The role of neuroinflammation and neuroimmune activation in persistent pain. Pain 90:1–6

Derkinderen P, Ledent C, Parmentier M, Girault JA (2001) Cannabinoids activate p38 mitogen-activated protein kinases through CB1 receptors in hippocampus. J Neurochem 77:957–960

Deutsch DG, Chin SA (1993) Enzymatic synthesis and degradation of anandamide, a cannabinoid receptor agonist. Biochem Pharmacol 46:791–796

Deutsch DG, Ueda N, Yamamoto S (2002) The fatty acid amide hydrolase (FAAH). Prostaglandins Leukot Essent Fatty Acids 66:201–210

Devane WA, Dysarz FA3, Johnson MR, Melvin LS, Howlett AC (1988) Determination and characterization of a cannabinoid receptor in rat brain. Mol Pharmacol 34:605–613

Devane WA, Hanus L, Breuer A, Pertwee RG, Stevenson LA, Griffin G, Gibson D, Mandelbaum A, Etinger A, Mechoulam R (1992) Isolation and structure of a brain constituent that binds to the cannabinoid receptor. Science 258:1946–1949

Di Marzo V, Deutsch DG (1998) Biochemistry of the endogenous ligands of cannabinoid receptors. Neurobiol Dis 5:386–404

Di Marzo V, Fontana A, Cadas H, Schinelli S, Cimino G, Schwartz JC, Piomelli D (1994) Formation and inactivation of endogenous cannabinoid anandamide in central neurons. Nature 372:686–691

Di Marzo V, Bisogno T, De Petrocellis L, Melck D, Martin BR (1999) Cannabimimetic fatty acid derivatives: the anandamide family and other endocannabinoids. Curr Med Chem 6:721–744

Di Marzo V, Bifulco M, De Petrocellis L (2004) The endocannabinoid system and its therapeutic exploitation. Nat Rev Drug Discov 9:771–784

Dinh TP, Carpenter D, Leslie FM, Freund TF, Katona I, Sensi SL, Kathuria S, Piomelli D (2002) Brain monoglyceride lipase participating in endocannabinoid inactivation. Proc Natl Acad Sci USA 99:10819–10824

Dinis P, Charrua A, Avelino A, Yaqoob M, Bevan S, Nagy I, Cruz F (2004) Anandamide-evoked activation of vanilloid receptor 1 contributes to the development of bladder hyperreflexia and nociceptive transmission to spinal dorsal horn neurons in cystitis. J Neurosci 24:11253–11263

Dogrul A, Gul H, Akar A, Yildiz O, Bilgin F, Guzeldemir E (2003) Topical cannabinoid antinociception: synergy with spinal sites. Pain 105:11–16

Dovrak M, Watkinson A, McGlone F, Rukwied R (2003) Histamine induced responses are attenuated by a cannabinoid receptor in human skin. Inflamm Res 52:238–245

Drew LJ, Harris J, Millns PJ, Kendall DA, Chapman V (2000) Activation of spinal cannabinoid 1 receptors inhibits C-fibre driven hyperexcitable neuronal responses and increases [35S]GTPgammaS binding in the dorsal horn of the spinal cord of noninflamed and inflamed rats. Eur J Neurosci 12:2079–2086

Egertova M, Elphick MR (2000) Localisation of cannabinoid receptors in the rat brain using antibodies to the intracellular C-terminal of CB1. J Comp Neurol 422:159–171

Egertova M, Giang DK, Cravatt BF, Elphick MR (1998) A new perspective on cannabinoid signalling: complementary localization of fatty acid amide hydrolase and CB1 receptor in brain. Proc R Soc Lond B Biol Sci 265:2081–2085

Egertova M, Cravatt BF, Elphick MR (2003) Comparative analysis of fatty acid amide hydrolase and cb1 cannabinoid receptor expression in the mouse brain: evidence of a widespread role for fatty acid amide hydrolase in regulation of endocannabinoid signaling. Neuroscience 119:481–496

Ellington HC, Cotter MA, Cameron NE, Ross RA (2002) The effect of cannabinoids on capsaicin-evoked calcitonin gene-related peptide (CGRP) release from the isolated paw skin of diabetic and non-diabetic rats. Neuropharmacology 42:966–975

Elmes SJR, Jhaveri MD, Smart D, Kendall DA, Chapman V (2004) Cannabinoid CB2 receptor activation inhibits mechanically evoked responses of wide dynamic range dorsal horn neurons in naive rats and in rat models of inflammatory and neuropathic pain. Eur J Pharmacol 20:2311–2320

Evans RM, Scott RH, Ross RA (2004) Multiple actions of anandamide on neonatal rat cultured sensory neurones. Br J Pharmacol 141:1223–1233

Farquhar-Smith WP, Rice AS (2003) A novel neuroimmune mechanism in cannabinoid-mediated attenuation of nerve growth factor-induced hyperalgesia. Anesthesiology 99:1391–1401

Farquhar-Smith WP, Rice ASC (2001) Administration of endocannabinoids prevents a referred hyperalgesia associated with inflammation of the urinary bladder. Anesthesiology 94:507–513

Farquhar-Smith WP, Egertova M, Bradbury EJ, McMahon SB, Rice ASC, Elphick MR (2000) Cannabinoid CB1 receptor expression in rat spinal cord. Mol Cell Neurosci 15:510–521

Farquhar-Smith WP, Jaggar SI, Rice ASC (2002) Attenuation of nerve growth factor-induced visceral hyperalgesia via cannabinoid CB1 and CB2-like receptors. Pain 97:11–21

Felder CC, Briley EM, Axelrod J, Simpson JT, Mackie K, Devane WA (1993) Anandamide, an endogenous cannabimimetic eicosanoid, binds to the cloned human cannabinoid receptor and stimulates receptor-mediated signal transduction. Proc Natl Acad Sci U S A 90:7656–7660

Finn DP, Jhaveri MD, Beckett SRG, Roe CH, Kendall DA, Marsden CA, Chapman V (2003) Effects of direct periaqueductal grey administration of a cannabinoid receptor agonist on nociceptive and aversive responses in rats. Neuropharmacology 45:594–604

Fowler CJ, Jacobsson SOP (2002) Cellular transport of anandamide, 2-arachidonoylglycerol and palmitoylethanolamide—target for drug development? Prostaglandins Leukot Essent Fatty Acids 66:193–200

Fox A, Kesingland A, Gentry C, McNair K, Patel S, Urban L, James IF (2001) The role of central and peripheral cannabinoid1 receptors in the antihyperalgesic activity of cannabinoids in a model of neuropathic pain. Pain 92:91–100

Fride E, Feigin C, Ponde DE, Breuer A, Hanus L, Arshavsky N, Mechoulam R (2004) (+)-Cannabidiol analogues which bind cannabinoid receptors but exert peripheral activity only. Eur J Pharmacol 506:179–188

Galiègue S, Mary S, Marchand J, Dussossoy D, Carriere D, Carayon P, Bouaboula M, Shire D, Le Fur G, Casellas P (1995) Expression of central and peripheral cannabinoid receptors in human immune tissues and leukocyte subpopulations. Eur J Pharmacol 232:54–61

Gaoni Y, Mechoulam R (1964) Isolation, structure and partial synthesis of an active constituent of hashish. J Am Chem Soc 86:1646–1647

Gebremedhin D, Lange AR, Campbell WB, Hillard CJ, Harder DR (1999) Cannabinoid CB1 receptor of cat cerebral arterial muscle functions to inhibit L-type Ca2+ channel current. Am J Physiol 276:H2085–H2093

Gerard CM, Mollereau C, Vassart G, Parmentier M (1991) Molecular cloning of a human cannabinoid receptor which is also expressed in testis. Biochem J 279:129–134

Giuffrida A, Parsons LH, Kerr TM, Rodriguez de Fonseca F, Navarro M, Piomelli D (1999) Dopamine activation of endogenous cannabinoid signalling in dorsal striatum. Nat Neurosci 2:358–363

Glass M, Dragunow M, Faull RL (1997) Cannabinoid receptors in the human brain: a detailed anatomical and quantitative autoradiographic study in the fetal, neonatal and adult human brain. Neuroscience 77:299–318

Greenwald MK, Stitzer ML (2000) Antinociceptive, subjective and behavioral effects of smoked marijuana in humans. Drug Alcohol Depend 59:261–275

Griffin G, Tao Q, Abood ME (2000) Cloning and pharmacological characterization of the rat CB2 cannabinoid receptor. J Pharmacol Exp Ther 292:886–894

Guhring H, Schuster J, Hamza M, Ates M, Kotalla CE, Brune K (2001) HU210 shows higher efficacy and potency than morphine after intrathecal administration in the mouse formalin test. Eur J Pharmacol 429:127–134

Gutierrez T, Nackley AG, Neely MH, Freeman KG, Edwards GL, Hohmann AG (2003) Effects of neurotoxic destruction of descending noradrenergic pathways on cannabinoid antinociception in models of acute and tonic nociception. Brain Res 987:176–185

Guylas AI, Cravatt BF, Bracey MH, Dinh TP, Piomelli D, Boscia F, Freund TF (2004) Segregation of two endocannabinoid-hydrolysing enzymes into pre- and postsynaptic compartments in the rat hippocampus, cerebellum and amygdala. Eur J Neurosci 20:441–458

Hájos N, Freund TF (2002) Distinct cannabinoid sensitive receptors regulate hippocampal excitation and inhibition. Chem Phys Lipids 121:73–82

Hájos N, Katona I, Naiem SS, Mackie K, Ledent C, Mody I, Freund TF (2000) Cannabinoids inhibit hippocampal GABAergic transmission and network oscillations. Eur J Neurosci 12:3239–3249

Hanus L, Breuer A, Tchilibon S, Shiloah S, Goldenburg D, Horowitz M, Pertwee RG, Ross RA, Mechoulam R, Fride E (1999) HU 308: a specific agonist for CB(2), a peripheral cannabinoid receptor. Proc Natl Acad Sci U S A 96:14228–14233

Harris J, Drew LJ, Chapman V (2000) Spinal anandamide inhibits nociceptive transmission via cannabinoid receptor activation in vivo. Neuroreport 12:2817–2818

Henquet C, Krabbendam L, Spauwen J, Kaplan C, Lieb R, Wittchen HU, van Os J (2005) Prospective cohort study of cannabis use, predisposition for psychosis, and psychotic symptoms in young people. Br Med J 330:11

Herkenham M, Lynn AB, Little MD, Johnson MR, Melvin LS, de Costa BR, Rice KC (1990) Cannabinoid receptor localization in brain. Proc Natl Acad Sci U S A 87:1932–1936

Herkenham M, Lynn AB, Johnson MR, Melvin LS, de Costa BR, Rice KC (1991) Characterization and localization of cannabinoid receptors in rat brain: a quantitative in vitro autoradiographic study. J Neurosci 11:563–583

Herzberg U, Eliav E, Bennett GJ, Kopin IJ (1997) The analgesic effects of R(+)-WIN55,212-2 mesylate, a high affinity cannabinoid agonist, in a rat model of neuropathic pain. Neurosci Lett 221:157–160

Hillard CJ (2000) Biochemistry and pharmacology of the endocannabinoids arachidonyl-ethanolamide and 2-arachidonylglycerol. Prostaglandins Other Lipid Mediat 61:3e18

Hohmann AG, Herkenham M (1998) Regulation of cannabinoid and mu opioid receptors in rat lumbar spinal cord following neonatal capsaicin treatment. Neurosci Lett 252:13–16

Hohmann AG, Herkenham M (1999a) Cannabinoid receptors undergo axonal flow in sensory nerves. Neuroscience 92:1171–1175

Hohmann AG, Herkenham M (1999b) Localization of central cannabinoid CB1 receptor messenger RNA in neuronal subpopulations of rat dorsal root ganglia: a double-label in situ hybridization study. Neuroscience 90:923–931

Hohmann AG, Martin WJ, Tsou K, Walker JM (1995) Inhibition of noxious stimulus-evoked activity of spinal cord dorsal horn neurons by the cannabinoid WIN55,212-2. Life Sci 56:2111–2118

Hohmann AG, Tsou K, Walker JM (1998) Cannabinoid modulation of wide dynamic range neurons in the lumbar dorsal horn of the rat by spinally administered WIN55,212. Neurosci Lett 257:119–122

Hohmann AG, Briley EM, Herkenham M (1999a) Pre- and postsynaptic distribution of cannabinoid and mu opioid receptors in rat spinal cord. Brain Res 822:17–25

Hohmann AG, Tsou K, Walker JM (1999b) Cannabinoid suppression of noxious heat-evoked activity in wide dynamic range neurons in the lumbar dorsal horn of the rat. J Neurophysiol 81:575–583

Hohmann AG, Farthing JN, Zvonok AM, Makriyannis A (2004) Selective activation of cannabinoid CB2 receptors suppresses hyperalgesia evoked by intradermal capsaicin. J Pharmacol Exp Ther 308:446–453

Hohmann AG, Suplita II RL, Bolton NM, Neely MH, Fegley D, Mangieri R, Krey JF, Walker JM, Holmes PV, Crystal JD, Duranti A, Tontini M, Tarzia G, Piomelli D (2005) An endocannabinoid mechanism for stress-induced analgesia. Nature 435:1108–1112

Howlett AC (1988) The CB1 cannabinoid receptor in the brain. Neurobiol Dis 5:405–416

Howlett AC, Barth F, Bonner TI, Cabral G, Casellas P, Devane WA, Felder CC, Herkenham M, Mackie K, Martin BR, Mechoulam R, Pertwee RG (2002) International Union of Pharmacology. XXVII. Classification of cannabinoid receptors. Pharmacol Rev 54:161–202

Ibrahim MM, Deng H, Zvonok A, Cockayne DA, Kwan J, Mata HP, Vanderah TW, Lai J, Porreca F, Makriyannis A, Malan TP Jr (2003) Activation of CB2 cannabinoid receptors by AM1241 inhibits experimental neuropathic pain: pain inhibition by receptors not present in the CNS. Proc Natl Acad Sci USA 100:10529–10533

Ibrahim MM, Porreca F, Lai J, Albrecht PJ, Rice FL, Khodortova A, Davar G, Makriyannis A, Vanderah TW, Mata HP, Malan TP Jr (2005) CB-2 cannabinoid receptor activation produces antinociception by stimulating peripheral release of endogenous opioids. Proc Natl Acad Sci USA 102:3039–3098

Ishac EJN, Jiang L, Lake KD, Varga K, Abood ME, Kunos G (1996) Inhibition of exocytotic noradrenaline release by presynaptic cannabinoid CB1 receptors on peripheral sympathetic nerves. Br J Pharmacol 118:2023–2028

Jaggar SI, Hasnie FS, Sellaturay S, Rice ASC (1998) The anti-hyperalgesic actions of the cannabinoid anandamide and the putative CB2 agonist palmitoylethanolamide investigated in models of visceral and somatic inflammatory pain. Pain 76:189–199

Járai Z, Wagner JA, Varga K, Lake KD, Compton DR, Martin BR, Zimmer AM, Bonner TI, Buckley NE, Mezey E, Razdan RK, Zimmer A, Kunos G (1999) Cannabinoid-induced mesenteric vasodilation through an endothelial site distinct from CB1 or CB2 receptors. Proc Natl Acad Sci U S A 96:14136–14141

Johanek LM, Simone DA (2004) Activation of peripheral cannabinoid receptors attenuates cutaneous hyperalgesia produced by a heat injury. Pain 109:432–442

Johanek LM, Simone DA (2005) Cannabinoid agonist, CP 55,940, prevents capsaicin-induced sensitization of spinal cord dorsal horn neurons. J Neurophysiol 93:989–997

Johanek LM, Heitmiller DR, Turner M, Nader N, Hodges J, Simone DA (2001) Cannabinoids attenuate capsaicin-evoked hyperalgesia through spinal and peripheral mechanisms. Pain 93:303–315

Jordt SE, Bautista DM, Chuang HH, McKemy DD, Zygmunt PM, Hogestatt ED, Mend ID, Julius D (2004) Mustard oils and cannabinoids excite sensory nerve fibres through the TRP channel ANKTM1. Nature 427:260–265

Karst M, Salim K, Burstein S, Conrad I, Hoy L, Schneider U (2003) Analgesic effect of the synthetic cannabinoid CT-3 on chronic neuropathic pain: a randomized controlled trial. JAMA 290:1757–1762

Katona I, Sperlagh B, Sik A, Kafalvi A, Vizi ES, Mackie K, Freund TF (1999) Presynaptically located CB1 cannabinoid receptors regulate GABA release from axon terminals of specific hippocampal interneurons. J Neurosci 19:4544–4558

Katona I, Rancz EA, Acsady L, Ledent C, Mackie K, Hajos N, Freund TF (2001) Distribution of CB1 cannabinoid receptors in the amygdala and their control of GABAergic transmission. J Neurosci 23:9506–9518

Kearn CS, Greenberg MJ, DiCamelli R, Kurzawa K, Hillard CJ (1999) Relationships between ligand affinities for the cerebellar cannabinoid receptor CB1 and the induction of GDP/GTP exchange. J Neurochem 72:2379–2387

Kehl LJ, Hamamoto DT, Wacnik PW, Croft DL, Norsted BD, Wilcox GL, Simone DA (2003) A cannabinoid agonist differentially attenuates deep tissue hyperalgesia in animal models of cancer and inflammatory muscle pain. Pain 103:175–186

Kelly S, Jhaveri DM, Sagar DR, Kendall DA, Chapman V (2003) Activation of peripheral cannabinoid CB1 receptors inhibits mechanically evoked responses of spinal neurons in non-inflamed rats and rats with hindpaw inflammation. Eur J Neurosci 18:2239–2243

Kemp T, Spike RC, Watt C, Todd AJ (1996) The mu opioid receptor (MOR1) is mainly restricted to neurones that do not contain GABA or glycine in the superficial dorsal horn of the rat spinal cord. Neuroscience 75:1231–1238

Khasabova IA, Simone DA, Seybold VS (2002) Cannabinoids attenuate depolarization-dependent Ca2+ influx in intermediate-size primary afferent neurons of adult rats. Neuroscience 115:613–625

Khasabova IA, Harding-Rose C, Simone DA, Seybold VS (2004) Differential effects of CB1 and opioid agonists on two populations of adult rat dorsal root ganglion neurons. J Neurosci 24:1744–1753

Ko MC, Woods JH (1999) Local administration of delta9-tetrahydrocannabinol attenuates capsaicin-induced thermal nociception in rhesus monkeys: a peripheral cannabinoid action. Psychopharmacology (Berl) 143:322–326

Kouznetsova M, Kelley B, Shen M, Thayer SA (2002) Desensitization of cannabinoid-mediated presynaptic inhibition of neurotransmission between rat hippocampal neurons in culture. Mol Pharmacol 61:477–485

Ledent C, Valverde O, Cossu G, Petitet F, Aubert JF, Beslot F, Bohme GA, Imperato A, Pedrazzini T, Roques BP, Vassart G, Fratta W, Parmentier M (1999) Unresponsiveness to cannabinoids and reduced addictive effects of opiates in CB1 receptor knockout mice. Science 283:401–404

Lever IJ, Malcangio M (2002) CB1 receptor antagonist SR141716A increases capsaicin-evoked release of Substance P from the adult mouse spinal cord. Br J Pharmacol 135:21–24

Li J, Daughters RS, Bullis C, Bengiamin R, Stucky MW, Brennan J, Simone DA (1999) The cannabinoid receptor agonist WIN55,212-2 blocks the development of hyperalgesia produced by capsaicin in rats. Pain 81:25–34

Liang CY, Huang CC, Hsu KS, Takahashi T (2004) Cannabinoid-induced presynaptic inhibition at the primary afferent trigeminal synapse of juvenile rat brainstem slices. J Physiol 555:85–96

Lichtman AH, Martin BR (1991) Spinal and supraspinal components of cannabinoid-induced antinociception. J Pharmacol Exp Ther 258:517–523

Lichtman AH, Hawkins EG, Griffin G, Cravatt BF (2002) Pharmacological activity of fatty acid amides is regulated, but not mediated, by fatty acid amide hydrolase in vivo. J Pharmacol Exp Ther 302:73–79

Lichtman AH, Shelton CC, Advani T, Cravatt BF (2004a) Mice lacking fatty acid amide hydrolase exhibit a cannabinoid receptor-mediated phenotypic hypoalgesia. Pain 109:319–327

Lichtman AH, Leung D, Shelton C, Saghatelian A, Hardouin C, Boger D, Cravatt BF (2004b) Reversible inhibitors of fatty acid amide hydrolase that promote analgesia: evidence for an unprecedented combination of potency and selectivity. J Pharmacol Exp Ther 311:441–448

Lim G, Sung B, Ji RR, Mao J (2003) Upregulation of spinal cannabinoid-1-receptors following nerve injury enhances the effects of Win 55,212-2 on neuropathic pain behaviors in rats. Pain 105:275–283

Lo VJ, Fu J, Astarita G, La Rana G, Russo R, Calignano A, Piomelli D (2005) The nuclear receptor peroxisome proliferator-activated receptor-alpha mediates the anti-inflammatory actions of palmitoylethanolamide. Mol Pharmacol 67:15–19

Lodzki M, Godin B, Rakou L, Mechoulam R, Gallily R, Touitou E (2003) Cannabidiol-transdermal delivery and anti-inflammatory effect in a murine model. J Control Release 93:377–387

Mackie K, Hille B (1992) Cannabinoids inhibit N-type calcium channels in neuroblastoma-glioma cells. Proc Natl Acad Sci USA 89:3825–3829

Mackie K, Devane WA, Hille B (1993) Anandamide, an endogenous cannabinoid, inhibits calcium currents as a partial agonist in N18 neuroblastoma cells. Mol Pharmacol 44:498–503

Mackie K, Lai Y, Westenbroek R, Mitchell R (1995) Cannabinoids activate an inwardly rectifying potassium conductance and inhibit Q-type calcium currents in AtT20 cells transfected with rat brain cannabinoid receptor. J Neurosci 15:6552–6561

Mailleux P, Vanderhaeghen JJ (1992) Distribution of neuronal cannabinoid receptor in the adult rat brain: a comparative receptor binding radioautography and in situ hybridization histochemistry. Neuroscience 48:655–668

Malan TP, Ibrahim MM, Deng H, Liu Q, Mata HP, Vanderah T, Porreca F, Makriyannis A (2001) CB2 cannabinoid receptor-mediated peripheral antinociception. Pain 93:239–245

Malan TP Jr, Ibrahim MM, Vanderah TW, Makriyannis A, Porreca F (2002) Inhibition of pain responses by activation of CB(2) cannabinoid receptors. Chem Phys Lipids 121:191–200

Malan TP, Ibrahim MM, Lai J, Vanderah T, Makriyannis A, Porreca F (2003) CB2 cannabinoid receptor agonists: pain relief without the psychoactive effects? Curr Opin Pharmacol 3:62–67

Malfait AM, Gallily R, Sumariwalla PF, Malik AS, Andreakos E, Mechoulam R, Feldmann M (2000) The nonpsychoactive cannabis constituent cannabidiol is an oral anti-arthritic therapeutic in murine collagen-induced arthritis. Proc Natl Acad Sci USA 97:9561–9566

Manning BH, Merin NM, Meng ID, Amaral DG (2001) Reduction in opioid- and cannabinoid-induced antinociception in Rhesus monkeys after bilateral lesions of the amygdaloid complex. J Neurosci 21:8238–8246

Manning BH, Martin WJ, Meng ID (2003) The rodent amygdala contributes to the production of cannabinoid-induced antinociception. Neuroscience 120:1157–1170

Manzanares J, Corchero J, Romero J, Fernandez-Ruiz JJ, Ramos JA, Fuentes JA (1999) Pharmacological and biochemical interactions between opioids and cannabinoids. Trends Pharmacol Sci 20:287–294

Mao J, Price DD, Lu J, Keniston L, Mayer DJ (2000) Two distinctive antinociceptive systems in rats with pathological pain. Neurosci Lett 280:13–16

Marsicano G, Wotjak CT, Azad SC, Bisogno T, Rammes G, Cascio MG, Hermann H, Tang J, Hofmann C (2002) The endogenous cannabinoid system controls extinction of aversive memories. Nature 418:530–534

Martin BR, Compton DR, Thomas BF, Prescott WR, Little PJ, Razdan RK, Johnson MR, Melvin LS, Mechoulam R, Ward SJ (1991) Behavioral, biochemical, and molecular modeling evaluations of cannabinoid analogs. Pharmacol Biochem Behav 40:471–478

Martin WJ, Tsou K, Walker JM (1998) Cannabinoid receptor-mediated inhibition of the rat tail-flick reflex after microinjection into the rostral ventromedial medulla. Neurosci Lett 242:33–36

Martin WJ, Gupta CM, Loo DS, Rohde DS, Basbaum AI (1999a) Differential effects of neurotoxic destruction of descending noradrenergic pathways on acute and persistent nociceptive processing. Pain 80:57–65

Martin WJ, Coffin PO, Attias E, Balinsky M, Tsou K, Walker JM (1999b) Anatomical basis for cannabinoid-induced antinociception as revealed by intracerebral microinjections. Brain Res 822:237–242

Martin WJ, Loo CM, Basbaum AI (1999c) Spinal cannabinoids are anti-allodynic in rats with persistent inflammation. Pain 82:199–205

Matsuda LA, Lolait SJ, Brownstein MJ, Young AC, Bonner TI (1990) Structure of a cannabinoid receptor and functional expression of the cloned cDNA. Nature 346:561–564

Matsuda LA, Bonner TI, Lolait SJ (1993) Localization of cannabinoid receptor mRNA in rat brain. J Comp Neurol 327:535–550

Mazzari S, Canella R, Petrelli L, Marcolongo G, Leon A (1996) N-(2-Hydroxyethyl)hexadecanamide is orally active in reducing edema formation and inflammatory hyperalgesia by down-regulating mast cell activation. Eur J Pharmacol 300:227–236

McAllister SD, Glass M (2002) CB(1) and CB(2) receptor-mediated signalling: a focus on endocannabinoids. Prostaglandins Leukot Essent Fatty Acids 66:161–171

Mechoulam R (2000) Looking back at cannabis research. Curr Pharm Des 6:1313–1322

Mechoulam R, Ben Shabat S, Hanus L, Ligumsky M, Kaminski NE, Schatz AR, Gopher A, Almog S, Martin BR, Compton DR, et al (1995) Identification of an endogenous 2-monoglyceride, present in canine gut, that binds to cannabinoid receptors. Biochem Pharmacol 50:83–90

Mechoulam R, Fride E, Ben-Shabat S, Meiri U, Horowitz M (1998) Endocannabinoids. Eur J Pharmacol 359:1–18

Melvin LS, Milne GM, Johnson MR, Subramaniam B, Wilken GH, Howlett AC (1993) Structure-activity relationships for cannabinoid receptor-binding and analgesic activity: studies of bicyclic cannabinoid analogs. Mol Pharmacol 44:1008–1015

Meng ID, Johansen JP (2004) Antinociception and modulation of rostral ventromedial medulla neuronal activity by local microinfusion of a cannabinoid receptor agonist. Neuroscience 124:685–693

Meng ID, Manning BH, Martin WJ, Fields HL (1998) An analgesic circuit activated by cannabinoids. Nature 395:381–383

Millns PJ, Chapman V, Kendall DA (2001) Cannabinoid inhibition of the capsaicin-induced calcium response in rat dorsal root ganglion neurones. Br J Pharmacol 132:969–971

Molina-Holgado F (2002) Cannabinoids promote oligodendrocyte progenitor survival: in-volvement of cannabinoid receptors and phosphatidylinositol-3 Kinase/Akt signalling. J Neurosci 22:9742–9753

Molina-Holgado F, Pinteaux E, Moore JD, Molina-Holgado E, Guaza C, Gibson RM, Rothwell NJ (2003) Endogenous interleukin-1 receptor antagonist mediates anti-inflammatory and neuroprotective actions of cannabinoids in neurons and glia. J Neurosci 23: 6470–6474

Monhemius R, Azami J, Green DL, Roberts MHT (2001) CB1 receptor mediated analgesia from the nucleus reticularis gigantocellularis pars alpha is activated in an animal model of neuropathic pain. Brain Res 908:67–74

Morisset V, Urban L (2001) Cannabinoid-induced presynaptic inhibition of glutamatinergic EPSCs in sustantia gelatinosa neurons of the rat spinal cord. J Neurophysiol 86:40–48

Moss DE, Johnson RL (1980) Tonic analgesic effects of delta 9 THC as measured with the formalin test. Eur J Pharmacol 61:313–315

Munro S, Thomas KL, Abu Shaar M (1993) Molecular characterization of a peripheral receptor for cannabinoids. Nature 365:61–65

Nackley AG, Makriyannis A, Hohmann AG (2003a) Selective activation of cannabinoid CB2 receptors suppresses spinal fos protein expression and pain behavior in a rat model of inflammation. Neuroscience 119:747–757

Nackley AG, Suplita II, Hohmann AG (2003b) A peripheral cannabinoid mechanism suppresses spinal fos protein expression and pain behavior in a rat model of inflammation. Neuroscience 117:659–670

Nackley AG, Zvonok AM, Makriyannis A, Hohmann AG (2004) Activation of cannabinoid CB2 receptors suppresses C-fiber responses and windup in spinal wide dynamic range neurons in the absence and presence of inflammation. J Neurophysiol 92:3562–3574

Naderi N, Shafaghi B, Khodayar MJ, Zarindast MR (2005) Interaction between gamma-aminobutyric acid GABA-B and cannabinoid CB1 receptors in spinal pain pathways in rat. Eur J Pharmacol 514:159–164

Naef M, Curatolo M, Petersen-Felix S, Arendt-Nielsen L, Zbinden A, Brenneisen R (2003) The analgesic effects of oral delta-nine-tetrahydrocannabinol (THC), morphine and THC-morphine combination in healthy subjects under experimental pain conditions. Pain 105:79–88

Nie J, Lewis DL (2001a) The proximal and distal C-terminal tail domains of the CB1 receptor mediate G protein coupling. Neuroscience 107:161–167

Nie J, Lewis DL (2001b) Structural domains of the CB1 cannabinoid receptor that contribute to constitutive activity and G-protein sequestration. J Neurosci 21:8758–8764

Notcutt W, Price M, Miller R, Newport S, Phillips C, Simmons S, Sansom C (2004) Initial experiences with medicinal extracts of cannabis for chronic pain: results from 34 'N of 1' studies. Anaesthesia 59:440–452

Noyes R, Brunk SF, Baram DA, Canter A (1975) The analgesic properties of delta-9-THC and codeine. Clin Pharmacol Ther 18:84–89

Offertaler L, Mo FM, Batkai S, Liu J, Begg M, Razdan RK, Martin BR, Bukoski RD, Kunos G (2003) Selective ligands and cellular effectors of a G protein-coupled endothelial cannabinoid receptor. Mol Pharmacol 63:699–705

Oka S, Yanagimoto S, Ikeda S, Gokoh M, Kishimoto S, Waku K, Ishima T,Sugiura T (2005) Evidence for the involvement of the cannabinoid CB2 receptor and its endogenous ligand 2-arachidonoylglycerol in 12-O-tetradecanoylphorbol-13-acetate-induced acute inflammation in mouse ear. J Biol Chem 280:18488–18497

Okamoto Y, Morishita J, Tsuboi K, Tonai T, Ueda N (2004) Molecular characterization of a phospholipase D generating anandamide and its congeners. J Biol Chem 279:5298–5305

Ong WY, Mackie K (1999) A light and electron microscopic study of the CB1 cannabinoid receptor in the primate spinal cord. J Neurocytol 28:39–45

Oshita K, Inoue A, Tang HB, Nakata Y, Kawamoto M, Yuge O (2005) CB1 cannabinoid receptor stimulation modulates transient receptor potential vanilloid receptor 1 activities in calcium influx and substance P release in cultured rat dorsal root ganglion cells. J Pharmacol Sci 97:377–385

Patton GC, Coffey C, Carlin JB, Degenhardt L, Lynskey M, Hall W (2002) Cannabis use and mental health in young people: cohort study. Br Med J 325:1195–1198

Pertwee RG (1997) Pharmacology of cannabinoid CB1 and CB2 receptors. Pharmacol Ther 74:129–180

Pertwee RG (2001) Cannabinoids and pain. Prog Neurobiol 63:569–611

Pestojamasp VK, Burstein SH (1998) Anandamide synthesis is induced by arachidonate mobilizing agonists in cells of the immune system. Biochim Biophys Acta 1394:249–260

Piomelli D, Beltramo M, Giuffrida A, Stella N (1998) Endogenous cannabinoid signaling. Neurobiol Dis 5:462–473

Presley RW, Menetrey D, Levine JD, Basbaum AI (1990) Systemic morphine suppresses noxious stimulus evoked Fos protein-like immunoreactivity in the rat spinal cord. J Neurosci 110:323–335

Price TJ, Helesic G, Parghi D, Hargreaves KM, Flores CM (2003) The neuronal distribution of cannabinoid receptor type 1 in the trigeminal ganglion of the rat. Neuroscience 120:155–162

Price TJ, Patwardhan A, Akopian AN, Hargreaves KM (2004) Cannabinoid receptor-independent actions of the aminoalkylindole WIN55212-2 on trigeminal sensory neurons. Br J Pharmacol 142:257–266

Puffenbarger R, Boothe AC, Cabral GA (2000) Cannabinoids inhibit LPS-inducible cytokine mRNA expression in rat microglial cells. Glia 29:58–69

Quartilho A, Mata HP, Ibrahim MM, Vanderah TW, Porreca F, Makriyannis A, Malan TP (2003) Inhibition of inflammatory hyperalgesia by activation of peripheral CB2 cannabinoid receptors. Anesthesiology 99:955–960

Raffa RB, Stone DJ, Hipp SJ (1999) Differential cholera-toxin sensitivity of supraspinal antinociception induced by the cannabinoid agonists delta9-THC, WIN 55,212-2 and anandamide in mice. Neurosci Lett 263:29–32

Randall MD, McCulloch AI, Kendall DA (1997) Comparative pharmacology of endothelium-derived hyperpolarizing factor and anandamide in rat isolated mesentery. Eur J Pharmacol 333:191–197

Rice ASC (2005) Cannabinoids. In: Koltzenburg M, McMahon SB (eds) Melzack and Wall: textbook of pain. Elsevier, London

Rice ASC, Brooks JW, Thompson SWN (2002) Spinal intrathecal administration of the cannabinoid WIN55,212-2 attenuates pain behaviour in the formalin model. 10th World Congress of Pain, Abstr 839:P109

Richardson JD, Aanonsen L, Hargreaves KM (1997) SR 141716A, a cannabinoid receptor antagonist, produces hyperalgesia in untreated mice. Eur J Pharmacol 319:R3–R4

Richardson JD, Aanonsen L, Hargreaves KM (1998a) Antihyperalgesic effects of spinal cannabinoids. Eur J Pharmacol 345:145–153

Richardson JD, Kilo S, Hargreaves KM (1998b) Cannabinoids reduce hyperalgesia and inflammation via interaction with peripheral CB1 receptors. Pain 75:111–119

Roberts LA, Christie MJ, Conor M (2002) Anandamide is a partial agonist at native vanilloid receptors in acutely isolated trigeminal sensory neurones. Br J Pharmacol 137:421–428

Rodella LF, Borsani E, Rezzani R, Ricci F, Buffoli B, Bianchi R (2005) AM404, an inhibitor of anandamide reuptake decreases Fos-immunoreactivity in the spinal cord of neuropathic rats after non-noxious stimulation. Eur J Pharmacol 508:139–146

Romero J, Hillard CJ, Calero M, Rabano A (2002) Fatty acid amide hydrolase localization in the human central nervous system: an immunohistochemical study. Mol Brain Res 100:85–93

Ross RA (2003) Anandamide and vanilloid TRPV1 receptors. Br J Pharmacol 140:790–801

Ross RA, Coutts AA, McFarlane SM, Anavi-Goffer S, Irving AJ, Pertwee RG, MacEwan DJ, Scott RH (2001) Actions of cannabinoid receptor ligands on rat cultured sensory neurones: implications for antinociception. Neuropharmacology 40:221–232

Ross RA, Evans RM, Scott RH (2004) Cannabinoids and sensory neurones. Curr Neuropharmacol 2:59–73

Rukwied R, Watkinson A, McGlone F, Dvorak M (2003) Cannabinoid agonists attenuate capsaicin-induced responses in human skin. Pain 102:283–288

Ryberg E, Vu HK, Larsson N, Groblewski T, Hjorth S, Elebring T, Sjogren S, Greasley PJ (2005) Identification and characterisation of a novel splice variant of the human CB1 receptor. FEBS Lett 579:259–264

Salim K, Schneider U, Burstein S, Hoy L, Karst M (2005) Pain measurements and side effect profile of the novel cannabinoid ajulemic acid. Neuropharmacology 48:1164–1171

Salio C, Fischer J, Franzoni MF, Mackie K, Kaneko T, Conrath M (2001) CB 1 cannabinoid and μ opioid receptor co-localization on postsynaptic targets in the rat dorsal horn. Neuroreport 12:3689–3692

Salio C, Fischer J, Franzoni MF, Conrath M (2002a) Pre- and postsynaptic localizations of the CB1 cannabinoid receptor in the dorsal horn of the rat spinal cord. Neuroscience 110:755–764

Salio C, Doly S, Fischer J, Franzoni MF, Conrath M (2002b) Neuronal and astrocytic localization of the cannabinoid receptor-1 in the dorsal horn of the rat spinal cord. Neurosci Lett 329:13–16

Samson MT, Small-Howard A, Shimoda LMN, Koblan-Huberson M, Stokes AJ, Turner H (2003) Differential roles of CB1 and CB2 cannabinoid receptors in mast cells. J Immunol 170:4953–4962

Sanudo-Pena MC, Strangman NM, Mackie K, Walker JM, Tsou K (1999) CB1 receptor localization in rat spinal cord and roots, dorsal root ganglion and peripheral nerve. Acta Pharmacol Sin 20:1115–1120

Scott DA, Wright CE, Angus JA (2004) Evidence that CB-1 and CB-2 cannabinoid receptors mediate antinociception in neuropathic pain in the rat. Pain 109:124–131

Seltzer Z, Dubner R, Yoram S (1990) A novel behavioural model of neuropathic pain disorders produced in rats by partial sciatic nerve injury. Pain 43:205–218

Shen M, Piser TM, Seybold VS, Thayer SA (1996) Cannabinoid receptor agonists inhibit glutamatergic synaptic transmission in rat hippocampal cultures. J Neurosci 16:4322–4334

Shire D, Carillon C, Kaghad M, Calandra B, Rinaldi Carmona M, Le Fur G, Caput D, Ferrara P (1995) An amino-terminal variant of the central cannabinoid receptor resulting from alternative splicing [published erratum appears in J Biol Chem 1996 Dec 27;271(52):33706]. J Biol Chem 270:3726–3731

Shire D, Calandra B, Rinaldi-Carmona M, Oustric D, Pessegue B, Bonnin-Cabanne O, Le Fur G, Caput D, Ferrara P (1996) Molecular cloning, expression and function of the murine CB2 peripheral cannabinoid receptor. Biochim Biophys Acta 1307:132–136

Siegling A, Hofmann HA, Denzer D, Mauler F, De Vry J (2001) Cannabinoid CB1 receptor upregulation in a rat model of chronic neuropathic pain. Eur J Pharmacol 415:R5–R7

Smart D, Gunthorpe MJ, Jerman JC, Nasir S, Gray J, Muir AI, Chambers JK, Randall AD, Davis JB (2000) The endogenous lipid anandamide is a full agonist at the human vanilloid receptor (hVR1). Br J Pharmacol 129:227–230

Smith FL, Fujimore K, Lowe J, Welch SP (1998) Characterisation of delta9 tetrahydro-cannabinol and anandamide antinociception in nonarthritic and arthritic rats. Pharmacol Biochem Behav 60:183–191

Smith PB, Martin BR (1992) Spinal mechanisms of delta 9-tetrahydrocannabinol-induced analgesia. Brain Res 578:8–12

Sokal DM, Elmes SJR, Kendall DA, Chapman V (2003) Intraplantar injection of anandamide inhibits mechanically-evoked responses of spinal neurones via activation of CB2 receptors in anaesthetised rats. Neuropharmacology 45:404–411

Solowij N, Stephens RS, Roffman RA, Babor T, Kadden R, Miller M, Christiansen K, McRee B, Vendetti J, et al (2002) Cognitive functioning of long-term cannabis users seeking treatment. JAMA 287:1123–1131

Ständer S, Schmelz M, Metze D, Luger T, Rukwied R (2005) Distribution of cannabinoid receptor 1 (CB1) and 2 (CB2) on sensory nerve fibres and adnexal structures in human skin. J Dermatol 38:177–188

Stella N, Piomelli D (2001) Receptor-dependent formation of endogenous cannabinoids in cortical neurones. Eur J Pharmacol 425:189–196

Stella N, Schweitzer P, Piomelli D (1997) A second endogenous cannabinoid that modulates long-term potentiation. Nature 388:773–778

Strangman NM, Walker JM (1999) Cannabinoid WIN 55,212-2 inhibits the activity-dependent facilitation of spinal nociceptive responses. J Neurophysiol 82:472–477

Sugiura T, Kondo S, Kishimoto S, Miyashita T, Nakane S, Kodaka T, Suhara Y, Takayama H, Waku K (2000) Evidence that 2-arachidonoylglycerol but not N-palmitoylethanolamine or anandamide is the physiological ligand for the cannabinoid CB2 receptor. Comparison of the agonistic activities of various cannabinoid receptor ligands in HL-60 cells. J Biol Chem 275:605–612

Sugiura T, Kobayashi S, Oka S, Waku K (2002) Biosynthesis and degradation of anandamide and 2-arachidonylglycerol and thieir possible physiological significance. Prostaglandins Leukot Essent Fatty Acids 66:173–192

Sun H, Xu J, Della Penna KB, Benz RJ, Kinose F, Holder DJ, Koblan KS, Gerhold DL, Wang H (2002) Dorsal horn-enriched genes identified by DNA microarray, in situ hybridization and immunohistochemistry. BMC Neurosci 3:11

Svendsen KB, Jensen TS, Bach FW (2004) Does the cannabinoid dronabinol reduce central pain in multiple sclerosis? Randomised double blind placebo controlled crossover trial. BMJ 329:253

Thomas EA, Cravatt BF, Danielson PE, Gilula NB, Sutcliffe JG (1997) Fatty acid amide hydrolase, the degradative enzyme for anandamide and oleamide, has selective distribution in neurons within the rat central nervous system. J Neurosci Res 50:1047–1052

Thorat SN, Bhargava HN (1994) Evidence for a bidirectional cross-tolerance between morphine and delta 9-tetrahydrocannabinol in mice. Eur J Pharmacol 260:5–13

Tognetto M, Amadesi S, Harrison S, Creminon C, Trevisani M, Carreras M, Matera M, Geppetti P, Bianchi A (2001) Anandamide excites central terminals of dorsal root ganglion neurons via vanilloid receptor-1 activation. J Neurosci 21:1104–1109

Tsou K, Lowitz KA, Hohmann AG, Martin WJ, Hathaway CB, Bereiter DA, Walker JM (1996) Suppression of noxious stimulus-evoked expression of FOS protein-like immunoreactivity in rat spinal cord by a selective cannabinoid agonist. Neuroscience 70:791–798

Tsou K, Brown S, Mackie K, Sanudo-Pena MC, Walker JM (1998) Immunohistochemical distribution of cannabinoid CB1 receptors in the rat central nervous system. Neuroscience 83:393–411

Tsuda M, Inoue K, Salter MW (2005) Neuropathic pain and spinal microglia: a big problem from molecules in 'small' glia. Trends Neurosci 28:101–107

Twitchell W, Brown S, Mackie K (1997) Cannabinoids inhibit N- and P/Q-type calcium channels in cultured rat hippocampal neurons. J Neurophysiol 78:43–50

Ulugol A, Karadag HC, Ipci Y, Tarner M, Dokmeci I (2004) The effect of WIN 55,212-2, a cannabinoid agonist, on tactile allodynia in diabetic rats. Neurosci Lett 371:167–170

Vaughan CW, McGregor IS, Christie MJ (1999) Cannabinoid receptor activation inhibits GABAergic neurotransmission in rostral ventromedial medulla neurons in vitro. Br J Pharmacol 127:935–940

Vaughan CW, Connor M, Bagley EE, Christie MJ (2000) Actions of cannabinoids on membrane properties and synaptic transmission in rat periaqueductal gray neurons in vitro. Mol Pharmacol 57:288–295

Wade DT, Robson P, House H, Makela P, Aram J (2003) A preliminary controlled study to determine whether whole-plant cannabis extracts can improve intractable neurogenic symptoms. Clin Rehabil 17:18–26

Walker JM, Huang SM, Strangman NM, Tsou K, Sanudo Pena MC (1999) Pain modulation by release of the endogenous cannabinoid anandamide. Proc Natl Acad Sci USA 96: 12198–12203

Wallace VCJ, Cottrell DF, Brophy PJ, Fleetwood-Walker SM (2003) Focal lysolecithin-induced demyelination of peripheral afferents results in neuropathic pain behavior that is attenuated by cannabinoids. J Neurosci 23:3221–3233

Walter L, Stella N (2004) Cannabinoids and neuroinflammation. Br J Pharmacol 141:775–785

Walter L, Franklin A, Witting A, Wade C, Xie Y, Kunos G, Mackie K, Stella N (2003) Nonpsychotropic cannabinoid receptors regulate microglial cell migration. J Neurosci 23:1398–1405

Ware MA, Doyle CR, Woods R, Lynch ME, Clark AJ (2003) Cannabis use for chronic noncancer pain: results of a prospective survey. Pain 102:211–216

Ware MA, Adams H, Guy GW (2005) The medicinal use of cannabis in the UK: results of a nationwide survey. Int J Clin Pract 59:291–295

Watkins LR, Milligan ED, Maier SF (2001) Spinal cord glia: new players in pain. Pain 93: 201–205

Watkins LR, Milligan ED, Maier SF (2003) Immune and glial involvement in physiological and pathological exaggerated pain states. Progress in Pain Research and Management, Proceedings of the 10th World Congress on Pain 24:369–385. IASP Press, Seattle

Welch SP, Eads M (1999) Synergistic interactions of endogenous opioids and cannabinoid systems. Brain Res 848:183–190

Woolridge E, Barton S, Samuel J, Osorio J, Dougherty A, Holdcroft A (2005) Cannabis use in HIV for pain and other medical symptoms. J Pain Symptom Manage 29:358–367

Yesilyurt O, Dogrul A, Gul H, Seyrek M, Kusmes O, Ozkan Y, Yildiz O (2003) Topical cannabinoid enhances topical morphine antinociception. Pain 105:303–308

Yu M, Ives D, Ramesha CS (1997) Synthesis of prostaglandin E2 ethanolamide from anandamide by cyclooxygenase-2. J Biol Chem 272:21181–21186

Zajicek J, Fox P, Sanders H, Wright D, Vickery J, Nunn A, Thompson A (2003) Cannabinoids for treatment of spasticity and other symptoms related to multiple sclerosis (CAMS study): multicentre randomised placebo-controlled trial. Lancet 362:1517–1526

Zammit S, Allebeck P, Andreasson S, Lundberg I, Lewis G (2002) Self reported cannabis use as a risk factor for schizophrenia in Swedish conscripts of 1969: historical cohort study. Br Med J 325:1199

Zhang J, Hoffert C, Khang V, Groblewski T, Ahmad S, O'Donnell D (2003) Induction of CB2 receptor expression in the rat spinal cord of neuropathic but not inflammatory chronic pain models. Eur J Pharmacol 17:2750–2754

Zimmer A, Zimmer AM, Hohmann AG, Herkenham M, Bonner TI (1999) Increased mortality, hypoactivity, and hypoalgesia in cannabinoid CB1 receptor knockout mice. Proc Natl Acad Sci USA 96:5780–5785

Zygmunt PM, Petersson J, Andersson DA, Chuang H, Sorgard M, Di Marzo V, Julius D, Hogestatt ED (1999) Vanilloid receptors on sensory nerves mediate the vasodilator action of anandamide. Nature 400:452–457

Part IV
Future Targets in Analgesia Research

HEP (2006) 177:309–328
© Springer-Verlag Berlin Heidelberg 2006

Adenosine and ATP Receptors

J. Sawynok

Department of Pharmacology, Dalhousie University, Halifax NS, B3H 1X5, Canada
jana.sawynok@dal.ca

1	**Introduction**	310
2	**P1 Receptors and Pain**	310
2.1	Peripheral Influences on Nociception	310
2.1.1	Adenosine A_1 Receptors	311
2.1.2	Adenosine A_{2A}, A_{2B}, and A_3 Receptors	311
2.2	Central Influences on Nociception	312
2.2.1	Adenosine A_1 Receptors	312
2.2.2	Adenosine A_{2A}, A_{2B}, and A_3 Receptors	314
2.3	Adenosine Receptor Knockouts and Pain	314
2.4	Clinical Studies and Implications	315
2.4.1	Potential for Development	315
2.4.2	Intrathecal Adenosine Analgesia	316
2.4.3	Intravenous Adenosine Analgesia	316
3	**P2 Receptors and Pain**	317
3.1	$P2X_3$ Receptors	317
3.2	$P2X_4$ Receptors	319
3.3	$P2X_7$ Receptors	319
3.4	P2Y Receptors	320
4	**Conclusions**	320
	References	321

Abstract Adenosine and ATP, via P1 and P2 receptors respectively, can modulate pain transmission under physiological, inflammatory, and neuropathic pain conditions. Such influences reflect peripheral and central actions and effects on neurons as well as other cell types. In general, adenosine A_1 receptors produce inhibitory effects on pain in a number of preclinical models and are a focus of attention. In humans, i.v. infusions of adenosine reduce some aspects of neuropathic pain and can reduce postoperative pain. For P2X receptors, there is a significant body of information indicating that inhibition of $P2X_3$ receptors may be useful for relieving inflammatory and neuropathic pain. More recently, data have begun to emerge implicating $P2X_4$, $P2X_7$ and P2Y receptors in aspects of pain transmission. Both P1 and P2 receptors may represent novel targets for pain relief.

Keywords Adenosine · ATP · Intravenous adenosine infusion · P2X receptors · P2Y receptors

1
Introduction

Both adenosine and ATP are able to influence nociceptive transmission by their functions as extracellular signaling molecules and actions on cell surface receptors. Adenosine acts at several P1 receptors (A_1, A_{2A}, A_{2B}, A_3), all of which are coupled to G proteins (Fredholm et al. 2001). Activation of adenosine receptors can influence nociception at peripheral, spinal, and supraspinal sites, and affect nociceptive, inflammatory, and neuropathic pain states (Sawynok 1998; Dickenson et al. 2000; Sawynok and Liu 2003). The role of adenosine A_1 receptors (A1Rs) in suppressing pain transmission is prominent, and adenosine receptors as a potential therapeutic target for the treatment of pain, either by directly acting agents (e.g., A1R agonists) or indirectly acting agents that increase endogenous adenosine availability (e.g., adenosine kinase inhibitors), have received considerable recent attention (Kowaluk and Jarvis 2000; McGaraughty et al. 2005). ATP acts on two families of receptors, the P2X ligand-gated ion channels and the P2Y metabotropic G protein-coupled receptor family (North 2002). $P2X_3$ receptors are selectively localized on sensory nerves, and have received much attention in the context of pain signaling and the potential therapeutic development of antagonists for such receptors (Jarvis and Kowaluk 2001; Jacobson et al. 2002; Kennedy et al. 2003). More recently, it has been recognized that $P2X_4$ receptors in the spinal cord may contribute to neuropathic pain (Tsuda et al. 2003), while $P2X_7$ receptors may influence inflammatory and neuropathic pain (Chessell et al. 2005). Furthermore, P2Y receptors may play a role in peripheral pain signaling. The purpose of the present chapter is to focus on recent developments that advance an understanding of the role of purines in nociception (see also Liu and Salter 2005).

2
P1 Receptors and Pain

2.1
Peripheral Influences on Nociception

Adenosine can produce different effects on peripheral pain signaling depending on the nature of the receptor involved, the localization of the receptor, and the tissue conditions (i.e., normal tissue, inflammation, or following nerve injury). Effects on adenosine A1Rs have received the most attention, as such actions lead to suppression of pain, and there is the potential for therapeutic agents to engage such mechanisms in producing analgesia.

2.1.1
Adenosine A₁ Receptors

The presence of A1Rs in dorsal root ganglia (Schulte et al. 2003) and trigeminal ganglion neurons (Carruthers et al. 2001) has now been visualized directly using immunohistochemistry. When sensory neurons are examined in vitro, adenosine A1Rs lead to reduced Ca^{2+} entry (Haas and Selbach 2000), decreased cyclic AMP generation, and decreased release of calcitonin gene-related peptide (CGRP) (Carruthers et al. 2001). In functional studies, the local peripheral inhibitory actions of A1R agonists administered locally to the rat hindpaw are most clearly observed as reduced mechanical hyperalgesia to inflammatory agents (Taiwo and Levine 1990; Aley et al. 1995) and reduced thermal hyperalgesia following nerve injury (Liu and Sawynok 2000). These peripheral antinociceptive actions have been attributed to decreased cyclic AMP production in sensory nerve endings (Taiwo and Levine 1990; Carruthers et al. 2001). Repeated administration of an A1R agonist produces tolerance and cross-tolerance and cross-dependence with other agents, and it was proposed that peripheral A1Rs exist as a complex with μ-opioid and α_2-adrenergic receptors (Aley and Levine 1997).

Endogenous adenosine can be released from sensory afferent nerves following their activation. Thus, capsaicin (which activates TRPV1 receptors selectively expressed on C-fibers; Liu et al. 2001), formalin (which leads to neurogenic and tissue inflammation; Liu et al. 2000) and glutamate (Liu et al. 2002) all increase peripheral extracellular levels of tissue adenosine as determined using peripheral microdialysis; in each case, this is inhibited by pretreatment with capsaicin. Inhibitory activity of this adenosine is revealed by the ability of a selective A1R antagonist to enhance formalin-evoked behaviors (Sawynok et al. 1998; Aumeerally et al. 2004). Peripheral administration of inhibitors of adenosine kinase also increase tissue levels of adenosine (Liu et al. 2000) and inhibit formalin-evoked responses (Sawynok et al. 1998) but not hypersensitivity to carrageenan inflammation (McGaraughty et al. 2001). Collectively, such observations indicate that inhibitory adenosine A1Rs on sensory afferents can be activated under certain conditions (i.e., mild intensities of stimulation, co-presence of certain mediators, nerve injury) by directly acting agonists, as well as by agents that increase the local tissue availability of extracellular adenosine, to produce a suppression of pain.

2.1.2
Adenosine A₂ₐ, A₂ᵦ, and A₃ Receptors

Adenosine A₂ₐ receptors are also present in the dorsal root ganglia of sensory neurons (Kaelin-Lang et al. 1998). In functional studies, local peripheral administration of A2AR agonists to the rat hindpaw leads to increased mechanical hyperalgesia (Taiwo and Levine 1990) and increased flinching in response to formalin (Doak and Sawynok 1995). Hyperalgesia is mediated by increases in cyclic AMP in the sensory nerve, which results in activation of protein kinase A, phosphorylation of Na^+ channels, increased currents, and sensory afferent activation (Gold et al. 1996). Adenosine A_{2B} and A_3 receptors are present on mast cells and can lead to enhanced pain signaling by increased release of mast cell mediators such as histamine and 5-hydroxytryptamine (Sawynok 1998). Local administration of agonists for A2ARs, A2BRs, and A3Rs also produces edema which involves mast cell degranulation (Sawynok et al. 2000; Esquisatto et al. 2001), while an A2R agonist enhances plasma extravasation when administered into the knee joint (Green et al. 1991). These cutaneous and joint effects are generally regarded as reflecting pro-inflammatory actions.

2.2
Central Influences on Nociception

2.2.1
Adenosine A₁ Receptors

The spinal administration of A1R agonists to rodents produces antinociception in models of nociceptive, inflammatory, and neuropathic pain, and such actions generally feature prominently in accounting for behavioral effects following systemic administration (Sawynok 1998; Dickenson et al. 2000). The involvement of A1Rs is confirmed by demonstrating antagonism of such actions by selective A1R antagonists (e.g., Lee and Yaksh 1996; Poon and Sawynok 1998; Gomes et al. 1999). Recently, immunohistochemical studies have shown that A1Rs are concentrated in laminae I and II of the dorsal horn of the spinal cord (Ackley et al. 2003; Schulte et al. 2003) and are present on intrinsic dorsal horn neurons (Schulte et al. 2003); this has also been demonstrated using electrophysiological approaches in vitro (Hugel and Schlichter 2003). Such studies confirm earlier reports which used autoradiographic approaches combined with selective lesions. While rhizotomy did not reveal a prominent presynaptic population of A1Rs on sensory nerve terminals (Geiger et al. 1984), there is some evidence for presynaptic receptors, as dorsal root ligation resulted in some accumulation of A1R immunoreactivity on the side close to the dorsal root ganglion (Schulte et al. 2003).

The main mechanisms implicated in spinal A1R-mediated antinociception include: (1) increased K^+ conductance and hyperpolarization of dorsal horn intrinsic neurons (Lao et al. 2001; Patel et al. 2001; Salter and Sollevi 2001), (2) inhibition of peptide release (substance P, CGRP) (Sjölund et al. 1997; Carruthers et al. 2001; Mauborgne et al. 2002), and (3) inhibition of glutamate release (Patel et al. 2001; Ackley et al. 2003; but see Yamamoto et al. 2003). A1R mechanisms also lead to a decreased release of γ-aminobutyric acid (GABA) from interneurons in the dorsal horn (Hugel and Schlichter 2003), but the net effect of such an action is likely to be stimulatory, and its contribution to suppression of pain is not readily apparent.

Spinal adenosine systems appear to exhibit a unique efficacy in models of hypersensitivity, such as neuropathic pain; this profile of activity is of considerable interest, given that neuropathic pain can be difficult to control pharmacologically. An initial study emphasized the potency of intrathecal (i.t.) adenosine analogs in reducing manifestations of hypersensitivity compared to nociceptive tests (Sosnowski and Yaksh 1989). Subsequent studies confirmed prominent activity in models of nerve injury with such analogs, and the potential for adenosine systems to represent a target in neuropathic pain conditions has been emphasized (Dickenson et al. 2000). Spinal administration of adenosine itself, while lacking activity in normal animals, leads to relief of hypersensitivity (mechanical allodynia) following nerve injury (Gomes et al. 1999); such efficacy was surprisingly long-lasting (i.e., to 24 h; Lavand'homme and Eisenach 1999). Altered pharmacokinetics did not appear to account for the duration of activity, and there was no change in the number of A1Rs or alteration in G protein coupling in the spinal cord following nerve injury (Bantel et al. 2002a, b). However, i.t. adenosine (via an A1R) enhances release of noradrenaline in vivo following nerve injury (but not in normal conditions; Bantel et al. 2003), and antiallodynic actions of adenosine are dependent on spinal adrenergic mechanisms following nerve injury (Gomes et al. 1999). Given the activity of α_2-adrenergic receptor agonists in nerve injury states, this may contribute to the efficacy of adenosine under such conditions. The mechanism underlying this essentially excitatory action mediated by an adenosine A1R is not clear in view of prominent inhibitory actions of A1Rs. However, this action emphasizes the potential complexity of A1R actions following nerve injury, where a number of spinal changes in nociceptive signaling occur (e.g., central sensitization, disinhibition, phenotype switch).

Spinal adenosine A1Rs can also be activated by agents which lead to increased endogenous levels of adenosine (i.e., inhibition of adenosine metabolism). Thus, i.t. delivery of prototype nucleoside inhibitors of adenosine kinase produces intrinsic antinociception or enhanced antinociception (induced by adenosine itself, or morphine which releases adenosine; Keil and DeLander 1994; Poon and Sawynok 1998). A series of novel non-nucleoside inhibitors of adenosine kinase (A-134974; A-286501, ABT-702) produces antinociception in inflammatory and neuropathic pain states following systemic administration (Kowaluk et al. 2000; McGaraughty et al. 2001, 2005; Zhu et al. 2001; Jarvis et al. 2002c). The antinociceptive actions of adenosine kinase inhibitors occur primarily at spinal sites, as intracerebroventricular (supraspinal) and intraplantar (peripheral) actions were weaker compared to i.t. delivery with neuropathic pain (Zhu et al. 2001). In an inflammatory model, peripheral sites were not implicated in analgesic actions (McGaraughty et al. 2001). Inhibition of adenosine metabolism results in enhanced extracellular tissue levels of adenosine in the spinal cord (Golembiowska et al. 1996), and this subsequently activates inhibitory spinal A1Rs (McGaraughty et al. 2005).

2.2.2
Adenosine A_{2A}, A_{2B}, and A_3 Receptors

Within the central nervous system, A2ARs exhibit a high expression in basal ganglia and the olfactory bulb but low levels in other brain regions, while A2BRs and A3Rs occur at very low levels (Fredholm et al. 2001). There are some reports that spinal (Lee and Yaksh 1996; Poon and Sawynok 1998) and supraspinal (Regaya et al. 2004) administration of CGS21680, an A2AR agonist, produces antinociception, but it is weakly active compared to A1R agonists and, in the absence of effects of selective A2AR antagonists, it is not clear if this receptor is indeed involved in such actions. Furthermore, spinal electrophysiological actions of CGS21680 are complex (Lao et al. 2001; Patel et al. 2001), and the receptors mediating its effects are far from clear.

Other approaches reveal additional influences on nociception. Thus, caffeine is a nonselective A1R, A2AR, and A2BR antagonist that exhibits analgesic and adjuvant analgesic effects (Sawynok 1998); as inhibition of A1Rs cannot account for such activity, the analgesic profiles of A2AR and A2BR antagonists have received attention. Antinociception (hot plate test) has been reported following spinal (but not systemic) administration of the A2AR antagonist SCH-58261 (Bastia et al. 2002). Furthermore, a series of A2BR antagonists was shown to produce antinociception (hot plate test) when administered systemically; as a structure that did not enter the central nervous system also exhibited activity, this action was attributed to a peripheral site of action (Abo-Salem et al. 2004). That same study observed that an A3R antagonist (PBS-10) produced hyperalgesia (hot plate) following systemic administration, but that study did not further explore this action in terms of central versus peripheral sites.

2.3
Adenosine Receptor Knockouts and Pain

Mouse strains lacking genes for A1Rs, A2ARs, and A3Rs have now been developed, and determining effects of gene deletions on thresholds to various forms of nociceptive stimulation has been helpful in appreciating their role in pain signaling (Fredholm et al. 2005). A1R knockout mice exhibited thermal hyperalgesia (tail flick) but there was no change to cold stimulation or mechanical thresholds (Johansson et al. 2001; Wu et al. 2005). The same pattern of changes was observed following carrageenan inflammation of the hindpaw, as well as a photochemically induced sciatic nerve ischemic injury (Wu et al. 2005). Such observations are consistent with some degree of tonic regulation of noxious heat, but not other modalities of stimulation, by A1Rs under various conditions. With respect to pharmacology, A1R knockout mice exhibited a reduced tail flick antinociception in response to i.t. administration of R-PIA (an A1R agonist) and i.t. morphine (releases adenosine in the spinal cord), confirming an involvement of adenosine receptors in spinal actions of morphine; there was, however, no change in the response to systemic morphine, which reflects supraspinal, as well as spinal, actions (Johansson et al. 2001; Wu et al. 2005).

In A2A knockout mice there was an increased reaction time to a number of thermal responses (tail flick, hot plate), indicating hypoalgesia (Ledent et al. 1997; Berrendero et al. 2003). This is generally consistent with the peripheral pain facilitatory effect of A2ARs noted above. Another study observed no change in thermal thresholds (tail immersion) or in antinociceptive responses to systemic morphine (μ-opioid receptor agonist); however, there was a reduced antinociceptive response to a δ-opioid receptor agonist, and an enhanced response to a κ-opioid receptor agonist (Bailey et al. 2002). These functional changes in opioid actions were proposed to reflect changes in opioid receptor patterns in the spinal cord, and perhaps changes in A2ARs in sensory nerves. No responses to inflammation or nerve injury have yet been reported in A2A knockout animals, but these are of interest due to the role of A2ARs in inflammation (Ohta and Sitkovsky 2001) and the emerging appreciation of the contribution of inflammation (peripheral and central) to neuropathic pain (Watkins and Maier 2002).

In A3R knockout mice there was no change in thermal or mechanical thresholds (Wu et al. 2002), although an increased latency in the hot plate test was noted in another report (Federova et al. 2003). Following carrageenan-induced inflammation in the hindpaw, heat hyperalgesia, plasma extravasation, and edema were reduced, indicating a pro-inflammatory role for A3Rs at peripheral sites (Wu et al. 2002). However, both pro- and antiinflammatory actions for A3Rs were inferred from observations in inflammatory cells in other studies using A3R knockout mice (Salvatore et al. 2000). Given the multiple influences of A3Rs on inflammation, effects on pain signaling have the potential to be complex and dependent on the pain condition and the degree of central and peripheral inflammation.

2.4
Clinical Studies and Implications

2.4.1
Potential for Development

Given the general ability of A1R agonists to reduce pain responses in a number of pain models following systemic delivery, adenosine receptors have been considered as a potential target for development as novel analgesics. However, A1R agonists also produced cardiovascular changes, suppression of locomotor activity, and hypothermia, and the systemic doses that produce such effects exhibit only a limited separation from those which produce antinociception. There is a broader separation between such actions for non-nucleoside adenosine kinase inhibitors, and this has led to an emphasis on the development of indirectly acting agents rather than directly acting agonists in the context of systemic delivery (Jarvis et al. 2002b; McGaraughty et al. 2005).

2.4.2
Intrathecal Adenosine Analgesia

Following preclinical reports that i.t. adenosine and A1R agonists produce antinociception, particularly in states of hypersensitivity, it has been of interest to evaluate the potential efficacy of spinally administered adenosine in humans. I.t. administration of adenosine (up to 2 mg) to human volunteers has been reported to reduce experimentally induced allodynia from mustard oil (Rane et al. 1998) and hyperalgesia and allodynia following intradermal capsaicin (Eisenach et al. 2002). In a double-blind study in patients with neuropathic pain, i.t. adenosine reduced the area of allodynia 2–24 h after injection (Eisenach et al. 2003), confirming earlier case reports (Belfrage et al. 1999). In contrast, i.t. adenosine had no effect on acute pain following noxious heat (Eisenach et al. 2002) or ongoing pain following hysterectomy (Rane et al. 2000). In view of limited efficacy (25% reduction in allodynia, no effect on ongoing pain), and the occurrence of back pain, a recent study concluded that i.t. adenosine was unlikely to be useful as a sole analgesic agent (Eisenach et al. 2003).

2.4.3
Intravenous Adenosine Analgesia

The systemic administration of adenosine to humans by i.v. infusions (usually 50–70 µg/kg per minute over 45–60 min) has been reported to produce some degree of pain relief in a number of settings. In healthy volunteers, i.v. adenosine infusions have led to analgesia in experimental pain involving cutaneous heat thresholds (Ekblom et al. 1995), ischemic pain (Segerdahl et al. 1994; Rae et al. 1999), allodynia induced by mustard oil (Segerdahl et al. 1995b) and cutaneous inflammatory pain (Sjölund et al. 1999). In clinical pain, i.v. adenosine reduced spontaneous and evoked pain in double-blind crossover trials involving peripheral neuropathic pain (Belfrage et al. 1995; Sjölund et al. 2001) and neuropathic pain of mixed etiology (with postsurgical/posttraumatic neuropathic pain as the most prevalent diagnosis; Lynch et al. 2003). The latter trial involved an enriched enrolment design in which 40/66 subjects (61%) were identified as adenosine responders in an initial open phase of the trial.

A curious feature of pain relief following i.v. administration of adenosine in neuropathic pain cases is that, on occasion, a single infusion leads to long-term pain relief (months) (estimated at 5%–10% in Segerdahl and Sollevi 1998; observed in 2/26 in Sjölund et al. 2001; and 3/62 in Lynch et al. 2003). It is interesting to note that following i.v. infusion of ATP, which is rapidly metabolized to adenosine, similar long-lasting pain relief has been noted in cases of postherpetic neuralgia with single (Hayashida et al. 2004) or multiple infusions of ATP (Moriyama et al. 2004).

Analgesic properties of i.v. infusions of adenosine also occur when adenosine is infused during surgery. In an earlier series of studies, Segerdahl and colleagues reported that i.v. infusion of adenosine (80μg/kg per minute) during surgery could reduce anesthetic requirements and/or the need for postoperative analgesics (Segerdahl et al. 1995a, 1996, 1997). In studies which compared i.v. adenosine infusions to i.v. remifentanil (a short-acting opioid) infusions, both agents provided cardiovascular stability during surgery, and use of adenosine led to less postsurgical pain and a decreased requirement for opioid analgesics (Zárate et al. 1999; Fukunaga et al. 2003). The Fukunaga et al. study reported the most dramatic difference (degree, duration to 48 h) and a lesser incidence of postoperative nausea, and this was attributed, potentially, to the higher doses of adenosine infused. Thus, Zárate et al. used 166 ± 17 μg/kg per minute for a mean total dose of 1,400 mg, while Fukunaga et al. used 292 ± 82 μg/kg per minute with a total dose of 2,500 mg.

Given that adenosine is rapidly metabolized (plasma half-life less than 10 s), it is unlikely that the prolonged analgesia that can occur following perioperative infusions is due to continued presence of unmetabolized adenosine. Analgesia may result from multiple influences including: (1) peripheral and central analgesia mediated by A1Rs on sensory afferent nerves and in the superficial dorsal horn (Sects. 2.1.1 and 2.2.1), (2) selective inhibitory effects of spinal A1Rs in sensitized states involving inflammation (Honore et al. 1998; Sorkin et al. 2003), and (3) peripheral antiinflammatory effects mediated by A2As and A3Rs within the tissue during surgery (Cronstein 1998; Sullivan and Linden 1998) leading to pre-emptive effects on pain. In comparisons with remifentanil, the possibility that remifentanil produces an acute tolerance that contributes to its pharmacological profile also needs to be considered.

3
P2 Receptors and Pain

3.1
P2X₃ Receptors

P2X receptors, which form cation-selective channels permeable to Na^+ and Ca^{2+}, mediate fast cell–cell signaling in excitable tissue; seven such receptors have been identified ($P2X_{1-7}$) (Khakh et al. 2001). $P2X_3$ receptors are selectively expressed on sensory afferent neurons, and the potential for these to represent a novel analgesic strategy has received considerable attention in recent years (Jarvis and Kowaluk 2001; Jacobson et al. 2002; Kennedy et al. 2003). Several types of observations support this focus of interest:

- Peripheral administration of ATP and $\alpha\beta$-methylene-ATP (a $P2X_3$ receptor agonist) leads to excitation of C-fibers (Dowd et al. 1998; Hamilton et al. 2001; Hilliges et al. 2002); such actions confirm extensive observations on cell bodies of dorsal root, trigeminal, and nodose ganglion neurons in vitro (North 2002).

- Peripheral administration of ATP and $\alpha\beta$-methylene-ATP leads to spontaneous pain behaviors, thermal hyperalgesia, and mechanical allodynia (Hamilton et al. 1999; Tsuda et al. 2000); these responses are enhanced by inflammation (formalin, carrageenan; Sawynok and Reid 1997; Hamilton et al. 1999) as well as noradrenaline (which is co-released with ATP from sympathetic neurons; Waldron and Sawynok 2004).

- Inflammation upregulates $P2X_3$ receptor expression and sensitizes $P2X_3$ receptor depolarization of sensory neurons (Xu and Huang 2002), while inflammation/inflammatory mediators lead to phosphorylation of $P2X_3$ receptors (Paukert et al. 2001; Dai et al. 2004).

- Nerve injury can lead to complex changes in $P2X_3$ receptor expression, with increases occurring in uninjured afferents and decreases in injured afferents (Tsuzuki et al. 2001; Kage et al. 2002; Kim et al. 2003). Functionally, following nerve injury, purinergic sensitization of sensory afferents is observed (Chen et al. 2001; Zhou et al. 2001), and this may involve an interaction with adrenergic mechanisms (Park et al. 2000).

- $P2X_3$ receptor knockdown using antisense oligonucleotides delivered spinally leads to reduced agonist-induced hyperalgesia (Dorn et al. 2004), inflammatory hyperalgesia (Barclay et al. 2002; Honore et al. 2002), and nerve injury-induced allodynia (Honore et al. 2002; Dorn et al. 2004).

- Studies with a non-nucleotide-selective $P2X_3$ receptor antagonist (A-317491) administered systemically indicate a reduction in inflammatory pain or hyperalgesia (formalin, carrageenan models) and in allodynia following spinal nerve ligation (Jarvis et al. 2002a). Both peripheral and spinal sites are involved in such actions, although spinal sites are more sensitive and exhibit a wider profile of activity (McGaraughty et al. 2003).

Collectively, these observations provide support for the exploration of $P2X_3$ receptor antagonists for relief of pain in inflammatory and neuropathic pain states.

3.2
P2X$_4$ Receptors

P2X$_4$ receptors are diffusely expressed in neuronal and non-neuronal tissues (Khakh et al. 2001). Microglia, which are responsive to various forms of central nervous system injury, are implicated in neuropathic pain, as peripheral nerve injury leads to hypertrophy, proliferation, and activation of microglia, and this is correlated with the development of behavioral hypersensitivity (Watkins and Maier 2002). P2X$_4$ receptors on spinal cord microglia were recently implicated in neuropathic pain on the basis of studies using P2X receptor antagonists. Thus, TNP-ATP, but not PPADS, reversed allodynia induced by spinal nerve injury, and from the pharmacological profile of these two agents it was inferred that P2X$_4$ receptors could regulate allodynia (Tsuda et al. 2003). Further observations that established this link were: (1) P2X$_4$ receptor expression, which is normally low in the naïve spinal cord, was increased in parallel with the time course of tactile allodynia; (2) antisense oligodeoxynucleotide targeting of P2X$_4$ receptors inhibited allodynia; (3) i.t. administration of cultured microglia, which had been stimulated in vitro with ATP, produced allodynia (Tsuda et al. 2003). Activation of P2X$_4$ receptors on microglia is proposed to lead to enhanced Ca^{2+} entry, p38 mitogen-activated protein kinase (MAPK) activation and release of diffusible factors (cytokines, chemokines) which then act on adjacent neurons to promote hypersensitivity responses (Inoue et al. 2005; Liu and Salter 2005).

In contrast to nerve injury, chronic inflammation induced by complete Freund's adjuvant does not lead to microglial activation (Rabchevsky et al. 1999) or P2X$_4$ receptor upregulation (Tsuda et al. 2003). However, spinal cord microglial activation does occur following injections of high concentrations of formalin (commonly used to provide a model of ongoing pain involving inflammation; this leads to long-lasting hyperalgesia) which may result from chemical damage to peripheral nerves (Fu et al. 2000). Spinal administration of suramin (a broad spectrum P2X and P2Y receptor antagonist) prevents both microglial activation and long-term hyperalgesia by high concentrations of formalin (Wu et al. 2004); it was speculated that spinal P2X$_4$ or P2Y receptors mediated the action of suramin.

3.3
P2X$_7$ Receptors

P2X$_7$ receptors, for which ATP has a relatively low affinity, are expressed on macrophages and microglia, and activation of these receptors leads to release of inflammatory cytokines (particularly interleukin-1β; North 2002). Following inflammation with complete Freund's adjuvant, P2X$_7$ receptor immunoreactivity is observed in a number of peripheral cell types including nerve terminals, endothelial cells, and macrophages (Dell'Antonio et al. 2002a). Oxidized ATP, a selective antagonist for $P2X_7$ receptors, can reduce hypersensitivity produced by complete Freund's adjuvant, but it is not clear which cell types mediate this response (Dell'Antonio et al. 2002a, b). While neuronal $P2X_7$ receptors have been proposed (Deuchars et al. 2001), this has been questioned recently (Sim et al. 2004).

A recent study using gene deletion of the $P2X_7$ receptor has demonstrated that, in mice lacking this receptor, inflammatory (adjuvant-induced model) and neuropathic (partial nerve ligation model) hypersensitivity is completely absent in response to both mechanical and thermal stimuli, although normal nociceptive processing is preserved (Chessell et al. 2005). Furthermore, gene deletion animals exhibited impaired release of interleukin-1β, as well as of other inflammatory mediators. Interestingly, $P2X_7$ receptors were shown to be upregulated in human dorsal root ganglia and injured nerves obtained from chronic pain patients (Chessell et al. 2005). It was proposed that drugs that block $P2X_7$ receptors could have the potential to produce broad-spectrum (inflammatory, neuropathic) analgesia.

3.4
P2Y Receptors

P2Y receptors (eight mammalian ones have been cloned: $P2Y_1$, $P2Y_2$, $P2Y_4$, $P2Y_6$, $P2Y_{11-14}$), which are nucleotide-preferring receptors, are coupled to G proteins leading to activation of a variety of intracellular pathways (Jacobson et al. 2002; Abbracchio et al. 2003). There is less information on possible roles of P2Y receptors in nociceptive signaling. However, dorsal root ganglia express $P2Y_1$ and $P2Y_2$ receptors and these may contribute to sensory nerve activation (Nakamura and Strittmatter 1996; Molliver et al. 2002; Stucky et al. 2004). $P2Y_1$ receptors are co-expressed with TRPV1 receptors (which have a widespread distribution on sensory afferents; Moriyama et al. 2003) and IB_4 (which selectively labels a subpopulation of sensory afferents; Ruan and Burnstock 2003). ATP may act at P2Y receptors to sensitize effects mediated by TRPV1 receptors, an action involving phosphorylation of the TRPV1 receptor (Tominaga et al. 2001). $P2Y_1$ receptors may play a role in neuropathic pain, as nerve axotomy leads to upregulation of these receptors in dorsal root ganglia and the dorsal spinal cord (Xiao et al. 2002; Yang et al. 2004). The potential of P2Y receptors playing a role in chronic pain states requires further elaboration.

4
Conclusions

Both P1 and P2 receptors provide attractive targets for the relief of chronic inflammatory and neuropathic pain. Adenosine has been given by i.v. infusions to humans to alleviate pain in neuropathic pain states, and it exhibits potential to be a useful adjunct to anesthesia. While development of selective A1R agonists may be limited by adverse effects, non-nucleoside inhibitors of adenosine kinase exhibit the potential to be useful in both inflammatory and neuropathic pain, and a number of such compounds are undergoing development. P2X$_3$ receptor antagonists, which target receptors selectively localized on sensory afferents, exhibit potential as analgesics and have received considerable attention. P2X$_4$ and P2X$_7$ receptors, with actions on microglia and immune cells, have been a more recent focus of attention but are also potential therapeutic targets for pain relief. Finally, an emerging appreciation of a potential role for P2Y receptors in pain signaling makes these worthy of further exploration. Collectively, this body of information indicates that multiple purine receptors exhibit considerable promise for development as analgesics for chronic pain states.

References

Abbracchio MP, Boeynaesm JM, Barnard EA, et al (2003) Characterization of the UDP-glucose receptor (renamed here the P2Y14 receptor) adds diversity to the P2Y receptor family. Trends Pharmacol Sci 24:52–55

Abo-Salem OM, Hayallah AM, Bilkei-Gorso A, et al (2004) Antinociceptive effects of novel A2B adenosine receptor antagonists. J Pharmacol Exp Ther 308:358–366

Ackley MA, Governo RJM, Cass CE, et al (2003) Control of glutamatergic neurotransmission in the rat spinal dorsal horn by the nucleoside transporter ENT1. J Physiol 548:507–517

Aley KO, Levine JD (1997) Multiple receptors involved in peripheral α2, μ and A1 antinociception, tolerance, and withdrawal. J Neurosci 17:735–744

Aley KO, Green PG, Levine JD (1995) Opioid and adenosine peripheral antinociception are subject to tolerance and withdrawal. J Neurosci 15:8031–8038

Aumeerally N, Allen G, Sawynok J (2004) Glutamate-evoked release of adenosine and regulation of peripheral antinociception. Neuroscience 127:1–11

Bailey A, Ledent C, Kelly M, et al (2002) Changes in spinal δ and κ systems in mice deficient in the A2A receptor gene. J Neurosci 22:9210–9220

Bantel C, Childers SR, Eisenach JC (2002a) Role of adenosine receptors in spinal G-protein activation after peripheral nerve injury. Anesthesiology 96:1443–1449

Bantel C, Tobin JR, Li X, et al (2002b) Intrathecal adenosine following spinal nerve ligation in rat. Short residence time in cerebrospinal fluid and no change in A1 receptor binding. Anesthesiology 96:103–108

Bantel C, Li X, Eisenach JC (2003) Intraspinal adenosine induces spinal cord norepinephrine release in spinal nerve-ligated rats but not in normal or sham controls. Anesthesiology 98:1461–1466

Barclay J, Patel S, Dorn G, et al (2002) Functional downregulation of P2X3 receptor subunit in rat sensory neurons reveals a significant role in chronic neuropathic and inflammatory pain. J Neurosci 22:8139–8147

Bastia E, Varani K, Manopoli A, et al (2002) Effects of A1 and A2A adenosine receptor ligands in mouse acute models of pain. Neurosci Lett 328:241–244

Belfrage M, Sollevi A, Segerdahl M, et al (1995) Systemic adenosine infusion alleviates spontaneous and stimulus evoked pain in patients with neuropathic pain. Anesth Analg 81:713–717

Belfrage M, Segerdahl M, Arnér S, et al (1999) The safety and efficacy of intrathecal adenosine in patients with chronic neuropathic pain. Anesth Analg 89:136–142

Berrendero F, Castañé A, Ledent C, et al (2003) Increase of morphine withdrawal in mice lacking A2A receptors and no changes in CB1/A2A double knockout mice. Eur J Neurosci 17:315–324

Carruthers AM, Sellers LA, Jenkins DW, et al (2001) Adenosine A1 receptor-mediated inhibition of protein kinase A-induced calcitonin gene-related peptide release from rat trigeminal neurons. Mol Pharmacol 59:1533–1541

Chen Y, Zhang YH, Zhao ZQ (2001) Novel purinergic sensitivity develops in injured sensory axons following sciatic nerve transection in rat. Brain Res 911:168–172

Chessell IP, Hatcher JP, Bountra C, et al (2005) Disruption of the P2X7 purinoceptor gene abolishes chronic inflammatory and neuropathic pain. Pain 114:386–396

Cronstein BN (1998) Adenosine and its receptors during inflammation. In: Serhan CN, Ward PA (eds) Molecular and cellular basis of inflammation. Humana Press, Totowa, pp 259–274

Dai Y, Fukuoka T, Wang H, et al (2004) Contribution of sensitized P2X receptors in inflamed tissue to the mechanical hypersensitivity revealed by phosphorylated ERK in DRG neurons. Pain 108:258–266

Dell'Antonio G, Quattrini A, Cin ED, et al (2002a) Relief of inflammatory pain in rats by local use of the selective P2X7 ATP receptor inhibitor, oxidized ATP. Arthritis Rheum 46:3378–3385

Dell'Antonio G, Quattrini A, Dal CE, et al (2002b) Antinociceptive effect of a new P2Z/P2X7 antagonist, oxidized ATP, in arthritic rats. Neurosci Lett 327:87–90

Deuchars SA, Atkinson L, Brooke RE, et al (2001) Neuronal P2X7 receptors are targeted to presynaptic terminals in the central and peripheral nervous systems. J Neurosci 21:7143–7152

Dickenson AH, Suzuki R, Reeve AJ (2000) Adenosine as a potential analgesic target in inflammatory and neuropathic pains. CNS Drugs 13:77–85

Doak GJ, Sawynok J (1995) Complex role of peripheral adenosine in the genesis of the response to subcutaneous formalin in the rat. Eur J Pharmacol 281:311–318

Dorn G, Patel S, Wotherspoon G, et al (2004) siRNA relieves chronic neuropathic pain. Nucleic Acids Res 32:e40

Dowd E, McQueen DS, Chessell IP, et al (1998) P2X receptor-mediated excitation of nociceptive afferents in the normal and arthritic rat knee joint. Br J Pharmacol 125:341–346

Eisenach JC, Hood DD, Curry R (2002) Preliminary efficacy assessment of intrathecal injection of an American formulation of adenosine in humans. Anesthesiology 96:29–34

Eisenach JC, Rauck RL, Curry R (2003) Intrathecal, but not intravenous adenosine reduces allodynia in patients with neuropathic pain. Pain 105:65–70

Ekblom A, Segerdahl M, Sollevi A (1995) Adenosine increases the cutaneous heat pain threshold in healthy volunteers. Acta Anaesthesiol Scand 39:717–722

Esquisatto LCM, Costa SKP, Camargo EA, et al (2001) The plasma protein extravasation induced by adenosine and its analogues in the rat dorsal skin: evidence for the involvement of capsaicin sensitive primary afferent neurones and mast cells. Br J Pharmacol 134:108–115

Federova IM, Jacobson MA, Basile A, et al (2003) Behavioral characterization of mice lacking the A3 receptor: sensitivity to hypoxic degeneration. Cell Mol Neurobiol 23:431–447

Fredholm BB, Ijzerman AP, Jacobson KA, et al (2001) International Union of Pharmacology. XXV. Nomenclature and classification of adenosine receptors. Pharmacol Rev 53:527–552

Fredholm BB, Chen JF, Masino SA, et al (2005) Actions of adenosine at its receptors in the CNS: insights from knockouts and drugs. Annu Rev Pharmacol Toxicol 45:385–412

Fu KY, Light AR, Maixner W (2000) Relationship between nociceptor activity, peripheral edema, spinal microglial activation and long-term hyperalgesia induced by formalin. Neuroscience 101:1127–1135

Fukunaga AF, Alexander GE, Stark CW (2003) Characterization of the analgesic actions of adenosine: comparison of adenosine and remifentanil infusions in patients undergoing major surgical procedures. Pain 101:129–138

Geiger JD, LaBella FS, Nagy JI (1984) Characterization and localization of adenosine receptors in rat spinal cord. J Neurosci 4:2303–2310

Gold MS, Reichling DB, Shuster MJ, et al (1996) Hyperalgesic agents increase a tetrodotoxin-resistant Na+ current in nociceptors. Proc Natl Acad Sci USA 93:1108–1112

Golembiowska K, White TD, Sawynok J (1996) Adenosine kinase inhibitors augment release of adenosine from spinal cord slices. Eur J Pharmacol 307:157–162

Gomes JA, Li X, Pan HL, et al (1999) Intrathecal adenosine interacts with a spinal noradrenergic system to produce antinociception in nerve-injured rats. Anesthesiology 91:1072–1079

Green PG, Basbaum AI, Helms C, et al (1991) Purinergic regulation of bradykinin-induced plasma extravasation and adjuvant-induced arthritis in the rat. Proc Natl Acad Sci USA 88:4162–4165

Haas HL, Selbach O (2000) Functions of neuronal adenosine receptors. Naunyn Schmiedebergs Arch Pharmacol 362:375–381

Hamilton SG, Wade A, McMahon SB (1999) The effects of inflammation and inflammatory mediators on nociceptive behaviour induced by ATP analogues in the rat. Br J Pharmacol 126:326–332

Hamilton SG, McMahon SB, Lewin GR (2001) Selective activation of nociceptors by P2X receptor agonists in normal and inflamed rat skin. J Physiol 534:437–445

Hayashida M, Sato K, Fukunaga A, et al (2004) Intravenous infusion of adenosine 5'-triphosphate alleviated a disabling postherpetic neuralgia. J Anesth 18:36–38

Hilliges M, Weidner C, Schmelz M, et al (2002) ATP responses in human C nociceptors. Pain 98:59–68

Honore P, Burovita J, Chapman V, et al (1998) UP 202–56, an adenosine analogue, selectively acts via A1 receptors to significantly decrease noxiously-evoked spinal c-Fos protein expression. Pain 75:281–293

Honore P, Kage K, Mijusa J, et al (2002) Analgesic profile of intrathecal P2X3 antisense oligonucleotide treatment in chronic inflammatory and neuropathic pain states in rats. Pain 99:11–19

Hugel S, Schlichter R (2003) Convergent control of synaptic GABA from rat dorsal horn neurones by adenosine and GABA autoreceptors. J Physiol 551:479–489

Inoue K, Tsuda M, Koizumi S (2005) ATP receptors in pain sensation: involvement of spinal microglia and P2X4 receptors. Purinerg Signal 1:95–100

Jacobson KA, Jarvis MF, Williams M (2002) Purine and pyrimidine P2 receptors as drug targets. J Med Chem 45:4057–4093

Jarvis MF, Kowaluk EA (2001) Pharmacological characterization of P2X3 homomeric and heteromeric channels in nociceptive signaling and behavior. Drug Dev Res 52:220–231

Jarvis MF, Burgard EC, McGaraughty S, et al (2002a) A-317491, a novel potent and selective non-nucleotide antagonist of P2X3 and P2X2/3 receptors reduced chronic inflammatory and neuropathic pain in the rat. Proc Natl Acad Sci USA 99:17179–17184

Jarvis MF, Mikusa J, Chu Kl, et al (2002b) Comparison of the ability of adenosine kinase inhibitors and adenosine receptor agonists to attenuate thermal hyperalgesia and reduce motor performance in rats. Pharmacol Biochem Behav 73:573–581

Jarvis MF, Yu H, McGaraughty S, et al (2002c) Analgesic and anti-inflammatory effects of A-286501, a novel orally active adenosine kinase inhibitor. Pain 96:107–118

Johansson B, Halldner L, Dunwiddie TV, et al (2001) Hyperalgesia, anxiety, and decreased hypoxic neuroprotection in mice lacking the adenosine A1 receptor. Proc Natl Acad Sci USA 98:9407–9412

Kaelin-Lang A, Lauterburg T, Burgunder JM (1998) Expression of adenosine A2A receptor gene in rat dorsal root and autonomic ganglia. Neurosci Lett 246:21–24

Kage K, Nifortos W, Zhu CZ, et al (2002) Alteration of dorsal root ganglion P2X3 receptor expression and function following spinal nerve ligation in the rat. Exp Brain Res 147: 511–519

Keil GJ, DeLander GE (1994) Adenosine kinase and adenosine deaminase inhibition modulate spinal adenosine- and opioid agonist-induced antinociception in mice. Eur J Pharmacol 271:37–46

Kennedy C, Assis TS, Currie AJ, et al (2003) Crossing the pain barrier: P2 receptors as targets for novel analgesics. J Physiol 553:683–694

Khakh BS, Burnstock G, Kennedy C, et al (2001) International Union of Pharmacology. XXIV. Current status of the nomenclature and properties of P2X receptors and their subunits. Pharmacol Rev 53:107–118

Kim C, Chung JM, Chung K (2003) Changes in the gene expression of six subtypes of P2X receptors in rat dorsal root ganglion after spinal nerve ligation. Neurosci Lett 337:81–84

Kowaluk EA, Jarvis MF (2000) Therapeutic potential of adenosine kinase inhibitors. Expert Opin Investig Drugs 9:551–564

Kowaluk EA, Mikusa J, Wismer CT, et al (2000) ABT-702 (4-amino-5-(3-bromophenyl)-7-(6-morpholino-pyridin-3-yl)pyrido[2,3-d}pyrimidine), a novel orally effective adenosine kinase inhibitor with analgesic and anti-inflammatory properties. II. In vivo characterization in the rat. J Pharmacol Exp Ther 295:1165–1174

Lao LJ, Kumamoto E, Luo C, et al (2001) Adenosine inhibits excitatory transmission to substantia gelatinosa neurons of the adult rat spinal cord through the activation of presynaptic A1 adenosine receptors. Pain 94:315–324

Lavand'homme PM, Eisenach JC (1999) Exogenous and endogenous adenosine enhance the spinal antiallodynic effects of morphine in a rat model of neuropathic pain. Pain 80:31–36

Ledent C, Vaugeois JM, Schiffmann SN, et al (1997) Aggressiveness, hypoalgesia and high blood pressure in mice lacking the adenosine A2A receptor. Nature 388:674–678

Lee YW, Yaksh TL (1996) Pharmacology of the spinal adenosine receptor which mediates the antiallodynic action of intrathecal adenosine agonists. J Pharmacol Exp Ther 277:1642–1648

Liu XJ, Salter MW (2005) Purines and pain mechanisms: recent developments. Curr Opin Investig Drugs 6:65–75

Liu XJ, Sawynok J (2000) Peripheral antihyperalgesic effects by adenosine A1 receptor agonists and inhibitors of adenosine metabolism in a rat neuropathic pain model. Analgesia 5:19–29

Liu XJ, White TD, Sawynok J (2000) Potentiation of formalin-evoked adenosine release by an adenosine kinase inhibitor and an adenosine deaminase inhibitor in the rat hind paw: a microdialysis study. Eur J Pharmacol 408:143–152

Liu XJ, White TD, Sawynok J (2001) Involvement of primary sensory afferents, postganglionic sympathetic nerves and mast cells in the formalin-evoked peripheral release of adenosine. Eur J Pharmacol 429:147–155

Liu XJ, White TD, Sawynok J (2002) Intraplantar injection of glutamate evokes peripheral adenosine in the rat hind paw: involvement of peripheral ionotropic glutamate receptors and capsaicin-sensitive sensory afferents. J Neurochem 80:562–570

Lynch ME, Clark AJ, Sawynok J (2003) Intravenous adenosine alleviates neuropathic pain: a double blind placebo controlled crossover trial using an enriched enrolment design. Pain 103:111–117

Mauborgne A, Polienor H, Hamon M, et al (2002) Adenosine receptor-mediated control of in vitro release of pain-related neuropeptides from the rat spinal cord. Eur J Pharmacol 441:47–55

McGaraughty S, Chu KL, Wismer CT, et al (2001) Effects of A-134974, a novel adenosine kinase inhibitor, on carrageenan-induced inflammatory hyperalgesia and locomotor activity in rats: evaluation of the sites of action. J Pharmacol Exp Ther 296:501–509

McGaraughty S, Wismer CT, Zhu CZ, et al (2003) Effects of A-317491, a novel and selective P2X3/P2X2/3 receptor antagonist, on neuropathic, inflammatory and chemogenic nociception following intrathecal and intraplantar administration. Br J Pharmacol 140:1381–1388

McGaraughty S, Cowart M, Jarvis MF, et al (2005) Anticonvulsant and antinociceptive actions of novel adenosine kinase inhibitors. Curr Top Med Chem 5:43–58

Molliver DC, Cook SP, Carlsten JA, et al (2002) ATP and UTP excite sensory neurons and induce CREB phosphorylation through the metabotropic receptor, P2Y2. Eur J Neurosci 16:1850–1860

Moriyama M, Kitamura A, Ikezaki H, et al (2004) Systemic ATP infusion improves spontaneous pain and tactile allodynia, but not tactile hyperesthesia, in patients with postherpetic neuralgia. J Anesth 18:177–180

Moriyama T, Iida T, Kobayashi K, et al (2003) Possible involvement of P2Y2 metabotropic receptors in ATP-induced transient receptor potential vanilloid receptor 1-mediated thermal hypersensitivity. J Neurosci 23:6058–6062

Nakamura F, Strittmatter SM (1996) P2Y1 purinergic receptors in sensory neurons: contribution to touch-induced impulse generation. Proc Natl Acad Sci USA 93:10465–10470

North RA (2002) Molecular physiology of P2X receptors. Physiol Rev 82:1013–1067

Ohta A, Sitkovsky M (2001) Role of G-protein-coupled adenosine receptors in downregulation of inflammation and protection from tissue damage. Nature 414:916–920

Park SK, Chung K, Chung JM (2000) Effects of purinergic and adrenergic antagonists in a rat model of painful peripheral neuropathy. Pain 87:171–179

Patel MK, Pinnock RD, Lee K (2001) Adenosine exerts multiple effects in dorsal horn neurones of the adult rat spinal cord. Brain Res 920:19–26

Paukert M, Osteroth R, Geisler HS, et al (2001) Inflammatory mediators potentiate ATP-gated channels through the P2X3 subunit. J Biol Chem 276:21077–21082

Poon A, Sawynok J (1998) Antinociception by adenosine analogs and inhibitors of adenosine metabolism in an inflammatory thermal hyperalgesia model in the rat. Pain 74:235–246

Rabchevsky AG, Degos JD, Dreyfus PA (1999) Peripheral injections of Freund's adjuvant in mice provoke leakage of serum proteins through the blood-brain barrier without inducing reactive gliosis. Brain Res 832:84–96

Rae CP, Mansfield MD, Dryden C, et al (1999) Analgesic effect of adenosine on ischaemic pain in human volunteers. Br J Anaesth 82:427–428

Rane K, Segerdahl M, Goiny M, et al (1998) Intrathecal adenosine administration. A phase I clinical safety study in healthy volunteers, with additional evaluation of its influence on sensory thresholds and experimental pain. Anesthesiology 89:1108–1115

Rane K, Sollevi A, Segerdahl M (2000) Intrathecal adenosine administration in abdominal hysterectomy lacks analgesic effect. Acta Anaesthesiol Scand 44:868–872

Regaya I, Pham T, Andretti N, et al (2004) Small conductance calcium-activated K+ channels, SkCa, but not voltage-gated K+ (Kv) channels, are implicated in the antinociception induced by CGS21680, a A2A adenosine receptor agonist. Life Sci 76:367–377

Ruan HZ, Burnstock G (2003) Localisation of P2Y1 and P2Y4 receptors in dorsal root, nodose and trigeminal ganglia of the rat. Histochem Cell Biol 120:415–426

Salter MW, Sollevi A (2001) Roles of purines in nociception. In: Abbracchio MP, Williams M (eds) Handbook of experimental pharmacology, vol 151. Springer, Berlin Heidelberg New York, pp 371–401

Salvatore CA, Tilley SL, Latour AM, et al (2000) Disruption of the A3 adenosine receptor gene in mice and its effect on stimulated inflammatory cells. J Biol Chem 275:4429–4434

Sawynok J (1998) Adenosine receptor activation and nociception. Eur J Pharmacol 347:1–11

Sawynok J, Liu XJ (2003) Adenosine in the spinal cord and periphery: release and regulation of pain. Prog Neurobiol 69:313–340

Sawynok J, Reid A (1997) Peripheral adenosine 5′-triphosphate enhances nociception in the formalin test via activation of purinergic P2X receptors. Eur J Pharmacol 330:115–121

Sawynok J, Reid A, Poon A (1998) Peripheral antinociceptive and anti-inflammatory properties of an adenosine kinase inhibitor and an adenosine deaminase inhibitor. Eur J Pharmacol 384:123–138

Sawynok J, Reid A, Liu XJ (2000) Involvement of mast cells, sensory afferents and sympathetic mechanisms in paw oedema induced by adenosine A1, A2B/3 receptor agonists. Eur J Pharmacol 395:47–50

Schulte G, Robertson B, Fredholm BB, et al (2003) Distribution of antinociceptive adenosine A1 receptors in the spinal cord dorsal horn, and relationship to primary afferents and neuronal subpopulations. Neuroscience 121:907–916

Segerdahl M, Sollevi A (1998) Adenosine and pain relief: a clinical overview. Drug Dev Res 45:151–158

Segerdahl M, Ekblom A, Sollevi A (1994) The influence of adenosine, ketamine, and morphine on experimentally induced ischemic pain in healthy volunteers. Anesth Analg 79:787–791

Segerdahl M, Ekblom A, Sandelin K, et al (1995a) Peroperative adenosine infusion reduces the requirements for isoflurane and postoperative analgesics. Anesth Analg 80:1145–1149

Segerdahl M, Ekblom A, Sjölund KF, et al (1995b) Systemic adenosine attenuates touch evoked allodynia induced by mustard oil in humans. NeuroReport 6:753–756

Segerdahl M, Persson E, Ekblom A, et al (1996) Peroperative adenosine infusion reduces isoflurane concentrations during general anesthesia for shoulder surgery. Acta Anaesthesiol Scand 40:792–797

Segerdahl M, Irestedt L, Sollevi A (1997) Antinociceptive effect of perioperative adenosine infusion in abdominal hysterectomy. Acta Anaesthesiol Scand 41:473–479

Sim JA, Young MT, Sung HY, et al (2004) Reanalysis of P2X7 receptor expression in rodent brain. J Neurosci 24:6307–6314

Sjölund KF, Sollevi A, Segerdahl M, et al (1997) Intrathecal adenosine analog administration reduces substance P in cerebrospinal fluid along with behavioral effects that suggest antinociception in rats. Anesth Analg 85:627–632

Sjölund KF, Segerdahl M, Sollevi A (1999) Adenosine reduces secondary hyperalgesia in two human models of cutaneous inflammatory pain. Anesth Analg 88:605–610

Sjölund KF, Belfrage M, Karlsten R, et al (2001) Systemic adenosine infusion reduces the area of tactile allodynia in neuropathic pain following peripheral nerve injury: a multi-centre, placebo-controlled study. Eur J Pain 5:199–207

Sorkin LS, Maruyama K, Boyle DL, et al (2003) Spinal adenosine agonist reduces c-fos and astrocyte activation in dorsal horn of rats with adjuvant-induced arthritis. Neurosci Lett 340:119–122

Sosnowski M, Yaksh TL (1989) Role of spinal adenosine receptors in modulating the hyperesthesia produced by spinal glycine receptor antagonism. Anesth Analg 69:587–592

Stucky CL, Medler KA, Molliver DC (2004) The P2Y agonist UTP activates cutaneous afferent fibers. Pain 109:36–44

Sullivan GW, Linden J (1998) Role of A2A adenosine receptors in inflammation. Drug Dev Res 45:103–112

Taiwo YO, Levine JD (1990) Direct cutaneous hyperalgesia induced by adenosine. Neuroscience 38:757–762

Tominaga M, Wada M, Masu M (2001) Potentiation of capsaicin receptor activity by metabotropic ATP receptors as a possible mechanism for ATP-evoked pain and hyperalgesia. Proc Natl Acad Sci USA 98:6951–6956

Tsuda M, Koizumi A, Shigemoto Y, et al (2000) Mechanical allodynia caused by intraplantar injection of P2X receptor agonist in rats: involvement of heteromeric P2X2/3 receptor signaling in capsaicin-insensitive primary afferent neurons. J Neurosci 20:1–9

Tsuda M, Shigemoto-Mogami Y, Koizumi S, et al (2003) P2X4 receptors induced in spinal microglia gate tactile allodynia after nerve injury. Nature 424:778–783

Tsuzuki K, Kondo E, Fukuoka T, et al (2001) Differential regulation of P2X3 mRNA expression by peripheral nerve injury in intact and injured neurons in the rat sensory ganglia. Pain 91:351–360

Waldron JB, Sawynok J (2004) Peripheral P2X receptors and nociception: interactions with biogenic amine systems. Pain 110:79–89

Watkins LR, Maier SF (2002) Beyond neurons: evidence that immune and glial cells contribute to pathological pain states. Physiol Rev 82:981–1011

Wu WP, Hao JX, Halldner-Henriksson L, et al (2002) Decreased inflammatory pain due to reduced carrageenan-induced inflammation in mice lacking adenosine A3 receptors. Neuroscience 114:523–527

Wu WP, Hao JX, Halldner L, et al (2005) Increased nociceptive response in mice lacking the adenosine A1 receptor. Pain 113:395–404

Wu Y, Willcockson HH, Maixner W, et al (2004) Suramin inhibits spinal cord microglial activation and long-term hyperalgesia induced by formalin injection. J Pain 5:48–55

Xiao HS, Huang QH, Zhang FX, et al (2002) Identification of gene expression profile of dorsal root ganglion in the rat peripheral axotomy model of neuropathic pain. Proc Natl Acad Sci USA 99:8360–8365

Xu GY, Huang LYM (2002) Peripheral inflammation sensitizes P2X receptor-mediated responses in rat dorsal root ganglion neurons. J Neurosci 22:93–102

Yamamoto S, Nakanishi O, Matsui T, et al (2003) Intrathecal adenosine A1 receptor agonist attenuates hyperalgesia without inhibiting spinal glutamate release in the rat. Cell Mol Neurobiol 23:175–185

Yang L, Zhang FX, Huang F, et al (2004) Peripheral nerve injury induces trans-synaptic modification of channels, receptors and signal pathways in rat dorsal spinal cord. Eur J Neurosci 19:871–883

Zárate E, Sá Rêgo MM, White PF, et al (1999) Comparison of adenosine and remifentanil infusions as adjuvants to desflurane anesthesia. Anesthesiology 90:956–963

Zhou J, Chung K, Chung JM (2001) Development of purinergic sensitivity in sensory neurons after peripheral nerve injury in the rat. Brain Res 915:161–169

Zhu CZ, Mikusa J, Chu KL, et al (2001) A-134974: a novel adenosine kinase inhibitor, relieves tactile allodynia via spinal sites of action in peripheral nerve injured rats. Brain Res 905:104–110

HEP (2006) 177:329–358

Ion Channels in Analgesia Research

J. N. Wood

Molecular Nociception Group, Biology Department, University College London, Gower
Street, London WC1E 6BT, UK
J.Wood@ucl.ac.uk

1	Introduction	330
2	Sodium Channels	332
2.1	$Na_v 1.3$	335
2.2	$Na_v 1.7$	336
2.3	$Na_v 1.8$	337
3	Splice Variants of Sodium Channels	339
4	Calcium Channels	341
5	Voltage-Gated Calcium Channels	341
6	Potassium Channels	343
7	Pacemaker Channels	345
8	Transient Receptor Potential Receptors	346
9	Acid-Sensing Ion Channels	348
10	HERG Channels	350
11	Target Validation of Ion Channels Using Transgenic Mice	350
12	Summary	351
	References	352

Abstract The distribution of ion channels in neurons associated with pain pathways is
becoming better understood. In particular, we now have insights into the molecular nature
of the channels that are activated by tissue-damaging stimuli, as well as the mechanisms
by which voltage-gated channels alter the sensitivity of peripheral neurons to change pain
thresholds. This chapter details the evidence that individual channels may be associated
with particular pain states, and describes genetic approaches to test the possible utility of
targeting individual channels to treat pain.

Keywords Voltage-gated sodium channels · Calcium channels · Potassium channels ·
HERG channels · TRP channels · Transgenic mice

1
Introduction

Because we know the entire sequence of the human genome we can now predict, clone, express and characterise all known and predicted ion channels and accessory subunits using heterologous expression systems. Molecular probes also enable us to define patterns of expression, altered transcriptional profiles in disease states, and splice variants. Armed with this information we can make an educated guess at which channels are likely to play an important role in somatosensation and pain pathways. Again, gene manipulation allows us to test the possible role of candidate target genes by means of small interfering (si)RNA blockade of translation or transgenic mouse studies. Thus, the post-genomic era is providing unprecedented technology and opportunities for pharmacologists to target subsets of cells and individual subtypes of receptors in order to understand more about and treat disease.

In the case of voltage-gated ion channels, an analysis of the relationship between the pore regions of expressed mammalian voltage-gated ion channels has resulted in the following useful analysis of the 'chanome' (Fig. 1) by Yu and Catterall (2004). Note the enormous diversity of potassium channels and the relationship between voltage-gated sodium, calcium, potassium and TRP (transient receptor potential) channels—receptors that have been implicated in a variety of sensory modalities and pain conditions. In this review we will concentrate on voltage-gated sodium and potassium channels, calcium channels, TRPs, acid-sensing ion channels (ASICs) and other channel subtypes, their role in pain transduction, and thus their potential as analgesic drug targets.

Although the global role of voltage-gated channels in electrical signalling might make one imagine that they would be unattractive as analgesic drug targets, recent studies have identified a selective role for subsets of sodium, calcium and potassium channels in setting pain thresholds. Thus, microarray analyses of altered gene expression in sensory neurons and the spinal cord following nerve injury have shown a number of altered sodium, calcium and potassium channel transcripts that may be associated with the pathophysiology of chronic pain (Xiao et al. 2002; Costigan et al. 2002; Wang et al. 2003). Consistent with this, drugs targeting sodium (mexiletine), calcium channels (ziconotide) and potassium channels (retigabine) have all been found to have analgesic actions either in man or animal models (or both).

Recapitulating inflammatory pain and the human peripheral nerve injuries that lead to neuropathic pain in animal models has proved extremely useful for mechanistic studies. Most models focus on partial nerve injury to sciatic or sural nerves, which allows altered hind-limb pain sensitivity to thermal and mechanical insults to be measured and compared with the uninjured contralateral paw.

A model of rodent neuropathic pain (Bennett model) relies upon the tight ligation of the sciatic nerve using thread soaked in chrome alum, which also

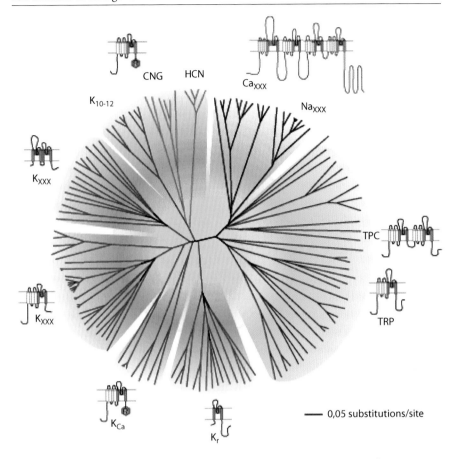

Fig. 1 The amino acid sequence relationship of pore regions in seven voltage-gated ion channel families. (For full details see Yu and Catterall 2004 and Yu et al. 2005)

imparts a low pH insult to the local tissue (Bennett et al. 1992). Kim et al. (1997) ligated tightly both L5 and L6 (or L5 alone) spinal nerves (Chung model), and compared the evoked behaviour with that found in the Bennett model. Both thermal and mechanical thresholds were affected, with a long-lasting hyperalgesia to noxious heat (at least 5 weeks) and mechanical allodynia (at least 10 weeks) of the affected foot. In addition there were behavioural signs of the presence of spontaneous pain. Seltzer (1990) ligated about half of the sciatic nerve close to the spinal cord. Within a few hours the rats developed guarding and licking behaviour of the ipsilateral hind paw, suggesting the presence of spontaneous pain. This continued for many months. There was a decrease in the withdrawal thresholds in response to repetitive Von Frey hair stimulation at the plantar side. Allodynia and mechanical hyperalgesia were apparent in this model, as was thermal hyperalgesia.

The spared nerve injury model (Decosterd and Woolf 2000) involves a lesion of two of the three terminal branches of the sciatic nerve (tibial and common peroneal nerves), leaving the remaining sural nerve intact. The spared nerve injury model is unique in restricting contact between intact and degenerating axons, allowing behavioural testing of the non-injured skin territories next to the denervated areas.

Erichsen and Blackburn-Munro (2002) investigated the pharmacological sensitivity of the sciatic nerve ligation (SNI) model to analgesic drugs, measuring reflex nociceptive responses to mechanical and cold stimulation after systemic administration of opioids, sodium channel blockers and other drugs. They found that morphine attenuated mechanical hypersensitivity and cold hypersensitivity. The sodium-channel blocker mexiletine relieved both cold allodynia and mechanical hyperalgesia, but the most distinct and prolonged effect was observed on mechanical allodynia. Gabapentin alleviated mechanical allodynia but had no effect on mechanical hyperalgesia.

The Chung model has also been characterised in terms of responses to different type of analgesic drugs that have some utility in the clinic (Abdi et al. 1998). Amitriptyline (an anti-depressant which also blocks sodium channels), gabapentin and lidocaine (a local anaesthetic) were effective in increasing the threshold for mechanical allodynia Amitriptyline and lidocaine reduced the rate of continuing discharges of injured afferent fibres, although gabapentin did not influence these discharges, presumably acting centrally. Analgesic drugs found serendipitously in the clinic (e.g. gabapentin) are effective in animal models, thus giving confidence to the conclusions drawn from animal experimentation.

2
Sodium Channels

Voltage-gated sodium channels comprise a family of ten structurally related genes that are expressed in spatially and temporally distinct patterns in the mammalian nervous system. Sodium channel blockers which act as anaesthetics at high concentrations are also well know for their analgesic actions at lower concentrations (Strichartz et al. 2002). Local anaesthetics seem to bind to and block sodium channels in a state-dependent manner. Thus, activation of the channels results in increased accessibility for these agents via the cytoplasmic vestibule of the channel, so that channels that are firing at high frequency are selectively inhibited (Fozzard et al. 2005). Such mechanisms are likely to operate in pain states where nociceptors are activated and are selectively targeted by low doses of local anaesthetics. Evidence of a role for sodium channels in various chronic pain situations has come from studies of neuronal excitability, analysis of patterns of expression of channel isoforms in animal models of neuropathic pain, and antisense and knock-out studies. Three sodium channels, $Na_V1.7$, $Na_V1.8$ and $Na_V1.9$, are selectively expressed within the peripheral nervous system, and these particular isoforms have attracted attention as analgesic drug targets. In addition, an embryonic channel $Na_V1.3$ and a β-subunit, β-3, have been found to be up-regulated in dorsal root ganglion (DRG) neurons in neuropathic pain states.

All sodium channel α-subunits consist of four homologous domains that form a single, voltage-gated aqueous pore. The α-subunits are greater than 75% identical over the amino-acid sequences comprising the transmembrane and extracellular domains. The α-subunits show distinct patterns of expression, and are associated with accessory β-subunits which modify channel properties and interact with cytoskeletal and extracellular matrix proteins. Despite the broadly similar properties of voltage-gated sodium channels, there is evidence for a specialised role of the various isoforms, highlighted for example by the different phenotypes of null mutant mice. For example, $Na_V1.2$ sodium channel knock-outs show severe hypoxia as a result of brain-stem apoptosis, and the $Na_V1.8$ channel plays a specialised role in pain pathways. Much attention has focussed on the regulation of expression of sodium channels in peripheral nociceptive neurons and the functional changes that are associated with various pain states (Fig. 2; Table 1).

Voltage-gated sodium channels provide the inward current that generates the upswing of an action potential in response to supra-threshold depolarisations of the membrane potential. At present, $Na_V1.1$ to $Na_V1.9$ have been characterised as voltage-gated sodium channels (Goldin 2001). A further sodium

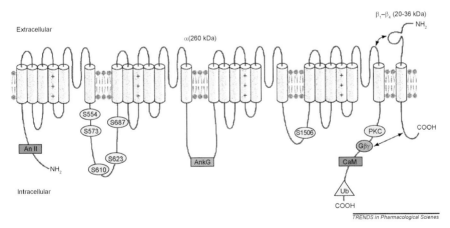

Fig. 2 The α- and β-subunits of Na_V channels. Sites at which Na_V channels are regulated are highlighted. S554, S573, S610, S623, S687 and S1506 residues within Na_V channels are phosphorylated by either protein kinase A (PKA) or PKC (or both ;see main text for further information). The *arrows* indicate possible interactions of different regions of the β-subunit with the α-subunit. Abbreviations: *An II*, annexin II; *AnkG*, ankyrin G; *CaM*, calmodulin; Gβγ, G protein β–γ complex; *Ub*, ubiquitin. (From Chahine et al. 2005)

Table 1 Mammalian voltage-gated sodium channels

Name	Gene	Distribution	DRG	TTX-S
$Na_v1.1$	(Type I) SCN1A	CNS Heart	+++	+
$Na_v1.2$	(Type II) SCN2A	CNS	+	+
$Na_v1.3$	(Type III) SCN3A	Fetal DRG	+	+
$Na_v1.4$	(SkM1) SCN4A	Muscle	−	+
$Na_v1.5$	(SkM2) SCN5A	Heart	+	
$Na_v1.6$	(NaCh6) SCN8A	DRG CNS	+	+
$Na_v1.7$	(PN1) SCN9A	DRG SCG	+++	+
$Na_v1.8$	(SNS) SCN10A	DRG	+++	
$Na_v1.9$	(NaN) SCN11A	DRG	++	
Na_vx	(NaG) SCN7A	Lung nerve	+	+

channel α-subunit has been cloned that lacks the amino acid sequence required for voltage gating. Watanabe et al. (2000) identified Na_X in the body-fluid regulating circumventricular organs of the brain. Behavioural data revealed that knock-out animals, when dehydrated, drink 300 mM NaCl solution in contrast to the avoidance behaviour demonstrated by dehydrated wild-type mice, leading Watanabe et al. (2000) to propose a role for Na_X in regulating salt intake behaviour. In support of this hypothesis, more recent data from the same group demonstrated that Na_X is gated by extracellular sodium concentration, with approximately 160 mM sodium producing a half maximal response (Hiyama et al. 2002).

Although the α-subunit alone is sufficient for the formation of a functional channel, the accessory β-subunits increase the efficiency of channel expression and are required for normal kinetics and voltage dependence of channel gating. In addition, β-subunits have an important role in the localisation of α-subunits (Malhotra et al. 2000).

Sodium channel α-subunits have a membrane topology consisting of a large intracellular N-terminal domain, four repeated homologous domains (DI, DII, DIII and DIV) containing six transmembrane regions (S1 to S6), a large intracellular loop between DII and DIII involved in sodium channel inactivation and a short intracellular C-terminus.

The loops between transmembrane region 5 and 6 (S5–S6 loop) contribute residues to the formation of the channel pore and are longer in DI and DIII than DII or DIV. The S5-S6 loop of DI provides residues important for the binding of the pore-blocking toxins saxitoxin (STX) and tetrodotoxin (TTX).

The accessory β-subunits are less well-conserved and significantly smaller, consisting of a large, immunoglobulin-like extracellular N-terminal domain required for functional expression and modulation of α-subunits, a single transmembrane region involved in modulating the voltage dependence of α-subunit steady state inactivation and a short intracellular C-terminal domain. Other accessory subunits that may modulate channel function have been reviewed (Malik-Hall et al. 2003).

Voltage-gated sodium channels can be pharmacologically classified into two main groups according to their sensitivity to TTX. $Na_V1.1$, 1.2, 1.3, 1.4, 1.6 and 1.7 are sensitive to TTX and are thus termed TTX-S, whereas $Na_V1.5$, 1.8 and 1.9 are relatively resistant to TTX and are thus termed TTX-R. An example of these two classes of current comes from whole cell electrophysiological recordings of dissociated adult rat DRG neurons. Here TTX has a K_d for TTX-S currents of approximately 300 pM compared to 100 μM for TTX-R currents composed of $Na_V1.8$ and $Na_V1.9$. $Na_V1.5$, although responsible for a TTX-R current, is more sensitive to TTX (IC_{50} 1 uM) than either $Na_V1.8$ or $Na_V1.9$.

TTX-R currents are mainly restricted to embryonic and denervated muscle and heart muscle ($Na_V1.5$) or small-diameter DRG neurons ($Na_V1.8$ and $Na_V1.9$). $Na_V1.8$ and $Na_V1.9$ are both expressed in sensory neurons and seem to play an import role in nociception and the setting of pain thresholds. $Na_V1.5$ has also been identified in a small number of sensory neurons. In experimental diabetes there is a significant up-regulation of messenger (m)RNA and protein for $Na_V1.3$, and $Na_V1.7$ and a down-regulation of $Na_V1.6$ and $Na_V1.8$ mRNA after the onset of allodynia (Hong et al. 2004). There is also an altered pattern of channel phosphorylation—the level of serine/threonine phosphorylation of $Na_V1.6$ and In $Na_V1.8$ increased in response to diabetes. Increased tyrosine phosphorylation of $Na_V1.6$ and $Na_V1.7$ was also observed in DRGs from diabetic rats. In most neuropathic pain models exemplified by axotomy, however, $Na_V1.8$ and 1.9 are down-regulated, whilst $Na_V1.3$ is induced (Waxman et al. 1994; Dib-Hajj et al. 1996, 1998).

2.1
$Na_V1.3$

$Na_V1.3$ is widely expressed in the adult CNS but is normally present at low levels in the adult peripheral nervous system. Axotomy or other forms of nerve damage lead to the re-expression of $Na_V1.3$ and the associated β-3 subunit in sensory neurons, but not in primary motor neurons (Waxman et al. 1994; Dib-Hajj et al. 1996; Hains et al. 2002). This event can be reversed in vitro and in vivo by treatment with high levels of exogenous glial-derived neurotrophic factor (GDNF). $Na_V1.3$ is known to recover (reprime) rapidly from inactivation (Cummins et al. 2001). Axotomy has been shown to induce the expression of rapidly repriming TTX-sensitive sodium channels in damaged neurons, and this event can also be reversed by the combined actions of GDNF and nerve growth factor (NGF) (Leffler et al. 2002). Concomitant with the reversal of $Na_V1.3$ expression by GDNF, ectopic action potential generation is diminished and thermal and mechanical pain-related behaviour in a rat chronic constrictive injury (CCI) model is reversed (Boucher et al. 2000). Moreover, $Na_V1.3$ is up-regulated in multi-receptive nociceptive dorsal horn neurons following experimental spinal cord injury. This up-regulation is associated with hyper-excitability of these nociceptive neurons and pain; antisense knock-down of $Na_V1.3$ attenuates the dorsal horn neuron hyperexcitability and the pain be-haviours in spinal-cord injured animals (Hains et al. 2003). It therefore seems plausible that $Na_V1.3$ re-expression may play a significant role in increasing neuronal excitability, thus contributing to neuropathic pain after nerve and spinal cord injury.

2.2
$Na_V1.7$

$Na_V1.7$, a peripheral nervous system-specific sodium channel isoform was first cloned from the pheochromocytoma PC12 cell line. Its presence at high levels in the growth cones of small-diameter neurons suggests that it is likely to play some role in the transmission of nociceptive information. Immunochemical studies of functionally defined sensory neurons in guinea-pigs supports the view that $Na_V1.7$ is associated with nociceptors. $Na_V1.7$ is expressed exclu-sively in peripheral, mainly small-diameter sensory and sympathetic neurons. $Na_V1.7$ global gene deletion leads to death shortly after birth, apparently as a consequence of failure to feed. This may reflect autonomic or enteric sensory neuron dysfunction.

Deleting the gene in a subset of sensory neurons that are predominantly nociceptive demonstrates that $Na_V1.7$ plays an important role in pain mecha-nisms, especially in the development of inflammatory pain. The specific deficits in acute mechano-sensation, rather than thermal sensitivity associated with the $Na_V1.7$ deletion, are striking. However, as TTX does not block mechani-cally activated currents in sensory neurons, $Na_V1.7$ must play a downstream role in mechano-transduction. $Na_V1.8$-nulls are also refractory to Randall–Sellito-induced mechanical insults. These data raise the possibility that sodium channels and mechano-sensitive channels are physically apposed at nociceptor terminals.

The roles of $Na_V1.7$ and 1.8 in pain pathways may be related. In the $Na_V1.8$-null mouse, NGF-induced thermal hyperalgesia is diminished, and there are small deficits in other inflammatory pain models. However, in the $Na_V1.8$-null, an up-regulation of $Na_V1.7$ mRNA has been noted, as well as an increase in TTX-S sodium current density. Thus, $Na_V1.7$ may compensate for the depletion of $Na_V1.8$. In contrast, deletion of $Na_V1.7$ is not compensated for by increased TTX-R current activity and leads to a dramatic phenotype in terms of inflammatory pain.

Peripheral changes in pain thresholds seem to involve several mechanisms including channel phosphorylation. NGF acting through TrkA-mediated ac-tivation of phospholipase C relieves phosphatidylinositol-4,5-bisphosphate

[PtdIns(4,5)P2] channel block of TRPV1; p38 mitogen-activated protein (MAP) kinase also plays a role in NGF-induced hyperalgesia. Carrageenan increases prostanoid levels that, acting through EP receptors, cause sodium channel phosphorylation involving protein kinase A (PKA). Complete Freund's adjuvant induces longer-term changes that are partially blocked by aspirin-like drugs. Remarkably, all these forms of inflammatory hyperalgesia are attenuated by deletion of $Na_V1.7$.

A number of possible mechanisms involving $Na_V1.7$ regulation may occur. $Na_V1.7$ is unlikely to be a target for kinase modulation in inflammatory pain; in vitro studies in Xenopus oocytes demonstrate a diminution in peak current density in response to PKA or protein kinase C (PKC) activation. $Na_V1.7$ contrasts with $Na_V1.8$, which shows increased peak current and an altered current voltage relationship consistent with nociceptor sensitisation and is relatively faster to reprime. The regulation of $Na_V1.7$ channel density, or localisation with respect to primary signal transducers at nociceptor terminals, could play a significant role in setting peripheral pain thresholds. NGF has already been shown to increase excitability of PC12 cells through increasing expression of $Na_V1.7$.

Primary erythermalgia, a chronic inflammatory disease that is inherited in a dominant form in man, maps to gain of function mutation in $Na_V1.7$ that lead to a lowered threshold of activation, demonstrating the utility of mouse models in understanding human pain conditions (Drenth et al. 2005).

2.3
$Na_V1.8$

$Na_V1.8$ is mainly expressed in nociceptive neurons (Akopian et al. 1996; Djouhri et al. 2003). This channel contributes a majority of the sodium current underlying the depolarising phase of the action potential in cells in which it is present (Renganathan et al. 2001). Functional expression of the channel is regulated by inflammatory mediators, including NGF, and both antisense and knock-out studies support a role for the channel in contributing to inflammatory pain (Khasar et al. 1998; Akopian et al. 1999). Antisense studies have also suggested a role for this protein in the development of neuropathic pain (Lai et al. 2002), and a deficit in ectopic action propagation has been described in the $Na_V1.8$-null mutant mouse (Roza et al. 2003). However, neuropathic pain behaviour at early time points seem to be normal in the $Na_V1.8$-null mutant mouse (Kerr et al. 2000), and studies of double knock-outs of $Na_V1.7$ and $Na_V1.8$ also demonstrate a normal neuropathic pain phenotype using the Chung model (Nassar et al. 2005).

Identification of annexin II/p11, which binds to $Na_V1.8$ and facilitates the insertion of functional channels in the cell membrane (Okuse et al. 2002), may provide a target that can be used to modulate the expression of $Na_V1.8$ and hence the level of $Na_V1.8$ current in nociceptive neurons.

Na$_V$1.9 is also expressed in nociceptive neurons (Dib-Hajj et al. 1998; Fang et al. 2003) and underlies a persistent sodium current with substantial overlap between activation and steady-state inactivation (Cummins et al. 1999) that has a probable role in setting thresholds of activation (Dib-Hajj et al. 2002; Baker et al. 2003), suggesting that blockade of Na$_V$1.9 might be useful for the treatment of pain. Conversely, it has been suggested that Na$_V$1.9 activators might alleviate pain because Na$_V$1.9 is down-regulated after axotomy (Dib-Hajj et al. 1998; Cummins et al. 2000); the resultant loss of the Na$_V$1.9 persistent current and its depolarising influence on resting potential (Cummins et al. 1999) might remove resting inactivation from other sodium channels (Cummins and Waxman 1997). Na$_V$1.9 null mutants show normal levels of neuropathic pain but have deficits in inflammatory pain. Normal level of expression seems to be dependent on the supply of NGF or GDNF (Cummins et al. 2000). Present evidence thus makes sodium channels highly attractive analgesic drug targets, but specific antagonists for Na$_V$1.3, 1.8 and 1.9 have yet to be tested in the clinic.

What determines the cell type expression of sodium channels in nociceptors? Although we do not have a comprehensive knowledge of any sodium channel promoter's structure and association with a particular transcription factor(s), we do have a number of insights into some aspects of sodium channel regulatory motifs. A short sequence found upstream of neuronal sodium channel genes named NRSE (neuron restricted silencing element) or RE-1 (repressor element 1) (Schoenherr and Anderson 1995; Kraner et al. 1992) regulates neuronal expression. Transcription factors that bound to the motif were found to act as inhibitors of gene expression in non-neuronal cells. These proteins were named REST (RE-1 silencing transcription factor), or NRSF (neuron-restrictive silencer factor). The inhibitory activity of the complex can be modulated by double stranded (ds)RNA molecules that have the same sequence as NRSE/RE-1 and are found in developing neuronal precursors. These regulatory RNA molecules are able to switch the repressor function of the complex to an activator role (Kuwabara et al. 2004). In this way the assumption of a neuronal phenotype seems to depend in part upon regulatory RNAs driving gene expression downstream of NRSE/RE-1 motifs. Sodium channels are known to be expressed at the very earliest stages of the appearance of a neuronal phenotype in the mouse. These studies highlight the significance of sodium channel expression in neuronal function throughout development (Albrieux et al. 2004).

Apart from the tissue-specific control of sodium channel expression most obviously demonstrated by the presence of neuronal and muscle isoforms, there is evidence that the relative levels of sodium channel transcripts vary in development. Early studies of the developing rat gave us the first indication that the type III sodium channel is prevalent in rat embryos and expressed at much lower levels in adult neuronal tissues, whilst the types 1 and 2 are expressed in variable patterns in adult tissues (Beckh et al. 1989). Interestingly, this pattern of expression does not seem to hold true in cynomolgus monkeys where Na$_V$1.3

is broadly expressed, albeit at low levels in both central and peripheral tissues in the adult (Raymond et al. 2004). Thus, the pattern of expression of human sodium channels may vary markedly from that described in detail in rodents. Felts et al. (1997) extended the rat development analysis with probes against $Na_V1.1$, 1.2, 1.3, 1.6 and 1.7 and showed a complex pattern of developmentally regulated channel expression in both peripheral and central neurons.

Accessory subunits that are assumed to be uniquely associated within voltage-gated sodium channels also show developmentally regulated patterns of expression. Shah et al. (2001) showed that in the developing rat the β-3 subunit was prevalent, and this subunit remained expressed in adult hippocampus and striatum. β-1 and -2 subunits were expressed after postnatal day 3 in the rat in central and peripheral tissues. The developmental pattern of expression of the β-2-like subunit β-4 (Yu et al. 2003) that is also expressed both centrally and peripherally has yet to be described. The functional significance of β-subunit expression for sodium channel kinetics properties and their tethering to extra-cellular signalling molecules has been explored extensively.

3
Splice Variants of Sodium Channels

A further level of complexity in the expression of sodium channels is created by the existence of splice variants of sodium channel α-subunits that may be regulated during development and by regulators of splicing choice in the adult. Because fly genetics is so advanced, more information is available about *Drosophila* splice choice sodium channel variants and their functional roles than the vertebrate equivalents. However, it seems reasonable to suppose that alternative splicing and RNA editing and transport may also have roles in regulating mammalian sodium channel function. In *Drosophila*, a mutation in a dsRNA helicase led to a lowering of expression of Para-encoded sodium channels. Reenan et al. (2000) showed that this was due to a failure to edit the Para transcript with adenosine to inosine substitutions, which apparently required the helicase for secondary structure modification of the mRNA transcript. At least three positions in the Para transcript are known to be edited (Hanrahan et al. 2000) by adenosine deaminase to give A to I substitutions, and these events are developmentally regulated.

The editing process requires a complementary sequence of intronic RNA to form secondary structure with the edited sequence in a similar manner to that demonstrated for mammalian glutamate receptors. Other editing events in cockroach sodium channels and *Drosophila para* have been correlated with dramatic functional changes. Liu et al. (2004) have shown that a U to C editing event resulting in a phenylalanine to serine modification can produce a sodium channel with persistent TTX-sensitive properties rather similar to currents identified in mammalian CNS neurons, raising the possibility that similar events could occur in mammals. Song et al. (2004) have catalogued further editing events that have functional consequences in terms of thresholds of activation and are developmentally regulated in the cockroach. Tan et al. (2002) have also found that alternatively spliced transcripts can have distinct pharmacological profiles as well as altered gating characteristics. They found alternative exons encoding transmembrane segments in DIII of a cockroach sodium channel, which had conserved splice sites across evolution in fish, flies, mice and men. The alternatively spliced forms were found in different tissues. One form with a premature stop codon occurred only in the peripheral nervous system whilst the two other functional forms differed in their sensitivity to pyrethroid insecticides such as δ-methrin. Remarkably, fetal mouse brain also contains transcripts of the SCN8A gene (Na$_V$1.6) that contains a stop codon at the same site as the fly genes predicting the production of two domain truncated sodium channel transcripts (Plummer et al. 1997). The role of these transcripts is unknown.

In mammals, mutually exclusive exon usage also occurs. The type III channel exists as an embryonic or adult spliced form with different exons that code for the S3 and S4 segments in DI of the rat channel. Despite the fact that the two exons both encode 29 amino acids, only a single amino acid residue is altered in these two alternative forms. Single amino acid changes may also occur through alternative 3′ splice site selection. Kerr et al. (2004) have found that both Na$_V$1.8 and Na$_V$1.5—two TTX-resistant sodium channels found in peripheral neurons—both exist as alternative forms containing an additional glutamine residue within the cytoplasmic loop linking DII and DIII of these channels. As well as alternative exon usage or amino acids insertions, transcripts encoding exon repeats have been identified in DRG neurons. The presence of a transcript with a three-exon repeat encoding Na$_V$1.8 is enhanced by treatment with NGF, suggesting that this neurotrophin may regulate trans-splicing events in these cells (Akopian et al. 1999). Once again the functional consequences of these conserved changes have yet to be established.

The regulation of splice choice in response to external signals is still little understood. Buchner et al. (2003), studying a modifier locus in different mouse lines that determines the lethality of a Na$_V$1.6 splice site mutation, discovered that the efficiency of action of a splice factor determined the amount of functional channel produced and hence the lethality of the original mutation. Thus, on a C57Bl6 background little correctly spliced mRNA was produced, causing a lethal phenotype, whilst on a wild-type background, 10% of the transcripts were correctly spliced, leading to a viable if dystonic phenotype.

Recent papers have suggested roles for sodium channels in regulating synaptic efficacy, as well as functions in immune system cells. Macrophages and microglia express Na$_V$1.6, a channel that is broadly expressed in the nervous system and which is functionally compromised in the naturally occurring *med* mutant that leads to dystonia. Interestingly, macrophage function is also inhibited in these animals. When microglia or macrophages are activated, Na$_V$1.6

expression is up-regulated, and this event seems to be important in terms of phagocytic activity, as the uptake of latex beads is partially blocked in med macrophages, or in normal macrophages treated with TTX. This suggests that voltage-gated sodium channels play an important functional role in immune system cell function. These kinds of unsuspected roles for voltage-gated channels may give rise to significant problems in attempts to use selective blockers as analgesic in chronic pain states.

4
Calcium Channels

Voltage-gated calcium channels comprise a single α-subunit and show strong structural homology with sodium channels, but the accessory subunits associated with these channel are much more complex. The functional calcium channel complexes contain four proteins: α1 (170 kDa), α2 (150 kDa), β (52 kDa), δ (17–25 kDa) and γ (32 kDa). Four α2δ subunit genes have now been cloned. Both the message and protein for the α2δ-1 subunit is highly expressed in sensory neurons but is also found almost ubiquitously in other tissues (Gong et al. 2001). All α2δ subunits have a predicted N-terminal signal sequence, indicating that the N-terminus is extracellular, with an intracellular C-terminus and potential transmembrane region. There are up to 14 conserved cysteines throughout the α2δ-1, 2 and 3 sequences, six of which are within δ, providing additional evidence that α2 and δ are disulphide-bonded. Following the identification of α2δ subunits as components of skeletal muscle calcium channels, they have also been shown to be associated with neuronal N- and P/Q-type channels. The α2δ-1 subunit has been shown to bind to extracellular regions including DIII on the $Ca_V1.2$ subunit (Felix et al. 1997).

5
Voltage-Gated Calcium Channels

High voltage-activated and low voltage-activated calcium channels are now known to comprise a number of cloned α-subunits (Peres-Reyes 2003). $Ca_V2.2$, $Ca_V2.3$ and $Ca_V3.2$ are now known to play an important role in pain sensation and are interesting analgesic drug targets.

The evidence of an important specialised role for certain voltage-gated calcium channels in the pathogenesis of neuropathic pain is strong. A variety of drugs targeted at calcium channel subtypes are effective analgesics, and mouse null mutants of N-type $Ca_V2.2$ calcium channels show dramatic diminution in neuropathic pain behaviour in response to both mechanical and thermal stimuli. Opioid peptides are known to inhibit the action of N-type calcium channels through post-translational mechanisms. In addition, two highly effective analgesic drugs used in neuropathic pain conditions selectively target calcium channel subtypes. The conotoxin ziconotide blocks $Ca_V2.2$ α-subunits, and the widely prescribed drug gabapentin binds with high affinity to α2δ subunits of calcium channels.

Gabapentin binds to high-affinity sites in the brain, and the target binding site has been identified as the α2δ-1 subunit. Transient transfection of cells with α2δ-1 increased the number of gabapentin binding sites (Gee et al. 1996). Subsequently, gabapentin has been found to bind to two isoforms of α2δ subunits (the α2δ-1 and α2δ-2 isoforms, but not α2δ-3 or α2δ-4) (Gee et al. 1996; Gong et al. 2001). The effects of gabapentin on native calcium currents are controversial, with some authors reporting small inhibitions of calcium currents in different cell types. Gabapentin could interfere with α2δ binding to the α1 subunit, thus destabilizing the heteromeric complex. Interestingly, α2δ1 up-regulation in neuropathic pain correlates well with gabapentin sensitivity (Luo et al. 2002), suggesting that the α2δ-1 isoform is the most likely site of action of gabapentin.

The up-regulation of α2-δ subunits does not occur in all animal models of neuropathic pain that result in allodynia. Luo et al. (2002) compared DRG and spinal cord α2δ-1 subunit levels and gabapentin sensitivity in allodynic rats with mechanical nerve injuries (sciatic nerve chronic constriction injury, spinal nerve transection, or ligation), a metabolic disorder (diabetes) or chemical neuropathy (vincristine neurotoxicity). Allodynia occurred in all types of nerve injury investigated, but DRG and/or spinal cord α2δ-1 subunit up-regulation and gabapentin sensitivity only co-existed in mechanical and diabetic neuropathies. This may partially explain why gabapentin is ineffective in some neuropathic pain patients. Recent studies with knock-in mice have demonstrated that gabapentin loses its effectiveness when it can no longer bind to a mutated form of α2δ-1, and the details of this work can be found in a patent application (Baron et al. 2005). Thus, the site of action of gabapentin/pregabalin seems resolved, but the mechanism of action is still uncertain.

Further support for calcium channels as useful drug targets in neuropathic pain comes from an analysis of the characteristics of the $Ca_V2.2$-null mutant mouse generated by Saegusa et al. (2001). The same authors (Saegusa et al. 2002) have compared the $Ca_V2.2$- and 2.3-null mutants in a variety of pain models. Despite the widespread expression of $Ca_V2.2$, it has proved possible to demonstrate major deficits in inflammatory and in particular neuropathic pain in this transgenic mouse using the Seltzer model. Thermal and mechanical thresholds were dramatically stabilized in this mutant mouse. The relationship between α2δ subunits and $Ca_V2.2$ has not been investigated in detail, so it is possible that gabapentin has sites of action on calcium channels other than $Ca_V2.2$—for example, T-type channels such as $Ca_V3.2$.

A role for $Ca_V2.2$ in chronic pain is consistent with a known analgesic role for N-type calcium channel blockers. Ziconotide, a toxin derived from marine snails, blocks $Ca_V2.2$ channels with high affinity and has been found to have analgesic actions in animal models and man. In a study of the anti-nociceptive properties of ziconotide, morphine and clonidine in a rat model of post-operative pain, heat hyperalgesia and mechanical allodynia were induced in the hind paw (Wang et al. 2000). Intrathecal ziconotide blocked established heat hyperalgesia in a dose-dependent manner and caused a reversible blockade of established mechanical allodynia. Intrathecal ziconotide was found to be more potent, longer acting, and more specific in its actions than intrathecal morphine in this model of post-surgical pain.

Brose (1997) found that intrathecal ziconotide provided complete pain relief with elimination of hyperaesthesia and allodynia in a dose dependent manner in a single patient suffering from intractable pain, although side-effects were experienced. This type of study has led to clinical use of ziconotide in the treatment of intractable pain in late stage cancer patients. Evidence that omega conotoxins also target P2X3 receptors (Lalo et al. 2001) suggests that ziconotide may act at a broader range of targets than first suspected.

Interestingly, a sensory neuron-specific splice variant of $Ca_V2.2$ has been identified in DRG neurons. Lipscombe and collaborators (Bell et al. 2004) showed that the DRG-specific exon, e37a, is preferentially present in $Ca_V2.2$ mRNAs expressed in neurons that contain nociceptive markers TRPV1 and $Na_V1.8$. Cell-specific inclusion of e37a correlated with the significantly larger N-type currents in nociceptive neurons, suggesting that splice-variant specific antagonists could have useful therapeutic effects. The situation in man has yet to be examined, however.

$Ca_V3.2$, a T-type calcium channel has also recently been found to play a role in pain. Antisense targeting $Ca_V3.2$ induced a knock-down of the $Ca_V3.2$ mRNA and protein expression as well as a large reduction of T-type calcium currents in nociceptive DRG neurons. Concomitantly, the antisense treatment resulted in major anti-nociceptive, anti-hyperalgesic and anti-allodynic effects, suggesting that $Ca_V3.2$ plays a major pronociceptive role in acute and chronic pain states. These antisense studies have also been confirmed by the generation and analysis of a knock-out mouse (Bourinet and Zamponi 2005).

6
Potassium Channels

Potassium channels act effectively as brakes on neurotransmission and excitability, allowing the flow of potassium ions out of the cell in response to a range of different stimuli. For example, some analgesic actions of opioids are mediated by the activation of calcium-dependent potassium channels. Potassium channels have been subdivided into four major subsets based on their structure and mode of gating. Voltage-gated channels are extraordinarily diverse—there are 12 different families, K_V1–K_V12, containing different individual members. However, all the voltage-gated channels comprise the classical six-transmembrane monomer that forms a tetrameric voltage-gated structure reminiscent of sodium and calcium channels (Fig. 3).

Evidence has been obtained that potassium channel transcripts are differentially regulated at the transcriptional level in animal models of neuropathic pain. Using RT-PCR, Ishikawa et al. (2002) found that, in a chronic constriction injury model of neuropathic pain, K_V1.2, 1.4, 2.2, 4.2 and 4.3 mRNA levels in the ipsilateral DRG were reduced to 63%–73% of the contralateral sides of the same animal at 3 days and to 34%–63% at 7 days following CCI. In addition, K_V1.1 mRNA levels declined to about 72% of the contralateral level at 7 days. No significant changes in K_V1.5, 1.6, 2.1, 3.1, 3.2, 3.5 and 4.1 mRNA levels were detectable in the ipsilateral DRG at either time. Interestingly, of the K_V channels present in DRG, K_V1.4 seems to be the main channel expressed in small-diameter sensory neurons, and the expression levels of this channel are much reduced in a Chung model of neuropathic pain (Rasband et al. 1999).

The calcium-activated potassium channel family comprises three subsets that have structural similarities with the K_V channels. They have been classified on the basis of their conductance into big, intermediate and small currents (BK, IK, SK). However, although voltage-dependent via some positive charges in the S4 domain, they are essentially opened by increases in cytoplasmic calcium concentrations through an interaction with a calmodulin binding domain found at the C-termini of these channels. They also differ from K_V channels in containing an additional N-terminal transmembrane domain that means the N-terminus is extracellular, unlike voltage-gated channels. Fascinatingly, Xie et al. (2005) have found that splice choice for the BK channel STREK exon is modulated through the actions of a CAM kinase response element, suggesting that neuronal excitability could be altered both directly though the actions of calcium on potassium channels, as well as indirectly by chang-

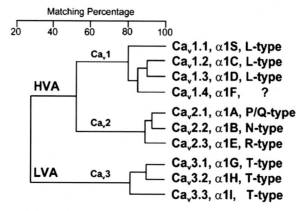

Fig. 3 Voltage-gated channels

ing the molecular structure of expressed ion channels through alternative splicing.

Two-pore K channels (K2P channels) comprise a dimer of the two transmembrane regions that form the functional pore with two P domains, and form functional dimers that are gated by a variety of stimuli. This area has recently been reviewed by Kim (2005). Sixteen K2P channel genes are expressed in a range of tissues and have the properties of leak K+ channels. They thus play a major role in setting resting membrane potential and regulating cell excitability. The stimuli that gate K2P channels are very diverse and include lipids, volatile anaesthetics, and heat, oxygen, acid and mechanical stimuli. Inward rectifier potassium channels retain just the two pore-forming subunits found in voltage-gated channels together with the potassium selective P loop and also form tetrameric structures that are, necessarily, voltage-independent. There is an enormous variety of these channels that have been classified into seven families. G protein-regulated potassium channels are gated by interactions with G protein $\beta\gamma$ subunits.

Recently a new set of K channels that are responsive to increased intracellular levels of sodium have also been identified (Bhattacharjee and Kaczmarek 2005), but their role in setting pain thresholds has not been explored.

Passmore et al. (2003) have provided evidence that KCNQ potassium currents (responsible for the M-current) may also play a role in setting pain thresholds. Retigabine potentiates M-currents and leads to a diminution of nociceptive input into the dorsal horn of the spinal cord in both neuropathic and inflammatory pain models in the rat. Thus, despite the enormous complexity of potassium channels, there is some possibility of targeting pain thresholds through activating potassium channels expressed on damage-sensing sensory neurons.

7
Pacemaker Channels

Cyclic nucleotide-regulated hyperpolarisation-activated cation channels (HCN channels) play an important role in cardiac function and are expressed within sensory neurons. Chaplan and collaborators (2003) have described a novel role for HCN channels in touch-related pain and spontaneous neuronal discharge originating in the damaged DRG. Nerve injury markedly increased pacemaker currents in large-diameter DRG neurons and resulted in pacemaker-driven spontaneous action potentials in the ligated nerve. Pharmacological blockade of HCN activity using the specific inhibitor ZD7288 reversed hypersensitivity to light touch and decreased the firing frequency of ectopic discharges originating in A-δ and A-β fibres by 90% and 40%. Targeting these channels appears problematic, however, given their other roles in the periphery.

8
Transient Receptor Potential Receptors

The TRP family of cation-selective channel subunits are encoded by 28 distinct genes, many of which exist as multiple splice variants. This class of channel was first identified in *Drosophila*, where the channel is involved in visual signalling. TRPs comprise seven sub-families that are structurally related, and form multimeric complexes that may involve heteromultimerisation both within and between different subsets. The structure of the channels (Fig. 4) includes six transmembrane domains reminiscent of the voltage-gated channels, and they do indeed seem to form tetrameric complexes. For historical reasons various aspect of TRP physiology have been extensively studied for some classes more than others. For example the TRPP subset, broadly expressed in neuronal and non-neuronal tissues, have been studied in tem of kidney function, because they are associated with polycystic kidney disease, TRPVs have been studied in terms of sensory neuron function, despite broad expression, because one of them is gated by chilli powder, whilst the calcium signalling community have focussed on TRPCs, which seem to be involved in calcium homeostasis and the replenishing of intracellular calcium stores. In fact, the range of ligands and stimuli, from mechanical and thermal to eicosanoids and environmental pollutants, is astonishing and makes these channels a fascinating topic of study for anyone interested in cellular signalling. Another curiosity of the TRP field is that the number of reviews written about this class of channel threatens to overtake the number of research papers published on their function.

In mammals the first TRP channels to be identified are known as the canonical TRPs or the TRPC family and comprise seven members. TRPC1 has been characterised as a mechano-sensor and is very broadly expressed; TRPC2 is exquisitely selectively expressed in the vomeronasal organ of rodents, and is essential for pheromone-induced normal mating behaviour and is absent in man. TRPC3, -6 and -7 are structurally similar, activated by diacylglycerol and implicated in calcium homeostasis, whilst TRPC4 and -5 are close relatives and are involved in ligands induced calcium signalling. In sensory neurons TRPC1, -3, -4, -5 and -6 are highly expressed (Fig. 4).

The identification of the capsaicin receptor as a member of another TRP class of so-called vanilloid receptors led to the classification of the TRPV family of receptors. There are six members of the TRPV class, the first four of which are expressed in sensory neurons, and which have been shown to have a potential role in thermoreception and mechano-sensation based on studies of heterologously expressed channels. The polymodal nature of responses to noxious stimuli demonstrated by the capsaicin receptor TRPV1, and the usefulness of capsaicin in treating some chronic pain syndromes suggested that members of this receptor class may play a role in chronic pain. There is indeed evidence that TRPV1 is up-regulated in the DRG neu-

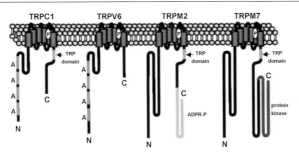

Fig. 4 The structural features of different sets of TRP channels. (Reproduced from Montiel 2004)

rons adjacent to those that have been damaged by spinal nerve ligation (Fukuoka et al. 2002) whilst being down-regulated in damaged neurons. The up-regulated TRPV1 expression seems to be associated with A-fibre sensory neurons (Hudson et al. 2001). These new receptors have been suggested to be important for the analgesic effects of capsaicin cream (Rashid et al. 2003). There are also claims that TRPV1 antagonists may be useful in treating neuropathic pain. Capsazepine, a non-competitive antagonist of TRPV1, markedly attenuated mechanical hyperalgesia in a guinea-pig sciatic nerve injury model (Walker et al. 2003), but this effect was absent in rodents.

Other TRPs also respond to noxious temperatures in an analogous manner to TRPV1. TRPM8 is activated by cold temperatures, whilst TRPV2 and TRPV4 are activated, like TRPV1, by high temperatures.

Genetic screens have also revealed a number of members of the TRP channel family to be candidate mechano-transducers. Fruit flies lacking the NompC channel showed a substantial loss of movement-evoked receptor potential in bristle mechano-receptor neurons, and NompC is also essential for normal hearing in zebrafish. Recently, Nan, a TRP-related protein expressed exclusively in chordotonal neurons in *Drosophila* was found to be required for mechano-transduction by these cells. Another family member, OSM-9, is required for detection of touch, osmolarity and olfactory stimuli in *Caenorhabditis elegans* (Colbert et al. 1997). The closest mammalian homologue of OSM-9, TRPV4, is activated by osmotically induced cell swelling, and a recent report (Suzuki et al. 2003) suggests it contributes to DRG mechanosensation. Animals lacking this channel showed diminished responses to pressure in electrophysiological and behavioural assays. Thus, TRP family members are good candidates for noxious mechano-sensors; however, few TRP channels, even TRPV1, are selectively expressed only in damage sensing neurons, raising the potential problem of side-effects with drugs targeting these channels.

9
Acid-Sensing Ion Channels

ASICs are voltage-independent H^+-gated ion channels belonging to the amiloride-sensitive DEG/ENac superfamily of receptor channels. Four genes encoding six different ASIC subunits have been cloned so far (ASIC1a, 1b, 2a, 2b, 3 and 4). ASIC1 and ASIC2 each have a splice variant, denoted "b", which differs from the "a" counterpart only by the N-terminus. Each ASIC subunit contains intracellular N- and C-termini, two transmembrane domains and a large extracellular loop containing cysteine-rich regions. The ASIC subunits can assemble to form functional homo- or heteromultimers that are mainly permeable to Na^+.

All ASIC subunits are expressed in DRG sensory neurons and have been implicated in a number of different physiological sensory processes such as nociception associated with tissue acidosis in inflammation and ischaemia (ASIC1 and ASIC3; Voilley et al. 2001; Chen et al. 2002), indirect regulation of cutaneous and visceral mechano-sensation (ASIC 1–3; Price et al. 2001; Page et al. 2004), sour taste (Ugawa et al. 2002), visual transduction (Ettaiche et al. 2004) and cochlear function (Peng et al. 2004). However, some ASIC subunits also show a wide distribution throughout the brain, where it has been suggested that they may be activated by the transient acidification that occurs in the synaptic cleft due to acidic vesicle exocytosis. Recently, 6 ASIC subunits cloned from the zebrafish were shown to be mainly expressed in the central nervous system, suggesting a conserved role across species in neuronal communication (Paukert et al. 2004). Supporting this hypothesis, several studies in knock-out mice have demonstrated a role for ASICs in long-term potentiation, learning, memory and fear behaviour (ASIC1 and 2; Wemmie et al. 2002, 2003, 2004). ASIC4 is broadly expressed in the nervous system but is not gated by protons and has no known function.

ASICs have also been implicated in pathophysiological states. ASIC1a is the main mediator of H^+-gated currents in hippocampal neurons (Wemmie et al. 2002; Alvarez de la Rosa et al. 2003). Ca^{2+} imaging in COS-7 cells transiently expressing ASIC1a recently demonstrated that homomeric ASIC1a channels are a major non-voltage-gated pathway for Ca^{2+} entry in cells (Yermolaieva et al. 2004). The same authors demonstrated that Ca^{2+} overload through ASIC1a channels makes a major contribution to hippocampal neuron damage in stroke. A role for ASIC1a in Ca^{2+} overload during brain ischaemia is consistent with the fact that lactic acid, an enhancer of ASIC currents (Immke and McCleskey 2001), and protons are both produced (by anaerobic glycolysis and ATP hydrolysis respectively) during ischaemia. In fact, it appears that the main source of Ca^{2+} entry occurring during ischaemia is not through ionotropic glutamate receptors but through ASIC1a channels, as ASIC1a blockade is a more efficient way to limit ischaemic damage than the use of glutamate antagonists (Xiong et al. 2004). Thus, apart from its acid-sensing function in various tissues,

ASIC1a activation may be a major factor in the biological events that lead to neuronal damage. Therefore, the search for drugs or factors regulating ASIC1a function has become potentially therapeutically important.

The mammalian ASICs are members of a channel superfamily involved in mechano-sensation in nematode worms (MEC-4 and MEC-10 mutants) and are highly expressed in sensory neurons (Waldmann and Lazdunski 1998). There are four identified genes encoding ASIC subunits, ASIC1–4, with two alternative splice variants of ASIC1 and -2 taking the number of known subunits to six. Although protons are the only confirmed activator of ASICs, the homology between ASICs and MEC channels, coupled to high levels of expression of ASICs in sensory neurons, has led to the hypothesis that these channels function in mechano-transduction (Lewin and Moshourab 2004). ASIC subunits are found at appropriate sites to contribute to mechano-sensation. However, studies show staining for ASIC subunits along the length of the fibres, not a specific enrichment at the terminals. Expression in sensory terminals is necessary for a role in the transduction of either acidic or mechanical stimuli. The finding that the majority of Aβ -fibre sensory terminals are immunoreactive for ASICs is at odds with the long-known observation that low-threshold mechano-receptors are not activated by low pH (see Lewin and Moshourab 2004). Thus, Welsh et al. (2001) have proposed that ASICs may exist, like MEC-4 and MEC-10, in a multiprotein transduction complex that through an unknown mechanism masks the proton sensitivity of these channels (Fig. 5).

Using the neuronal cell body as a model of the sensory terminal, mechanically activated currents in DRG neurons have been characterized (Drew et al. 2004). Neurons from ASIC2- and ASIC3-null mutants were compared with wild-type controls. Neuronal subpopulations generated distinct responses to mechanical stimulation consistent with their predicted in vivo phenotypes. In

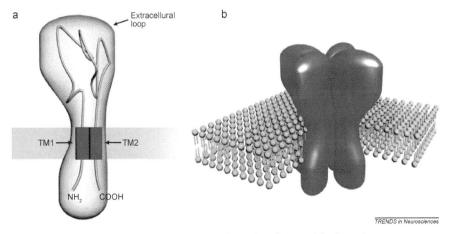

Fig. 5a, b Schematic structure of ASIC channels. (Taken from Krishtal 2003)

particular, there was a striking relationship between action potential duration and mechano-sensitivity as has been observed in vivo. Putative low-threshold mechano-receptors exhibited rapidly adapting mechanically activated currents. Conversely, when nociceptors responded they displayed slowly or intermediately adapting currents that were smaller in amplitude than responses of low-threshold mechano-receptor neurons. No differences in current amplitude or kinetics were found between ASIC2 and/or ASIC3-null mutants and controls. These findings are consistent with another ion channel type being important in DRG mechano-transduction. Lazdunski's group also investigated the effect of ASIC2 gene knock-out in mice on hearing, cutaneous mechano-sensation and visceral mechano-nociception. Their data also failed to support a role of ASIC2 in mechano-sensation (Roza et al. 2004).

Despite the mounting evidence that ASICs are not important for mechano-sensation, and the discovery of a number of unexpected functions for these channels, it does appear that in some pain states, for example in visceral pain or in ischaemic heart pain, ASICs may play an important role. However, given their multiple functions, they may not be ideal analgesic drug targets.

10
HERG Channels

HERG channels are heart channels related to the *Drosophila* ether-a-go-go potassium channels. A structurally diverse range of drugs seems to act as blockers of this channel, resulting in prolongation of cardiac muscle repolarisation which manifests itself with a prolonged Q-T interval. Premature action potential generation can result in ventricular tachyarrhythmias (torsades de pointes) which may cause lethal ventricular fibrillation.

Sanguinetti et al. (2005) used site-directed mutagenesis to identify several residues of the HERG channel that comprise a common drug binding site. A number of residues located in the S6 domain (Tyr652, Phe656) and the base of the pore helix (Thr623, Ser624, Val625) were important sites of interaction for structurally different drugs. The reason why so many drugs seem to block HERG channels is related to the external atrium of the channel, and so early-stage screening to weed out compounds that interact with and block HERG channels is an essential part of the drug development process, and has halted the progress of many compounds that appeared to be promising ion channel blockers.

11
Target Validation of Ion Channels Using Transgenic Mice

Many ion channels have been implicated in pain pathways because of, for example, their tissue-specific pattern of expression. In the absence of specific antagonists, genetic approaches to target validation may be useful. Dissecting the role of potential targets in regulating pain thresholds has often relied upon the use of antisense oligonucleotides, the specific down-regulation of mRNA using siRNA and the generation of mice with targeted mutations.

Each of these approaches has advantages and disadvantages. Antisense technology is cheap, but specificity is a problem, as high concentrations of oligonucleotide may have some cellular toxicity, and may also target structurally related transcripts. SiRNA technology is still being developed, but has already revolutionised C. elegans genetics, where the specificity of siRNA action and the catalytic nature of RNA degradation mean that very low concentrations of dsRNA can be employed. SiRNA is effective in vitro and in vivo in primary sensory neurons, where a 21-bp complementary dsRNA can be used to specifically degrade cognate RNA sequences through the formation of a complex with ribonucleases. SiRNA acts transiently and catalytically and may not lead to long-lived RNA degradation (part of its attraction), but for animal models where neuropathic pain is modelled over a period of weeks this is a major difficulty. Null mutants do not share this problem, but the problems of developmental compensatory mechanisms and death during development have often provided obstacles to interpretation of phenotype. It is also desirable to generate mice where tissue-specific deletions can be carried out, and ideally postnatal activation of Cre recombinase should be possible.

Thanks to the work of Sauer and collaborators (Le and Sauer 1999), who have exploited the recombinase activity of a bacteriophage enzyme Cre to delete DNA sequences that are flanked by lox-P sites recognized by this enzyme, it has proved possible to generate tissue-specific null mutants This powerful technology is likely to be applied increasingly over the next few years, and together with siRNA promises to speed up target validation strategies in animal models of neuropathic pain. DRG-specific Cre-recombinase mice have been made, and an increasing number of floxed target genes are also now available for tissue-specific gene deletion studies.

12
Summary

We now have a clear idea of the vast repertoire of signalling molecules that are activated by tissue-damaging stimuli, and the voltage-gated channels that are responsible for electrical signalling and, eventually, the perception of pain. However, splice variants, post-translational modifications and altered properties due to association with regulatory molecules all may confound the drug development process that usually relies on cell-based high-throughput screening and tests in animal models. There are nevertheless good reasons for optimism, as the first set of new analgesic drugs acting on individual channels defined over the past decade (for example $Na_V1.8$ and P2X3 antagonists) start to progress through the drug development pipeline, and genetic studies in both mice and man narrow down the potentially significant channels to validated and effective targets.

Acknowledgements We thank our colleagues for helpful insights and suggestions. Our work is supported by the MRC, the BBSRC and the Wellcome Trust.

References

Abdi S, Lee DH, Chung JM (1998) The anti-allodynic effects of amitriptyline, gabapentin, and lidocaine in a rat model of neuropathic pain. Anesth Analg 87:1360–1366

Abe M, Kurihara T, Han W, Shinomiya K, Tanabe T (2002) Changes in expression of voltage-dependent ion channel subunits in dorsal root ganglia of rats with radicular injury and pain. Spine 27:1517–1524

Akopian AN, Sivilotti L, Wood JN (1996) A tetrodotoxin-resistant voltage-gated sodium channel expressed by sensory neurons. Nature 379:257–262

Akopian AN, Souslova V, England S, Okuse K, McMahon S, Boyce S, Dickenson AH, Wood JN (1999) The TTX-R sodium channel SNS has a specialized function in pain pathways. Nat Neurosci 2:541–5489

Albrieux M, Platel JC, Dupuis A, Villaz M, Moody WJ (2004) Early expression of sodium channel transcripts and sodium current by cajal-retzius cells in the preplate of the embryonic mouse neocortex. J Neurosci 24:1719–1725

Altier C, Zamponi GW (2004) Targeting Ca^{2+} channels to treat pain: T-type versus N-type. Trends Pharmacol Sci 25:465–470

Baker MD, Chandra SY, Ding Y, Waxman SG, Wood JN (2003) GTP-induced tetrodotoxin-resistant Na+ current regulates excitability in mouse and rat small diameter sensory neurones. J Physiol 548:373–382

Baron SP, Hidayetoglu DL, Offord JD, Ti-Zhi S (2005) United States Patent Application 20050144659 Warner-Lambert Company, 2800 Plymouth Rd, Ann Arbor, MI 48105 US

Beckh S, Noda M, Lubbert H, Numa S (1989) Differential regulation of three sodium channel messenger RNAs in the rat central nervous system during development. EMBO J 8: 3611–3616

Bell TJ, Thaler C, Castiglioni AJ, Helton TD, Lipscombe D (2004) Cell-specific alternative splicing increases calcium channel current density in the pain pathway. Neuron 41: 127–138

Bennett GJ, Xie YK (1988) A peripheral mononeuropathy in rat that produces disorders of pain sensation like those seen in man. Pain 33:87–107

Bhattacharjee A, Kaczmarek LK (2005) For K+ channels, Na+ is the new Ca^{2+}. Trends Neurosci 28:422–428

Black JA, Cummins TR, Yoshimura N, de Groat WC, Waxman SG (2003) Tetrodotoxin-resistant sodium channels Na(v)1.8/SNS and Na(v)1.9/NaN in afferent neurons innervating urinary bladder in control and spinal cord injured rats. Brain Res 963:132–138

Boucher TJ, Okuse K, Bennett DL, Munson JB, Wood JN, McMahon SB (2000) Potent analgesic effects of GDNF in neuropathic pain states. Science 290:124–127

Bourinet E, Zamponi GW (2005) Voltage gated calcium channels as targets for analgesics. Curr Top Med Chem 5:539–546

Bourinet E, Alloui A, Monteil A, Barrere C, Couette B, Poirot O, Pages A, McRory J, Snutch TP, Eschalier A, Nargeot J (2005) Silencing of the $Ca_v3.2$ T-type calcium channel gene in sensory neurons demonstrates its major role in nociception. EMBO J 24:315–324

Brose WG, Gutlove DP, Luther RR, Bowersox SS, McGuire D (1997) Use of intrathecal SNX-111, a novel, N-type, voltage-sensitive, calcium channel blocker, in the management of intractable brachial plexus avulsion pain. Clin J Pain 13:256–259

Buchner DA, Trudeau M, Meisler MH (2003) SCNM1, a putative RNA splicing factor that modifies disease severity in mice. Science 301:967–969

Calderone V, Testai L, Martinotti E, Del Tacca M, Breschi MC (2005) Drug-induced block of cardiac HERG potassium channels and development of torsade de pointes arrhythmias: the case of antipsychotics. J Pharm Pharmacol 57:151–161

Chahine M, Ziane R, Vijayaragavan K, Okamura Y (2005) Regulation of Na v channels in sensory neurons. Trends Pharmacol Sci 26:496–502

Chaplan SR, Guo HQ, Lee DH, Luo L, Liu C, Kuei C, Velumian AA, Butler MP, Brown SM, Dubin AE (2003) Neuronal hyperpolarization-activated pacemaker channels drive neuropathic pain. J Neurosci 23:1169–1178

Chen CC, Zimmer A, Sun WH, Hall J, Brownstein MJ, Zimmer A (2002) A role for ASIC3 in the modulation of high-intensity pain stimuli. Proc Natl Acad Sci U S A 99:8992–8997

Costigan M, Befort K, Karchewski L, Griffin RS, D'Urso D, Allchorne A, Sitarski J, Mannion JW, Pratt RE, Woolf CJ (2002) Replicate high-density rat genome oligonucleotide microarrays reveal hundreds of regulated genes in the dorsal root ganglion after peripheral nerve injury. BMC Neurosci 3:16

Cummins TR, Waxman SG (1997) Down-regulation of tetrodotoxin-resistant sodium currents and up-regulation of a rapidly repriming tetrodotoxin-sensitive sodium current in small spinal sensory neurons following nerve injury. J Neurosci 17:3503–3514

Cummins TR, Dib-Hajj SD, Black JA, Akopian AN, Wood JN, Waxman SG (1999) A novel persistent tetrodotoxin-resistant sodium current in SNS-null and wild-type small primary sensory neurons. J Neurosci 19:RC43

Cummins TR, Black JA, Dib-Hajj SD, Waxman SG (2000) GDNF up-regulates expression of functional SNS and NaN sodium channels and their currents in axotomized DRG neurons. J Neurosci 20:8754–8761

Cummins TR, Aglieco F, Renganathan M, Herzog RI, Dib-Hajj SD, Waxman SG (2001) $Na_v1.3$ sodium channels: rapid repriming and slow closed-state inactivation display quantitative differences following expression in a mammalian cell line and in spinal sensory neurons. J Neurosci 21:5952–5961

Decosterd I, Woolf CJ (2000) Spared nerve injury: an animal model of persistent peripheral neuropathic pain. Pain 87:149–158

Dib-Hajj S, Black JA, Felts P, Waxman SG (1996) Down-regulation of transcripts for Na channel SNS in spinal sensory neurons following axotomy. Proc Natl Acad Sci U S A 93:14950–14954

Dib-Hajj S, Black JA, Cummins TR, Waxman SG (2002) NaN/$Na_v1.9$: a sodium channel with unique properties. Trends Neurosci 25:253–259

Dib-Hajj SD, Tyrrell L, Black JA, Waxman SG (1998) NaN, a novel voltage-gated Na channel preferentially expressed in peripheral sensory neurons and down-regulated following axotomy. Proc Natl Acad Sci U S A 95:8963–8968

Dib-Hajj SD, Rush AM, Cummins TR, Hisama FM, Novella S, Tyrrell L, Marshall L, Waxman SG (2005) Gain-of-function mutation in $Na_v1.7$ in familial erythromelalgia induces bursting of sensory neurons. Brain 128:1847–1854

Djouhri L, Fang X, Okuse K, Wood JN, Berry CM, Lawson S (2003) The TTX-resistant sodium channel $Na_V1.8$: expression and correlation with membrane properties in rat nociceptive primary afferent neurons. J Physiol 550:739–752

Drenth JP, te Morsche RH, Guillet G, Taieb A, Kirby RL, Jansen JB (2005) SCN9A mutations define primary erythermalgia as a neuropathic disorder of voltage gated sodium channels. J Invest Dermatol 124:1333–1338

Erichsen HK, Blackburn-Munro G (2002) Pharmacological characterisation of the spared nerve injury model of neuropathic pain. Pain 98:151–161

Ettaiche M, Guy N, Hofman P, Lazdunski M, Waldmann R (2004) Acid-sensing ion channel 2 is important for retinal function and protects against light-induced retinal degeneration. J Neurosci 24:1005–1012

Fang X, Djouhri L, Black JA, Dib-Hajj SD, Waxman SG, Lawson SN (2002) The presence and role of the TTX resistant sodium channel $Na_V1.9$ (NaN) in nociceptive primary afferent neurons. J Neurosci 22:7425–7433

Felix R, Gurnett CA, De Waard M, Campbell KP (1997) Dissection of functional domains of the voltage-dependent Ca^{2+} channel alpha2delta subunit. J Neurosci 17:6884–6891

Felts PA, Yokoyama S, Dib-Hajj S, Black JA, Waxman SG (1997) Sodium channel alpha-subunit mRNAs I, II, III, NaG, Na6 and hNE (PN1): different expression patterns in developing rat nervous system. Brain Res Mol Brain Res 45:71–82

Fozzard HA, Lee PJ, Lipkind GM (2005) Mechanism of local anesthetic drug action on voltage-gated sodium channels. Curr Pharm Des 11:2671–2686

Fukuoka T, Tokunaga A, Tachibana T, Dai Y, Yamanaka H, Noguchi K (2002) VR1, but not P2X(3), increases in the spared L4 DRG in rats with L5 spinal nerve ligation. Pain 99:111–120

Gee NS, Brown JP, Dissanayake VU, Offord J, Thurlow R, Woodruff GN (1996) The novel anticonvulsant drug, gabapentin (Neurontin), binds to the alpha2delta subunit of a calcium channel. J Biol Chem 271:5768–5776

Goldin AL (2001) Resurgence of sodium channel research. Annu Rev Physiol 63:871–894

Gong HC, Hang J, Kohler W, Li L, Su TZ (2001) Tissue-specific expression and gabapentin-binding properties of calcium channel alpha2delta subunit subtypes. J Membr Biol 184:35–43

Hains BC, Klein JP, Saab CY, Craner MJ, Black JA, Waxman SG (2003) Upregulation of sodium channel $Na_V1.3$ and functional involvement in neuronal hyperexcitability associated with central neuropathic pain after spinal cord injury. J Neurosci 23:8881–8892

Hanrahan CJ, Palladino MJ, Ganetzky B, Reenan RA (2000) RNA editing of the *Drosophila para* Na(+) channel transcript. Evolutionary conservation and developmental regulation. Genetics 155:1149–1160

Hiyama TY, Watanabe E, Ono K, Inenaga K, Tamkun MM, Yoshida S, Noda M (2002) Na(x) channel involved in CNS sodium-level sensing. Nat Neurosci 5:511–512

Hong S, Morrow TJ, Paulson PE, Isom LL, Wiley JW (2004) Early painful diabetic neuropathy is associated with differential changes in tetrodotoxin-sensitive and -resistant sodium channels in dorsal root ganglion neurons in the rat. J Biol Chem 279:29341–29350

Hudson LJ, Bevan S, Wotherspoon G, Gentry C, Fox A, Winter J (2001) VR1 protein expression increases in undamaged DRG neurons after partial nerve injury. Eur J Neurosci 13:2105–2114

Immke DC, McCleskey EW (2003) Protons open acid-sensing ion channels by catalyzing relief of Ca^{2+} blockade. Neuron 37:75–84

Ishikawa K, Tanaka M, Black JA, Waxman SG (1999) Changes in expression of voltage-gated potassium channels in dorsal root ganglion neurons following axotomy. Muscle Nerve 22:502–507

Kerr BJ, Souslova V, McMahon SB, Wood JN (2001) A role for the TTX-resistant sodium channel Na$_v$ 1.8 in NGF-induced hyperalgesia, but not neuropathic pain. Neuroreport 12:3077–3080

Kerr NC, Holmes FE, Wynick D (2004) Novel isoforms of the sodium channels Na$_v$1.8 and Na$_v$1.5 are produced by a conserved mechanism in mouse and rat. J Biol Chem 279:24826–24833

Khasar SG, Gold MS, Levine JD (1998) A tetrodotoxin-resistant sodium current mediates inflammatory pain in the rat. Neurosci Lett 256:17–20

Kim CH, Oh Y, Chung JM, Chung K (2001) The changes in expression of three subtypes of TTX sensitive sodium channels in sensory neurons after spinal nerve ligation. Brain Res Mol Brain Res 95:153–161

Kim D (2005) Physiology and pharmacology of two-pore domain potassium channels. Curr Pharm Des 11:2717–2736

Kim DS, Choi JO, Rim HD, Cho HJ (2002) Downregulation of voltage-gated potassium channel alpha gene expression in dorsal root ganglia following chronic constriction injury of the rat sciatic nerve. Brain Res Mol Brain Res 105:146–152

Kim KJ, Yoon YW, Chung JM (1997) Comparison of three rodent neuropathic pain models. Exp Brain Res 113:200

Kraner SD, Chong JA, Tsay HJ, Mandel G (1992) Silencing the type II sodium channel gene: a model for neural-specific gene regulation. Neuron 9:37–44

Krishtal O (2003) The ASICs: signaling molecules? Modulators? Trends Neurosci 26:477–483

Kuwabara T, Hsieh J, Nakashima K, Taira K, Gage FH (2004) A small modulatory dsRNA specifies the fate of adult neural stem cells. Cell 116:779–793

Lai J, Gold MS, Kim CS, Bian D, Ossipov MH, Hunter JC, Porreca F (2002) Inhibition of neuropathic pain by decreased expression of the tetrodotoxin-resistant sodium channel, Na$_v$1.8. Pain 95:143–152

Lalo UV, Pankratov YV, Arndts D, Krishtal OA (2001) Omega-conotoxin GVIA potently inhibits the currents mediated by P2X receptors in rat DRG neurons. Brain Res Bull 54:507–512

Le Y, Sauer B (2001) Conditional gene knockout using Cre recombinase. Mol Biotechnol 17:269–275

Leffler A, Cummins TR, Dib-Hajj SD, Hormuzdiar WN, Black JA, Waxman SG (2002) GDNF and NGF reverse changes in repriming of TTX-sensitive Na(+) currents following axotomy of dorsal root ganglion neurons. J Neurophysiol 88:650–658

Lewin GR, Moshourab R (2004) Mechanosensation and pain. J Neurobiol 61:30–44

Liu Z, Song W, Dong K (2004) Persistent tetrodotoxin-sensitive sodium current resulting from U-to-C RNA editing of an insect sodium channel. Proc Natl Acad Sci U S A 101:11862–11867

Luo ZD, Calcutt NA, Higuera ES, Valder CR, Song YH, Svensson CI, Myers RR (2002) Injury type-specific calcium channel alpha 2 delta-1 subunit up-regulation in rat neuropathic pain models correlates with antiallodynic effects of gabapentin. J Pharmacol Exp Ther 303:1199–1205

Malhotra JD, Kazen-Gillespie K, Hortsch M, Isom LL (2000) Sodium channel beta subunits mediate homophilic cell adhesion and recruit ankyrin to points of cell-cell contact. J Biol Chem 275:11383–11388

Malik-Hall M, Wood JN, Okuse K (2003) Voltage-gated sodium channels. In: Moss SJ, Henley J (eds) Receptor and ion channel trafficking. Oxford University Press, Oxford, pp 3–28

Mogil JS, Wilson SG, Bon K, Lee SE, Chung K, Raber P, Pieper JO, Hain HS, Belknap JK, Hubert L, Elmer GI, Chung JM, Devor M (1999) Heritability of nociception I: responses of 11 inbred mouse strains on 12 measures of nociception. Pain 80:67–82

Montell C (2005) The TRP superfamily of cation channels. Sci STKE 272:re3

Nassar MA, Levato A, Stirling LC, Wood JN (2005) Neuropathic pain develops normally in mice lacking both $Na_v1.7$ and $N_{av}1.8$. Mol Pain 1:24

Nicholson B (2000) Gabapentin use in neuropathic pain syndromes. Acta Neurol Scand 101:359–371

Oberwinkler J, Lis A, Giehl KM, Flockerzi V, Philipp SE (2005) Alternative splicing switches the divalent cation selectivity of TRPM3 channels. J Biol Chem 280:22540–22548

Okuse K, Malik-Hall M, Baker MD, Poon WYL, Kong H, Chao MV, Wood JN (2002) Annexin II light chain regulates sensory neuron-specific sodium channel expression. Nature 47:653–656

Page AJ, Brierley SM, Martin CM, Martinez-Salgado C, Wemmie JA, Brennan TJ, Symonds E, Omari T, Lewin GR, Welsh MJ, Blackshaw LA (2004) The ion channel ASIC1 contributes to visceral but not cutaneous mechanoreceptor function. Gastroenterology 127:1739–1747

Passmore GM, Selyanko AA, Mistry M, Al-Qatari M, Marsh SJ, Matthews EA, Dickenson AH, Brown TA, Burbidge SA, Main M, Brown DA (2003) KCNQ/M currents in sensory neurons: significance for pain therapy. J Neurosci 23:7227–7236

Paukert M, Sidi S, Russell C, Siba M, Wilson SW, Nicolson T, Grunder S (2004) A family of acid-sensing ion channels from the zebrafish: widespread expression in the central nervous system suggests a conserved role in neuronal communication. J Biol Chem 279:18783–18791

Peng BG, Ahmad S, Chen S, Chen P, Price MP, Lin X (2004) Acid-sensing ion channel 2 contributes a major component to acid-evoked excitatory responses in spiral ganglion neurons and plays a role in noise susceptibility of mice. J Neurosci 24:10167–10175

Perez-Reyes E (2003) Molecular physiology of low-voltage-activated t-type calcium channels. Physiol Rev 83:117–161

Price MP, McIlwrath SL, Xie J, Cheng C, Qiao J, Tarr DE, Sluka KA, Brennan TJ, Lewin GR, Welsh MJ (2001) The DRASIC cation channel contributes to the detection of cutaneous touch and acid stimuli in mice. Neuron 32:1071–1083

Rasband MN, Park EW, Vanderah TW, Lai J, Porreca F, Trimmer JS (2001) Distinct potassium channels on pain-sensing neurons. Proc Natl Acad Sci U S A 98:13373–13378

Rashid MH, Inoue M, Kondo S, Kawashima T, Bakoshi S, Ueda H (2003) Novel expression of vanilloid receptor 1 on capsaicin-insensitive fibers accounts for the analgesic effect of capsaicin cream in neuropathic pain. J Pharmacol Exp Ther 304:940–948

Reenan RA, Hanrahan CJ, Barry G (2000) The mle(napts) RNA helicase mutation in Drosophila results in a splicing catastrophe of the para Na+ channel transcript in a region of RNA editing. Neuron 25:139–149

Renganathan M, Cummins TR, Waxman SG (2001) Contribution of $Na_v1.8$ sodium channels to action potential electrogenesis in DRG neurons. J Neurophysiol 86:629–640

Rowbotham MC, Twilling L, Davies P, Taylor K, Mohr D, Reisner L (2003) Oral opioid therapy for chronic peripheral and central neuropathic pain. N Engl J Med 348:1223–1232

Roza C, Laird JM, Souslova V, Wood JN, Cervero F (2003) The tetrodotoxin-resistant Na+ channel $Na_v1.8$ is essential for the expression of spontaneous activity in damaged sensory axons of mice. J Physiol 550:921–926

Saegusa H, Kurihara T, Zong S, Kazuno A, Matsuda Y, Nonaka T, Han W, Toriyama H, Tanabe T (2001) Suppression of inflammatory and neuropathic pain symptoms in mice lacking the N-type Ca^{2+} channel. EMBO J 20:2349–2356

Saegusa H, Matsuda Y, Tanabe T (2002) Effects of ablation of N- and R-type Ca(2+) channels on pain transmission. Neurosci Res 43:1–7

Sanguinetti MC, Chen J, Fernandez D, Kamiya K, Mitcheson J, Sanchez-Chapula JA (2005) Physicochemical basis for binding and voltage-dependent block of hERG channels by structurally diverse drugs. Novartis Found Symp 266:159–166

Schafers M, Sorkin LS, Geis C, Shubayev VI (2003) Spinal nerve ligation induces transient upregulation of tumor necrosis factor receptors 1 and 2 in injured and adjacent uninjured dorsal root ganglia in the rat. Neurosci Lett 347:179–182

Schoenherr CJ, Anderson DJ (1995) The neuron-restrictive silencer factor (NRSF): a coordinate repressor of multiple neuron-specific genes. Science 267:1360–1363

Seltzer Z, Dubner R, Shir Y (1990) A novel behavioral model of neuropathic pain disorders produced in rats by partial sciatic nerve injury. Pain 43:205–218

Shah BS, Gonzalez MI, Bramwell S, Pinnock RD, Lee K, Dixon AK (2001) Beta3, a novel auxiliary subunit for the voltage gated sodium channel is upregulated in sensory neurones following streptozocin induced diabetic neuropathy in rat. Neurosci Lett 309:1–4

Sindrup SH, Jensen TS (1999) Efficacy of pharmacological treatments of neuropathic pain: an update and effect related to mechanism of drug action. Pain 83:389–400

Sleeper AA, Cummins TR, Dib-Hajj SD, Hormuzdiar W, Tyrrell L, Waxman SG, Black JA (2000) Changes in expression of two tetrodotoxin-resistant sodium channels and their currents in dorsal root ganglion neurons after sciatic nerve injury but not rhizotomy. J Neurosci 20:7279–7289

Strichartz GR, Zhou Z, Sinnott C, Khodorova A (2002) Therapeutic concentrations of local anaesthetics unveil the potential role of sodium channels in neuropathic pain. Novartis Found Symp 241:189–201

Suzuki M, Mizuno A, Kodaira K, Imai M (2003) Impaired pressure sensation in mice lacking TRPV4. J Biol Chem 278:22664–22668

Tan J, Liu Z, Nomura Y, Goldin AL, Dong K (2002) Alternative splicing of an insect sodium channel gene generates pharmacologically distinct sodium channels. J Neurosci 22:5300–5309

Ugawa S, Ueda T, Ishida Y, Nishigaki M, Shibata Y, Shimada S (2002) Amiloride-blockable acid-sensing ion channels are leading acid sensors expressed in human nociceptors. J Clin Invest 110:1185–1190

Voilley N, de Weille J, Mamet J, Lazdunski M (2001) Nonsteroid anti-inflammatory drugs inhibit both the activity and the inflammation-induced expression of acid-sensing ion channels in nociceptors. J Neurosci 21:8026–8033

Waldmann R, Lazdunski M (1998) H(+)-gated cation channels: neuronal acid sensors in the NaC/DEG family of ion channels. Curr Opin Neurobiol 8:418–424

Wang H, Sun H, Della PK, Benz R, Xu J, Gerhold D, Holder D, Koblan K (2002) Chronic neuropathic pain is accompanied by global changes in gene expression and shares pathobiology with neurodegenerative diseases. Neuroscience 114:529–546

Wang YX, Pettus M, Gao D, Phillips C, Scott Bowersox S (2000) Effects of intrathecal administration of ziconotide, a selective neuronal N-type calcium channel blocker, on mechanical allodynia and heat hyperalgesia in a rat model of postoperative pain. Pain 84:151–158

Waxman SG, Kocsis JK, Black JA (1994) Type III sodium channel mRNA is expressed in embryonic but not adult spinal sensory neurons, and is re-expressed following axotomy. J Neurophysiol 72:466–471

Waxman SG, Cummins TR, Dib-Hajj S, Fjell J, Black JA (1999) Sodium channels, excitability of primary sensory neurons, and the molecular basis of pain. Muscle Nerve 22:1177–1187

Wemmie JA, Chen J, Askwith CC, Hruska-Hageman AM, Price MP, Nolan BC, Yoder PG, Lamani E, Hoshi T, Freeman JH Jr, Welsh MJ (2002) The acid-activated ion channel ASIC contributes to synaptic plasticity, learning, and memory. Neuron 34:463–477

Wemmie JA, Askwith CC, Lamani E, Cassell MD, Freeman JH Jr, Welsh MJ (2003) Acid-sensing ion channel 1 is localized in brain regions with high synaptic density and contributes to fear conditioning. J Neurosci 23:5496–5502

Wemmie JA, Coryell MW, Askwith CC, Lamani E, Leonard AS, Sigmund CD, Welsh MJ (2004) Overexpression of acid-sensing ion channel 1a in transgenic mice increases acquired fear-related behavior. Proc Natl Acad Sci U S A 101:3621–3626

Xiao HS, Huang QH, Zhang FX, Bao L, Lu YJ, Guo C, Yang L, Huang WJ, Fu G, Xu SH, Cheng XP, Yan Q, Zhu ZD, Zhang X, Chen Z, Han ZG, Zhang X (2002) Identification of gene expression profile of dorsal root ganglion in the rat peripheral axotomy model of neuropathic pain. Proc Natl Acad Sci U S A 99:8360–8365

Xie J, Jan C, Stoilov P, Park J, Black DL (2005) A consensus CaMK IV-responsive RNA sequence mediates regulation of alternative exons in neurons. RNA 11:1825–1834

Xiong ZG, Chu XP, Simon RP (2006) Ca^{2+}-permeable acid-sensing ion channels and ischemic brain injury. J Membr Biol 209:59–68

Yermolaieva O, Leonard AS, Schnizler MK, Abboud FM, Welsh MJ (2004) Extracellular acidosis increases neuronal cell calcium by activating acid-sensing ion channel 1a. Proc Natl Acad Sci U S A 101:6752–6757

Yoon YW, Lee DH, Lee BH, Chung K, Chung JM (1999) Different strains and substrains of rats show different levels of neuropathic pain behaviors. Exp Brain Res 129:167–171

Yu FH, Catterall WA (2004) The VGL-chanome: a protein superfamily specialized for electrical signaling and ionic homeostasis. Sci STKE 253:re15

Yu FH, Yarov-Yarovoy V, Gutman GA, Catterall WA (2005) Overview of molecular relationships in the voltage-gated ion channel superfamily. Pharmacol Rev 57:387–395

HEP (2006) 177:359–389
© Springer-Verlag Berlin Heidelberg 2006

Protein Kinases as Potential Targets for the Treatment of Pathological Pain

R.-R. Ji[1] (✉) · Y. Kawasaki[1] · Z.-Y. Zhuang[1] · Y.-R. Wen[1] · Y.-Q. Zhang[2]

[1]Department of Anesthesiology, Brigham and Women's Hospital, Harvard Medical School, 75 Francis Street, MRB 604, Boston MA, 02115, USA
rrji@zeus.bwh.harvard.edu

[2]Institute of Neurobiology, Fudan University, 220 Han Dan Road, Shanghai 200433, China

1	Pathological Pain and Neural Plasticity	360
1.1	Physiological and Pathological Pain	360
1.2	Neural Plasticity: Peripheral and Central Sensitization	361
2	Protein Kinases and Pain Sensitization	362
2.1	Serine-Threonine Protein Kinases	364
2.2	Tyrosine Kinases	366
2.3	Mitogen-Activated Proteins Kinases (MAPKs)	367
2.3.1	ERK/MAPK (p44/42 MAPK) Pathway	367
2.3.2	p38 MAPK Pathway	370
2.3.3	JNK/MAPK Pathway	372
3	Mechanisms of Pain Sensitization by Protein Kinases	372
3.1	Peripheral Mechanisms	372
3.1.1	Induction of Peripheral Sensitization: Posttranslational Regulation	372
3.1.2	Maintenance of Peripheral Sensitization: Transcriptional and Translational Regulation	373
3.2	Spinal Mechanisms	374
3.2.1	Induction of Central Sensitization: Posttranslational Regulation	374
3.2.2	Maintenance of Central Sensitization: Transcriptional Regulation	375
3.3	Brain Mechanisms	377
3.4	Glial and Immuno–Mechanisms	378
4	Protein Kinase Inhibitors in Clinical Studies	380
5	Summary	381
References		382

Abstract Pathological pain or clinical pain refers to tissue injury-induced inflammatory pain and nerve injury-induced neuropathic pain and is often chronic. Pathological pain is an expression of neural plasticity that occurs both in the peripheral nervous system (e.g., primary sensory nociceptors), termed peripheral sensitization, and in the central nervous system (e.g., dorsal horn and brain neurons), termed central sensitization. Our insufficient understanding of mechanisms underlying the induction and maintenance of injury-induced neuronal plasticity hinders successful treatment for pathological pain.

The human genome encodes 518 protein kinases, representing one of the largest protein families. There is growing interest in developing protein kinase inhibitors for the treatment of a number of diseases. Although protein kinases were not favored as targets for analgesics, studies in the last decade have demonstrated important roles of these kinases in regulating neuronal plasticity and pain sensitization. Multiple protein kinases have been implicated in peripheral and central sensitization following intense noxious stimuli and injuries. In particular, mitogen-activated protein kinases (MAPKs), consisting of extracellular signal-regulated kinase (ERK), p38, and c-Jun N-terminal kinase (JNK), are downstream to many kinases and are activated in primary sensory and dorsal horn neurons by nociceptive activity, growth factors and inflammatory mediators, contributing to the induction and maintenance of pain sensitization via posttranslational, translational, and transcriptional regulation. MAPKs are also activated in spinal glial cells (microglia and astrocytes) after injuries, leading to the synthesis of inflammatory mediators/neuroactive substances that act on nociceptive neurons, enhancing and prolonging pain sensitization. Inhibition of multiple kinases has been shown to attenuate inflammatory and neuropathic pain in different animal models. Development of specific inhibitors for protein kinases to target neurons and glial cells will shed light on the development of new therapies for debilitating chronic pain.

Keywords Neural plasticity · MAP kinases · Phosphorylation · Primary sensory neurons · Spinal cord · Glia

1
Pathological Pain and Neural Plasticity

1.1
Physiological and Pathological Pain

During evolution, living organisms develop a specialized apparatus called a nociceptor, detecting harmful stimuli from the environment. Intense noxious stimulation of high-threshold nociceptors will elicit a pain sensation. Nociception is initiated from the action potential generated in the peripheral nociceptor terminal, conducted via thin unmyelinated C fibers and myelinated Aδ fibers to the spinal cord dorsal horn, thalamus, and cortex. This acute pain sensation in normal conditions is called physiological pain, and has a protective role that warns of potential tissue damage in response to a noxious stimulus. Many pain transduction molecules have recently been identified, including the thermal receptors TRVP1 (transient receptor potential ion channel family; also called vanilloid receptor 1, VR1), TRPV2, TRPM8, and TRPA1, the mechanoreceptors DEG (degenerin), DRASIC (dorsal root acid-sensing ion channel), and TREK-1 (TWIK-related K^+ channel-1), and the chemical receptor P2X3 (Scholz and Woolf 2002).

In contrast to physiological pain, pathological pain or clinical pain is caused by tissue and nerve injuries. Pathological pain is usually chronic and mainly divided into inflammatory pain and neuropathic pain. Inflammatory pain is a pain related to peripheral tissue damage/inflammation (e.g., arthritis pain). In animal models this pain is usually produced by injection of irritative substances such as formalin, carrageenan, or complete Freund's adjuvant (CFA) into a hindpaw or joint of rats and mice (Stein et al. 1988), with a duration ranging from hours to days and weeks. Neuropathic pain is a pain caused by damage or dysfunction of the peripheral nervous system (PNS) and CNS. In animal models neuropathic pain is often induced by a partial lesion of the sciatic nerve and its branches in rats and mice, and this pain can last for many weeks to several months (Bennett and Xie 1988; Kim and Chung 1992; Decosterd and Woolf 2000). In addition, animal models have been developed for cancer pain and postoperative pain (incisional pain), which share some features with inflammatory and neuropathic pain but also have their distinct characteristics (Brennan et al. 1996; Mantyh et al. 2002). Pathological pain is typically characterized by hyperalgesia (increased responsiveness to noxious stimuli) and allodynia (painful responses to normally innocuous stimuli), as well as by spontaneous pain. Pain hypersensitivity is not only produced in the injured tissue or territory (innervated by the injured nerve), but also spread to the adjacent noninjured regions or the extra-territory.

1.2
Neural Plasticity: Peripheral and Central Sensitization

Pathological pain is caused by altered sensitivity in both the PNS and CNS. It is an expression of neural plasticity, an adaptation of nervous system in response to external stimuli. This plasticity also occurs in other parts of the nervous system during learning and memory and drug addiction (Ji et al. 2003).

During tissue injury and inflammation, inflammatory mediators (IFMs) such as prostaglandin E_2 (PGE$_2$), 5-HT, bradykinin, ATP, protons, nerve growth factor (NGF), lipids, and proinflammatory cytokines interleukin-1β (IL-1β) and tumor necrosis factor-α (TNF-α) are released from inflammatory cells, nerve terminals, and surrounding non-neural tissues, or from damaged axons and their enclosing Schwann cells. The soma and axons of primary sensory neurons express receptors for these IFMs, and activation of the receptors leads to the activation of multiple intracellular signaling pathways, increasing the sensitivity and excitability of nociceptors. A sensitivity increase in the PNS (e.g., primary sensory neurons) is called peripheral sensitization. Various types of ion channels such as TRPV1, TRPV2, TRPM8, DEG, P2X3, acid-sensitive channel (ASIC), and tetrodotoxin (TTX)-resistant sodium channels (TTX$_R$, including Na$_V$1.8 and 1.9), are expressed in primary sensory neurons in the dorsal root ganglion (DRG) or trigeminal ganglion. The sensitivity of these channels can be regulated by IFMs. Current studies focus on TRPV1 and TTX$_R$, which are known to be essential for the induction of peripheral sensitization and pain hypersensitivity (Julius and Basbaum 2001).

Activation of peripheral nociceptors by high-threshold and persistent noxious stimuli (heat, mechanical, electrical) or by IFM (chemical stimuli) also results in an activity- or use-dependent neuronal plasticity in the CNS. This plasticity modifies the performance of nociceptive pathway by enhancing and prolonging the responses to subsequent peripheral stimuli. These changes in the spinal cord, as well as in the brain, are referred to central sensitization (Woolf and Salter 2000). Although central sensitization is often but not always initiated by peripheral sensitization, it is responsible for the pain after injury by normally innocuous low-threshold afferent inputs (allodynia) and the spread of pain hypersensitivity to regions beyond injured tissue. In chronic pain conditions, when injury-induced peripheral sensitization becomes less significant after wound healing, central sensitization could still be self-maintained, contributing importantly to the persistence of chronic pain. Current studies on central sensitization focus on dorsal horn neurons. Spontaneous activity is generated in primary sensory neurons after tissue injury, leading to the release of the neurotransmitter glutamate from central terminals of these neurons and subsequent activation of postsynaptic glutamate receptors in dorsal horn neurons. While glutamate AMPA (S-alpha-amino-3-hydroxy-5-methyl-4-isoxazolepropionic acid) receptor is important for normal synaptic transmission, N-methyl-D-aspartate (NMDA) receptor is essential for synaptic plasticity after tissue injury, underlying central sensitization. Further, injury also releases the neuropeptide substance P and the neurotrophin BDNF (brain-derived neurotrophic factor), acting on neurokinin-1 (NK-1) and tyrosine kinase receptor (TrkB), respectively in dorsal horn neurons, also contributing to central sensitization (Woolf and Salter 2000; Ji et al. 2003).

2
Protein Kinases and Pain Sensitization

Nearly 50 years ago, protein phosphorylation was identified as a regulatory mechanism for the control of glycogen metabolism. It took many years before its general significance came to be appreciated. Protein kinases almost regulate every aspect of cell life from growth to death. They mediate most of the signal transduction in eukaryotic cells by regulating substrate activity via phosphorylation. Protein kinases are among the largest families of genes and have been intensively studied. The human genome encodes 518 protein kinases, accounting for 1.7% of all human genes (Manning et al. 2002). These kinases share a catalytic domain conserved in sequence and structure but also notably different in how their catalysis is regulated. The ATP binding pocket together with less-conserved surrounding pockets has been the focus of inhibitor design. Multiple protein kinases have been implicated in pain sensitization (Table 1). Importantly, inhibitors of protein kinases do not affect physiological pain: the normal pain threshold in response to mechanical or thermal stimulus remains unchanged. The serine-threonine kinases consist of most protein kinases, and many of serine-threonine kinases are involved in pain regulation (Table 1). There are also 90 tyrosine kinases in the human

Table 1 A list of protein kinases that are known to be involved in inflammatory pain (IP), neuropathic pain (NP), peripheral sensitization (PS), and central sensitization (CS). See Sects. 2.1–2.3 for more details

	IP	NP	PS	CS
Ser/Thr kinases				
PKA	Yes	Yes	Yes	Yes
PKA, R1β	Yes	No	Yes	Yes
PKB (AKT)	N.T.	N.T.	Yes	Yes
PKC	Yes	Yes	Yes	Yes
PKCε	Yes	Yes	Yes	N.T.
PKCγ	Yes	Yes	N.T.	Yes
PKG	Yes	N.T.	Yes	Yes
PKG-I	Yes	N.T.	N.T.	Yes
CaM kinase II	Yes	Yes	Yes	Yes
MEK/ERK1/2	Yes	Yes	Yes	Yes
p38 MAPK	Yes	Yes	Yes	Yes
p38-β	N.T.	N.T.	N.T.	Yes
JNK /MAPK	N.T.	Yes	N.T.	N.T.
Rho kinase (ROCK)	Yes	Yes	N.T.	N.T.
IκB kinase (IKK)	Yes	Yes	N.T.	N.T.
Casein kinase 2	Yes	N.T.	N.T.	Yes
Cdk5	N.T.	N.T.	N.T.	Yes
Tyrosine kinases				
TrK A	Yes	Yes	Yes	N.T.
TrK B	Yes	Yes	N.T.	Yes
EphB	Yes	N.T.	N.T.	Yes
Src	N.T.	N.T.	N.T.	Yes
Other kinases				
PI3K	N.T.	N.T.	Yes	Yes

N.T., not tested

genome including receptor tyrosine kinases and nonreceptor tyrosine kinases (Manning et al. 2002); several tyrosine kinases are implicated in pain facilitation. In particular, we will discuss the roles of mitogen-activated protein kinases (MAPKs) in regulating pathological pain (see Sect. 2.3), because there is increasing evidence suggesting that this family of serine/threonine kinases is critical for the induction and maintenance of pain hypersensitivity after injuries (Ji and Woolf 2001).

2.1
Serine-Threonine Protein Kinases

Protein Kinase A (PKA) This is one of the most classic kinases. Although protein
kinase A (PKA) is typically activated by cyclic AMP (cAMP), cAMP's actions
are not exclusively mediated by PKA. cAMP could activate Epac, a guanine
nucleotide exchange factor, leading to the activation of p44/42 MAPK and the
ε-isoform of PKC. PKA has been strongly implicated in peripheral and central
sensitization. The adenyl cyclase–cAMP–PKA pathway mediates sensitization
of the peripheral terminals of nociceptors induced by PGE$_2$, a major inflammatory mediator (Aley and Levine 1999). PKA is also required for the second
phase nociceptive response to formalin and capsaicin-produced mechanical
allodynia, two pain models that are thought to result from central sensitization
(Coderre and Yashpal 1994; Sluka and Willis 1997). PKA also contributes to
the sensitization of spinal-thalamic projection neurons in the lamina I of the
spinal cord following tissue injury (Willis 2002). These NK-1-expressing projection neurons are essential for injury-induced pain hypersensitivity (Mantyh et al. 1997). In mice with a null mutation of the neuronal-specific isoform
of PKA's type I regulatory subunit (RIβ), a selective deficit is found in the
development of inflammation and tissue injury-produced pain (Malmberg
et al. 1997a).

Protein Kinase C PKC is activated by diacylglycerol (DAG) and Ca^{2+}. There is
substantial evidence supporting a role of spinal PKC in regulating pain hypersensitivity in different pain models (Mao et al. 1992; Coderre 1992; Sluka
and Willis 1997). PKC is also required for the sensitization of spinal-thalamic
projection neurons in the lamina I following intense C fiber stimulation (Willis
2002). There is an increase in spinal cord membrane-bound PKC following
nerve injury (Mao et al. 1992). In particular, the γ-isoform of PKC is expressed predominantly in inner lamina II neurons of the dorsal horn; there
is reduced neuropathic and inflammatory pain but preserved acute nociceptive pain in mice lacking PKCγ (Malmberg et al. 1997b). PKCγ expression is
further induced in the spinal cord by inflammation and nerve injury (Martin et al. 1999). The ε-isoform of PKC, in contrast, is expressed in primary
sensory neurons and plays a major role in peripheral sensitization of nociceptor terminals in inflammatory and neuropathic pain conditions (Khasar
et al. 1999).

Calcium/Calmodulin-Dependent Kinase This kinase (CaMK-II) has been intensively studied in hippocampal neurons and plays an essential role in synaptic
plasticity and learning and memory. The active form of αCaMK-II autophosphorylated at threonine 286, a critical site for CaMK-II activation, has been
shown to enhance excitatory synaptic transmission in dorsal horn neurons
(Kolaj et al. 1994). The superficial dorsal horn is densely stained with an

anti-αCaMK-II antibody (Fang et al. 2002; Zeitz et al. 2004). Recent studies show that CaMK-II is required for central sensitization and neuropathic pain sensitization (Fang et al. 2002; Garry et al. 2003). Disruption of CaMK-II's docking to the NMDA receptor may be important for the activation of this receptor and the subsequent sensitization of pain behavior after nerve injury (Garry et al. 2003). However, in mice with a point mutation in the αCaMK-II gene at threonine 286, inflammatory pain and neuropathic pain remain unchanged (Zeitz et al. 2004). The role of another isoform, CaMK-IV, in pain regulation is unclear, although it is expressed in 30% of DRG neurons and implicated in the activation of cAMP-response element binding protein (CREB), an important transcription factor for many neuronal genes (Ji et al. 1996).

Protein Kinase G (PKG) Ca^{2+} influx through the NMDA receptor activates the nitric oxide/cGMP/PKG pathway. Neuronal nitric oxide synthase (NOS) is Ca^{2+}/calmodulin-dependent. Nitric oxide (NO) serves as a diffusible and retrograde messenger. The major target of NO in the CNS appears is a soluble guanylyl cyclase (sGC) leading to the production of cyclic guanosine monophosphate (cGMP) and subsequent activation of PKG (Meller and Gebhart 1993). Nerve injury upregulates NOS in DRG neurons (Zhang et al. 1993). PKG appears to play a role in peripheral and central sensitization (Meller and Gebhart 1993; Sluka and Willis 1997; Aley et al. 1998). PKG-I is expressed in the spinal cord, and mice lacking PKG-I show reduced inflammatory hyperalgesia with preservation of acute thermal nociception (Tegeder et al. 2004a). In *Aplysia* sensory neurons, PKG-I couples to the ERK (extracellular signal-regulated kinase) pathway and contributes to axotomy-induced long-term hyperexcitability (Sung et al. 2004).

Other Kinases The transcription factor nuclear factor NF-κB plays an important role in inflammatory responses by inducing the transcription of genes encoding many inflammatory mediators. NF-κB is normally retained in cytoplasm by IκB inhibitor proteins. The phosphorylation of IκB by its kinase, IKK, results in IκB degradation. IκB degradation enables nuclear translocation of NF-κB for gene transcription. Specific inhibition of IKK is shown to reduce both inflammatory and neuropathic pain (Tegeder et al. 2004b). Rho kinase (ROCK) is regarded as a promising drug target for neurological disorders (Mueller et al. 2005). ROCK inhibitors were shown to suppress inflammatory and neuropathic pain (Inoue et al. 2004; Tatsumi et al. 2005). Casein kinase 2 (CK2) is a widely expressed protein kinase and involved in central sensitization and inflammatory pain (Li et al. 2005). Although cyclin-dependent kinase 5 (Cdk5) is typically involved in cell division, recent evidence also suggests a role of this kinase in regulating neural plasticity in the brain. Intrathecal administration of roscovitine, a Cdk5 inhibitor, attenuates formalin-induced nociceptive response in rats (Wang et al. 2005).

Finally, it is worth discussing phosphatidylinositol 3-kinase (PI3K) and the PI3K pathway. Although PI3K is a lipid kinase that phosphorylates the D-3 position of phosphatidylinositol lipids to produce $PI(3,4,5)P_3$, acting as a membrane-embedded second messenger (Toker and Cantley 1997), PI3K behaves like a protein kinase. Another reason to include PI3K is that the downstream protein kinase Akt (protein kinase B) is a serine/threonine kinase and is postulated to mediate most of PI3K's effects. Activation of Akt is typically used to examine the activation of PI3K pathway (Zhuang et al. 2004). PI3K is a major pathway activated by growth factors; therefore, NGF can strongly activate the PI3K pathway in DRG neurons. PI3K is also activated in DRG neurons by C fiber activator capsaicin due to intracellular Ca^{2+} increase. PI3K inhibitors prevent heat hyperalgesia by both NGF and capsaicin. The PI3K is especially important for the induction of heat hyperalgesia (Zhuang et al. 2004).

2.2
Tyrosine Kinases

Receptor Tyrosine Kinases The receptors for growth factors are tyrosine kinases that are autophosphorylated upon ligand binding. In particular, NGF and BDNF mediate their effects largely via TrkA and TrkB, respectively. Although NGF is required for the survival of sensory neurons during fetal development, it is not necessary for the survival of mature sensory neurons. Rather it maintains the phenotype of sensory neurons in the adult. NGF plays an essential role in peripheral sensitization; local and systemic injection of NGF produces hyperalgesia. Although BDNF is synthesized in primary sensory neurons, it can be released from central terminals in the spinal cord following intense noxious stimulation and plays an important role in central sensitization. Intrathecal infusion of a scavenger for TrkA and TrkB (BDNF receptor) or a general Trk inhibitor k252a reduces both inflammatory and neuropathic pain (McMahon et al. 1995; Mannion et al. 1999; Ji and Strichartz 2004). A recent study has also shown that receptor tyrosine kinase EphB is required for central sensitization and the development of inflammatory pain (Battaglia et al. 2003).

Non-receptor Tyrosine Kinases Among this large group of signaling molecules, the Src family is the best known, which includes Src, Fyn, Lck, Lyn, and Yes. Src is activated by receptor tyrosine kinases as well as by G protein-coupled receptor (GPCR) and PKC. Activation of Src is implicated in p44/42 MAPK activation (Kawasaki et al. 2004). Salter and his collaborators have shown an important role of Src in regulating the activity of NMDA receptors, an essential mediator of central sensitization (Salter and Kalia 2004). Thus, Src inhibitor was shown to suppress central sensitization (Guo et al. 2002). It is not clear whether other nonreceptor tyrosine kinases also contribute to pain sensitization.

2.3
Mitogen-Activated Proteins Kinases (MAPKs)

The MAPKs are a family of evolutionarily conserved molecules that play a critical role in cell signaling. This family includes three major members—extracellular signal-regulated kinase (ERK or p44/42 MAPK), p38, and c-Jun N-terminal kinase (JNK)—that represent three different signaling cascades. MAPKs transduce a broad range of extracellular stimuli into diverse intracellular responses by both transcriptional and nontranscriptional regulation (Widmann et al. 1999). Early studies indicated a critical role of ERK in regulating mitosis, proliferation, differentiation, and survival of mammalian cells during development. Recent evidence shows that ERK also plays an important role in neuronal plasticity and inflammatory responses in the adult. p38 and JNK are typically activated by cellular stress (ultraviolet irradiation, osmotic shock, heat shock), lipopolysaccharide (LPS), and certain proinflammatory cytokines such as TNF-α and IL-1β (Widmann et al. 1999; Ji and Woolf 2001). Therefore, these two kinases, especially JNK, are also called stress-activated protein kinase (SAPK), contributing importantly to inflammatory responses and neuronal degeneration. All the family members are activated by different upstream MAPK kinases (MKKs). The corresponding MKKs for ERK, p38, and JNK are MKK1/2 (also called MEK1/2), MKK3/6, MKK4/7. The ERK5 is the least-known member of MAPK family and is activated by MKK5. MKKs are activated by MAPK kinase kinase. Studies on MAPKs greatly benefit from specific inhibitors available to explore the function of each pathway and from phosphorylation-specific antibodies available to investigate the activation of each pathway. Like other kinase inhibitors, MAPK inhibitors do not affect basal pain perception.

2.3.1
ERK/MAPK (p44/42 MAPK) Pathway

ERK is the first and the most studied member of the MAPK family. It was originally identified as a primary effector of growth factor receptor signaling, a cascade that involves sequential activation of Ras, Raf (MAPK kinase kinase), MEK (MAPK kinase), and ERK (MAPK). However, the activation of the ERK cascade is not restricted to growth factor signaling. ERK is activated by persistent neural activity and pathological stimuli. A growing body of evidence demonstrates an involvement of ERK in neuronal plasticity, such as learning and memory, as well as pain hypersensitivity (Widmann et al. 1999; Ji and Woolf 2001; Ji et al. 2003).

Activation of ERK in Primary Sensory Neurons There is an activity-dependent ERK activation in DRG neurons. Depolarization of adult DRG neuronal cultures induces a very rapid and transient ERK phosphorylation (pERK). This transient pERK induction is also observed in vivo following peripheral noxious stimuli, reaching peak at 2 min and almost returning to the baseline after 10 min (Dai et al. 2002). In addition to neuronal activity, NGF, capsaicin, and epinephrine can all activate ERK in a subset of DRG neurons. ERK is not only induced in the soma of DRG neurons but also in peripheral axons of DRG neurons (Dai et al. 2002; Zhuang et al. 2004). Intraplantar injection of capsaicin increases pERK-labeled nerve fibers in the epidermis within 2 min. Inhibition of the ERK pathway by MEK inhibitors attenuates heat hyperalgesia by capsaicin and NGF as well as mechanical hyperalgesia by epinephrine (Aley et al. 2001; Dai et al. 2002; Zhuang et al. 2004). ERK is likely to mediate heat hyperalgesia by inducing TRPV1 sensitization (Dai et al. 2002; Zhuang et al. 2004).

Activation of ERK in Dorsal Horn Neurons We have shown that ERK activation in spinal dorsal horn neurons is nociceptive activity-dependent (Ji et al. 1999). Injection of the C fiber nociceptor activator capsaicin into a hindpaw of rats induces a remarkable ERK phosphorylation. pERK is induced in dorsal horn neurons as early as 1 min after C fiber activation. This activation exactly follows the rule of spinal topographic organization: pERK-labeled neurons are found in the medial superficial dorsal horn of the spinal cord on the stimulated side where primary nociceptive afferents from the hindpaw terminate. The pERK can only be induced by thermal noxious (heat and cold) and mechanical noxious (prick) stimulus, but not by innocuous stimulus (light touch) (Ji et al. 1999). It appears that the duration of noxious stimulation is also important; a very brief noxious stimulation (<10 s) may not induce pERK. Noxious stimulation also induces ERK activation in the trigeminal spinal nucleus (Huang et al. 2000).

Moreover, pERK can be induced in a spinal cord slice preparation, where different types of afferent fibers in the attached dorsal root can be electrically stimulated (Ji et al. 1999; Lever et al. 2003). A bath application of capsaicin to spinal slices, which will activate TRPV1 receptors in presynaptic C fiber terminals to stimulate the release of neurotransmitter acting on postsynaptic receptor, strongly activates ERK in superficial dorsal horn neurons in spinal slices (Fig. 1a, b). Using this simple and reliable in vitro (or ex vivo) model, we have investigated the molecular mechanisms involved in the regulation of C fiber-induced ERK activation (Kawasaki et al. 2004). We found that multiple neurotransmitter receptors, including NMDA, AMPA, and metabotropic glutamate receptors, substance P NK-1 receptor, and TrkB receptor all contribute to C fiber-evoked ERK activation (Kawasaki et al. 2004; Fig. 1c).

To investigate the functional significance of ERK activation, a MEK (ERK kinase) inhibitor (PD98059) was tested in the formalin model, where injection of diluted formalin into a hindpaw of rats elicits a pain behavior lasting for an hour. Intrathecal injection of PD98059 blocks the central sensitization-

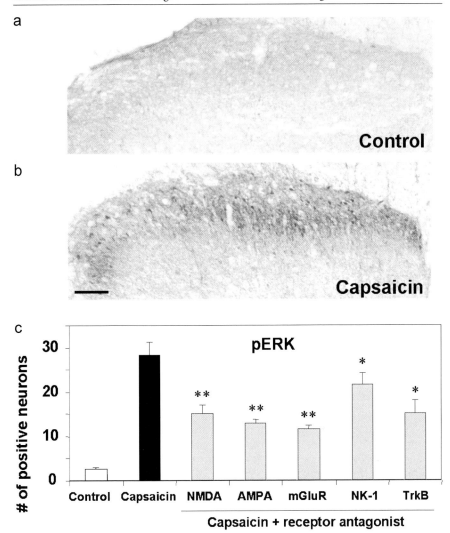

Fig. 1a–c ERK activation in the superficial dorsal horn of spinal slices as indicated by phospho ERK (pERK) immunostaining. **a** There are very few pERK-labeled neurons in the control slices. **b** A bath application of capsaicin (3 µM, 5 min) induces pERK in many neurons in the stimulated slices. Scale, 50 µm. **c** This panel shows the number of pERK-positive neurons in the laminae I–II of spinal slices after capsaicin stimulation in the presence of different receptor antagonists. Capsaicin-induced pERK is reduced by blocking NMDA (MK-801, 100 µM), AMPA (CNQX, 20 µM), mGluR (CPCCOEt, 1 µM), NK-1 (GR205171A, 100 µM), and TrkB receptors (k252a 100 nM). *, $p<0.05$; **, $p<0.01$, compared to capsaicin group, ANOVA. Mean±SEM ($n=5$). (See Kawasaki et al. 2004 for more details)

mediated second phase of the painful response to formalin injection (Ji et al. 1999). After this initial study, multiple studies in different animal models from different labs have confirmed that the ERK pathway contributes importantly to the development of central sensitization (Karim et al. 2001; Galan et al. 2003; Kawasaki et al. 2004; Yu and Chen 2005; Yu and Yezierski 2005). Injection of CFA into a hindpaw produces persistent (>2 weeks) inflammatory pain. CFA also induces sustained ERK activation in dorsal horn neurons, whereas capsaicin and formalin only induce transient ERK activation (Ji et al. 1999; Ji et al. 2002a). Intrathecal infusion of the MEK inhibitor U0126 reduces the late phase of inflammatory pain. This delayed action of ERK is likely to be caused by transcriptional regulation (Ji et al. 2002a). MEK inhibitors are also shown to alleviate neuropathic pain (Obata and Noguchi 2004; Zhuang et al. 2005).

Although overall pERK induction is persistent after CFA inflammation, the peak induction only lasts a few hours. The duration of ERK activation is controlled by phosphatases. pERK could be inactivated by MKP-1 (MAP kinase phosphatase-1) and PP2A (protein phosphatase 2A). Neuronal activity not only induces ERK activation but also rapidly increases the expression of immediate early gene MKP-1. Intrathecal injection of okadaic acid, a general PP2A inhibitor, enhances central sensitization by prolonging capsaicin-induced mechanical hyperalgesia and allodynia. Phosphatase inhibitor might prolong capsaicin-induced ERK activation, resulting in prolonged pain facilitation (Zhang et al. 2003; Ji and Strichartz 2004).

pERK Expression as a Marker for Nociceptive Activity and as an Assay for Screening Analgesic Compounds The expression of the immediate early-gene *c-fos* has been extensively used as a marker for demonstrating the activity of spinal nociceptive neurons (Hunt et al. 1987; Presley et al. 1990). Like the expression of c-Fos protein, pERK expression can also serve as a marker for neuronal activity following nociceptive input. Compared to c-Fos expression, pERK expression is more rapid and transient, following neuronal activity more closely. Importantly, pERK expression is functional, contributing critically to dorsal horn neuron sensitization. The function of ERK activation can be easily assessed by blocking this activation with specific MEK inhibitors. Further, pERK expression can be reliably studied in spinal slice preparation. Since many slices (>10) can be obtained from spinal lumbar enlargement of one rat and C fiber can be easily stimulated by bath capsaicin, pERK expression by capsaicin in spinal slices can be used for the screening of potential analgesic drugs (Ji 2004). Interestingly, pERK can be induced by tactile stimulation (touch) after nerve injury, which may underlie tactile allodynia after neuropathic pain.

2.3.2
p38 MAPK Pathway

p38 is typically activated by cellular stress and inflammatory mediators. p38 activation can also be activity-dependent. Systematic p38 inhibitors produce antiinflammatory effects in animal models (Ji and Woolf 2001). Interestingly, phospholipase A2 (PLA2) is downstream to p38. The activation of PLA2 leads to the generation of arachidonic acid for prostaglandin production, eliciting pain (Svensson et al. 2005). Activated p38 is also translocated to the nucleus phosphorylating the transcriptional factors and induces gene expression. The biosynthesis of TNF-α and IL-1β, as well as many other inflammatory mediators, is positively regulated by p38 (Ji and Woolf 2001).

p38 Activation in the DRG and Spinal Cord Phospho-p38 (p-p38), the active form of p38, is normally expressed in 10%–15% of DRG neurons that are primary C fiber nociceptors (Ji et al. 2002b; Obata et al. 2004). p38 is activated in DRG neurons following peripheral inflammation and nerve injuries (Kim et al. 2002; Ji et al. 2002b; Jin et al. 2003; Schafers et al. 2003; Obata and Noguchi 2004). However, total p38 (nonphosphorylated and phosphorylated) levels do not increase after injury, indicating that the increase in p-p38 is caused by increased phosphorylation, rather than elevated substrate (Ji et al. 2002b). After nerve injury, p38 is activated not only in DRG neurons with axonal injury, but also in adjacent neurons without axonal injury (Obata et al. 2004). While TNF-α contributes to an early activation of p38 after nerve injury, NGF, via retrograde transport, is important for persistent p38 activation after inflammation and nerve injury (Ji et al. 2002b; Schafers et al. 2003; Obata et al. 2004). Unlike ERK, p38 is not activated in spinal cord neurons in either control or pathological pain conditions (Jin et al. 2003; see further discussion in Sect. 3.4).

p38 and Pathological Pain The pyridinyl imidazole compounds SB203580, SB202190, and PD169316 are regarded as specific inhibitors for p38. SB203580 is the most frequently used p38 inhibitor. It does not inhibit the phosphorylation of p38 MAPK, but rather binds to the ATP pocket in the enzyme, inhibiting activity of the enzyme. CNI-1493 is a potent antiinflammatory agent and was initially used as a monocyte synthesis inhibitor to block glial activation and later recognized as a p38 inhibitor (Milligan et al. 2003). FR167653 is another p38 inhibitor. Unlike SB203580, CNI-1493 and FR167653 can block the phosphorylation of p38 (Koistinaho and Koistinaho 2002; Obata et al. 2004). To examine whether p38 activation in the DRG is involved in the generation of inflammatory pain, SB203580 was administered into the intrathecal space to target p38 activity in the DRG. This inhibitor reduced inflammation-induced heat hyperalgesia and suppressed CFA-induced TRPV1 upregulation, but had no effect on CFA-induced inflammation (Ji et al. 2002b). Intrathecal injection of p38 inhibitors SD-282 and SB203580 also reduced substance P- and NMDA-induced pain hypersensitivity and suppressed COX-2 upregulation and PGE$_2$ release in the spinal cord (Svensson et al. 2003a; Svensson et al. 2003b). p38 inhibitor can also alleviate neuropathic pain. Intrathecal SB203580 prevents the development mechanical allodynia after spinal nerve ligation (Jin et al. 2003; Schafers et al. 2003; Tsuda et al. 2004). SB203580, CNI-1493, FR167653, and SD-282 further reverses neuropathic pain after spinal nerve ligation, sciatic inflammatory neuropathy (SIN), and diabetic neuropathy (Jin et al. 2003; Milligan et al. 2003; Obata et al. 2004; Sweitzer et al. 2004). The mechanisms of p38 regulation of pain sensitization are discussed in Sects. 3.1 and 3.4.

2.3.3
JNK/MAPK Pathway

JNK is the least studied member of MAPK family regarding its role in pain regulation. JNK can be activated by cell stress such as heat shock, direct DNA damage, and generation of reactive oxygen species and plays an important role in the induction of apoptosis. JNK has three isoforms: JNK1, JNK2, and JNK3, and JNK3 is closely correlated with neuronal function. Activated JNK phosphorylates the transcription factors c-Jun and ATF-2 (Widmann et al. 1999). Nerve injury induces JNK activation in DRG neurons (Obata et al. 2004; Zhuang et al. 2006). JNK is also induced in glial cells in the spinal cord by nerve lesion. Intrathecal injection of the JNK inhibitor SP600125 and D-JNKI-1 could prevent and reverse neuropathic pain (Ma and Quirion 2002; Obata et al. 2004; Zhuang et al. 2006; also see Sect. 3.4).

3
Mechanisms of Pain Sensitization by Protein Kinases

3.1
Peripheral Mechanisms

3.1.1
Induction of Peripheral Sensitization: Posttranslational Regulation

As discussed in Sect. 1.2, TRPV1 and TTX_R sodium channels are expressed in nociceptive primary sensory neurons and play a pivotal role in the induction of peripheral sensitization (Fig. 2). TRPV1 is essential for the generation of heat hyperalgesia. Inflammatory heat hypersensitivity following bradykinin, NGF, CFA, and carrageenan is significantly reduced in TRPV1 knockout mice (Caterina et al. 2000; Chuang et al. 2001). TTX_R sodium channels are crucial for the generation of hyperexcitability of sensory neurons. Knockdown of $Na_V1.8$ with antisense oligodeoxynucleotides results in decreased inflammatory pain and neuropathic pain (Porreca et al. 1999). Hypersensitivity of TRPV1 and TTX_R following stimulation of inflammatory mediators underlies the induction of peripheral sensitization (Julius and Basbaum 2001).

Several protein kinases such as PKA, PKC, CaMK-II, PI3K and ERK are implicated in TRPV1 sensitization. PKA and PKC are also involved in regulating the sensitivity of TTX_R. A membrane translocation of PKCε appears to be important for its activation of TTX_R. The PI3K pathway could contribute to peripheral sensitization by inducing the trafficking and membrane insertion

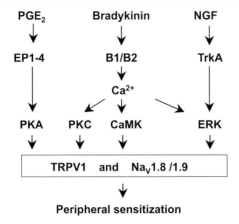

Fig. 2 Induction of peripheral sensitization by protein kinases in nociceptors. Following tissue injury, inflammatory mediators PGE$_2$, bradykinin, and NGF activate corresponding G protein-coupled receptors EP1–4 and B1/B2, and tyrosine kinase receptor TrkA on nociceptor terminals, axons, and soma, leading to the activation of PKA, PKC, CaMK-II, and ERK. These protein kinases increase the sensitivity of TRPV1 and TTX-resistant sodium channels Na$_v$1.8/1.9 by posttranslational regulation, causing peripheral sensitization

of critical ion channels (Gold et al. 1998; Julius and Basbaum 2001; Ji and Strichartz 2004; Zhuang et al. 2004). Since the action of these kinases could happen within minutes and occur in nociceptor terminals, it should involve posttranslational regulation of protein kinases.

3.1.2
Maintenance of Peripheral Sensitization: Transcriptional and Translational Regulation

Tissue and nerve injuries induce gene transcription and protein synthesis in primary sensory neurons in the DRG, contributing to persistent pain hypersensitivity. For example, peripheral inflammation increases the transcription of substance P, calcitonin gene-related protein (CGRP), and BDNF. After nerve injury, these genes are also induced in noninjured DRG neurons that are adjacent to injured DRG neurons. NGF is believed to be critical for the expression of these genes (reviewed in Ji and Strichartz 2004). Since p38 and ERK can be activated by NGF; these two MAPKs appear to mediate NGF-induced expression of substance P, CGRP, and BDNF via the transcription factor CREB. The cAMP-response element (CRE) sites are found in many genes expressed in the DRG including substance P, CGRP, and BDNF (Ji and Strichartz 2004).

In addition to transcriptional regulation, MAPK also mediates gene expression via translational regulation. Peripheral inflammation and NGF induce increase in TRPV1 protein levels but not in TRPV1 messenger RNA (mRNA) levels in the DRG. CFA increases p-p38 and TRPV1 expression in C fiber nociceptors, and p-p38 is heavily colocalized with NGF receptor TrkA and TRPV1. Further, intrathecal inhibition of p38 blocked inflammation-induced upregulation of TRPV1. p38 is likely to regulate the translation of TRPV1 via translation initiation factor eIF-4E in a NGF-dependent way (Ji et al. 2002b). NGF levels increase in the inflamed paw after CFA injection. NGF is taken up by nerve terminals and retrogradely transported to neuronal soma in the DRG, inducing p38 activation and TRPV1 translation. Finally, TRPV1 is anterogradely transported from DRG cell body to peripheral nerve terminals, contributing to persistent inflammatory heat hyperalgesia (Ji et al. 2002b). The NGF–p38–TRPV1 cascade in also important for heat hyperalgesia after nerve injury, in which NGF is produced from injured axons after Wallerian degeneration and taken up by adjacent intact axons (Obata et al. 2004).

3.2
Spinal Mechanisms

3.2.1
Induction of Central Sensitization: Posttranslational Regulation

Glutamate is a predominant excitatory neurotransmitter in all nociceptors. Mild noxious stimulation generates fast excitatory postsynaptic potentials, lasting milliseconds. This fast synaptic transmission is mediated by ionotropic glutamate AMPA and kainate receptors. Additional activation of intracellular signaling cascades is required for the development of central sensitization (Woolf and Salter 2000; Ji and Woolf 2001).

Activation of second messenger systems, especially protein kinases, can phosphorylate AMPA and NMDA receptors via posttranslational regulation, enhancing synaptic transmission and producing central sensitization (Fig. 3). For example, a PKC-mediated phosphorylation of NMDA receptor in dorsal horn neurons removes its voltage-dependent Mg^{2+} block, which in turn enables glutamate to generate a greater inward current through the NMDA ion channel at resting membrane potentials (Chen and Huang 1992). Tyrosine kinase Src enhances NMDA current via phosphorylation of NR2A/B subunit of NMDA receptor. The tyrosine phosphorylation appears to increase channel open time and kinetics. Noxious simulation and inflammation induce the phosphorylation of NMDA receptor subunits in dorsal horn neurons (Zou et al. 2000; Guo et al. 2002; Salter and Kalia 2004). CaMK and PKA have been implicated in the phosphorylation of AMPA receptors, leading to an increase of AMPA current (Ji et al. 2003).

Recently it was shown that painful stimulation induces trafficking and insertion of AMPA receptor subunits to the plasma membrane of spinal cord neurons (Galan et al. 2004). CaMK and ERK appear to mediate membrane insertion of AMPA receptors during synaptic plasticity. ERK could also regulate the activity of $K_v4.2$ potassium channels, increasing the excitability of dor-

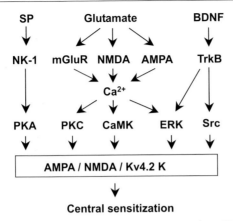

Fig. 3 Induction of central sensitization by protein kinases in dorsal horn neurons. Injury-evoked spontaneous activity induces the release of the neurotransmitters glutamate and the neuromodulators substance P and BDNF from primary afferents in the dorsal horn, activating corresponding ionotropic NMDA and AMPA receptors, metabotropic mGluR receptors, and tyrosine kinase TrkB receptors, leading to subsequent activation of PKA, PKC, CaMK-II, ERK, and Src in postsynaptic dorsal horn neurons. These protein kinases increase the sensitivity of AMPA and NMDA receptors and suppress the activity of $K_v4.2$ potassium channels by posttranslational regulation, causing central sensitization

sal horn neurons (Hu et al. 2003). In addition to posttranslational regulation, nociceptive activity also induces a rapid increase of CaMK-II protein (within 10 min), which may involve translational regulation (Fang et al. 2002).

3.2.2
Maintenance of Central Sensitization: Transcriptional Regulation

Intense noxious stimulation, inflammation, and nerve injury produce an increase in the expression of immediate early genes (e.g., *c-fos, Zif268, Cox-2*) and later response genes (e.g., prodynorphin, NK-1, and TrkB) in the dorsal horn of spinal cord. A continuous production of the protein products of these genes could maintain central sensitization (reviewed in Ji et al. 2003). Upon activation, pERK is translocated to the nucleus of dorsal horn neurons. ERK activation is likely to maintain pain hypersensitivity via regulating gene expression. Inhibition of ERK activation blocks inflammation-induced upregulation of *c-fos*, prodynorphin, NK-1, as well as CREB phosphorylation (Ji et al. 2002a; Kawasaki et al. 2004). pERK is shown to activate CREB via a CREB kinase RSK2 (Fig. 4). CREB-binding site CRE has been identified in the promoter regions of numerous genes expressed in the dorsal horn, including those mentioned above. It is of particular interest that ERK activation is downstream to many other kinases, such as PKA, PKC, PI3K, Trk, and Src (Kawasaki et al. 2004; Fig. 4). Convergence of multiple signal pathways on ERK activation indicates a pivotal role of the ERK pathway in intracellular signal transduction.

Recently the concept for the "memory of pain" has been proposed to explain the persistence of pain. Studies on neural plasticity in the spinal cord and in the hippocampus reveal similar mechanisms for central sensitization

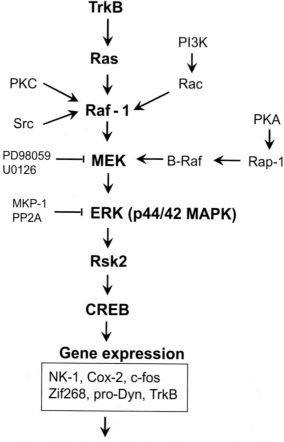

Fig. 4 Maintenance of central sensitization by protein kinases in dorsal horn neurons. ERK is classically activated by the Ras–Raf–MEK pathway following stimulation of growth factor receptors (TrkB). Several kinases such as PKA, PKC, Src, and PI3K can converge on ERK activation. Meanwhile, ERK is inhibited by the phosphatases MKP-1 and PP2A. MEK is inhibited by the inhibitors PD98059 and U0126. Upon phosphorylation, pERK activates the transcription factor CREB via CREB kinase Rsk2, leading to the transcription of CRE-mediated genes including immediate early genes *Zif268*, *Cox-2*, *c-fos* and late response genes *NK-1*, *TrkB*, and *prodynorphin* in dorsal horn neurons. Central sensitization is maintained by the protein products of these genes

and long-term potentiation (LTP), which are believed to underlie generation of pain hypersensitivity and memory, respectively (Sandkuhler 2000; Willis 2002; Ji et al. 2003). LTP is also induced in dorsal horn neurons following intense noxious stimulation (Sandkuhler 2000). Whereas long-term memory requires gene transcription, short-term memory only requires posttranslational modifications. This same dichotomy appears to apply to central sensitization-mediated pain hypersensitivity: persistent pain (chronic pain) but not acute pain requires gene transcription (Ji et al. 2003). In particular, the transcription factor CREB is believed to play an essential role in long-term neuronal plasticity in both hippocampal and dorsal horn neurons. CREB can maintain long-term neural plasticity not only by inducing gene transcription but also by forming new synapses (Lonze and Ginty 2002).

3.3
Brain Mechanisms

In addition to dorsal horn neurons, central sensitization also develops in rostroventral medial medulla (RVM) neurons, amygdala neurons, and cingulate cortex neurons following tissue injury (Urban and Gebhart 1999; Porreca et al. 2002). Inflammation induces phosphorylation of AMPA receptor (GluR1) in the RVM, in a PKC- and CaMK-dependent manner, which may regulate descending facilitation (Guan et al. 2004). The spino–parabrachio–amygdaloid pathway is implicated in nociception. Tissue injury induces an enhanced NMDA receptor function in rat amygdala neurons via PKA activation (Bird et al. 2005). The PKA pathway in the anterior cingulate cortex (ACC) also contributes to inflammatory pain, since calcium-dependent adenylate cyclase AC1 and AC8 are highly expressed in the ACC and inflammatory pain is attenuated in AC1 and AC8 knockout mice. The action of AC1 and AC8 appears to be mediated by the cAMP–PKA–CREB pathway (Wei et al. 2002a). Neuronal activity in the ACC could influence nociceptive transmission in the dorsal horn of the spinal cord by activating the endogenous facilitatory system.

Pain experience includes not only a sensory-discriminative component describing the quality, intensity, and spatiotemporal characteristics of the sensation, but also an emotional-affective component, referring to the unpleasantness or aversion of sensation. Emotional distress could be the most disruptive and undesirable feature of painful experiences. Physiological arousal and hypervigilance to pain cause a negative affect, such as fear, anxiety, anger, worry, aversion, and depression, which in turn could alter pain sensation. While current studies focus primarily on the sensory component of pain, mechanisms underlying the affective dimension of pain have recently received more attention. ACC is a part of the brain's limbic system and plays an important role in affect. ACC neurons respond to noxious stimuli with very large, often whole-body receptive fields, and acquire responses to environmental cues that predict a painful stimulus (Koyama et al. 1998). Formalin-induced conditioned place avoidance (F-CPA, noxious conditioning) has been established as an animal model to examine affective pain and pain-associated memory. Lesions of ACC in animals produce severe deficits in avoidance conditioning (Johansen et al. 2001).

Molecular mechanisms underlying learning and memory have been intensively investigated in hippocampal neurons. It has been demonstrated that PKA, ERK, and CaMK can all converge on CREB phosphorylation, leading to long-term memory via gene transcription (Lonze and Ginty 2002). These mechanisms may also contribute to affective pain and pain-associated memory in ACC neurons. Activation of NMDA receptors results in Ca^{2+} influx and is required for formalin-induced affective pain (Lei et al. 2004). Ca^{2+}-dependent CaMK-IV is required for CREB activation in the ACC by noxious shock and for fear memory, but behavioral responses to acute noxious stimuli or tissue inflammation may not require CaMK-IV (Wei et al. 2002b). ERK activation has been implicated in several forms of learning and memory, including fear conditioning, spatial learning, conditioned taste aversion, etc. We found that pain-related aversion (F-CPA) induced ERK activation in the ACC, and that microinjection of the MEK inhibitor PD98059 in the ACC significantly inhibited affective pain as well as CREB phosphorylation following F-CPA (Zhang et al. 2005). These results indicate that the ERK/CREB signaling pathway, which has been implicated in the sensory component of pain in spinal neurons, may also participate in affective pain in ACC neurons.

3.4
Glial and Immuno–Mechanisms

Studies on pathological pain mostly focus on the responses of the neurons and neuronal-specific mechanisms of hypersensitivity and chronicity. However, glial cells express various receptors for neurotransmitters and neuromodulators (Watkins et al. 2001; Ji and Strichartz 2004). There is accumulating evidence indicating a role of spinal glial cells in the pathogenesis of pain. Both microglia and astrocytes are activated in inflammatory and neuropathic pain conditions. Multiple mediators such as proinflammatory cytokines (e.g., IL-1β, IL-6, and TNF-α) and inflammatory enzymes (e.g., iNOS, COX-1, and COX-2) are synthesized in spinal astrocytes and microglia (DeLeo and Yezierski 2001; Watkins et al. 2001). There is increased synthesis of these mediators in activated glia following injuries; all of them are shown to produce pain sensitization. Spinal injection of the glial toxin fluorocitrate, glial modulator propentofylline, or nonspecific microglial inhibitor minocycline has been shown to reduce inflammatory and neuropathic pain (Meller et al. 1994; Watkins et al. 1997; Sweitzer et al. 2001; Raghavendra et al. 2003). In particular, several receptors such as ATP receptor P2X4, chemokine receptors CCR2 and CX3CR1, and Toll-like receptor TLR-4 are expressed in spinal microglia after nerve injury. Blockade of these receptors results in a reduction of neuropathic pain (Abbadie et al. 2003; Tsuda et al. 2003; Verge et al. 2004; Tanga et al. 2005).

It is not very clear how activation of these receptors in microglia leads to pain sensitization. We have proposed that activation of MAPKs may mediate pro-nociceptive effects of these receptors (Ji and Strichartz 2004). Nerve injury induces a drastic and widespread activation of p38 MAPK in the spinal cord. This activation begins at 12 h and peaks 3 days after nerve injury, in parallel with the time course of microglial activation. Moreover, p-p38 is completely colocalized with OX-42 (CD-11b), a hall marker for microglia (Jin et al. 2003). Inhibition of p38 activation in microglia attenuates nerve injury-induced me-

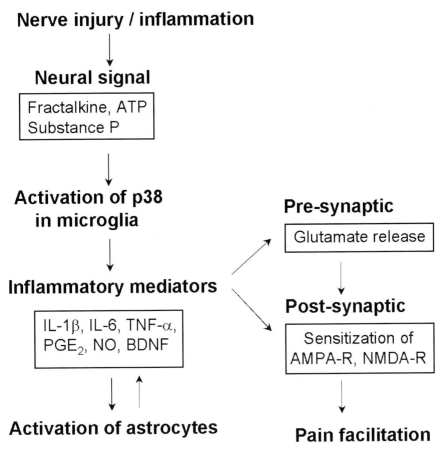

Fig. 5 Microglial regulation of pain facilitation via p38 MAPK. Inflammation and nerve injury release the signaling molecules fractalkine, ATP, and substance P from primary afferents, leading to p38 activation in spinal microglia. p38 activation results in the synthesis of multiple inflammatory mediators (e.g., IL-1β, IL-6, TNF-α, PGE$_2$, NO), enhancing and prolonging pain facilitation via both presynaptic (glutamate release) and postsynaptic (AMPA and NMDA receptor sensitization) mechanisms. Microglia may also synthesize neuromodulator BDNF to sensitize postsynaptic dorsal horn neurons

chanical allodynia (Jin et al. 2003; Tsuda et al. 2005). p38 activation in microglia is likely to induce the synthesis of inflammatory mediators as well as neuro-modulator BDNF. The release of these neuroactive substances could diffuse to synaptic regions and sensitize pain transmission neurons via both presy-naptic and postsynaptic mechanisms (Fig. 5). In addition to p38, ERK is also activated in spinal microglia after nerve lesion and contributes to neuropathic pain (Zhuang et al. 2005).

Compared to rapid activation of microglia, injury induces a delayed but per-sistent activation of astrocytes, suggesting a particular role of astroglia in the persistence of chronic pain. Nerve injury induces persistent activation of JNK in spinal astrocytes (Ma and Quirion 2002; Zhuang et al. 2006). Importantly, this activation is requried for the maintenance of neuropathic pain (Zhuang et al. 2006). Further, ERK is activated in spinal astrocytes at late times of nerve injury and contributes to late maintenance of neuropathic pain (Zhuang et al. 2005). Therefore, MAPKs could mediate different phases of chronic pain by regulating the activity of different subtypes of glial cells.

In addition to spinal glial cells, MAPKs can also be activated in glial cells in the sciatic nerve (Schwann cells) and DRG (satellite cells), as well as in inflammatory cells infiltrating the damaged tissue after injuries, increasing the sensitivity of sensory neurons by producing inflammatory mediators (Ji and Strichartz 2004).

4
Protein Kinase Inhibitors in Clinical Studies

A number of diseases including cancer, diabetes, and inflammation are as-sociated with perturbation of protein kinase-mediated signal transduction. Chromosomal mapping has shown that 244 kinases map to disease loci or can-cer amplicons (Manning et al. 2002). Many kinase inhibitors are developed to treat cancer in clinical trials. These include receptor tyrosine kinas inhibitors (e.g., EGF receptor inhibitors) and several MEK inhibitors such as CI-1040, PD0325901, and ARRY-142886, and Raf inhibitor BAY 43-9006 (Cohen 2002; Sebolt-Leopold and Herrera 2004). In the cancer field, protein kinase inhibitors are proving to be well-tolerated compared with conventional chemotherapeu-tic treatments. The MEK inhibitor PD184352 was shown to inhibit the growth of colon cancer that was implanted into mice, without causing obvious ad-verse side effects over several months treatment (Sebolt-Leopold et al. 1999). The lack of significant side effects of MEK inhibitors is surprising since the ERK cascade has been implicated in many cell processes including cell growth. However, the essential roles of the ERK cascade in proliferation and differen-tiation are only required during development, and this pathway might be far less crucial for normal function in adults. Since cancer pain is so devastating (Mantyh et al. 2002), MEK inhibitors could be assessed for anticancer pain effects while being tested for antitumor effects in clinical trials.

Several p38 MAPK inhibitors including SB281838, BIRB0796, Ro320-1195, and SCIO-469 are in clinical trials for rheumatoid arthritis (Cohen 2002; Watkins and Maier 2003; Nikas and Drosos 2004). Given the important role of p38 MAPK in several pathological pain conditions, these inhibitors should also be tested for clinical pain, if they are well tolerated. JNK pathway is essential for regulating neurotoxicity and apoptosis. CEP-1347, an inhibitor for the JNK upstream kinase MLK (mixed lineage kinase) was in clinical trial for neurodegenerative diseases (Cohen 2002). Given the fact that neuropathic pain is also regarded as a neurodegenerative condition and JNK inhibition attenuates neuropathic pain (Zhuang et al. 2006), CEP-1347 or JNK inhibitor (e.g., D-JNKI-1) could also be tested for neuropathic pain in clinical studies.

In addition to MAPK inhibitors, wortmannin, a selective inhibitor for PI3K pathway, is in clinical trials for the treatment of osteoporosis (Noble et al. 2004). Inhibitors for Rho kinase (ROCK) such as HA1077 (AT877, fasudil) are used to treat cerebral vasospasm. Indirubin is a CDK5 inhibitor used to treat neurodegenerative disorders (Noble et al. 2004). Since all the kinases are implicated in pain facilitation, these inhibitors could be potentially useful for the management of clinical pain.

Many specific protein kinase inhibitors that cannot be used as drugs for reasons of toxicity, pharmacology, or solubility—such as the MEK inhibitors PD98059 and SB203580—could be useful reagents for basic research. While current efforts on developing protein kinase inhibitors focus on small molecules, membrane permeable peptide inhibitors could provide another efficient way to block the function of protein kinases. Recently, a peptide JNK inhibitor, derived from JNK binding domain of JNK-interacting protein-1 (JIP-1), was designed to block selectively the access of JNK to c-Jun and other substrates by a competitive mechanism. A TAT sequence (transporter sequence) is linked to the peptide, making the peptide membrane permeable. This highly specific peptide inhibitor is an extremely potent neuroprotectant both in vitro and in vivo (Borsello et al. 2003; Borsello and Bonny 2004). It is also highly effective in suppressing neuropathic pain symptoms after nerve injury (Zhaung et al. 2006). Studies on kinase regulation of pathological pain will greatly benefit from the development of specific and potent kinase inhibitors.

5
Summary

There are over 500 protein kinases in the human genome. More than 20 protein kinase inhibitors are in clinical trials, and many others have entered clinical trials without their structure being disclosed, and a great many more are still in preclinical studies. Protein kinases are becoming the second largest group of drug targets after GPCRs, accounting for 20%–30% of drug discovery activity in many pharmaceutical companies. There is increasing evidence suggesting that protein kinases play essential roles in regulating various kinds of pathological pain in animal models. Although many protein kinase inhibitors are in clinical trials for treating different diseases, especially cancer, they are not specifically being tested for clinical pain.

Animal studies have shown that kinase inhibitors do not affect basal pain perception, indicating that protein kinases are not very active in normal conditions. Although several kinases such as ERK, PI3K, and Cdk5 are important for cell growth during development, they play different roles in the adult by regulating neural plasticity. Importantly, protein kinases are activated after tissue injuries and contribute to the induction and maintenance of pathological pain by posttranslational, translational, and transcriptional regulation. Therefore, protein kinase inhibitors are different from traditional analgesics such as morphine. Instead of raising pain thresholds, they are antihyperalgesic and antiallodynic by "normalizing" pain sensitivity.

There is growing interest in MAPK cascades in the field of pain research for the following reasons:

– There are specific antibodies available to detect the activation of ERK, p38, and JNK. Potentially, phosphorylated MAPKs could be used as biomarkers for pathological pain.

– Compared to other kinases, there are relatively specific inhibitors available to study the function of MAPK pathways.

– MAPK pathways appear to be downstream to many other kinases.

– Multiple MAPK inhibitors are in clinical trials for treating different diseases.

Chronic pain (persistent pathological pain) has affected hundreds of millions people in the world. Although pathological pain is an expression of neural plasticity manifesting as peripheral and central sensitization, the activation of glial cells enhance and prolong neuronal sensitization. Since traditional painkillers were mainly designed to target neurons and are only partially effective, the development of glial- or neural/glial-targeting protein kinase inhibitors (e.g., MAPK inhibitors) could lead to more effective treatments for chronic pain.

References

Abbadie C, Lindia JA, Cumiskey AM, Peterson LB, Mudgett JS, Bayne EK, DeMartino JA, MacIntyre DE, Forrest MJ (2003) Impaired neuropathic pain responses in mice lacking the chemokine receptor CCR2. Proc Natl Acad Sci U S A 100:7947–7952

Adwanikar H, Karim F, Gereau RW (2004) Inflammation persistently enhances nocifensive behaviors mediated by spinal group I mGluRs through sustained ERK activation. Pain 111:125–135

Aley KO, Levine JD (1999) Role of protein kinase A in the maintenance of inflammatory pain. J Neurosci 19:2181–2186

Aley KO, McCarter G, Levine JD (1998) Nitric oxide signaling in pain and nociceptor sensitization in the rat. J Neurosci 18:7008–7014

Aley KO, Martin A, McMahon T, Mok J, Levine JD, Messing RO (2001) Nociceptor sensitization by extracellular signal-regulated kinases. J Neurosci 21:6933–6939

Battaglia AA, Sehayek K, Grist J, McMahon SB, Gavazzi I (2003) EphB receptors and ephrin-B ligands regulate spinal sensory connectivity and modulate pain processing. Nat Neurosci 6:339–340

Bennett GJ, Xie YK (1988) A peripheral mononeuropathy in rat that produces disorders of pain sensation like those seen in man. Pain 33:87–107

Bird GC, Lash LL, Han JS, Zou X, Willis WD, Neugebauer V (2005) Protein kinase A-dependent enhanced NMDA receptor function in pain-related synaptic plasticity in rat amygdala neurones. J Physiol 564:907–921

Borsello T, Bonny C (2004) Use of cell-permeable peptides to prevent neuronal degeneration. Trends Mol Med 10:239–244

Borsello T, Clarke PG, Hirt L, Vercelli A, Repici M, Schorderet DF, Bogousslavsky J, Bonny C (2003) A peptide inhibitor of c-Jun N-terminal kinase protects against excitotoxicity and cerebral ischemia. Nat Med 9:1180–1186

Brennan TJ, Vandermeulen EP, Gebhart GF (1996) Characterization of a rat model of incisional pain. Pain 64:493–501

Caterina MJ, Leffler A, Malmberg AB, Martin WJ, Trafton J, Petersen-Zeitz KR, Koltzenburg M, Basbaum AI, Julius D (2000) Impaired nociception and pain sensation in mice lacking the capsaicin receptor. Science 288:306–313

Chen L, Huang LY (1992) Protein kinase C reduces Mg2+ block of NMDA-receptor channels as a mechanism of modulation. Nature 356:521–523

Chuang HH, Prescott ED, Kong H, Shields S, Jordt SE, Basbaum AI, Chao MV, Julius D (2001) Bradykinin and nerve growth factor release the capsaicin receptor from PtdIns(4,5)P2-mediated inhibition. Nature 411:957–962

Coderre TJ (1992) Contribution of protein kinase C to central sensitization and persistent pain following tissue injury. Neurosci Lett 140:181–184

Coderre TJ, Yashpal K (1994) Intracellular messengers contributing to persistent nociception and hyperalgesia induced by L-glutamate and substance P in the rat formalin pain model. Eur J Neurosci 6:1328–1334

Cohen P (2002) Protein kinases—the major drug targets of the twenty-first century? Nat Rev Drug Discov 1:309–315

Dai Y, Iwata K, Fukuoka T, Kondo E, Tokunaga A, Yamanaka H, Tachibana T, Liu Y, Noguchi K (2002) Phosphorylation of extracellular signal-regulated kinase in primary afferent neurons by noxious stimuli and its involvement in peripheral sensitization. J Neurosci 22:7737–7745

Decosterd I, Woolf CJ (2000) Spared nerve injury: an animal model of persistent peripheral neuropathic pain. Pain 87:149–158

DeLeo JA, Yezierski RP (2001) The role of neuroinflammation and neuroimmune activation in persistent pain. Pain 90:1–6

Fang L, Wu J, Lin Q, Willis WD (2002) Calcium-calmodulin-dependent protein kinase II contributes to spinal cord central sensitization. J Neurosci 22:4196–4204

Galan A, Cervero F, Laird JM (2003) Extracellular signaling-regulated kinase-1 and -2 (ERK 1/2) mediate referred hyperalgesia in a murine model of visceral pain. Brain Res Mol Brain Res 116:126–134

Galan A, Laird JM, Cervero F (2004) In vivo recruitment by painful stimuli of AMPA receptor subunits to the plasma membrane of spinal cord neurons. Pain 112:315–323

Garry EM, Moss A, Delaney A, O'Neill F, Blakemore J, Bowen J, Husi H, Mitchell R, Grant SG, Fleetwood-Walker SM (2003) Neuropathic sensitization of behavioral reflexes and spinal NMDA receptor/CaM kinase II interactions are disrupted in PSD-95 mutant mice. Curr Biol 13:321–328

Gold MS, Levine JD, Correa AM (1998) Modulation of TTX-R INa by PKC and PKA and their role in PGE2-induced sensitization of rat sensory neurons in vitro. J Neurosci 18:10345–10355

Guan Y, Guo W, Robbins MT, Dubner R, Ren K (2004) Changes in AMPA receptor phosphorylation in the rostral ventromedial medulla after inflammatory hyperalgesia in rats. Neurosci Lett 366:201–205

Guo W, Zou S, Guan Y, Ikeda T, Tal M, Dubner R, Ren K (2002) Tyrosine phosphorylation of the NR2B subunit of the NMDA receptor in the spinal cord during the development and maintenance of inflammatory hyperalgesia. J Neurosci 22:6208–6217

Hu HJ, Glauner KS, Gereau RW (2003) ERK integrates PKA and PKC signaling in superficial dorsal horn neurons. I. Modulation of A-type K+ currents. J Neurophysiol 90:1671–1679

Huang WJ, Wang BR, Yao LB, Huang CS, Wang X, Zhang P, Jiao XY, Duan XL, Chen BF, Ju G (2000) Activity of p44/42 MAP kinase in the caudal subnucleus of trigeminal spinal nucleus is increased following perioral noxious stimulation in the mouse. Brain Res 861:181–185

Hunt SP, Pini A, Evan G (1987) Induction of c-fos-like protein in spinal cord neurons following sensory stimulation. Nature 328:632–634

Inoue M, Rashid MH, Fujita R, Contos JJ, Chun J, Ueda H (2004) Initiation of neuropathic pain requires lysophosphatidic acid receptor signaling. Nat Med 10:712–718

Ji RR (2004) Mitogen-activated protein kinases as potential targets for pain killers. Curr Opin Investig Drugs 5:71–75

Ji RR, Strichartz G (2004) Cell signaling and the genesis of neuropathic pain. Sci STKE 2004:reE14

Ji RR, Woolf CJ (2001) Neuronal plasticity and signal transduction in nociceptive neurons: implications for the initiation and maintenance of pathological pain. Neurobiol Dis 8:1–10

Ji RR, Shi TJ, Xu ZQ, Zhang Q, Sakagami H, Tsubochi H, Kondo H, Hokfelt T (1996) Ca2+/calmodulin-dependent protein kinase type IV in dorsal root ganglion: colocalization with peptides, axonal transport and effect of axotomy. Brain Res 721:167–173

Ji RR, Baba H, Brenner GJ, Woolf CJ (1999) Nociceptive-specific activation of ERK in spinal neurons contributes to pain hypersensitivity. Nat Neurosci 2:1114–1119

Ji RR, Befort K, Brenner GJ, Woolf CJ (2002a) ERK MAP kinase activation in superficial spinal cord neurons induces prodynorphin and NK-1 upregulation and contributes to persistent inflammatory pain hypersensitivity. J Neurosci 22:478–485

Ji RR, Samad TA, Jin SX, Schmoll R, Woolf CJ (2002b) p38 MAPK activation by NGF in primary sensory neurons after inflammation increases TRPV1 levels and maintains heat hyperalgesia. Neuron 36:57–68

Ji RR, Kohno T, Moore KA, Woolf CJ (2003) Central sensitization and LTP: do pain and memory share similar mechanisms? Trends Neurosci 26:696–705

Jin SX, Zhuang ZY, Woolf CJ, Ji RR (2003) p38 mitogen-activated protein kinase is activated after a spinal nerve ligation in spinal cord microglia and dorsal root ganglion neurons and contributes to the generation of neuropathic pain. J Neurosci 23:4017–4022

Johansen JP, Fields HL, Manning BH (2001) The affective component of pain in rodents: direct evidence for a contribution of the anterior cingulate cortex. Proc Natl Acad Sci U S A 98:8077–8082

Julius D, Basbaum AI (2001) Molecular mechanisms of nociception. Nature 413:203–210

Karim F, Wang CC, Gereau RW (2001) Metabotropic glutamate receptor subtypes 1 and 5 are activators of extracellular signal-regulated kinase signaling required for inflammatory pain in mice. J Neurosci 21:3771–3779

Kawasaki Y, Kohno T, Zhuang ZY, Brenner GJ, Wang H, Van Der MC, Befort K, Woolf CJ, Ji RR (2004) Ionotropic and metabotropic receptors, protein kinase A, protein kinase C, and Src contribute to C-fiber-induced ERK activation and cAMP response element-binding protein phosphorylation in dorsal horn neurons, leading to central sensitization. J Neurosci 24:8310–8321

Khasar SG, Lin YH, Martin A, Dadgar J, McMahon T, Wang D, Hundle B, Aley KO, Isenberg W, McCarter G, Green PG, Hodge CW, Levine JD, Messing RO (1999) A novel nociceptor signaling pathway revealed in protein kinase C epsilon mutant mice. Neuron 24:253–260

Kim SH, Chung JM (1992) An experimental model for peripheral neuropathy produced by segmental spinal nerve ligation in the rat. Pain 50:355–363

Kim SY, Bae JC, Kim JY, Lee HL, Lee KM, Kim DS, Cho HJ (2002) Activation of p38 MAP kinase in the rat dorsal root ganglia and spinal cord following peripheral inflammation and nerve injury. Neuroreport 13:2483–2486

Koistinaho M, Koistinaho J (2002) Role of p38 and p44/42 mitogen-activated protein kinases in microglia. Glia 40:175–183

Kolaj M, Cerne R, Cheng G, Brickey DA, Randic M (1994) Alpha subunit of calcium/calmodulin-dependent protein kinase enhances excitatory amino acid and synaptic responses of rat spinal dorsal horn neurons. J Neurophysiol 72:2525–2531

Koyama T, Tanaka YZ, Mikami A (1998) Nociceptive neurons in the macaque anterior cingulate activate during anticipation of pain. Neuroreport 9:2663–2667

Lei LG, Sun S, Gao YJ, Zhao ZQ, Zhang YQ (2004) NMDA receptors in the anterior cingulate cortex mediate pain-related aversion. Exp Neurol 189:413–421

Lever IJ, Pezet S, McMahon SB, Malcangio M (2003) The signaling components of sensory fiber transmission involved in the activation of ERK MAP kinase in the mouse dorsal horn. Mol Cell Neurosci 24:259–270

Li X, Shi X, Liang DY, Clark JD (2005) Spinal CK2 regulates nociceptive signaling in models of inflammatory pain. Pain 115:182–190

Lonze BE, Ginty DD (2002) Function and regulation of CREB family transcription factors in the nervous system. Neuron 35:605–623

Ma W, Quirion R (2002) Partial sciatic nerve ligation induces increase in the phosphorylation of extracellular signal-regulated kinase (ERK) and c-Jun N-terminal kinase (JNK) in astrocytes in the lumbar spinal dorsal horn and the gracile nucleus. Pain 99:175–184

Malmberg AB, Brandon EP, Idzerda RL, Liu H, McKnight GS, Basbaum AI (1997a) Diminished inflammation and nociceptive pain with preservation of neuropathic pain in mice with a targeted mutation of the type I regulatory subunit of cAMP-dependent protein kinase. J Neurosci 17:7462–7470

Malmberg AB, Chen C, Tonegawa S, Basbaum AI (1997b) Preserved acute pain and reduced neuropathic pain in mice lacking PKCgamma. Science 278:279–283

Manning G, Whyte DB, Martinez R, Hunter T, Sudarsanam S (2002) The protein kinase complement of the human genome. Science 298:1912–1934

Mannion RJ, Costigan M, Decosterd I, Amaya F, Ma QP, Holstege JC, Ji RR, Acheson A, Lindsay RM, Wilkinson GA, Woolf CJ (1999) Neurotrophins: peripherally and centrally acting modulators of tactile stimulus-induced inflammatory pain hypersensitivity. Proc Natl Acad Sci U S A 96:9385–9390

Mantyh PW, Rogers SD, Honore P, Allen BJ, Ghilardi JR, Li J, Daughters RS, Lappi DA, Wiley RG, Simone DA (1997) Inhibition of hyperalgesia by ablation of lamina I spinal neurons expressing the substance P receptor. Science 278:275–279

Mantyh PW, Clohisy DR, Koltzenburg M, Hunt SP (2002) Molecular mechanisms of cancer pain. Nat Rev Cancer 2:201–209

Mao J, Price DD, Mayer DJ, Hayes RL (1992) Pain-related increases in spinal cord membrane-bound protein kinase C following peripheral nerve injury. Brain Res 588:144–149

Martin WJ, Liu H, Wang H, Malmberg AB, Basbaum AI (1999) Inflammation-induced up-regulation of protein kinase Cgamma immunoreactivity in rat spinal cord correlates with enhanced nociceptive processing. Neuroscience 88:1267–1274

McMahon SB, Bennett DL, Priestley JV, Shelton DL (1995) The biological effects of endogenous nerve growth factor on adult sensory neurons revealed by a trkA-IgG fusion molecule. Nat Med 1:774–780

Meller ST, Gebhart GF (1993) Nitric oxide (NO) and nociceptive processing in the spinal cord. Pain 52:127–136

Meller ST, Dykstra C, Grzybycki D, Murphy S, Gebhart GF (1994) The possible role of glia in nociceptive processing and hyperalgesia in the spinal cord of the rat. Neuropharmacology 33:1471–1478

Milligan ED, Twining C, Chacur M, Biedenkapp J, O'Connor K, Poole S, Tracey K, Martin D, Maier SF, Watkins LR (2003) Spinal glia and proinflammatory cytokines mediate mirror-image neuropathic pain in rats. J Neurosci 23:1026–1040

Mueller BK, Mack H, Teusch N (2005) Rho kinase, a promising drug target for neurological disorders. Nat Rev Drug Discov 4:387–398

Nikas SN, Drosos AA (2004) SCIO-469 Scios Inc. Curr Opin Investig Drugs 5:1205–1212

Noble ME, Endicott JA, Johnson LN (2004) Protein kinase inhibitors: insights into drug design from structure. Science 303:1800–1805

Obata K, Noguchi K (2004) MAPK activation in nociceptive neurons and pain hypersensitivity. Life Sci 74:2643–2653

Obata K, Yamanaka H, Kobayashi K, Dai Y, Mizushima T, Katsura H, Fukuoka T, Tokunaga A, Noguchi K (2004) Role of mitogen-activated protein kinase activation in injured and intact primary afferent neurons for mechanical and heat hypersensitivity after spinal nerve ligation. J Neurosci 24:10211–10222

Porreca F, Lai J, Bian D, Wegert S, Ossipov MH, Eglen RM, Kassotakis L, Novakovic S, Rabert DK, Sangameswaran L, Hunter JC (1999) A comparison of the potential role of the tetrodotoxin-insensitive sodium channels, PN3/SNS and NaN/SNS2, in rat models of chronic pain. Proc Natl Acad Sci U S A 96:7640–7644

Porreca F, Ossipov MH, Gebhart GF (2002) Chronic pain and medullary descending facilitation. Trends Neurosci 25:319–325

Presley RW, Menetrey D, Levine JD, Basbaum AI (1990) Systemic morphine suppresses noxious stimulus-evoked Fos protein-like immunoreactivity in the rat spinal cord. J Neurosci 10:323–335

Raghavendra V, Tanga F, DeLeo JA (2003) Inhibition of microglial activation attenuates the development but not existing hypersensitivity in a rat model of neuropathy. J Pharmacol Exp Ther 306:624–630

Salter MW, Kalia LV (2004) Src kinases: a hub for NMDA receptor regulation. Nat Rev Neurosci 5:317–328

Sandkuhler J (2000) Learning and memory in pain pathways. Pain 88:113–118

Schafers M, Svensson CI, Sommer C, Sorkin LS (2003) Tumor necrosis factor-alpha induces mechanical allodynia after spinal nerve ligation by activation of p38 MAPK in primary sensory neurons. J Neurosci 23:2517–2521

Scholz J, Woolf CJ (2002) Can we conquer pain? Nat Neurosci 5 Suppl:1062–1067

Sebolt-Leopold JS, Herrera R (2004) Targeting the mitogen-activated protein kinase cascade to treat cancer. Nat Rev Cancer 4:937–947

Sebolt-Leopold JS, Dudley DT, Herrera R, Van Becelaere K, Wiland A, Gowan RC, Tecle H, Barrett SD, Bridges A, Przybranowski S, Leopold WR, Saltiel AR (1999) Blockade of the MAP kinase pathway suppresses growth of colon tumors in vivo. Nat Med 5:810–816

Sluka KA, Willis WD (1997) The effects of G-protein and protein kinase inhibitors on the behavioral responses of rats to intradermal injection of capsaicin. Pain 71:165–178

Stein C, Millan MJ, Herz A (1988) Unilateral inflammation of the hindpaw in rats as a model of prolonged noxious stimulation: alterations in behavior and nociceptive thresholds. Pharmacol Biochem Behav 31:455–451

Sung YJ, Walters ET, Ambron RT (2004) A neuronal isoform of protein kinase G couples mitogen-activated protein kinase nuclear import to axotomy-induced long-term hyperexcitability in Aplysia sensory neurons. J Neurosci 24:7583–7595

Svensson CI, Hua XY, Protter AA, Powell HC, Yaksh TL (2003a) Spinal p38 MAP kinase is necessary for NMDA-induced spinal PGE(2) release and thermal hyperalgesia. Neuroreport 14:1153–1157

Svensson CI, Marsala M, Westerlund A, Calcutt NA, Campana WM, Freshwater JD, Catalano R, Feng Y, Protter AA, Scott B, Yaksh TL (2003b) Activation of p38 mitogen-activated protein kinase in spinal microglia is a critical link in inflammation-induced spinal pain processing. J Neurochem 86:1534–1544

Svensson CI, Lucas KK, Hua XY, Powell HC, Dennis EA, Yaksh TL (2005) Spinal phospholipase A(2) in inflammatory hyperalgesia: role of the small, secretory phospholipase A(2). Neuroscience 133:543–553

Sweitzer SM, Schubert P, DeLeo JA (2001) Propentofylline, a glial modulating agent, exhibits antiallodynic properties in a rat model of neuropathic pain. J Pharmacol Exp Ther 297:1210–1217

Sweitzer SM, Medicherla S, Almirez R, Dugar S, Chakravarty S, Shumilla JA, Yeomans DC, Protter AA (2004) Antinociceptive action of a p38alpha MAPK inhibitor, SD-282, in a diabetic neuropathy model. Pain 109:409–419

Tanga FY, Nutile-McMenemy N, DeLeo JA (2005) The CNS role of Toll-like receptor 4 in innate neuroimmunity and painful neuropathy. Proc Natl Acad Sci U S A 102:5856–5861

Tatsumi S, Mabuchi T, Katano T, Matsumura S, Abe T, Hidaka H, Suzuki M, Sasaki Y, Minami T, Ito S (2005) Involvement of Rho-kinase in inflammatory and neuropathic pain through phosphorylation of myristoylated alanine-rich C-kinase substrate (MARCKS). Neuroscience 131:491–498

Tegeder I, Del Turco D, Schmidtko A, Sausbier M, Feil R, Hofmann F, Deller T, Ruth P, Geisslinger G (2004a) Reduced inflammatory hyperalgesia with preservation of acute thermal nociception in mice lacking cGMP-dependent protein kinase I. Proc Natl Acad Sci U S A 101:3253–3257

Tegeder I, Niederberger E, Schmidt R, Kunz S, Guhring H, Ritzeler O, Michaelis M, Geisslinger G (2004b) Specific Inhibition of IkappaB kinase reduces hyperalgesia in inflammatory and neuropathic pain models in rats. J Neurosci 24:1637–1645

Toker A, Cantley LC (1997) Signalling through the lipid products of phosphoinositide-3-OH kinase. Nature 387:673–676

Tsuda M, Shigemoto-Mogami Y, Koizumi S, Mizokoshi A, Kohsaka S, Salter MW, Inoue K (2003) P2X4 receptors induced in spinal microglia gate tactile allodynia after nerve injury. Nature 424:778–783

Tsuda M, Mizokoshi A, Shigemoto-Mogami Y, Koizumi S, Inoue K (2004) Activation of p38 mitogen-activated protein kinase in spinal hyperactive microglia contributes to pain hypersensitivity following peripheral nerve injury. Glia 45:89–95

Tsuda M, Inoue K, Salter MW (2005) Neuropathic pain and spinal microglia: a big problem from molecules in "small" glia. Trends Neurosci 28:101–107

Urban MO, Gebhart GF (1999) Supraspinal contributions to hyperalgesia. Proc Natl Acad Sci U S A 96:7687–7692

Verge GM, Milligan ED, Maier SF, Watkins LR, Naeve GS, Foster AC (2004) Fractalkine (CX3CL1) and fractalkine receptor (CX3CR1) distribution in spinal cord and dorsal root ganglia under basal and neuropathic pain conditions. Eur J Neurosci 20:1150–1160

Wang CH, Chou WY, Hung KS, Jawan B, Lu CN, Liu JK, Hung YP, Lee TH (2005) Intrathecal administration of roscovitine inhibits Cdk5 activity and attenuates formalin-induced nociceptive response in rats. Acta Pharmacol Sin 26:46–50

Watkins LR, Maier SF (2003) Glia: a novel drug discovery target for clinical pain. Nat Rev Drug Discov 2:973–985

Watkins LR, Martin D, Ulrich P, Tracey KJ, Maier SF (1997) Evidence for the involvement of spinal cord glia in subcutaneous formalin induced hyperalgesia in the rat. Pain 71:225–235

Watkins LR, Milligan ED, Maier SF (2001) Glial activation: a driving force for pathological pain. Trends Neurosci 24:450–455

Wei F, Qiu CS, Kim SJ, Muglia L, Maas JW, Pineda VV, Xu HM, Chen ZF, Storm DR, Muglia LJ, Zhuo M (2002a) Genetic elimination of behavioral sensitization in mice lacking calmodulin-stimulated adenylyl cyclases. Neuron 36:713–726

Wei F, Qiu CS, Liauw J, Robinson DA, Ho N, Chatila T, Zhuo M (2002b) Calcium calmodulin-dependent protein kinase IV is required for fear memory. Nat Neurosci 5:573–579

Widmann C, Gibson S, Jarpe MB, Johnson GL (1999) Mitogen-activated protein kinase: conservation of a three-kinase module from yeast to human. Physiol Rev 79:143–180

Willis WD (2002) Long-term potentiation in spinothalamic neurons. Brain Res Brain Res Rev 40:202–214

Woolf CJ, Salter MW (2000) Neuronal plasticity: increasing the gain in pain. Science 288:1765–1769

Yu CG, Yezierski RP (2005) Activation of the ERK1/2 signaling cascade by excitotoxic spinal cord injury. Brain Res Mol Brain Res 138:244–255

Yu YQ, Chen J (2005) Activation of spinal extracellular signaling-regulated kinases by intraplantar melittin injection. Neurosci Lett 381:194–198

Zeitz KP, Giese KP, Silva AJ, Basbaum AI (2004) The contribution of autophosphorylated alpha-calcium-calmodulin kinase II to injury-induced persistent pain. Neuroscience 128:889–898

Zhang X, Verge V, Wiesenfeld-Hallin Z, Ju G, Bredt D, Synder SH, Hokfelt T (1993) Nitric oxide synthase-like immunoreactivity in lumbar dorsal root ganglia and spinal cord of rat and monkey and effect of peripheral axotomy. J Comp Neurol 335:563–575

Zhang X, Wu J, Fang L, Willis WD (2003) The effects of protein phosphatase inhibitors on nociceptive behavioral responses of rats following intradermal injection of capsaicin. Pain 106:443–451

Zhang YQ, Zhao ZQ, Ji RR (2005) Emotional distress and related memory of pain: a neuro-biological review. Nerosci Bull 21:10–17

Zhuang ZY, Xu H, Clapham DE, Ji RR (2004) Phosphatidylinositol 3-kinase activates ERK in primary sensory neurons and mediates inflammatory heat hyperalgesia through TRPV1 sensitization. J Neurosci 24:8300–8309

Zhuang ZY, Gerner P, Woolf CJ, Ji RR (2005) ERK is sequentially activated in neurons, microglia, and astrocytes by spinal nerve ligation and contributes to mechanical allodynia in this neuropathic pain model. Pain 114:149–159

Zhuang ZY, Wen YR, Zhang DR, Borsello T, Bonny C, Strichartz GR, Decosterd I, Ji RR (2006) A peptide c-Jun N-terminal kinase (JNK) inhibitor blocks mechanical allodynia after spinal nerve ligation: respective roles of JNK activation in primary sensory neurons and spinal astrocytes for neuropathic pain development and maintenance. J Neurosci 26:3551–3560

Zou X, Lin Q, Willis WD (2000) Enhanced phosphorylation of NMDA receptor 1 subunits in spinal cord dorsal horn and spinothalamic tract neurons after intradermal injection of capsaicin in rats. J Neurosci 20:6989–6997

Part V
Pain Management Beyond Pharmacotherapy

HEP (2006) 177:393–413
© Springer-Verlag Berlin Heidelberg 2006

Placebo and Endogenous Mechanisms of Analgesia

F. Benedetti

Department of Neuroscience, Clinical and Applied Physiology Programme,
University of Turin Medical School, Corso Raffaello 30, 10125 Turin, Italy
fabrizio.benedetti@unito.it

1	Endogenous Mechanisms of Analgesia	394
2	The Placebo Effect	395
2.1	Methodology to Reveal Real Placebo Effects	395
2.2	The Role of Expectation, Motivation and Conditioning	396
3	The Neurobiology of the Placebo Effect	398
3.1	Opioid Mechanisms	398
3.2	Non-opioid Mechanisms	401
4	The Uncertainty Principle in Clinical Trials	403
5	Hidden Administration of Painkillers	404
6	Harnessing Placebo Effects to the Patient's Advantage	406
6.1	The Therapist–Patient Interaction	406
6.2	Reducing Drug Intake	407
7	Conclusions	408
	References	408

Abstract The discovery of the endogenous systems of analgesia has produced a large amount of research aimed at investigating their biochemical and neurophysiological mechanisms and their neuroanatomical localization. Nevertheless, the neurobiological acquisitions on these mechanisms have not been paralleled by behavioural correlates in humans—in other words, by the understanding of when and how these endogenous mechanisms of analgesia are activated. Until recent times one of the most studied behavioural correlates of endogenous analgesia was stress-induced analgesia, in which the activation of endogenous opioid systems is known to be involved. By contrast, today the placebo analgesic effect represents one of the best-described situations in which this endogenous opioid network is naturally activated in humans. Therefore, not only is placebo research helpful towards improving clinical trial design and medical practice, but it also provides us with a better understanding of the endogenous mechanisms of analgesia.

Keywords Placebo · Endogenous opioids · Expectation · Conditioning · Clinical trials

1
Endogenous Mechanisms of Analgesia

Placebo administration has been found to activate the endogenous mechanisms of analgesia, and today the placebo effect represents one of the most interesting models to help us understand when and how these mechanisms are activated (Petrovic et al. 2002; Wager et al. 2004; Colloca and Benedetti 2005). As most of our knowledge about placebo analgesia is based on opioid mechanisms, particular attention has been paid to the endogenous opioid systems. However, non-opioid mechanisms are also involved in placebo analgesia (Colloca and Benedetti 2005), although nothing is known about them. A recent comprehensive review of the endogenous mechanisms of analgesia by Millan (2002) clearly shows the complexity of this endogenous network, which includes both opioid and non-opioid systems. Thus, the opioid systems represent a first step towards understanding the intricate mechanisms underlying the placebo analgesic effect.

Opioid receptors can be found throughout the brain, brainstem and spinal cord (Pfeiffer et al. 1982; Wamsley et al. 1982; Atweh and Kuhar 1983; Sadzot et al. 1991; Fields and Basbaum 1999; Fields 2004). These receptors may exert analgesic effects through different mechanisms (Jensen 1997), such as modulation at the spinal level and/or control of cortical and brainstem regions. The modulation of the spinal cord is one of the best described (Fields and Basbaum 1999; Fields 2004). The opioid system in the brainstem comprises different regions like the periaqueductal grey (PAG), the parabrachial nuclei (PBN) and the rostral ventromedial medulla (RVM) (Fields and Basbaum 1999; Fields 2004). Although the opioid receptors are less characterized in the cortex, autoradiographic studies indicate high concentrations of opioid receptors in the cingulate cortex and prefrontal cortex (Wamsley et al. 1982; Pfeiffer et al. 1982; Sadzot et al. 1991), and one of the highest levels of opioid receptor binding has been found in the anterior cingulate cortex (ACC) (Vogt et al. 1993). Studies performed by means of positron emission tomography (PET) and the radioactive opioid ^{11}C-diprenorphine confirm previous animal and human autoradiography findings (Jones et al. 1991; Willoch et al. 1999, 2004). In addition, opioid receptor agonists such as remifentanil and fentanyl have been shown to act on several regions known to be involved in pain processing and containing high concentrations of opioid receptors (Firestone et al. 1996; Adler et al. 1997; Casey et al. 2000; Wagner et al. 2001; Petrovic et al. 2002).

One of the main problems of this endogenous opioid network is to understand when and how it is involved in analgesic effects. For example, it has long been known that fear and stress play an important role in the activation of the endogenous opioid system (Willer and Albe-Fessard 1980; Fanselow 1994). It has also been hypothesized that several other contexts may be important for the activation of the endogenous opioid systems (Fields and Basbaum 1999; Price 1999). In this regard, today the placebo response is probably the best-described situation in which this endogenous opioid network is naturally activated in humans (Colloca and Benedetti 2005). Therefore, placebo research is also important for the understanding of the endogenous mechanisms of analgesia.

2
The Placebo Effect

2.1
Methodology to Reveal Real Placebo Effects

The placebo effect is the effect that follows the administration of an inert medical treatment (the placebo), be it pharmacological or not. In order for a placebo effect to be demonstrated, several other phenomena have to be ruled out (Table 1), as the placebo itself is not always the cause of the effect that is observed (Benedetti and Colloca 2004; Colloca and Benedetti 2005; Pollo and Benedetti 2004). For example, most painful conditions show a spontaneous variation in pain intensity that is known as natural history (Fields and Levine 1984). If a subject takes a placebo just before his pain starts decreasing, he may believe that the placebo is effective although that decrease would have occurred anyway. This is not a placebo effect but a misinterpretation of the cause–effect relationship. Regression to the mean represents another example. This is a statistical phenomenon in which individuals tend to receive their initial pain assessment when pain is near its greatest intensity, but their pain level is likely to be lower when they return for a second assessment (Davis 2002). In this case also, the improvement cannot be attributed to any intervention they might have undergone. A further source of confusion is represented by false-positive errors made by the patient according to signal detection theory (Allan and Siegel 2002). In other words, a patient may erroneously detect a symptomatic relief in response to an inert treatment. The ambiguity of the symptom intensity may also lead to biases following verbal suggestion of benefit. Sometimes it is a co-intervention, such as the mechanical stimulation produced by the insertion of a needle to inject an inert solution, which is responsible for the reduction of pain (Pollo and Benedetti 2004). All these examples show that, although an improvement may occur after the administration of a placebo, the placebo is not necessarily the cause of the effect that is observed.

In a clinical trial all these factors are present. Therefore, clinical trials do not represent a good model to study and to understand the mechanisms of the placebo effect. For example, it has been shown that many results obtained in the clinical trial setting (Hrobjartsson and Gotzsche 2001) differ from those obtained in the laboratory setting where strictly controlled conditions are adopted (Vase et al. 2002). In the laboratory setting, for instance, it is possible to compare a no-treatment group with a placebo group so that the spontaneous

Table 1 Causes that may induce pain reduction after placebo administration in a clinical trial, and methods for their identification

Possible cause of pain reduction after placebo administration	Methods for its identification
Spontaneous remission	Group that receives no treatment
Regression to the mean	Group that receives no treatment or experimentally controlled pain
Symptom ambiguity and bias	Objective measurements
Desire to please the experimenter	Objective measurements
Co-intervention (e.g. mechanical stimulation due to needle insertion to inject saline)	Correct experimental design
Complex cognitive functions (expectation, anticipation) (Real placebo effect)	Exclusion of the above causes and experimental design
Pavlovian conditioning (Real placebo effect)	Exclusion of the above causes and experimental design

remission of the symptom can be identified. The difference between the no-treatment group and the placebo group represents the real placebo effect. In the laboratory setting other confounding variables can be controlled as well (Benedetti and Colloca 2004; Colloca and Benedetti 2005), like regression to the mean, which can be ruled out by using experimental pain. Likewise, symptom detection ambiguity and subjects' biases can be eliminated through the measurement of objective physiological parameters. Finally, the effects of a co-intervention can be identified by using the appropriate experimental model.

The term placebo effect is generally considered to be different from placebo response. The former has been used to refer to any improvement in the condition of a group of subjects that has received a placebo. By contrast, the latter refers to the change in an individual caused by a placebo manipulation. However, these two terms can be used interchangeably.

2.2
The Role of Expectation, Motivation and Conditioning

When all the factors described above have been ruled out, the real placebo response is a psychobiological phenomenon whereby several brain mechanisms can be identified (Table 1). It is important to realize that the administration of a placebo involves the complex psychosocial context around the patient, such as the doctor's words, the hospital environment, the sight of a therapeutic apparatus and the like. Therefore, the study of the placebo effect is basically the study of the psychosocial context that surrounds the patient.

It has long been known that the placebo effect involves both cognitive factors and conditioning mechanisms. On the one hand the deceptive administration of a placebo treatment can lead the subjects to believe that the treatment is effective, such that the anticipation and expectation of analgesia lead to a significant placebo analgesic effect (Amanzio and Benedetti 1999; Benedetti et al. 1999b; Price et al. 1999; Pollo et al. 2001). Some studies show that different verbal instructions lead to different expectations and thus to different responses, and this plays a fundamental role in the placebo effect (Kirsch 1985; Kirsch and Weixel 1988; Kirsch 1990, 1999; Price and Fields 1997; Pollo et al. 2001). This occurs not only with placebos but even with active drugs such as epinephrine (Schachter and Singer 1962), amphetamine and chloral hydrate (Lyerly et al. 1964), and carisoprodol (Flaten et al. 1999). In other words, a typical drug effect can sometimes be reduced if the subjects are misinformed on the action of the drug and, similarly, new side-effects can be elicited with the appropriate verbal instructions. Motivation and desire for pain relief has also been found to play a role in placebo analgesia (Price and Fields 1997; Vase et al. 2003).

The context around a therapy may act not only through expectation and conscious anticipatory processes. There are some lines of evidence indicating that, at least in some circumstances, the placebo response is a conditioned response due to repeated associations between a conditioned stimulus (e.g. shape and colour of pills and tablets) and an unconditioned stimulus (the active substance inside the pills and tablets) (Gleidman et al. 1957; Herrnstein 1962; Siegel 1985, 2002; Ader 1997; Voudouris et al. 1989, 1990; Wickramasekera 2001). In this case, it is the context itself that is the conditioned stimulus. However, even by considering a typical conditioning procedure, it has been shown that a conditioned placebo response can result from conditioning but is actually mediated by expectancy (Montgomery and Kirsch 1997). In fact, conditioning would lead to the expectation that a given event will follow another event, and this occurs on the basis of the information that the conditioned stimulus provides about the unconditioned stimulus (Reiss 1980; Rescorla 1988).

A recent study has investigated some physiological functions that are affected by placebos through anticipatory conscious processes and some other functions that undergo an unconscious mechanism of conditioning (Benedetti et al. 2003b). For example, verbally induced expectations of either analgesia or hyperalgesia antagonize completely the effects of a conditioning procedure in experimentally induced pain. By contrast, verbally induced expectations of either an increase or decrease of growth hormone (GH) and cortisol do not have any effect on the secretion of these hormones. However, if a pre-conditioning is performed with sumatriptan, a serotonin agonist that stimulates GH and inhibits cortisol secretion, a significant GH increase and cortisol decrease can be found in plasma after placebo administration. These findings indicate that verbally induced expectations have no effect on hormonal secretion whereas they affect pain. This suggests that placebo responses are mediated by conditioning when unconscious physiological functions, like hormonal secretion, are involved, whereas they are mediated by expectation when conscious physiological processes, like pain, come into play. Thus the placebo effect is a phenomenon that can be learned either consciously or unconsciously, depending on the system that is involved.

3
The Neurobiology of the Placebo Effect

The recent explosion of research on the neurobiological mechanisms of the placebo effect is paying dividends, as we are beginning to understand the cascade of events that occur following the administration of a placebo along with verbal suggestions of clinical benefit (Fig. 1). Most of our neurobiological knowledge comes from the field of pain and analgesia, and several lines of evidence suggest that placebo administration activates the endogenous mechanisms of analgesia described in Sect. 1. Today we know that placebo analgesia is mediated by both opioid and non-opioid mechanisms, depending on different factors.

3.1
Opioid Mechanisms

An important step in understanding the mechanisms of placebo-induced analgesia was made in the clinical setting when Levine et al. (1978) provided evidence that placebo analgesia is mediated by endogenous opioids. Other studies subsequently further confirmed this hypothesis (Grevert et al. 1983; Levine and Gordon 1984; Benedetti 1996). In addition, cholecystokinin was found to inhibit placebo-induced analgesia, as cholecystokinin antagonists are capable of potentiating the placebo analgesic effect (Benedetti et al. 1995, 1996). In fact, cholecystokinin is an anti-opioid peptide which antagonizes endogenous opioid neuropeptides, so that its blockade results in the potentiation of opioid effects (Benedetti 1997).

Fields and Levine (1984) were the first to hypothesize that the placebo response may be subdivided into opioid and non-opioid components. In fact, they suggested that different physical, psychological and environmental situations could affect the endogenous opioid systems differently. This problem was recently addressed by Amanzio and Benedetti (1999), who showed that both expectation and a conditioning procedure could result in placebo analgesia. The former is capable of activating opioid systems whereas the latter activates specific sub-systems. In fact, if the placebo response is induced by means of strong expectation cues, it can be blocked by the opioid antagonist naloxone.

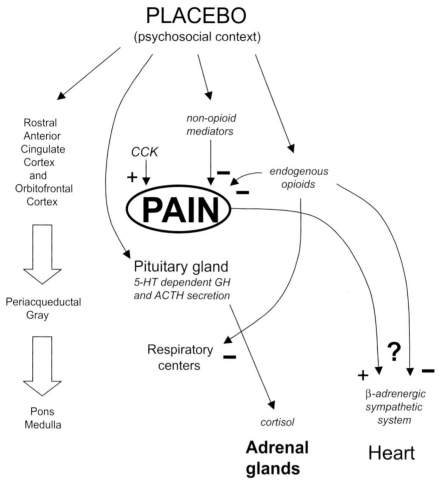

Fig. 1 Events that might occur following the administration of a placebo along with verbal suggestions of analgesia. A descending pain inhibitory network that involves the rostral anterior cingulate cortex, the orbitofrontal cortex, the periaqueductal grey and the pons/medulla is activated. Endogenous opioids might inhibit pain through this descending network and/or other mechanisms. The endogenous opioids also act at the level of the respiratory centres. The β-adrenergic sympathetic system is also inhibited during placebo analgesia, but the mechanism is not known (it might involve either reduction of the pain itself or direct action of endogenous opioids). Non-opioid mechanisms also play a role. Cholecystokinin (*CCK*) counteracts the effects of the endogenous opioids thus antagonizing placebo analgesia. Placebo can also affect serotonin-dependent hormone secretion, mimicking the effect of the analgesic drug sumatriptan. *GH*, growth hormone; *ACTH*, adrenocorticotropic hormone; *5HT*, serotonin

Conversely, if the placebo response is induced by means of a prior conditioning with a non-opioid drug, it is naloxone-insensitive.

Regional placebo analgesic responses can be obtained in different parts of the body (Montgomery and Kirsch 1996; Price et al. 1999), and these responses are naloxone-reversible (Benedetti et al. 1999b). If four noxious stimuli are applied to the hands and feet and a placebo cream is applied to one hand only, pain is reduced only on the hand where the placebo cream had been applied. This effect is blocked by naloxone, suggesting that the placebo-activated endogenous opioids have a somatotopic organization (Benedetti et al. 1999b). An additional study supporting the involvement of endogenous opioids in placebo analgesia was performed by Lipman et al. (1990) in chronic pain patients. These authors found that those patients who responded to placebo showed higher concentrations of endorphins in the cerebrospinal fluid compared with those patients who did not respond.

A likely candidate for the mediation of placebo-induced analgesia is the opioid neuronal network described in Sect. 1 (Fields and Price 1997; Fields and Basbaum 1999; Price 1999). A recent brain imaging study that used PET supports this hypothesis (Petrovic et al. 2002). These authors found that both a placebo and the rapidly acting opioid agonist remifentanil affect similar regions in the cerebral cortex and in the brainstem, thus indicating a related mechanism in placebo-induced and opioid-induced analgesia. In particular, the administration of a placebo induced the activation of the rostral anterior cingulate cortex (rACC) and the orbitofrontal cortex (OrbC). Moreover, there was a significant co-variation in activity between the rACC and the lower pons/medulla, and a sub-significant co-variation between the rACC and the PAG, thus suggesting that the descending rACC/PAG/brainstem pain-modulating circuit is involved in placebo analgesia. In another study using functional magnetic resonance imaging (fMRI), it was also found that brain activation patterns in the prefrontal cortex changed in anticipation to analgesia following placebo administration (Wager et al. 2004).

Placebo-activated endogenous opioids have also been shown to produce a typical side-effect of opioids, that is, respiratory depression (Benedetti et al. 1998; Benedetti et al. 1999a). After repeated administrations of analgesic doses of buprenorphine in the post-operative phase, which induces a mild decrease of ventilation, a placebo is capable of mimicking the same respiratory depressant response. This respiratory placebo response can be blocked by naloxone, indicating that it is mediated by endogenous opioids. Thus, placebo-activated opioid systems act not only on pain mechanisms but also on the respiratory centres.

The involvement of other systems during placebo analgesia is further supported by recent work in which the sympathetic and parasympathetic control of the heart were analysed during placebo analgesia (Pollo et al. 2003). In the clinical setting, it was found that the placebo analgesic response to a noxious stimulus was accompanied by a reduced heart rate response. In order to investigate this effect from a pharmacological viewpoint, the same effect was reproduced in the laboratory setting. It was found that the opioid antagonist naloxone completely antagonized both placebo analgesia and the concomitant reduced heart rate response, whereas the β-blocker propranolol antagonized the placebo heart rate reduction but not placebo analgesia. By contrast, both placebo responses were present during muscarinic blockade with atropine, indicating no involvement of the parasympathetic system. A spectral analysis of the heart rate variability for the identification of the sympathetic and parasympathetic components showed that the β-adrenergic low-frequency spectral component was reduced during placebo analgesia, an effect that was reversed by naloxone. These findings indicate that opioid-mediated placebo analgesia also affects the cardiovascular system, although we do not know whether the placebo-activated endogenous opioids inhibit the sympathetic system directly or—through the reduction of pain—indirectly.

3.2
Non-opioid Mechanisms

Recently, some non-opioid mechanisms have begun to be explored, although nothing is known about non-opioid mediators of placebo analgesia. In fact, the release of neurotransmitters, like dopamine, has been identified in other illnesses such as Parkinson's disease. Nonetheless, it is important to emphasize that the integration between the findings in the field of pain and those obtained in other pathological conditions is necessary and essential to better understand the intricate mechanisms of the placebo effect.

As described in Sect. 2.2, by using the analgesic drug sumatriptan, a serotonin agonist of the $5\text{-HT}_{1B/1D}$ receptors that stimulates GH and inhibits cortisol secretion, it was shown that a conditioning procedure is capable of producing hormonal placebo responses. In fact, if a placebo is given after repeated administrations of sumatriptan, a placebo GH increase and a placebo cortisol decrease can be found (Benedetti et al. 2003b). Interestingly, verbally induced expectations of increase/decrease of GH and cortisol did not have any effect on the secretion of these hormones. Therefore, whereas hormone secretion is not affected by expectations, it is affected by a conditioning procedure. Although we do not know whether these placebo responses are really mediated by serotonin, a pharmacological pre-conditioning appears to affect serotonin-dependent hormone secretion. These new findings may help investigate non-opioid mechanisms in placebo analgesia.

The verbal instructions that induce expectations may have either a hopeful and trust-inducing meaning, eliciting a placebo effect, or a fearful and stressful meaning, inducing a nocebo effect (Hahn 1985, 1997; Benedetti and Amanzio 1997; Moerman 2002a, b). In a study performed in post-operative patients (Benedetti et al. 1997), negative expectations were induced by injecting an inert substance along with the suggestion that pain was going to increase.

In fact, pain increased and this increase was prevented by the CCK antagonist proglumide. This indicates that expectation-induced hyperalgesia of these patients was mediated, at least in part, by CCK. The effects of proglumide were not antagonized by naloxone, which suggests that endogenous opioids were not involved. Since CCK plays a role in anxiety and negative expectations themselves are anxiogenic, these results suggest that proglumide acted on a CCK-dependent increase of anxiety during the verbally induced negative expectations. Although this study analysed a nocebo procedure, the involvement of CCK in the nocebo effect might help better clarify the modulation of pain by both positive and negative expectations.

The release of endogenous substances following a placebo procedure is a phenomenon which is not confined to the field of pain, but it is also present in motor disorders such as Parkinson's disease. As occurs with pain, in this case patients are given an inert substance (placebo) and are told that it is an anti-Parkinsonian drug that produces an improvement in their motor performance. Both clinical improvements (Shetty et al. 1999; Goetz et al. 2000; Pollo et a. 2002) and changes in the single-neuron firing pattern (Benedetti et al. 2004) have been found after placebo administration in Parkinson's patients. A study used PET in order to assess the competition between endogenous dopamine and ^{11}C-raclopride for D_2/D_3 receptors, a method that allows identification of endogenous dopamine release (de la Fuente-Fernandez et al. 2001). This study shows that placebo-induced expectation of motor improvement activates endogenous dopamine in the striatum of Parkinsonian patients, thus indicating that endogenous substances other than opioids may be involved in the placebo response in other illnesses. De la Fuente-Fernandez and Stoessl (2002) argue that the expectation-induced release of dopamine in Parkinson's disease is related to reward mechanisms. According to these authors, dopamine release by expectation of reward, in this case the expectation of clinical benefit, could represent a common biochemical substrate in many pathological situations, including pain. It is worth noting that there is an important interaction between dopamine and opioid systems, and that endogenous opioids are also involved in reward mechanisms (de la Fuente-Fernandez and Stoessl 2002).

Very recently, the neural mechanisms of placebo treatments have also been studied in depression, although these studies need further research and confirmation because they did not include appropriate control groups. Depressed patients who received a placebo treatment showed both electrical and metabolic changes in the brain. In the first case, placebos induced electroencephalographic changes in the prefrontal cortex of patients with major depression, particularly in the right hemisphere (Leuchter et al. 2002). In the second case, changes in brain glucose metabolism were measured by using PET in subjects with unipolar depression. Placebo treatments were associated with metabolic increases in the prefrontal, anterior cingulate, premotor, parietal, posterior insula, and posterior cingulate cortex, and metabolic decreases in the subgenual cingulate cortex, para-hippocampus and thalamus (Mayberg et al. 2002).

Interestingly, these regions also were affected by the selective serotonin reuptake inhibitor fluoxetine, a result that suggests a possible role for serotonin in placebo-induced antidepressant effects.

Therefore, although very little is known on the role of non-opioid mediators in placebo analgesia, the investigation of the placebo effect in other illnesses demonstrates that other neurotransmitters—like CCK, serotonin and dopamine—may contribute to the modulation of the placebo responses in different circumstances and pathological conditions.

4
The Uncertainty Principle in Clinical Trials

On the basis of the findings described above, it appears clear that different substances may be released in the patient's brain during the expectation of clinical benefit. For example, endogenous opioids are activated during expectation of analgesia. Can a drug interfere with these neuromediators of expectation? If yes, what is the effect?

In 1995 we ran a clinical trial in which the CCK antagonist proglumide was better than placebo, and placebo was better than no-treatment in relieving post-operative pain (Benedetti et al. 1995). According to classical clinical trial methodology, these results would indicate that proglumide is a good painkiller acting on the pain pathways, whereas placebo reduces pain by inducing expectations of analgesia. However, this conclusion proved to be erroneous, as a hidden injection of proglumide—a procedure whereby subjects are completely unaware that a treatment is being administered—was totally ineffective. If proglumide were a real painkiller acting on the pain pathways, its painkilling effects should have occurred anyway, regardless of the hidden injection. Therefore, the likely interpretation of the mechanism of action of proglumide is that it does not act on pain pathways at all, but rather on expectation pathways, thus enhancing the placebo analgesic response. In other words, proglumide induces a reduction of pain if, and only if, it is associated with a placebo procedure. Today we know that proglumide is not a painkiller, but it acts on placebo-activated opioid mechanisms.

This trial shows that sometimes it is difficult to understand the real action of a drug. In other words, as the patient's expectations of clinical benefit may induce a release of endogenous substances, virtually any drug may act on these expectation-activated biochemical events, thus confounding the interpretation of the data. As shown in Fig. 2, this represents a sort of uncertainty principle whereby we can never be certain about the mechanism of action of a therapeutic agent (Colloca and Benedetti 2005). As we have no a priori knowledge of which substances act on pain pathways and which on expectation mechanisms, it is sometimes extremely difficult to say whether a drug is a real painkiller. This uncertainty cannot be solved with the standard clinical trial design.

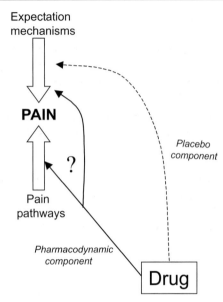

Fig. 2 The uncertainty principle in clinical trials. When a drug is injected, we cannot be sure where its pharmacodynamic effects take place. It can act either on the pain pathways or on placebo-activated expectation mechanisms

5
Hidden Administration of Painkillers

A partial solution to the uncertainty principle in clinical trials is represented by the hidden injection of drugs. In this condition, patients do not know that any drug is being injected; the expectation mechanisms are, so to speak, silent.

So far the placebo effect has been studied by simulating a treatment through the administration of a placebo, in order to eliminate the specific effects of the therapy itself. Recently, this approach has been changed completely by eliminating the placebo component and maintaining the specific effects of the treatment. In order to eliminate the context around a medical treatment the patient is made completely unaware that a medical therapy is being carried out. This can be done by administering drugs through computer-controlled machines (Gracely et al. 1983; Levine et al. 1981; Levine and Gordon 1984; Amanzio et al. 2001). In this situation, the patient does not know that any drug is being injected. For example, in post-operative pain following the extraction of the third molar, Levine et al. (1981) and Levine and Gordon (1984) found that a hidden injection of a 6- to 8-mg dose of morphine corresponds to an open injection of saline solution in full view of the patient (placebo). In other words, telling the patient that a painkiller is being injected (actually a placebo) is as potent as 6–8 mg of morphine. These authors concluded that an open injection of morphine in full view of the patient, which represents usual medical practice, is more effective than a hidden one because in the latter the placebo component is absent.

An analysis of the differences between open and hidden injections in the post-operative setting has been recently performed for four widely used painkillers: buprenorphine, tramadol, ketorolac and metamizol (Amanzio et al. 2001). The open administration was performed by a doctor at the bedside, and the patient was told that the injection was a powerful analgesic and that the pain was going to decrease in a few minutes. By contrast, the hidden injection of the same analgesic dose was performed by an automatic infusion machine that started delivering the painkiller without any doctor or nurse in the room. Thus, these patients were completely unaware that an analgesic therapy had been started. In a first analysis, it was found that the analgesic dose needed to reduce the pain by 50% (AD_{50}) was much higher when the infusion was carried out covertly than when it was carried out overtly, indicating that a hidden administration is less effective than an open one.

In a second analysis, it was found that the time course of post-operative pain was significantly different between open and hidden injections. In fact, during the first hour after the injection, pain ratings were much higher with a hidden injection than with an open one. In the same study (Amanzio et al. 2001), the difference between open and hidden injections was also investigated in the laboratory setting by inducing experimental ischaemic arm pain in healthy volunteers. As occurred in the clinical setting, it was found that a hidden injection of the non-opioid painkiller ketorolac was less effective than an open one. Most interesting, in these controlled experimental conditions the opiate antagonist naloxone was capable of reducing the open-hidden difference. This suggests that an open injection in full view of the patient activates the endogenous opioid systems which in turn enhance the effects of the injected painkiller. Therefore, the endogenous opioid mechanisms described above are likely to be present also in the routine therapist-patient relationship.

An extensive study has recently been performed in which treatments for different conditions like pain, anxiety, Parkinson's disease, tachycardia and bradycardia were given either overtly or covertly (Benedetti et al 2003a; see also Colloca et al. 2004 for a review). As far as pain is concerned, this study not only confirms the previous studies (Levine et al. 1981; Levine and Gordon 1984; Amanzio et al. 2001) but it also adds important clinical implications to the open-hidden paradigm. For example, in this study (Benedetti et al. 2003a) the open-hidden interruption of an analgesic therapy with morphine was investigated, and it was found that the relapse of pain occurred faster and the pain intensity was larger with an open interruption of morphine compared with a hidden one, which indicates that the hidden interruption prolonged the analgesic effect. Again, it is worth pointing out that the same results were found in anxiety, Parkinson's disease and heart rate changes (Benedetti et al. 2003a; see also Colloca et al. 2004 for a review). Therefore, pain and analgesia are not a special case.

Another example of the difference between the effects of expected and unexpected treatments is represented by a recent study by Volkow et al. (2003). The effects of methylphenidate on brain glucose metabolism, measured by ^{18}F-deoxyglucose-PET, were compared in cocaine abusers who did and did not expect to receive the drug. The effect of methylphenidate was approximately 50% greater in patients who expected the drug than those who did not. In other words, unexpected methylphenidate induced smaller metabolic changes in the brain, indicating that expectation enhances the pharmacological effects.

Although the difference between an open and a hidden injection cannot be called a placebo effect, as no placebo is administered, it strongly indicates the importance of the psychosocial context surrounding a therapy or, as suggested by Price (2001) and Vase et al. (2002), of the patient's perception that a therapy is being received. In particular, the real pharmacodynamic effect of a drug is likely to be represented by the outcome following the hidden administration, free of any psychological contamination.

6
Harnessing Placebo Effects to the Patient's Advantage

6.1
The Therapist–Patient Interaction

As the placebo effect is strongly induced by verbal suggestions, and indeed most of the studies described above used verbal suggestions to elicit placebo responses, a better understanding of the placebo effect is likely to improve the therapist–patient interaction. In other words, we are beginning to understand how the doctor's words affect the patient's brain (Benedetti 2002).

The powerful effect of the therapist–patient relationship and of the context surrounding the therapeutic setting has long been known and, accordingly, clinicians have used the appropriate words and attitudes with their patients. For example, Thomas (1987) found that positive and negative consultations in general practice have an important impact on patients who present with minor illness. Likewise, Kaplan et al. (1989) found that blood pressure, blood sugar, functional status and overall health status were consistently related to specific aspects of physician–patient communication. Although many other studies have shown that the doctor–patient relationship plays an important role in the outcome of illness (Stewart et al. 1979; Stewart 1995; Starfield et al. 1981; Gracely et al. 1985; Greenfield et al. 1985; Bass et al. 1986), the underlying mechanisms are not always clear. For example, a better interaction between the doctor and the patient might lead to a better compliance with the drug regimens (Inui et al. 1976). However, the symbolic and emotional impact of doctors and other aspects of medical contexts on the patient certainly have a crucial role (Brody 1988). This is also shown by the fact that diagnostic tests, which have nothing to do with therapy, reduce short-term disability (Sox et al. 1981).

On the basis of the recent neurobiological acquisitions concerning the placebo effect, today we can assert that words and attitudes of doctors, and more in general of the medical personnel, are capable of changing the biochemistry of the patient's brain and, in some circumstances, may help her recover from a symptom. In this regard, some ethical considerations are necessary, particularly with regard to placebos.

For example, in an article by Bok (1974), the administration of a placebo is seen as an unethical procedure since it necessarily involves some degree of deception, thus damaging the institution of medicine and contributing to the erosion of confidence and trust in medical staff and caregivers (see also Bok 2002). Rawlinson (1985) justifies such deception by using the concept of paternalism and benevolent deception, in which the physician's purpose is not actually to deceive but to cure. Rawlinson (1985) also asserts that one of the effects of illness is an undermining of the patient's autonomy, and the physician must restore this loss, even through the use of benevolent paternalism and deception. Of course, the use of benevolent deception in routine medical practice requires some rules: for example, that it never be employed for the convenience of the caregiver, that it be used only in cases where there is substantial evidence that it is necessary, or that the doctor determine whether any physical or psychological condition for which other treatments are indicated would be masked by the placebo itself.

Despite the ethical debate on the use of placebos in medical practice, a good therapist–patient relationship is always necessary and important. Therefore, by considering the reduced effects of a hidden treatment, the therapist should always strive to enhance the patient's expectations of the therapeutic outcome by using the appropriate words and attitudes.

6.2
Reducing Drug Intake

It is also important to stress that the ethical debate on the use of placebos in clinical practice needs to consider that the mechanisms of the placebo effect can be harnessed to the patient's advantage. For example, there is some experimental evidence that placebo administration can reduce the intake of narcotics.

In one study, post-operative patients were treated with buprenorphine on request for three consecutive days, and with a concurrent basal infusion of saline solution (Pollo et al. 2001). However, the symbolic meaning of this saline basal infusion varied in three different groups of patients. The first group was told that the infusion was a re-hydrating solution (natural history or no-treatment group), the second was told that it could be either a potent analgesic or a placebo (classic double-blind administration), and the third group was told that the infusion was a potent painkiller (deceptive administration). The placebo effect of the saline basal infusion was measured by recording the doses of buprenorphine requested over the 3-day treatment period. It is important to point out that the double-blind group received uncertain verbal instructions ("It can be either an inert substance or a painkiller"), whereas the deceptive administration group received certain instructions ("It is a painkiller"). There was a decrease in buprenorphine intake with the double-blind administration and even more so with the deceptive administration of the saline basal infusion. In fact, the reduction of buprenorphine requests in the double-blind group was as large as 20.8% compared with the natural history group, and the reduction in the deceptive administration group was even larger (33.8%).

It should be noted that the time-course of pain was the same in the three groups over the 3-day period of treatment. Thus, the same analgesic effect was obtained with different doses of buprenorphine. Although further experimental and clinical work is needed, this study clearly shows that those patients who are under the effect of strong expectations of analgesia request fewer drugs than those who are not.

7
Conclusions

The placebo effect has passed from a nuisance in clinical research to an important target of scientific inquiry. There are at least three points that have been clarified by using the placebo response as a model. First, the endogenous mechanisms of analgesia appear to come into play in different circumstances, but certainly a cognitive brain network plays a crucial role in the expectation and anticipation phase of analgesia. Second, in the interpretation of clinical trial outcomes, particular attention should be paid to the possibility that injected drugs do not have any specific effect, but rather they could act on expectation-activated endogenous substances (the uncertainty principle). Third, the hidden (unexpected) administration of medical treatments have shown that the knowledge about a therapy affects the therapeutic outcome, and highlights the important role of communication between the therapist and his or her patient.

References

Ader R (1997) The role of conditioning in pharmacotherapy. In: Harrington A (ed) The placebo effect: an interdisciplinary exploration. Harvard University Press, Cambridge, pp 138–165
Adler LJ, Gyulai FE, Diehl DJ, Mintun MA, Winter PM, Firestone LL (1997) Regional brain activity changes associated with fentanyl analgesia elucidated by positron emission tomography. Anesth Analg 84:120–126

Allan LG, Siegel S (2002) A signal detection theory analysis of the placebo effect. Eval Health Prof 25:410–420

Amanzio M, Benedetti F (1999) Neuropharmacological dissection of placebo analgesia: expectation-activated opioid systems versus conditioning-activated specific sub-systems. J Neurosci 19:484–494

Amanzio M, Pollo A, Maggi G, Benedetti F (2001) Response variability to analgesics: a role for non-specific activation of endogenous opioids. Pain 90:205–215

Atweh F, Kuhar MJ (1983) Distribution and physiological significance of opioid receptors in the brain. Br Med Bull 39:47–52

Bass MJ, Buck C, Turner L, Dickie G, Pratt G, Campbell Robinson H (1986) The physician's actions and the outcome of illness in family practice. J Fam Pract 23:43–47

Benedetti F (1996) The opposite effects of the opiate antagonist naloxone and the cholecystokinin antagonist proglumide on placebo analgesia. Pain 64:535–543

Benedetti F (1997) Cholecystokinin type-A and type-B receptors and their modulation of opioid analgesia. News Physiol Sci 12:263–268

Benedetti F (2002) How the doctor's words affect the patient's brain. Eval Health Prof 25:369–386

Benedetti F, Amanzio M (1997) The neurobiology of placebo: from endogenous opioids to cholecystokinin. Prog Neurobiol 52:109–125

Benedetti F, Colloca L (2004) Placebo-induced analgesia: methodology, neurobiology, clinical use, and ethics. Rev Analg 7:129–143

Benedetti F, Amanzio M, Maggi G (1995) Potentiation of placebo analgesia by proglumide. Lancet 346:1231

Benedetti F, Amanzio M, Casadio C, Oliaro A, Maggi G (1997) Blockade of nocebo hyperalgesia by the cholecystokinin antagonist proglumide. Pain 70:431–436

Benedetti F, Amanzio M, Baldi S, Casadio C, Cavallo A, Mancuso M, Ruffini E, Oliaro A, Maggi G (1998) The specific effects of prior opioid exposure on placebo analgesia and placebo respiratory depression. Pain 75:313–319

Benedetti F, Amanzio M, Baldi S, Casadio C, Maggi G (1999a) Inducing placebo respiratory depressant responses in humans via opioid receptors. Eur J Neurosci 11:625–631

Benedetti F, Arduino C, Amanzio M (1999b) Somatotopic activation of opioid systems by target-directed expectations of analgesia. J Neurosci 19:3639–3648

Benedetti F, Maggi G, Lopiano L, Lanotte M, Rainero I, Vighetti S, Pollo A (2003a) Open versus hidden medical treatments: the patient's knowledge about a therapy affects the therapy outcome. Prev Treatment. http://journals.apa.org/prevention/volume6/toc-jun-03.html. Cited 30 Apr 2006

Benedetti F, Pollo A, Lopiano L, Lanotte M, Vighetti S, Rainero I (2003b) Conscious expectation and unconscious conditioning in analgesic; motor and hormonal placebo/nocebo responses. J Neurosci 23:4315–4323

Benedetti F, Colloca L, Torre E, Lanotte M, Melcarne A, Pesare M, Bergamasco B, Lopiano L (2004) Placebo-responsive Parkinson patients show decreased activity in single neurons of subthalamic nucleus. Nat Neurosci 7:587–588

Bok S (1974) The ethics of giving placebos. Sci Am 231:17–23

Bok S (2002) Ethical issues in use of placebo in medical practise and clinical trials. In: Guess HA, Kleinman A, Kusek JW, Engel LW (eds) The science of the placebo: toward an interdisciplinary research agenda. BMJ Books, London, pp 63–73

Brody H (1988) The symbolic power of the modern personal physician: the placebo response under challenge. J Drug Issues 29:149–161

Casey KL, Svensson P, Morrow TJ, Raz J, Jone C, Minoshima S (2000) Selective opiate modulation of nociceptive processing in the human brain. J Neurophysiol 84:525–533

Colloca L, Benedetti F (2005) Placebos and painkillers: is mind as real as matter? Nat Rev Neurosci 6:545–552

Colloca L, Lopiano L, Lanotte M, Benedetti F (2004) Overt versus covert treatment for pain, anxiety and Parkinson's disease. Lancet Neurol 3:679–684

Davis CE (2002) Regression to the mean or placebo effect? In: Guess HA, Kleinman A, Kusek JW, Engel LW (eds) The science of the placebo: toward an interdisciplinary research agenda. BMJ Books, London, pp 158–166

de la Fuente-Fernandez R, Stoessl AJ (2002) The biochemical bases for reward: implications for the placebo effect. Eval Health Prof 25:387–398

de la Fuente-Fernandez R, Ruth TJ, Sossi V, Schulzer M, Calne DB, Stoessl AJ (2001) Expectation and dopamine release: mechanism of the placebo effect in Parkinson's disease. Science 293:1164–1166

Fanselow MS (1994) Neural organization of the defensive behavior system responsible for fear. Psychon Bull Rev 1:429–438

Fields H (2004) State-dependent opioid control of pain. Nat Rev Neurosci 5:565–575

Fields HL, Basbaum AI (1999) Central nervous system mechanisms of pain modulation. In: Wall PD, Melzack R (eds) Textbook of pain. Churchill Livingstone, Edinburgh, pp 309–329

Fields HL, Levine JD (1984) Placebo analgesia—a role for endorphins? Trends Neurosci 7:271–273

Fields HL, Price DD (1997) Toward a neurobiology of placebo analgesia. In: Harrington A (ed) The placebo effect: an interdisciplinary exploration. Harvard University Press, Cambridge, pp 93–116

Firestone LL, Gyulai F, Mintun M, Adler LJ, Urso K, Winter PM (1996) Human brain activity response to fentanyl imaged by positron emission tomography. Anesth Analg 82:1247–1251

Flaten MA, Simonsen T, Olsen H (1999) Drug-related information generates placebo and nocebo responses that modify the drug response. Psychosom Med 61:250–255

Gleidman LH, Grantt WH, Teitelbaum HA (1957) Some implications of conditional reflex studies for placebo research. Am J Psychiatry 113:1103–1107

Goetz CG, Leurgans S, Raman R, Stebbins GT (2000) Objective changes in motor function during placebo treatment in Parkinson's disease. Neurology 54:710–714

Gracely RH, Dubner R, Wolskee PJ, Deeter WR (1983) Placebo and naloxone can alter postsurgical pain by separate mechanisms. Nature 306:264–265

Gracely RH, Dubner R, Deeter WR, Wolskee PJ (1985) Clinicians' expectations influence placebo analgesia. Lancet 1:43

Greenfield S, Kaplan S, Ware JE (1985) Expanding patient involvement in care. Ann Intern Med 102:520–528

Grevert P, Albert LH, Goldstein A (1983) Partial antagonism of placebo analgesia by naloxone. Pain 16:129–143

Hahn RA (1985) A sociocultural model of illness and healing. In: White L, Tursky B, Schwartz GE (eds) Placebo: theory, research, and mechanisms. Guilford Press, New York, pp 167–195

Hahn RA (1997) The nocebo phenomenon: scope and foundations. In: Harrington A (ed) The placebo effect: an interdisciplinary exploration. Harvard University Press, Cambridge, pp 56–76

Herrnstein RJ (1962) Placebo effect in the rat. Science 138:677–678

Hrobjartsson A, Gotzsche PC (2001) Is the placebo powerless? N Engl J Med 344:1594–1602

Inui TS, Yourtee EL, Williamson JW (1976) Improved outcomes in hypertension after physician tutorials. Ann Intern Med 84:646–651

Jensen TS (1997) Opioids in the brain: supraspinal mechanisms in pain control. Acta Anaesthesiol Scand 41:123–132

Jones AK, Qi LY, Fujirawa T, Luthra SK, Ashburner J, Bloomfield P, Cunningham VJ, Itoh M, Fukuda H, Jones T (1991) In vivo distribution of opioid receptors in man in relation to the cortical projections of the medial and lateral pain systems measured with positron emission tomography. Neurosci Lett 126:25–28

Kaplan SH, Greenfield S, Ware JE Jr (1989) Assessing the effects of physiscian-patient interactions on the outcomes of chronic disease. Med Care 27 Suppl 3:S110–S127

Kirsch I (1985) Response expectancy as a determinant of experience and behavior. Am Psychol 40:1189–1202

Kirsch I (1990) Changing expectations: a key to effective psychotherapy. Brooks-Cole, Pacific Grove

Kirsch I (ed) (1999) How expectancies shape experience. American Psychological Association, Washington

Kirsch I, Weixel LJ (1988) Double-blind versus deceptive administration of a placebo. Behav Neurosci 102:319–323

Leuchter AF, Cook IA, Witte EA, Morgan M, Abrams M (2002) Changes in brain function of depressed subjects during treatment with placebo. Am J Psychiatry 159:122–129

Levine JD, Gordon NC (1984) Influence of the method of drug administration on analgesic response. Nature 312:755–756

Levine JD, Gordon NC, Fields HL (1978) The mechanisms of placebo analgesia. Lancet 2:654–657

Levine JD, Gordon NC, Smith R, Fields HL (1981) Analgesic responses to morphine and placebo in individuals with postoperative pain. Pain 10:379–389

Lipman JJ, Miller BE, Mays KS, Miller MN, North WC, Byrne WL (1990) Peak B endorphin concentration in cerebrospinal fluid: reduced in chronic pain patients and increased during the placebo response. Psychopharmacology (Berl) 102:112–116

Lyerly SB, Ross S, Krugman AD, Clyde DJ (1964) Drugs and placebos: the effects of instructions upon performance and mood under amphetamine sulphate and chloral hydrate. J Abnorm Soc Psychol 68:321–327

Mayberg HS, Silva AJ, Brannan SK, Tekell JL, Mahurin RK, McGinnis S, Jerabek PA (2002) The functional neuroanatomy of the placebo effect. Am J Psychiatry 159:728–737

Millan MJ (2002) Descending control of pain. Prog Neurobiol 66:355–474

Moerman DE (2002a) Meaningful dimensions of medical care. In: Guess HA, Kleinman A, Kusek JW, Engel LW (eds) The science of the placebo: toward an interdisciplinary research agenda. BMJ Books, London, pp 77–107

Moerman DE (2002b) Meaning, medicine and the placebo effect. Cambridge University Press, Cambridge

Montgomery GH, Kirsch I (1996) Mechanisms of placebo pain reduction: an empirical investigation. Psychol Sci 7:174–176

Montgomery GH, Kirsch I (1997) Classical conditioning and the placebo effect. Pain 72: 107–113

Petrovic P, Kalso E, Petersson KM, Ingvar M (2002) Placebo and opioid analgesia—imaging a shared neuronal network. Science 295:1737–1740

Pfeiffer A, Pasi A, Mehraein P, Herz A (1982) Opiate receptor binding sites in human brain. Brain Res 248:87–96

Pollo A, Benedetti F (2004) Neural mechanisms of placebo-induced analgesia. In: Price DD, Bushnell MC (eds) Psychological methods of pain control: basic science and clinical perspectives. IASP Press, Seattle,pp 171–186

Pollo A, Amanzio M, Arslanian A, Casadio C, Maggi G, Benedetti F (2001) Response expectancies in placebo analgesia and their clinical relevance. Pain 93:77–84

Pollo A, Torre E, Lopiano L, Rizzone M, Lanotte M, Cavanna A, Bergamasco B, Benedetti F (2002) Expectation modulates the response to subthalamic nucleus stimulation in Parkinsonian patients. NeuroReport 13:1383–1386

Pollo A, Rainero I, Vighetti S, Benedetti F (2003) Placebo analgesia and the heart. Pain 102:125–133

Price DD (1999) Psychological mechanisms of pain and analgesia. IASP Press, Seattle

Price DD (2001) Assessing placebo effects without placebo groups: an untapped possibility? Pain 90:201–203

Price DD, Fields HL (1997) The contribution of desire and expectation to placebo analgesia: implications for new research strategies. In: Harrington A (ed) The placebo effect: an interdisciplinary exploration. Harvard University Press, Cambridge, pp 117–137

Price DD, Milling LS, Kirsch I, Duff A, Montgomery GH, Nicholls SS (1999) An analysis of factors that contribute to the magnitude of placebo analgesia in an experimental paradigm. Pain 83:147–156

Rawlinson MC (1985) Truth-telling and paternalism in the clinic: philosophical reflection on the use of placebo in medical practice. In: White L, Tursky B, Scwartz GE (eds) Placebo: theory, research, and mechanisms. Guilford Press, New York, pp 403–416

Reiss S (1980) Pavlovian conditioning and human fear: an expectancy model. Behav Ther 11:380–396

Rescorla RA (1988) Pavlovian conditioning: it is not what you think it is. Am Psychol 43:151–160

Sadzot B, Price JC, Mayberg HS, Douglass KH, Dannals RF, Lever JR, Ravert HT, Wilson AA, Wagner HN Jr, Feldman MA (1991) Quantification of human opiate receptor concentration and affinity using high and low specific activity and diprenorphine and positron emission tomography. J Cereb Blood Flow Metab 11:204–219

Schachter S, Singer JE (1962) Cognitive, social and physiological determinants of emotional states. Psychol Rev 69:379–399

Shetty N, Friedman JH, Kieburtz K, Marshall FJ, Oakes D (1999) The placebo response in Parkinson's disease. Parkinson study group. Clin Neuropharmacol 22:207–212

Siegel S (1985) Drug-anticipatory responses in animals. In: White L, Tursky B, Schwartz GE (eds) Placebo: theory, research, and mechanisms. Guilford Press, New York, pp 288–305

Siegel S (2002) Explanatory mechanisms for placebo effects: Pavlovian conditioning. In: Guess HA, Kleinman A, Kusek JW, Engel LW (eds) The science of the placebo: toward an interdisciplinary research agenda. BMJ Books, London, pp 133–157

Sox HC, Margulies I, Sox CH (1981) Psychologically mediated effects of diagnostic tests. Ann Intern Med 95:680–685

Starfield B, Wray C, Hess K, Gross R, Birk PS, D'Lugoff BC (1981) The influence of patient-practitioner agreement on outcome of care. Am J Public Health 71:127–132

Stewart MA (1995) Effective physician-patient communication and health outcomes: a review. Can Med Assoc J 152:1423–1433

Stewart MA, McWhinney IR, Buck CW (1979) The doctor-patient relationship and its effect upon outcome. J R Coll Gen Pract 29:77–82

Thomas KB (1987) General practice consultations: is there any point in being positive? Br Med J 294:1200–1202

Vase L, Riley JL 3rd, Price DD (2002) A comparison of placebo effects in clinical analgesic trials versus studies of placebo analgesia. Pain 99:443–452

Vase L, Robinson ME, Verne GN, Price DD (2003) The contribution of suggestion, expectancy and desire to placebo effect in irritable bowel syndrome patients. Pain 105:17–25

Vogt BA, Sikes RW, Vogt LJ (1993) Anterior cingulate cortex and the medial pain system. In: Vogt BA, Gabriel M (eds) Neurobiology of cingulate cortex and limbic thalamus: a comprehensive handbook. Birkhäuser, Boston, pp 313–344

Volkow ND, Wang GJ, Ma Y, Fowler JS, Zhu W, Maynard L, Telang F, Vaska P, Ding YS, Wong C, Swanson JM (2003) Expectation enhances the regional brain metabolic and the reinforcing effects of stimulants in cocaine abusers. J Neurosci 23:11461–11468

Voudouris NJ, Peck CL, Coleman G (1989) Conditioned response models of placebo phenomena: further support. Pain 38:109–116

Voudouris NJ, Peck CL, Coleman G (1990) The role of conditioning and verbal expectancy in the placebo response. Pain 43:121–128

Wager TD, Rilling JK, Smith EE, Sokolik A, Casey KL, Davidson RJ, Kosslyn SM, Rose RM, Cohen JD (2004) Placebo-induced changes in fMRI in the anticipation and experience of pain. Science 303:1162–1166

Wagner KJ, Willoch F, Kochs EF, Siessmeier T, Tölle TR (2001) Dose-dependent regional cerebral blood flow changes during remifentanil infusion in humans. A positron emission tomography study. Anesthesiology 94:732–739

Wamsley JK, Zarbin MA, Young WS, Kuhar MJ (1982) Distribution of opiate receptors in the monkey brain: an autoradiographic study. Neuroscience 7:595–613

Wickramasekera I (2001) The placebo efficacy study: problems with the definition of the placebo and the mechanisms of placebo efficacy. Adv Mind Body Med 17:309–312

Willer JC, Albe-Fessard D (1980) Electrophysiological evidence for a release of endogenous opiates in stress-induced "analgesia" in man. Brain Res 198:419–426

Willoch F, Tolle TR, Wester HJ, Munz F, Petzold A, Schwaiger M, Conrad B, Bartenstein P (1999) Central pain after pontine infarction is associated with changes in opioid receptor binding: a PET study with 11C-diprenorphine. AJNR Am J Neuroradiol 20:686–690

Willoch F, Schindler F, Wester HJ, Empl M, Straube A, Schwaiger M, Conrad B, Tolle TR (2004) Central poststroke pain and reduced opioid receptor binding within pain processing circuitries: a [11C]diprenorphine PET study. Pain 108:213–220

HEP (2006) 177:415–427
© Springer-Verlag Berlin Heidelberg 2006

Limitations of Pharmacotherapy: Behavioral Approaches to Chronic Pain

H. Flor (✉) · M. Diers

Department of Clinical and Cognitive Neuroscience, University of Heidelberg, Central Institute of Mental Health, J 5, 68159 Mannheim, Germany
flor@zi-mannheim.de

1	Introduction	416
2	The Role of Learning Mechanisms and Psychological Factors in Chronic Pain	416
2.1	Operant Learning	416
2.2	Respondent Learning Mechanisms	417
2.3	Cognitive Factors in Chronic Pain	418
2.4	Pain and Affect	419
2.5	A Biobehavioral Perspective	420
2.6	Memory for Pain	420
3	Psychological Treatment of Chronic Pain	421
3.1	Operant Behavioral Treatment	421
3.2	Cognitive-Behavioral Treatment of Chronic Pain	421
3.3	Biofeedback and Relaxation	422
3.4	Innovative Treatment of Chronic Pain: Changing Pain Memories	423
3.5	Interdisciplinary Treatment Of Chronic Pain	425
4	Conclusions	426
References		427

Abstract Pharmacotherapy is most appropriate in acute pain, whereas in chronic pain states behavioral approaches or a combination of behavioral treatment and pharmacotherapy is more appropriate. In this chapter we first describe the role of learning and memory as well as other psychological factors in the development of chronic pain and emphasize that chronic pain must viewed as the result of a learning process with resulting central neuroplastic changes. We then describe operant behavioral and cognitive-behavioral treatments as well as biofeedback and relaxation techniques and present innovative treatment procedures aimed at altering central pain memories. We complete the section with a discussion of combined behavioral and pharmacological approaches and an interdisciplinary view.

Keywords Operant conditioning in acute and chronic pain · Learning · Memory · Physical training · Cognitive and behavioral therapeutic approaches · Multidisciplinary rehabilitation

1
Introduction

Pharmacotherapy of chronic pain has several limitations. First, the drug does not always target the region in the central nervous system where the main effect should be but will occupy all receptors, thus leading to unwanted general and side effects. Second, analgesic medication is as much prone to tolerance and loss of efficacy as other drugs, and especially opioids can themselves induce hyperalgesia over time (Angst and Clark 2006). Third, long-term analgesic medication can be associated with learning processes that enhance the amount of medication consumed and can drive patients into dependence and lead to cognitive and other neuropsychological deficits (Buntin-Mushock et al. 2005). Moreover, in chronic states of pain the initial cause of the pain is often no longer relevant and other—in many cases central—factors may now be causal for the pain that is experienced. In this chapter we will give an overview of the behavioral and learning-related factors that contribute to chronic pain, including their neural correlates, and will then describe behavioral as well as combined behavioral and pharmacological approaches that can address these factors and can overcome some of the limitations of pharmacotherapy.

2
The Role of Learning Mechanisms and Psychological Factors in Chronic Pain

2.1
Operant Learning

A new era in thinking about pain began with Fordyce's (1976) description of the role of operant factors in chronic pain. In the operant formulation, behavioral manifestations of pain rather than pain per se are central. It is suggested that when an individual is exposed to a stimulus that causes tissue damage, the immediate response is withdrawal and attempts to escape from noxious sensations. This may be accomplished by avoidance of activity believed to cause or exacerbate pain, help seeking to reduce symptoms, and so forth. These behaviors are observable and, consequently, subject to the principles of operant conditioning, i.e., they respond to contingencies of reward and punishment.

The operant view proposes that acute "pain behavior" such as limping to protect a wounded limb from producing additional nociceptive input may come under the control of external contingencies of reinforcement and thus develop into a chronic pain problem. Pain behavior (e.g., complaining, inactivity) may be positively reinforced directly, for example, by attention form a spouse or healthcare provider. Pain behavior may also be maintained by the escape from noxious stimulation by the use of drugs or rest, or the avoidance of undesirable activities such as work. In addition, "well behavior" (e.g., activity, working) may not be sufficiently reinforcing and the more rewarding pain behaviors may therefore be maintained. The pain behavior originally elicited by organic factors may come to occur, totally or in part, in response to reinforcing environmental events. Because of the consequences of specific behavioral responses, it is proposed that pain behaviors may persist long after the initial cause of the pain is resolved or greatly reduced. The operant conditioning model does not concern itself with the initial cause of pain. Rather it considers pain as an internal subjective experience that may be maintained even after an initial physical basis of pain has resolved. Operant conditioning can lead to increased inactivity and invalidity and also plays an important role in the increase of medication levels since the intake of medication—especially on a prn basis when there are high pain levels—may be viewed as a consequence of a negative reinforcement process (a negative consequence, the pain, is removed by medication intake). Not only observable pain behaviors but also verbal expressions of pain and physiological variables may come under the control of the contingencies of reinforcement.

2.2
Respondent Learning Mechanisms

Factors contributing to chronicity that have previously been conceptualized in terms of operant learning may also be initiated and maintained by respondent conditioning (Gentry and Bernal 1977). In the typical classical conditioning paradigm, a previously neutral variable (conditioned stimulus, CS), when paired with a biologically significant stimulus (unconditioned stimulus, US) comes to elicit a conditioned response (CR) that resembles the response to the unconditioned stimulus, the unconditioned response (UR). For example, if a certain movement has been associated with pain, just thinking about the movement may already elicit fear and muscle tension (previously elicited by pain) and may then motivate avoidance behaviors. Lethem et al. (1983) have suggested that once an acute pain problem exists, fear of motor activities that the patient expects to result in pain may develop and motivate avoidance of activity. Nonoccurrence of pain is a powerful reinforcer for reduction of activity and thus the original respondent conditioning may be followed by an operant learning process whereby the nociceptive stimuli and the associated responses need no longer be present for the avoidance behavior to occur. In acute pain states it may be useful to reduce movement, and consequently avoiding pain, to accelerate the healing process. Pain related to sustained muscle contractions might, however, also be conceptualized as a US in the case where no acute injury was present and sympathetic activation and tension increases might be viewed as URs that may elicit more pain, and conditioning might proceed in the same fashion as outlined above. Thus, although the original association between pain and pain-related stimuli results in anxiety regarding these stimuli, with time the expectation of pain related to activity may lead to avoidance of adaptive behaviors even if the nociceptive stimuli and the related sympathetic activation are no longer present. Fear of pain and activity may become conditioned to an expanding number of situations. Avoided activities may involve simple motor behaviors, but also work, leisure, and sexual activity. In addition to the avoidance learning, pain may be exacerbated and maintained in these encounters with potentially pain-increasing situations due to the anxiety-related sympathetic activation and muscle tension increases that may occur in anticipation of pain and also as a consequence of pain. Thus, psychological factors may directly affect nociceptive stimulation and need not be viewed as only reactions to pain. Vlaeyen and Linton (2000) have shown that fear avoidance is a major predictor of chronic pain and disability.

2.3
Cognitive Factors in Chronic Pain

Cognitive-behavioral models of chronic pain emphasize that the evaluation of the pain experience by the patient greatly determines the amount of pain that is experienced as well as its negative consequences (Turk et al. 1983). General assumptions that characterize the cognitive-behavioral perspective are: (1) people are active processors of information and not passive reactors; (2) thoughts (e.g., appraisals, expectancies) can elicit or modulate mood, affect physiological processes, influence the environment, and serve as the impetus for behavior. Conversely, mood, physiology, environmental factors, and behavior can influence thought processes; (3) behavior is reciprocally determined by the person and environmental factors; (4) people can learn more adaptive ways of thinking, feeling, and behaving; and (5) people are capable and should be involved as active agents in change of maladaptive thoughts, feelings, and behaviors.

From the cognitive-behavioral perspective, people suffering from chronic pain are viewed as having negative expectations about their own ability to control certain motor skills such as performing specific physical activities (e.g., climbing stairs, lifting objects) that are attributed to one overwhelming factor, namely, a chronic pain syndrome. Moreover, chronic pain patients tend to believe that they have a limited ability to exert any control over their pain. Such negative, maladaptive appraisals about the situation and personal efficacy may reinforce the experience of demoralization, inactivity, and overreaction to nociceptive stimulation. A great deal of research has been directed toward identifying cognitive factors that contribute to pain and disability. These have consistently demonstrated that patients' attitudes, beliefs, expectancies about their plight, themselves, their coping resources and the healthcare system affect their reports of pain, activity, disability, and response to treatment. A number of studies have used experimental pain stimuli and demonstrated that the conviction of personal control can ameliorate the experience of experimentally induced nociception. Moreover, the type of thoughts employed during exposure to painful stimulation has been related to pain tolerance and pain intensity ratings. Catastrophic thoughts have been associated with lower pain tolerance and higher ratings of pain intensity. In contrast, coping thoughts have been related to higher pain tolerance and lower pain intensity ratings. Once beliefs and expectancies (cognitive schemata) about a disease are formed they become stable and are very difficult to modify. Patients tend to avoid experiences that could invalidate their beliefs and they guide their behavior in accordance with these beliefs even in situations where the belief is no longer valid (no corrective feedback is received to discredit this belief). For example, feeling some muscular pain following activity may be caused by lack of muscle strength and general deconditioning and not by additional tissue damage. Imaging studies have shown that cognitive factors modify the central processing of pain and that attention can increase and distraction can decrease brain activation related to pain.

2.4
Pain and Affect

The affective factors associated with pain include many different emotions, but they are primarily negative in quality. Anxiety and depression have received the greatest amount of attention in chronic pain patients; however, anger has recently received considerable interest as an important emotion in chronic pain patients. Research suggests that from 40% to 50% of chronic pain patients suffer from depression (Bair et al 2003). There have been extensive and fruitless debates concerning the causal relationship between depression and pain. In the majority of cases, depression appears to be the patients' reaction to their plight. The presence of depression is closely related to the feelings of loss of control and helplessness often associated with pain. Several investigators have also found a close association between fear of pain and dysfunctional coping. In addition, high comorbidity between anxiety disorders and pain seems to be present. Muscular hyperreactivity to stress seems to be closely associated with fear of pain. Anger has been widely observed in individuals with chronic pain. The internalization of angry feelings seems to be strongly related to measures of pain intensity, perceived interference, and reported frequency of pain behaviors. Anger and hostility are closely associated with pain in persons with lower back pain. Frustrations related to persistence of symptoms, limited information on etiology, and repeated treatment failures along with anger toward employers, the insurance industry, the healthcare system, family members, and themselves, also contribute to the general dysphoric mood of these patients. The impact of anger and frustration on exacerbation of pain and treatment acceptance has not received adequate attention. It would be reasonable to expect that the presence of anger may serve as an aggravating factor, associated with increasing autonomic arousal and blocking motivation and acceptance of treatments oriented toward rehabilitation and disability management rather than cure, which are often the only treatments available for chronic pain.

2.5
A Biobehavioral Perspective

A biobehavioral or a diathesis-stress model of chronic pain needs to consider the factors discussed above and their mutual interrelationships in the explanation of chronic pain. The existence of a physiological disposition or diathesis is one important component. This predisposition is related to a reduced threshold for nociceptive stimulation and can be determined by genetic factors and acquired through early learning experiences. For example, Mogil (1999) showed that large genetic variations in individual pain sensitivity exist. Very impressive evidence for the role of early traumatic experience comes from the work of Anand et al. (1999) who showed that minor noxious experience in neonate rats leads to dramatic alterations (sensitization) in nociceptive processing in the adult organism. A further component of the biobehavioral model is a response stereotypy of a particular bodily system such as exaggerated muscular responses of the lower back muscle to stress and pain that is based both on the diathesis and on aversive experiences present at the time of the development of the response. These aversive stimuli may include personal or work stress or problematic occupational conditions and will lead not only to painful responses but also to avoidance behaviors and associated maladaptive cognitive and affective processes. The cognitive evaluation of these external or internal stimuli is of great importance in the pain response as discussed above. The focus of the biobehavioral perspective is thus on the patient and not just on the symptoms or the underlying pathology, and this focus also requires that the treatment of the patients be tailored not only to medical factors but that it incorporates psychosocial variables that may often be predominant in states of chronic pain.

2.6
Memory for Pain

An important maintaining factor in this chronicity process is the development of central neuroplastic changes or pain memories. These pain-related memories may be explicit (open to conscious awareness) or implicit (not conscious such as habits) and may subsequently guide the patient's experience and behaviors. For example, pain patients have a tendency to remember preferentially negative and pain-related life events and show a deficit in the retrieval of positive memories. The experience of chronic pain also leads to the development of somatosensory pain memories, for example, an expanded representation of the affected body part in primary somatosensory cortex and other areas related to the processing of pain. This expanded cortical representation is accompanied by increased sensitivity to both painful and nonpainful stimuli and may be further enhanced by learning processes or attention to painful stimulation. An even more dramatic example of a learned memory for pain has been found in phantom limb pain patients (Flor et al. 1995). In upper extremity amputees the magnitude of the phantom limb pain was found to be proportional to the amount of reorganization in primary somatosensory cortex, namely, the shift of the cortical mouth representation into the area where the amputated limb was formerly represented. The brain obviously maintains a memory of the former input to the deafferented area and subsequently stimulation stemming from areas adjacent to the deafferented zone elicits sensations and pain in the now absent limb. Phantom pain and cortical reorganization are absent in congenital amputees, suggesting a major role for learning. Neuroplastic learning-related changes outlast the time of nociceptive stimulation and can produce extensive and enduring alterations of nociceptive processing that have to be taken into account in effective treatment planning.

3
Psychological Treatment of Chronic Pain

3.1
Operant Behavioral Treatment

Patients who show high levels of pain behaviors and are incapacitated by their pain should profit from operant behavioral treatment. The goals of this treatment are the increase of activity levels and healthy behaviors related to work, leisure time, and family as well as medication reduction and management and the change of the behavior of significant others (cf., Fordyce 1976). The overall goal is to reduce disability by reducing pain and increasing healthy behaviors. Medication is switched from a prn basis to a fixed time schedule, where medication is given at certain times of the day to avoid negative reinforcement learning from occurring. Similar principles are applied to the enhancement of activity and the reduction of inactivity and invalidity. This approach has been found to be effective in patients with chronic back pain as well as other pain syndromes. Figure 1 shows data on the treatment of fibromyalgia in an operant protocol (Thieme et al. 2003).

3.2
Cognitive-Behavioral Treatment of Chronic Pain

The cognitive-behavioral model of chronic pain emphasizes the role of cognitive, affective and behavioral factors in the development and maintenance of chronic pain. The central tenet of cognitive-behavioral treatment is to reduce feelings of helplessness and uncontrollability and to establish a sense of

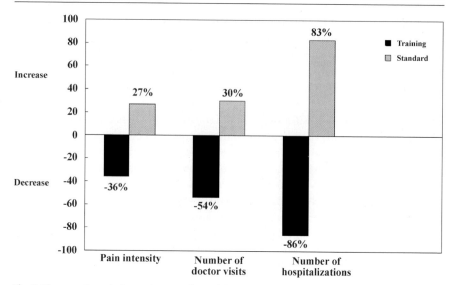

Fig. 1 Changes in pain intensity, number of doctor visits, and number of hospital visits in an operant behavioral compared to a standard medical treatment for chronic fibromyalgia syndrome. (Based on Thieme et al. 2003)

control over pain in the patients. This is achieved by the modification of pain-eliciting and maintaining behaviors, cognitions, and emotions. The cognitive-behavioral approach teaches patients various techniques to effectively deal with episodes of pain. Pain-related cognitions are changed by cognitive restructuring and pain coping strategies such as attention diversion, use of imagery, or relaxation that increase self-efficacy. Several studies have examined the efficacy of cognitive-behavioral pain management, which must be considered as a very effective treatment of chronic pain (e.g., Turk and Okifuji 2002).

3.3
Biofeedback and Relaxation

Biofeedback refers to the modification of a normally nonconscious bodily process (e.g., skin temperature, muscle tension) by making the bodily process perceptible to the patient. The respective physiological signal is measured and amplified and fed back to the patients by the use of a computer that translates variations in bodily processes into visual, auditory, or tactile signals. Seeing or hearing one's blood pressure or muscle tension enables a person to self-regulate it. The most common type of biofeedback for chronic pain is muscle tension or electromyographic (EMG) biofeedback, which was found to be effective for several chronic musculoskeletal pain syndromes (e.g., Flor et al. 1992; see Fig. 2). For migraine headache, temperature, blood flow of the temporal artery, or slow cortical potentials have been fed back with good

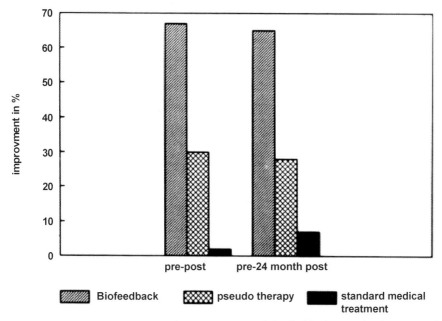

Fig. 2 Changes in pain intensity after treatment with biofeedback, pseudo therapy, and a standard medical treatment for chronic back pain

results. Similar positive data are available for Raynaud's disease with respect to temperature feedback. Another respondent method uses various types of relaxation training among which progressive muscle relaxation seems to be especially suited for the treatment of chronic musculoskeletal pain.

3.4
Innovative Treatment of Chronic Pain: Changing Pain Memories

The discussion in the preceding sections suggests that the alteration of somatosensory pain memories might be an influential method to reduce both chronic musculoskeletal and neuropathic pain. This could be achieved by altering the peripheral input that enters the brain region that coded a pain memory, e.g., by using EMG or temperature biofeedback or by employing a sensory simulation protocol that provides relevant correlated sensory input to the respective brain region. It would also be possible to directly alter the brain response to pain by providing feedback of event-related potential components or EEG rhythms or even blood oxygenation level-dependent changes in functional magnetic resonance imaging (fMRI). Most of these methods have not yet been tested in a systematic manner and their effects on cortical reorganization are so far unknown. Alternatively, pharmacological interventions could be used that prevent or reverse the establishment of central memory traces.

In phantom limb pain, it was assumed that the pain is maintained by cortical alterations fed by peripheral random input. In this case the provision of correlated input into the amputation zone might be an effective method to influence phantom limb pain. fMRI was used to investigate the effects of prosthesis use on phantom limb pain and cortical reorganization. Patients who systematically used a myoelectric prosthesis that provides sensory and visual as well as motor feedback to the brain showed much less phantom limb pain and cortical reorganization than patients who used either a cosmetic or no prosthesis. The relationship between phantom limb pain and use of a myoelectric prosthesis was entirely mediated by cortical reorganization (Lotze et al. 1999). When cortical reorganization was controlled for, phantom limb pain and prosthesis use were no longer associated. This suggests that sensory input to the brain region that formerly represented the now absent limb may be beneficial in reducing phantom limb pain. These studies were performed in chronic phantom limb pain patients. An early fitting and training with a myoelectric prosthesis would probably be of great value not only in the rehabilitation of amputees but also in preventing or reversing phantom limb pain.

These assumptions were further confirmed in an intervention study where the patients received feedback on sensory discrimination of the residual limb. Eight electrodes were attached to the residual limb and provided high-intensity nonpainful electric stimulation of varying intensity and location that led to the experience of intense phantoms (Flor et al. 2001). The patients were trained to discriminate the location or the frequency of the stimulation (in alternating trials) and received feedback on the correct responses. The training was conducted for 90 min per day and was spread over a period of 2 weeks (10 days of training). Compared to a medically treated control group (receiving an equal amount of attention) the trained patients showed significantly better discrimination ability on the stump. They also experienced a more than 60% reduction of phantom limb pain and a significant reversal of cortical reorganization with a shift of the mouth representation back to its original location. The alterations in discrimination ability, pain, and cortical reorganization were highly significantly correlated.

In a related study asynchronous tactile stimulation of the mouth and hand region was used over a period of several weeks. This training was based on the idea that synchronous stimulation leads to fusion and asynchronous stimulation leads to a separation of cortical representation zones. In this case it was postulated that input from the mouth representation that would now activate the region that formerly represented the now-amputated hand and arm would be eliminated and with it the phantom phenomena that would be projected to the amputated limb. This intervention also showed a reduction in phantom limb pain and cortical reorganization (Huse et al. 2001).

Moseley (2004) used a tripartite program for patients with complex regional pain syndrome (CRPS). This program contained a hand laterality recognition task (recognizing a pictured hand to be left or right), imagined movements of the affected hand, and mirror therapy (adoption of the hand posture shown on a picture with both hands in a mirror box while watching the reflection of the unaffected hand). After a 2-week treatment, pain scores were significantly reduced (see Fig. 3). McCabe et al. (2003) also found a reduction in pain ratings during and after mirrored visual feedback of movement of the unaffected limb in complex regional pain syndrome. These studies suggest that modification of input into the affected brain region may alter pain sensation.

3.5
Interdisciplinary Treatment Of Chronic Pain

Psychological treatment of chronic pain is usually performed in an interdisciplinary setting that includes medical interventions, physiotherapy, and social measures that are often combined to a multimodal approach. The problem with multimodal approaches is that some parts of the treatments may counteract each other and that it is difficult to assess the contribution of the individual components. Rather than combining an array of diverse intervention strategies, it might be more fruitful to aim for a differential indication of various treatment components based on pain-related characteristics of the patients. For example, Turk et al. (1998) found that persons characterized by high levels of dysfunction responded better to an interdisciplinary pain treatment program

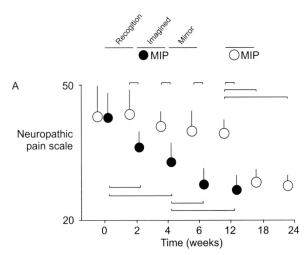

Fig. 3 Mean (*circles*) and standard error of the mean (*vertical bars*) for Neuropathic Pain Scale (NPS) scores for the motor imagery program (MIP) group (*filled circles*) and control group (*open circles*) during the experimental period (weeks 0–12) and after cross-over of the control group (weeks 12–24). MIP consisted of 2 weeks each of recognition of hand laterality (recognition), imagined hand movements (imagined), and mirror movements (mirror). *Horizontal bars* indicate significance ($p<0.05$) on post hoc Scheffé tests. (From Moseley 2004)

for fibromyalgia syndrome that those who were interpersonally distressed. Another important aspect of psychological pain management is motivating the patients for a psychological approach. This is often difficult since they may be concerned that the referral to a mental health professional implies that their pain is "not real," they are exaggerating, the pain they feel is really "all in their head," or their pain is a psychological and therefore not a physical problem. Furthermore, many pain sufferers fear that a referral for psychological intervention implies that they can no longer be helped by the traditional healthcare system and that they are being abandoned as "hopeless cases." They may view the referral as requiring that they prove that they do have legitimate reasons for their reported symptoms. These people usually believe that psychological assessment is not relevant to their problem, when they know that there must be a known physical basis for their symptoms. The patient may believe that cure of the disease or elimination of the symptoms or physical limitations is all that is required or why they are being referred to a psychologist or psychiatrist. This requires a motivational phase prior to treatment that familiarizes the patients with the multidimensional view of chronic pain and motivates them to view a psychological approach as a chance to alter their attitude toward their pain and a first step toward improvement. Interesting new perspectives focus on the combination of behavioral and pharmacological interventions. For example, Dinse et al. (2003) have shown that the effects of sensory discrimination training can be enhanced or reduced if the training is combined with amphetamine or an N-methyl-D-aspartate (NMDA) receptor antagonist. Likewise, Ressler et al. (2004) showed that the effects of exposure therapy for aversive fear memories could be enhanced by combining the treatment with a partial NMDA receptor agonist. We are currently testing if the combination of behavior therapy with a cannabinoid treatment is more effective than behavioral treatment alone in the extinction of pain memories.

4
Conclusions

This chapter focused on the role of learning mechanisms and psychological factors in the development and maintenance of chronic pain. Different psychological treatments of chronic pain were discussed with a focus on innovative treatments of chronic pain designed to change pain memories. Future work should investigate the combination of behavioral and pharmacological interventions. We closed this chapter with an overview of the interdisciplinary treatment of chronic pain.

References

Anand KJ, Coskun V, Thrivikraman KV, Nemeroff CB, Plotsky PM (1999) Long-term behavioral effects of repetitive pain in neonatal rat pups. Physiol Behav 66:627–637

Angst MS, Clark JD (2006) Opioid-induced hyperalgesia: a qualitative systematic review. Anesthesiology 104:570–587

Bair MJ, Robinson RL, Katon W, Kroenke K (2003) Depression and pain comorbidity: a literature review. Arch Intern Med 163:2433–2434

Buntin-Mushock C, Phillip L, Moriyama K, Palmer PP (2005) Age-dependent opioid escalation in chronic pain patients. Anesth Analg 100:1740–1745

Dinse HR, Ragert P, Pleger B, Schwenkreis P, Tegenthoff M (2003) Pharmacological modulation of perceptual learning and associated cortical reorganization. Science 301:91–94

Flor H, Fydrich T, Turk DC (1992) Efficacy of multidisciplinary pain treatment centers: a meta-analytic review. Pain 49:221–230

Flor H, Elbert T, Wienbruch C, Pantev C, Birbaumer N, Larbig W, Taub E (1995) Phantom-limb pain as a perceptual correlate of cortical reorganization following arm amputation. Nature 375:482–484

Flor H, Denke C, Schaefer M, Gruesser S (2001) Effect of sensory discrimination training on cortical reorganisation and phantom limb pain. Lancet 357:1763–1764

Fordyce GL (1976) Behavioral concepts in chronic pain illness. Mosby, St. Louis

Fordyce GL, Shelton JL, Dundore DE (1982) The modification of avoidance learning pain behaviors. J Behav Med 5:405–414

Gentry J, Bernal K (1977) Chronic pain. In: Williams RB, Gentry WD (eds) Behavioral approaches to medical treatment. Ballinger, Cambridge, pp 173–182

Huse E, Preissl H, Larbig W, Birbaumer N (2001) Phantom limb pain. Lancet 358:1015

Lethem J, Slade PD, Troup JD, Bentley G (1983) Outline of a fear-avoidance model of exaggerated pain perception. Behav Res Ther 21:401–408

Lotze M, Grodd W, Birbaumer N, Erb M, Huse E, Flor H (1999) Does use of a myoelectric prosthesis prevent cortical reorganization and phantom limb pain? Nat Neurosci 2:501–502

McCabe CS, Haigh RC, Ring EF, Halligan PW, Wall PD, Blake DR (2003) A controlled pilot study of the utility of mirror visual feedback in the treatment of complex regional pain syndrome (type 1). Rheumatology 42:97–101

Mogil JS (1999) The genetic mediation of individual differences in sensitivity to pain and its inhibition. Proc Natl Acad Sci U S A 96:7744–7751

Moseley GL (2004) Graded motor imagery is effective for long-standing complex regional pain syndrome: a randomised controlled trial. Pain 108:192–198

Ressler KJ, Rothbaum BO, Tannenbaum L, Anderson P, Graap K, Zimand E, Hodges L, Davis M (2004) Cognitive enhancers as adjuncts to psychotherapy: use of D-cycloserine in phobic individuals to facilitate extinction of fear. Arch Gen Psychiatry 61:1136–1144

Thieme K, Gromnica-Ihle E, Flor H (2003) Operant behavioral treatment of fibromyalgia: a controlled study. Arthritis Rheum 49:314–320

Turk DC, Okifuji A (2002) Psychological factors in chronic pain: evolution and revolution. J Consult Clin Psychol 70:678–690

Turk DC, Meichenbaum DH, Genest M (1983) Pain and behavioral medicine: a cognitive-behavioral perspective. Guilford, New York

Turk DC, Okifuji A, Sinclair JD, Starz TW (1998) Interdisciplinary treatment for fibromyalgia syndrome: clinical and statistical significance. Arthritis Care Res 11:186–195

Vlaeyen JW, Linton SJ (2000) Fear-avoidance and its consequences in chronic musculoskeletal pain: a state of the art. Pain 85:317–332

Subject Index

$\alpha_2\delta$ binding   149
$\alpha_2\delta$ protein   149
$\alpha_2\delta$ subunit   159
δ opioid receptor   19
γ-Aminobutyric acid (GABA)   18
κ opioid receptor   19
μ opioid receptor   19
5-lipoxygenase   87
5HT3 receptor   165

Aβ afferents   6
Aβ fibres   7
Aδ fibres   6
aceclofenac   76
acetylcholine   18, 252, 253, 255
acid sensing ion channel (ASIC)   9
action potentials   96
– differential blockade   98, 112
– – size principle   98
– generation   98
– K$^+$ channel blockade   101
acute pain   253
ADAPT   85
adenosin
– A$_1$ receptors   311, 312
– A$_{2A}$ receptors   311, 314
– A$_3$ receptors   311, 314
– peripheral influences   310
adenosine (and pain)
– clinical studies   316, 317
– intrathecal analgesia   313, 316
– intravenous analgesia   316
– knockout   314
adrenergic receptor   12
agonist   236
agranulocytosis   81
allodynia   4, 228, 232, 234, 235, 241
aminophenazone   79, 81
amitriptyline   166, 169, 170

amygdala   15, 226, 230, 233, 236
anandamide   66
aniline derivates   73
aniline derivatives   78, 79
antagonist   242
anterior cingulate cortex   23, 233
anti-convulsant drugs   148–150
anti-depressants   146, 164, 165
anti-epileptic drugs (AEDs)   148
APC   85, 86
APPROVe   85
arthritis   236
aspirin   68, 72–74, 77, 78, 81, 84–86
ATP   17
ATP receptor   18
autonomic reflexes   6

Bradykinin   198
bradykinin   10
– B$_1$ receptor   202
– B$_1$ receptors   199
– B$_2$ receptor   199
– bradyzide   202
– cross species differences   199
– des-[Arg^{10}] kallidin   198
– des-[Arg^9] bradykinin   198
– FR173657   202
– HOE 140 or icatibant   202
– inducer of B$_1$ receptor expression   200
– kallidin   198
– kallikreins   198
– kinin receptor antagonists   202
– kinin receptors and pathophysiology   199
– kinins   198
– NVP-SAA164   203
– R-954   203
– SSR240612   203
– transgenic animals   201

– WIN64338   202
bradykinin receptor   10
brain-derived neurotrophic factor
    (BDNF)   20
buprenorphine   400, 405, 407, 408

C fibres   6
C-FOS   14
calcitonin gene-related peptide
    (CGRP)   5
calcium channel   19
– L-type   20
– N-type   19
– P/Q-type   19
– T-type   20
calcium channels   149, 159
cancer pain   5, 238
capsaicin   9
Carbamazepine   151
carbamazepine   145
carbamazepine (CBZ)   147
CBZ   152
CCK_B receptor   22
celecoxib   82–86
central neuropathic pain   5
central sensitization   7, 230, 231, 236
CGRP   192
– adrenomedullin   192
– amylin   192
– amylin 22–52   196
– BIBN4096   197
– calcitonin   192
– CGRP 8–37   196
– CGRP Receptors   195
– CGRPα and β   192
– cizolirtine   197
– Clinical association   193
– CREB   195
– CRLR   195
– cyclic AMP (cAMP)   195
– evidence for a role in pain and headache
    192
– intracellular calcium   195
– multi-subunit complexity   195
– pathogenesis of migraine headache
    194
– RAMP1   195
– RCP   195
– salivary CGRP   194
– SB-273779   197

– strain-dependent CGRP expression
    193
– studies with CGRP receptor antagonists
    196
CGRP receptor   20
cholecystokinin   398
cholecystokinin (CCK)   18, 402, 403
cholinergic
– muscarinic   252, 257–259
– nicotinic   252, 257, 258
cholinesterase inhibitors   256, 258
chronic pain   5
CLASS   84, 85
clinical trial   237, 395, 403, 408
clonidine   253, 254
complex regional pain syndrome   240
conditioning   397, 398, 400, 401
cortex   14, 226, 233
corticotropin-releasing hormone (CRH)
    18
COX-1   67
– physiological functions   66, 67
COX-2   67
– physiological functions   67, 84–86
– regulation of expression   66, 70, 78
– role in hyperalgesia   71
– selectivity   72, 76, 81
COX-3   80
cyclic AMP   66, 71
cyclic AMP (cAMP)   10
cyclic guanosine monophosphate
    (cGMP)   10
cytokines   11

deep dorsal horn   14
depression   402
descending facilitation   21
descending inhibition   6
descending inhibitory neurons (DINs)
    252, 254
descending tracts   6
dexmedetomidine   252, 254
diabetic neuropathy   146, 150, 156
diacylglycerol   10
diclofenac   73, 74, 76, 82–84, 86, 87
diffuse noxious inhibitory control
    (DNIC)   21
diflunisal   75, 76
dipyrone   79, 81
dopamine   401–403

dorsal columns   15
dorsal horn   70, 71
dorsal root ganglion (DRG) neuron   6
dorsolateral funiculus   15
DRG neuron   6
dynorphin   19

ectopic discharges   7
endomorphin-1   19
endomorphin-2   19
EP receptor   10
EP_2 receptor   71, 87
ethosuximide   162
etoricoxib   82–84
excitability   223, 242
expectation   397, 398, 403, 404, 406, 408
expectations   401, 402

fenoprofen   76
fibromyalgia   238
flurbiprofen   74, 76
FOS protein   14

G protein-coupled inwardly rectifying
    potassium (GIRK)   253–255, 257, 258
GABA   259
$GABA_A$ receptor   18
$GABA_B$ receptor   18
gabapentin   145, 147
galanin   19
GBP   148, 156, 158, 160, 162
glia   378
– astrocytes   380
– microglia   378
glia cell   19
glutamate   17
glutamate receptor   20
glycine   18
glycinergic neurotransmission   71
GPCRs   102
– G_{11} 103
– G_q 102

Head zone   14
hyperalgesia   4, 68, 70, 71, 225–228,
    231–235, 241

ibuprofen   72–74, 78, 86, 87
imipramine   166–168
impulse propagation

– margin of safety   101
incisional pain   5
indomethacin   73, 74, 76, 82
inflammation   7, 233
inflammatory   230–232, 234–236,
    238–240, 242
inflammatory hyperalgesia   9
inflammatory mediators   8
insula   23
ion channels
– redistribution   104

ketoprofen   73, 74, 76
ketorolac   405
kinins   183

lamina I   13
lamina II   13
lamina III   13
lamina IV   13
lamina V   13
lamotrigine   145, 155–157, 160
lateral thalamocortical system   15
leu-enkephalin   19
leukotrienes   87
licofelone   87
lidocaine   112
limbic system   23
local anaestetics
– toxicity   110
local anaesthetic blockade
– Ca^{2+} channels   100
– HCN channels   100
– K^+ channels   100
local anaesthetics
– capsaicin   107
– inflammation   103, 104
– NMDA   109
– phospholipase C (PLC)   102
– signaling pathways   102
– state-dependent binding   99
– stereoselectivity   99
– transmitter release   101
local anesthetics   96
locus coeruleus (LC)   254
locus coeruleus (LC)   254, 258
long-term depression (LTD)   16
long-term potentiation (LTP)   16
lornoxicam   72, 74, 76
low back pain   5

lumiracoxib   82–85

MAPK   108
– ERK   108, 111
– p38   111
margin of safety
– for AP propagation   98
mechanical hyperalgesia   10
medial thalamocortical system   23
mefenamic acid   74, 76
meloxicam   75, 77
membrane stabilizers   148
met-enkephalin   19
metamizol   405
mexiletine   145
microsomal prostaglandin E synthase I
    87
mitogen-activiated protein kinase
    (MAPK)
– ERK/MAPK   367
– JNK/MAPK   372
– p38/MAPK   370
modulated receptor   99
monoamines   163
morphine   404, 405
muscarinergic receptor   18
muscarinic   259

N-methyl-D-aspartate (NMDA)
    receptor   17
Na$^+$
– TTX-sensitive (S)   9
Na$^+$ channel
– TTX-resistant (R)   9
nabumetone   75
naloxone   398, 400–402, 405
naproxen   75, 76, 85, 87
natural history   395, 407, 408
nerve growth factor (NGF)   11
nerve injury   7
neural plasticity   360
– central sensitization   362
– peripheral sensitization   361
neuralgias   238
neurogenic inflammation   5
neurokinin A (NKA)   18
neurokinin-1 (NK-1) receptors   18
neuronal Ca^{2+} 110
neuropathic   230–232, 234, 235,
    237–240, 242, 252

neuropathic pain   4, 5, 145, 146, 156
– HCN channels   100
neuropathy   17, 239, 240
neuropeptide Y (NPY)   11
neuropeptides   182, 183
– bradykinin   182
– calcitonin gene-related peptide (CGRP)
    182
– calcitonin/calcitonin gene-related
    peptide   182
– CGRP   183
– galanin   183
– knock-out mice   184
– neurokinin A   183
– neuropeptide Y   183
– peptide   183
– peptides   182, 183
– receptors for neuropeptides   184
– specific receptor antagonist drugs
    182
– substance P   182, 183
– tachykinin   182
– transgenic animals   184
– vasoactive intestinal polypeptide (VIP)
    183
neuropeptides and kinins   181
– calcitonin gene-related peptide (CGRP)
    181
– peptides   181
– substance P   181
neurotensin   18
neurotoxicity   241
neurotoxicity of LA
– Ca^{2+} 111
neurotransmission   218, 242
neurotrophins   11
nitric oxide   87
NMDA activation   226
NMDA receptor
– subunits   20
NNT   150, 168
NO   12
nocebo   401, 402
nociceptin   19
nociception   5, 234
– nociceptive processing   225
nociceptive   224, 226, 227, 229, 232, 236,
    242
nociceptive motor reflexes   6
nociceptive processing   229

nociceptive system   5
nociceptive-specific neuron   14
nociceptor   5, 68, 70, 71
– activation   8
– chemosensitivity   6
– initially mechano-insensitive   7
– ion channels   8
– joint   6
– joint nerve   7
– muscle   6
– polymodal   5
– receptor   8
– sensitization   8
– silent   7
– skin   6
– skin nerve   7
– visceral nerves   7
– visceral organs   6
norepinephrine   252, 253
NSAIDs   66–68, 72, 73, 76–78, 80, 81,
    84–87
nucleus paragigantocellularis lateralis
    21
nucleus raphe magnus (NRM)   21
nucleus reticularis gigantocellularis   21
numbers needed to treat (NNTs)   147

Off-cell   21
On-cell   21
opioid   19, 393, 402, 405
opioids   11, 398, 400, 401, 403
orphanin fluoroquinolone (FQ)
    receptor   19
oxcarbazepine   153

P2X receptors (and pain)
– P2X3 receptors   317
– P2X4 receptors   319
– P2X7 receptors   319
PAG   229, 233, 236
pain   4, 228, 231
– acute   252, 254, 257
– chronic   5, 252, 256, 257
– hyperalgesia   226, 254, 255
– inflammatory   254, 258, 259
– neuropathic   252, 258, 259
– nociceptive   4
painful diabetic neuropathy   158
paracetamol   68, 78, 79, 81
parecoxib   82, 83, 85, 86

Parkinson   401, 402, 405
periaqueductal gray   226
periaqueductal grey   6, 252
periaqueductal grey matter (PAG)   21
peripheral sensitization   230
PGB   148, 161
phantom limb   238
pharmacogenetics   253
pharmacogenomics   253
phenazone   68, 79, 80
phenytoin   150, 151
phospholipase C   10
piroxicam   73, 75, 77
pituitary adenylate cyclase-activating
    polypeptide (PACAP)   18
pK_a value   68, 72
plasticity   237
polymodal nociceptor   7
post-herpetic neuralgia (PHN)   146
postoperative pain   238
prefrontal cortex   23
pregabalin   145, 147
presynaptic
– receptor glutamate   109
primary afferent   224, 225, 227
primary hyperalgesia   21
primary nociceptive neurons   5
proglumide   402, 403
propyphenazone   79, 81
prostacyclin   67, 77, 85, 87
prostaglandin   78, 80
prostaglandin E_2 (PGE_2)   9
prostaglandins   66, 68, 70, 71, 86
protein kinases   359
– serine-threonine protein kinases   364
– tyrosine kinases   366
pyrazolinone derivates   73, 79
pyrazolinone derivatives   80

receptor
– agonist   222, 223, 229, 230, 234,
    235, 242
– antagonist   219, 222, 224, 231,
    233–235, 237–241
– G protein   222
– ligand   219
– transmission   219
receptors   231
regression to the mean   395
rofecoxib   82–84, 86

rostral ventromedial medulla   6, 226
rostral ventromedial medulla (RVM)
    21
RVM   233

salicylic acid   72, 74, 77, 78
S-alpha-amino-3-hydroxy-5-methyl-
    4-isoxazolepropionic acid (AMPA)
    receptor   17
secondary hyperalgesia   21
selective serotonin reuptake inhibitors
    (SSRIs)   147
serine-threonine protein kinases
– calcium/calmodulin-dependent kinase
    (CaMK)   364
– protein kinase A (PKA)   364
– protein kinase C (PKC)   364
– protein kinase G (PKG)   365
serine-threonune protein kinases
– mitogen-activiated protein kinase
    (MAPK)   367
serotonin   252, 259, 397, 401, 403
serotonin/NA reuptake inhibitors
    (SNRIs)   147
SI Cortex   23
signal transduction pathways   106
– ERK   105
SII Cortex   23
silent nociceptor   7
sodium channels   96, 148, 150, 154, 155
somatosensory cortex   23
– SI   23
– SII   23
somatostatin   11
somatostatin receptor   11
spinal cord   7
– dorsal horn   225, 231
– spinal dorsal horn   228
spinal cord injury   158, 161, 238, 240
spino-amygdalar pathway   15
spino-cervical tract (SCT)   15
spino-parabrachio-amygdalar pathway
    15
spinohypothalamic tract   15
spinomesencephalic tract (SMT)   15
spinoreticular tract (SRT)   15
spinothalamic tract (STT)   15
stimulus transduction   8
substance P   185
– aprepitant (MK-0869)   186

– chronic pain conditions   189
– CI-1021   186
– CJ-11,974   191
– Clinical Trials with NK_1 Receptor
    Antagonists   189
– CP-96,345   186
– CP-99,994   186
– GR205171   187
– L-733,060   186
– L-743,310   186
– L-760,735   187
– LY303870   186
– migraine headache   190
– NK_1 receptor antagonists   185
– NK_1 receptor knock-out (–/–) mice
    187
– NK_1 receptors   185
– RP-67,580   187
– RP67580   186
– RPR 100,893   186
– saporin toxin conjugated to
    substance P   191
– SDZ NKT 343   186
– TAK-637   187
substance P (SP)   5
superficial dorsal horn   14
sympathetic fibres   12
synaptic plasticity   233

TARGET   84, 85
TCAs   167, 168
tenoxicam   75, 77
tetrodotoxin-resistant sodium channels
    70, 71
thalamic   233
thalamus   23, 226, 230
therapist–patient interaction   406, 407
thermal hyperalgesia   9
threshold   97
thrombomodulin   86
thromboxanes   67, 77, 85
thyrotropin-releasing hormone (TRH)
    18
tolerance   237, 239
topiramate   157
tramadol   405
transient receptor potential vanilloid 1
    70
transient receptor protein (TRP)   9
transmission   221, 223, 228, 230, 236

– G protein   222
– neurotransmission   226, 228
transmitter   218
tricyclic anti-depressants (TCAs)   147
TRPA1 receptor   9
TRPM8 receptor   9
TRPV1   106
TRPV1 receptor   9
TRPV2 receptor   9
TRPV3 receptor   9
TRPV4 receptor   9
tyrosine kinases
– non-receptor tyrosine kinases   366
– receptor tyrosine kinases   366

valdecoxib   82, 83, 85, 86
valproic acid   153, 154

vasoactive intestinal polypeptide (VIP)
    18
venlafaxine   170
ventral horn   14
ventral posterior lateral (VPL) nucleus
    15
VIGOR   84
vocalization   237
voltage-dependent calcium channel   19
voltage-gated Na^+ channel   9

Wallerian degeneration   8
wide dynamic range neuron   14
wind-up   16

Y1 receptor   19
Y2 receptor   19